SHEEP MEDICINE

PHILIP R SCOTT
BVM&S MPhil DVM&S CertCHP DSHP FRCVS DiplECBHM ILTM
Royal (Dick) School of Veterinary Studies
Large Animal Hospital
University of Edinburgh
Roslin, Midlothian, UK

MANSON PUBLISHING/THE VETERINARY PRESS

ISBN: 1–84076–049–4
ISBN: 978–1–84076–049–1

A CIP catalogue record for this book is available from the British Library.

For full details of all Manson Publishing Ltd titles please write to:
Manson Publishing Ltd, 73 Corringham Road, London NW11 7DL, UK.
Tel: +44(0)20 8905 5150
Fax: +44(0)20 8201 9233
Email: manson@mansonpublishing.com
Website: www.mansonpublishing.com

Commissioning editor: Jill Northcott
Project manager: Paul Bennett
Copy-editor: Peter Beynon
Cover and book design: Cathy Martin, Presspack Computing Ltd
Layout: DiacriTech, Chennai, India
Colour reproduction: Tenon & Polert Colour Scanning Ltd, Hong Kong
Printed by: Grafos SA, Barcelona, Spain

Contents

PREFACE 4

ABBREVIATIONS 5

GLOSSARY 6

Chapter 1: Introduction 7

Chapter 2: Husbandry 12

Chapter 3: Reproductive System
Part 1: Female Reproductive System 33
Part 2: Male Reproductive System 72

Chapter 4: Neonatal Lamb Diseases 83

Chapter 5: Digestive System 99

Chapter 6: Cardiorespiratory System
Part 1: Thorax 137
Part 2: Cardiovascular System 161

Chapter 7: Neurological Diseases 165

Chapter 8: Musculoskeletal System 199

Chapter 9: Urinary System 232

Chapter 10: The Skin 243

Chapter 11: Eye Diseases 265

Chapter 12: Mammary Gland 271

Chapter 13: Metabolic Disorders and Trace Element Deficiencies 279

Chapter 14: Parasitic Diseases 297

Chapter 15: Anaesthesia 315

Chapter 16: Miscellaneous Diseases 320

Appendix: Practice Newsletters 324

INDEX 328

Preface

The major objective of this book is to describe, with the aid of a large number of high-quality images, how to investigate, treat and control the important diseases of sheep encountered by veterinarians in general practice, taking full account of welfare implications and the economic limitations of commercial sheep farming.

Drawing on the knowledge gained from his own clinical investigations of sheep disease problems, and in collaboration with colleagues, the author has published extensively in scientific journals worldwide over the past 25 years. The practical applications of these clinical studies are highlighted throughout the book; for example, the use of extradural anaesthesia under farm operating conditions; the clinical application of cerebrospinal fluid collection and analysis in neurological disease cases; and the diagnostic value of ultrasonography. These are aspects of ovine clinical medicine that rarely feature in textbooks. The diagnosis, treatment, prognosis, control and, where appropriate, postmortem features of sheep diseases are described. Wherever possible the images will take the reader through all stages of the disease process, highlighting clinical features important in the diagnosis. A unique aspect of this book is that the welfare sections are backed by the author's own large-scale survey data, which allow comment and discussion on the animal welfare implications of each disease.

The book has been written for veterinary practitioners and for veterinary students undertaking their clinical rotations. Many of the techniques and treatments described may be new to busy practitioners who do not find the time to read scientific journals. The book will also appeal to animal scientists, agricultural advisers and, more generally, to progressive farmers/sheep owners intent on providing the best available care for their sheep.

This book must be read against a background of little or no improvement over the last four decades in disease prevalence, mortality rates and welfare standards on the majority of sheep farms worldwide, despite great scientific advances. The text focuses on the veterinarian's clinical examination and inspection of husbandry practices, and the subsequent practical and cost-effective advice. In New Zealand, for example, over the past decade the national lambing performance has increased by nearly 20% due to a complex variety of factors in which veterinary input has played no small part. Such general information is rarely published in discipline-specific scientific journals, and for this reason only key references are listed. Readers are directed to the CAB International Animal Health and Production Compendium 2003 for an extended bibliography on each disease condition (www.cabicompendium.org; also available via www.animalscience.com).

The chapters are mainly based on specific body systems and, where appropriate, they open with a suggested approach to the clinical examination of that system. This systematic approach is most applicable to the nervous and respiratory systems.

Many of the chapters conclude with exercises featuring typical clinical cases. The reader is given the history and clinical findings and any laboratory and ancillary test results. He/she is then guided through the common differential diagnoses, suggested specific diagnosis and treatment. This will enable the reader to determine whether he/she has understood the chapter before progressing to the next body system. This approach will be most useful for students but it may be equally applicable to practitioners who attend sheep only occasionally.

Contributions, comments, suggestions and corrections by readers will be gratefully received by the author via www.mansonpublishing.com and included with due acknowledgement in any future publication. It is only through the free exchange of such knowledge and experience that improvements in the veterinary care of sheep can be achieved and, most importantly, applied more widely.

Philip Scott

Abbreviations

AGIT	agar gel immunodiffusion test
AST	aspartate aminotransferase
BCS	body condition score
BDV	border disease virus
bpm	beats per minute
BUN	blood urea nitrogen
BVD	bovine virus diarrhoea
BZ	benzimidazole
CFT	complement fixation test
CLA	caseous lymphadenitis
CN	cranial nerve
CNS	central nervous system
CPD	contagious pustular dermatitis
CSF	cerebrospinal fluid
DM	dry matter
EAE	enzootic abortion of ewes
EDTA	ethylenediamine tetra-acetic acid
ELISA	enzyme-linked immunosorbent assay
ENTV	enzootic nasal tumour virus
epg	eggs per gram
EU	European Union
FAT	fluorescent antibody test
FMD	foot and mouth disease
FSE	focal symmetrical encephalomalacia
GGT	gamma glutamyltransferase
GLDH	glutamate dehydrogenase
Hb	haemoglobin
IKC	infectious keratoconjunctivitis
JSRV	jaagsiekte retrovirus
L3	third stage larva
LM	levamisole/morantel
MBC	minimal bactericidal concentration
ME	metabolizable energy
MJ	megajoules
MLC	Meat and Livestock Commission
MMA	methylmalonic acid
MVV	maedi-visna virus
NEFA	non-esterified fatty acid
NSAID	non-steroidal anti-inflammatory drug
OPP	ovine progressive pneumonia
OPT	ovine pregnancy toxaemia
PBS	phosphate buffered saline
PCV	packed cell volume
PEM	polioencephalomalacia
PLD	phospholipase D (toxoid)
RBC	red blood cell
SCC	squamous cell carcinoma
SPA	sheep pulmonary adenomatosis
T3	tri-iodothyronine
T4	thyroxine
UK	United Kingdom
USA	United States of America
WBC	white blood cell
ZN	Ziehl-Neelsen (stain)

Glossary

bruxism gnashing, grinding or clenching of teeth

enthesis the site of attachment of a muscle or ligament to bone

enthesitis a term that has been broadly used to describe a traumatic disease occurring at the insertion of a muscle, tendon, ligament or articular capsule where recurring concentration of stress provokes inflammation with a strong tendency towards fibrosis and calcification (enthesophyte formation)

gimmer a ewe hogg becomes a gimmer after its first clipping; a gimmer becomes a ewe after it lambs

ginglymus a joint that allows movement in one plane

hogg a ewe lamb becomes a hogg after the autumn lamb sales

metaphylactic/metaphylaxis treatment of all animals in a group when some show signs of disease

Mules 'operation' the removal of strips of skin from the perineal area of lambs so as to increase the area of wool-less skin and confer a lower susceptibility to fly strike

odontoprisis same as bruxism

quidding dropping of food from the mouth while in the process of eating

snacker feed dispenser pulled behind a tractor or quad bike

wether a castrated ram lamb after the autumn sales

1 Introduction

MARKET FLUCTUATIONS AND VETERINARY SERVICES

In recent years the sheep industry worldwide has suffered dramatic fluctuations in prices for prime lambs, breeding replacements and cull ewes. For example, UK market prices for fat lambs and breeding sheep fell during the foot and mouth disease (FMD) epidemic of 2001 but have shown good signs of recovery since 2003. Faced with uncertain returns from their livestock enterprises, farmers try to reduce variable costs and, in consequence, veterinary services come under close scrutiny.

INTENSIFICATION

The intensification of sheep production over the past 20 years has typically resulted in a threefold increase in the number of breeding ewes for which a single shepherd is responsible. While such intensification has often involved housing sheep during late gestation, which permits higher welfare standards by affording protection from adverse weather and early detection of problems, with prompt remedial action being taken, research data[1] have shown no reduction in mortality rates of ewes and neonatal lambs.

A review of flock production data reveals some harsh statistics. The perinatal lamb mortality rate has remained static at 15–25% over the past 40 years despite major advances in veterinary science, and the annual ewe mortality rate has remained at 5–7% over the same period. For a major sheep-producing country whose adult sheep population is approximately 16–20 million, a 1% disease incidence represents a very significant number of sheep.

PRODUCTION STATISTICS VERSUS BEST PRACTICE

Production statistics alone can mask undesirable management practices. For example, most intensively managed flocks depend on prophylactic antibiotics, administered to lambs within the first few hours of life, to prevent watery mouth disease (endotoxaemia caused by *Escherichia coli*), which was previously controlled by good husbandry practices. On certain farms polyarthritis caused by *Streptococcus dysgalactiae* is controlled by the metaphylactic injection of procaine penicillin to lambs before they are 48 hours old. The promotion of farmer/veterinarian collaboration must be based on the adoption of best management practices, which may prove more costly with respect to staff time.

RECENT SURVEY DATA

During 1999 a questionnaire was sent to 350 sheep farms served by three veterinary practices to determine the extent of veterinary involvement on those sheep enterprises. Replies were received from 183 farmers, with an average farm size of 120 hectares and 491 ewes. The resulting data are referred to throughout this book to highlight the important sheep diseases in the UK and identify opportunities for veterinary intervention and supervision. The implications of these data will be of relevance to veterinarians in all sheep-producing countries.

Management practices

A total of 99 farmers (54.1%) in the survey used ultrasound scanning to determine fetal numbers. Reference is made to this management tool in the section detailing late gestation nutrition (see Chapter 2: Placental development, p. 16).

Only 21 of the farmers (11.5%) had asked their veterinarian to collect blood samples to determine flock nutritional and/or mineral status. Accurate assessment of late gestation ewe nutrition is the single most valuable veterinary input to the sheep enterprise (see Chapter 2: Fetal growth and development, p. 16). These data indicate that there is great potential for veterinarians to offer advice regarding ewe nutrition during late gestation. The reader is directed to the article written by Russel[2].

Vaccinations

Surprisingly, 16.4% of sheep farmers in the survey did not vaccinate their ewes against clostridial diseases, which represents a basic failing of their flock health programme. It is essential that veterinarians develop a more effective flock management strategy with their clients. Vaccination against clostridial diseases is cheap, effective and an essential component of all flock health programmes.

Vaginal prolapse

The number of ewes with vaginal prolapse was 892 (1.0%) and 136 farms (74.3%) experienced more than one case. Sadly, only 94 of the vaginal prolapses (10.5%) received veterinary attention.

Assisted lambings

The number of ewes in the survey with assisted deliveries was 4,313 (4.8% of total births) but only 289 (6.7%) of them were presented to a veterinarian. More encouragingly, 102 of the farmers (55.7%) took one or more ewes with dystocia to their veterinarian.

Twenty-seven out of 81 farmers (33%) quoted too high professional fees as the major reason for not seeking help with dystocia cases, and 31% of the farmers considered themselves to be as competent as their veterinarian in correcting a dystocia.

Caesarean section

Caesarean section was performed in 104 (35.9%) of the 289 ewes presented to a veterinarian for correction of dystocia. A success rate of 82.7% was reported for surgery compared to 96.2% for those ewes with dystocia arising from malposition/malposture where the lambs were delivered *per vaginam*. This relatively low success rate for caesarean sections could be attributed to trauma of the reproductive tract prior to surgery.

Uterine prolapse

One hundred and ninety-three cases of uterine prolapse (0.21% of ewes at risk) were reported. Of these only 41 ewes were presented to a veterinarian, with a success rate of 75.6%. The other 152 ewes were treated by the farmer and the mortality rate was 45.3%.

Metabolic diseases

Pregnancy toxaemia

During late gestation, 494 ewes (0.55%) on 79 farms were affected with ovine pregnancy toxaemia (OPT, twin lamb disease). Five farmers took a total of nine ewes to the veterinary surgery for treatment. The other 485 ewes were treated by the farmer and only 22.3% survived.

Hypocalcaemia

Hypocalcaemia was reported on 54 farms, with 325 sheep affected (0.4%), but only two farmers requested veterinary attention. Only 38.6% of ewes treated by the farmer survived.

Hypomagnesaemia

Surprisingly, 246 ewes were diagnosed as suffering from hypomagnesaemia. One farmer took four ewes to his veterinarian. Only 31 ewes (12.8%) survived after treatment by the farmer.

Interpretation of metabolic diseases statistics

The statistics listed above highlight concerns regarding the prevention, diagnosis and treatment of suspected metabolic disease in sheep. They also indicate a potential area for veterinary intervention (e.g. practice newsletters, client meetings and farm advisory visits). Hypocalcaemia responds very well to timely treatment; the poor success rate achieved by farmers raises serious doubts about the diagnosis and the appropriateness of the therapy. Hypomagnesaemia is uncommon in sheep. It is possible that farmers confuse 'staggers', a colloquial name for hypocalcaemia in sheep, with hypomagnesaemia and treat recumbent ewes with subcutaneous magnesium solutions only.

WELFARE

There has been little discussion by practising veterinarians of welfare standards on their clients' sheep farms. For example, papers have been published detailing electrolyte concentrations and cortisol measurements during and after long distance road journeys brought about by the trade in live sheep, and describing castration and tail docking of young lambs (**1**), but there are few papers by veterinarians concerned about the welfare standards and level of obstetrical care on many of their clients' farms (**2**), where sheep suffering dystocia often do not receive veterinary attention.

Many aspects of sheep farming should be reviewed in relation to the Five Freedoms[3], and these are applicable worldwide:

- **Freedom from hunger and thirst:** by ready access to fresh water and a diet to maintain full health and vigour (**3**).
- **Freedom from discomfort:** by providing an appropriate environment including shelter and a comfortable resting area (**4**).
- **Freedom from pain, injury or disease:** by prevention or by rapid diagnosis and treatment (**2, 5**).
- **Freedom to express normal behaviour:** by providing sufficient space (**6**), proper facilities and company of the animals' own kind.
- **Freedom from fear and distress:** by ensuring conditions and treatment to avoid mental suffering.

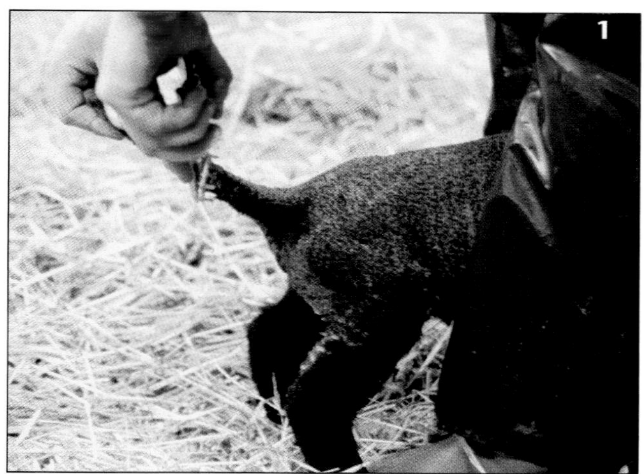
1 Is castration and tail docking in young lambs the major welfare concern in sheep farming?

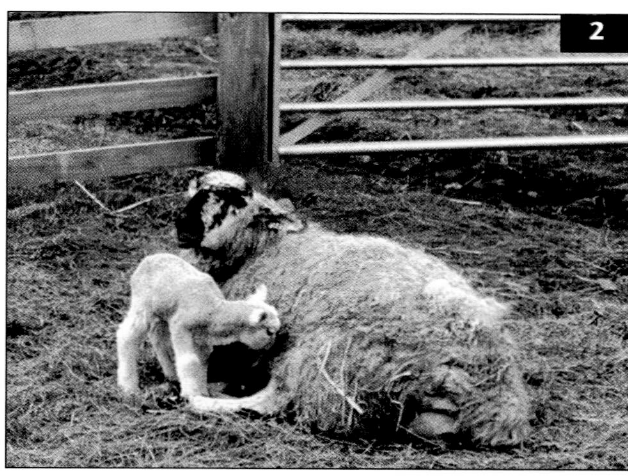
2 What is the level of care of obstetrical problems?

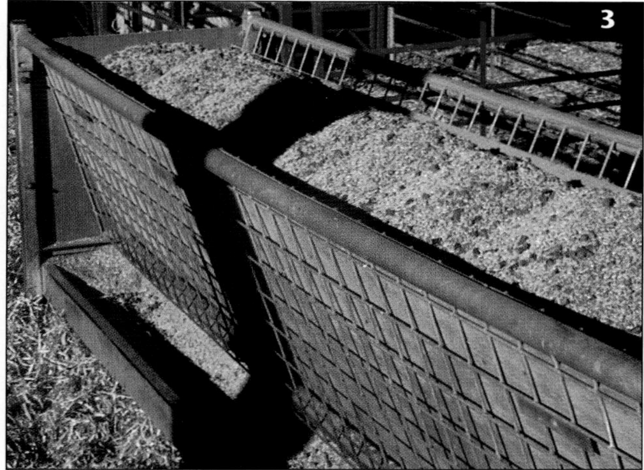
3 Does this diet maintain full health and vigour? Do sheep adapt to such dietary restrictions?

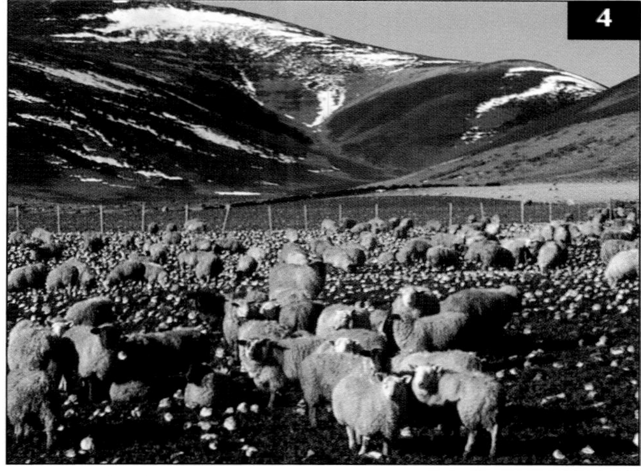
4 Does this husbandry system provide shelter and a comfortable resting area?

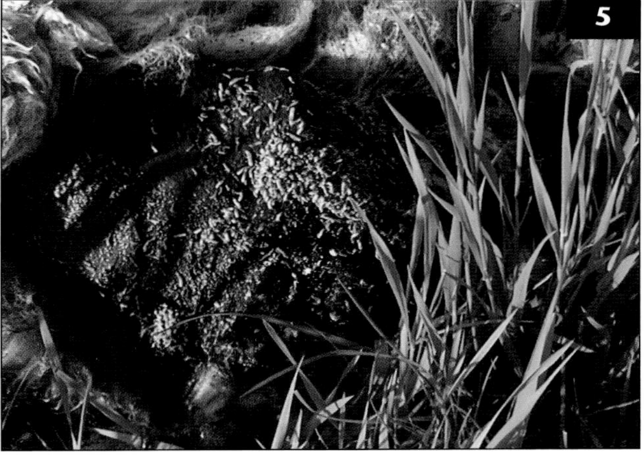
5 Has there been diligent stockmanship in this case of cutaneous myiasis?

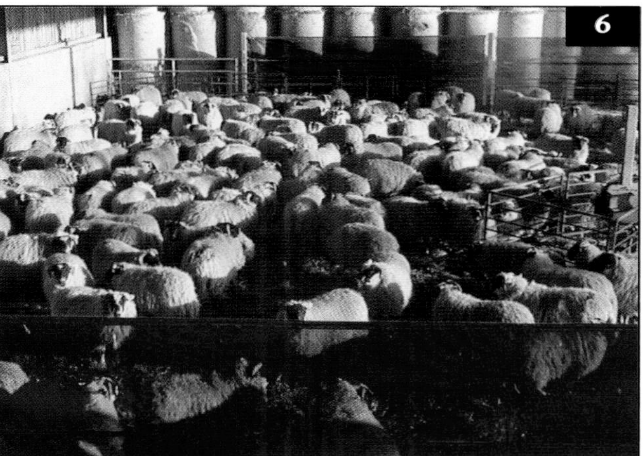
6 Is there provision of sufficient space?

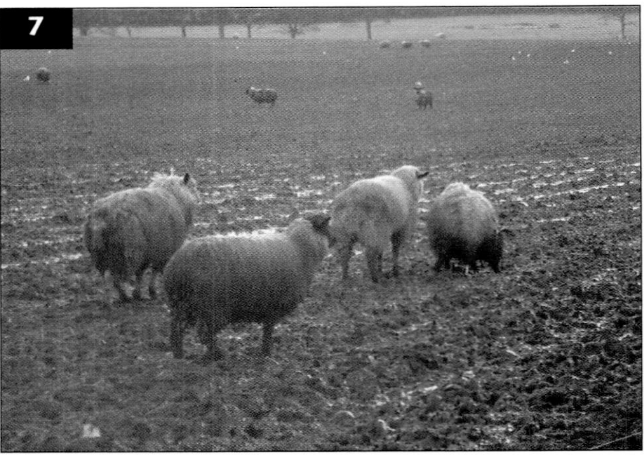
7 Does this represent responsible management?

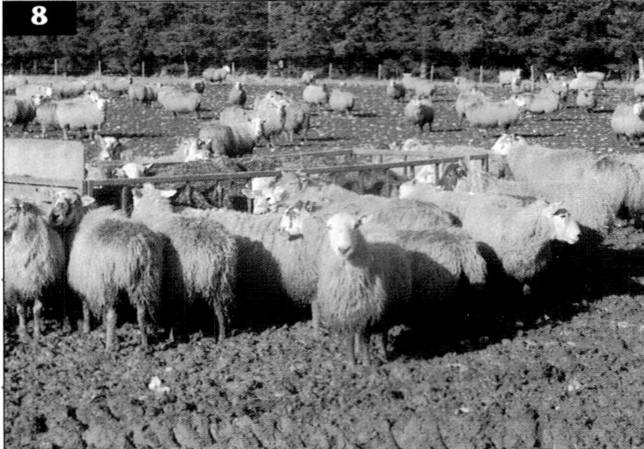
8 Caring and responsible planning and management for heavily pregnant ewes?

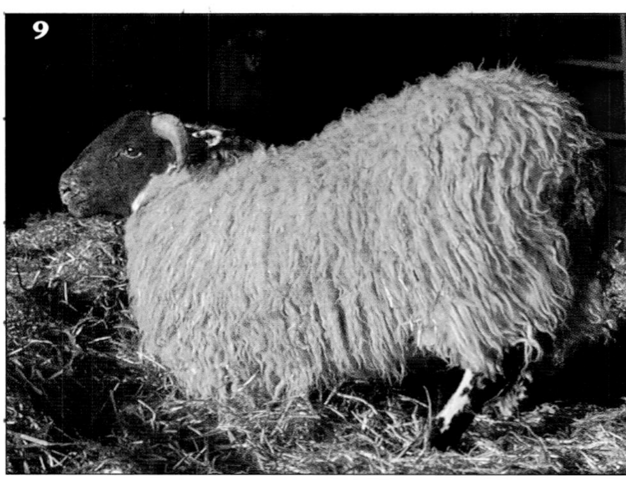
9 Environmental design leading to virulent footrot?

The Codes of Recommendations for the Welfare of Livestock: Sheep[4] provide a succinct and perceptive interpretation of these Five Freedoms and are applicable worldwide. The Codes state that:

'In acknowledging these freedoms, those who have care of livestock should practise:

- Caring and responsible planning and management (**7**, **8**).
- Skilled, knowledgeable and conscientious stockmanship (**2**, **5**).
- Appropriate environmental design (**6**, **9**).
- Considerate handling and transport.
- Humane slaughter.'

ECONOMICS

The most significant single influence on the welfare of any flock is the shepherd, who should develop and carry out an effective routine for continuing care. The most significant single influence on the husbandry skills of the shepherd should be his/her veterinarian. Tragically, the most significant single influence on the welfare of sheep is economics. However dedicated and caring the shepherd, decisions are too often based on cost:benefit factors. Veterinarians need to make a more vigorous contribution to discussions on the future of farming and the countryside. Unfortunately, veterinary care and attention will only be sought when there is a perceived financial incentive; therefore, any publication detailing sheep medicine and focusing on welfare standards must outline basic farm economics.

The economic calculations in this book are based on veterinary practice pricing structures and market values for sheep in the UK. There will be variations from year to year both between veterinary practices and between sheep production systems worldwide, but such costs must not be ignored.

At the most basic level, the cost of a caesarean section may often exceed the value of the ewe. Conversely, giving extra feed during late gestation in a 500-ewe flock could result in an extra 100 lambs and a 15% increase in the total sale value. The economics section for each disease is discussed in relation to the section detailing welfare implications.

CONCLUSION

The care and welfare of sheep, particularly in the UK, has deteriorated over the past few years, caused largely by the poor economic returns from sheep farming. Farmers are now attempting to lamb ewes rather than pay for a caesarean section. Ewes with dystocia have been shot rather than incur the expense of veterinary attention. The data listed above highlight opportunities for the veterinary practitioner.

It is probable that all flocks will soon require an individual flock health plan to enable membership of various farm assurance schemes. Unfortunately, such schemes will be operated to satisfy various food safety issues imposed by retailers and not determined by the veterinary profession for the improved care and welfare of sheep. The following chapters describe the common diseases of sheep and their treatment, control and prevention, while remaining aware of the welfare and economic implications of the recommended treatments.

REFERENCES

1 *Meat and Livestock Commission Sheep Yearbooks*. Meat and Livestock Commission, Milton Keynes.
2 Russel A (1985) Nutrition of the pregnant ewe. *In Practice* 7, 23–28.
3 UK Farm Animal Welfare Council's Five Freedoms (1993) *Second Report on Priorities for Research and Development in Farm Animal Welfare*. Ministry of Agriculture, Fisheries and Food, London.
4 Issued by the Scottish Parliament (16/02/2001).

2 Husbandry

Flock management varies greatly worldwide and it is beyond the scope of this book to detail all production systems. This chapter describes intensive flock management in a country such as the UK, where the major target is the seasonal production per ewe of two 40 kg lambs, of good conformation by 4–8 months of age, achieved largely from pasture.

HANDLING FACILITIES

Ewes pass through handling facilities 12–20 times per annum. It is therefore essential that the facilities function well and are in good repair. They should be roofed (**10, 11**) to afford protection for the sheep and the shepherd during adverse weather. A concrete base and galvanized metal partitions (**11**) allows thorough cleaning and disinfection of the facilities at the end of the day's work. Such precautions are essential when large numbers of sheep are handled over a few days. Infections such as caseous lymphadenitis and contagious pustular dermatitis can persist on surfaces for weeks and be transmitted between groups of sheep.

During the handling process the ewes should move around through 180° so that they head out of the pens in the direction from which they came (**11, 12**), thus giving the sheep the impression that they are returning to the field ('escaping'). The pens should have solid sides to a level above the height of the sheep (**13**). With such a design the sheep cannot see through the pen partitions and they are neither distracted nor frightened when moving through the facilities. In this way the sheep will head towards daylight (**14**) and move smoothly through the handling pens. Sheep quickly become familiar with a quiet and relaxed handling system where the shepherd's patience is rewarded by smooth progression through the pens. The presence of dogs around the handling pens invariably disrupts the smooth flow of sheep and increases workload unnecessarily, stressing both sheep and shepherd.

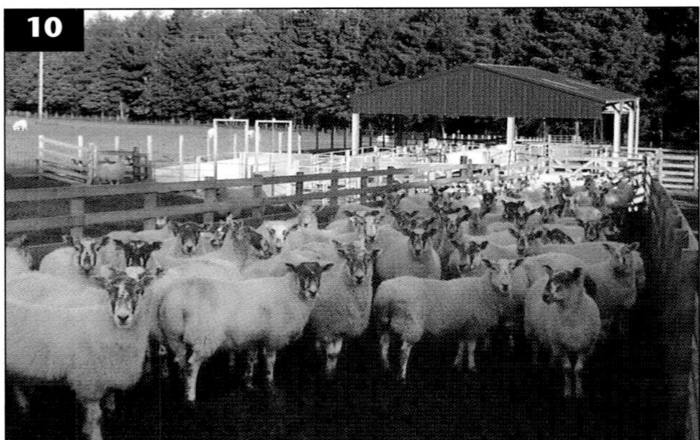

10 Covered sheep handling facility. Note the 180° circuit taken by the sheep.

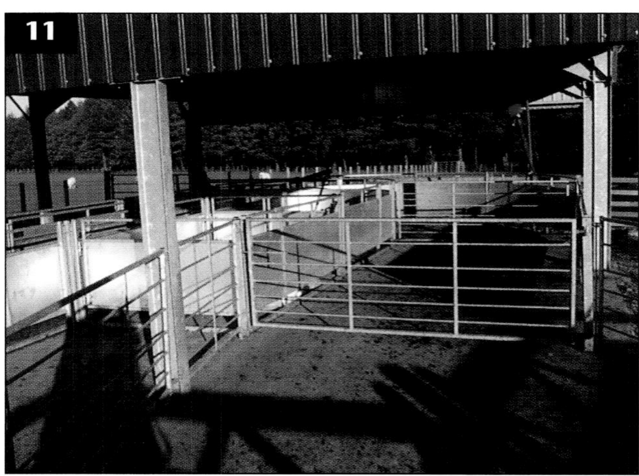

11 Sheep handling facility. There is a concrete floor and solid galvanized metal sidewalls.

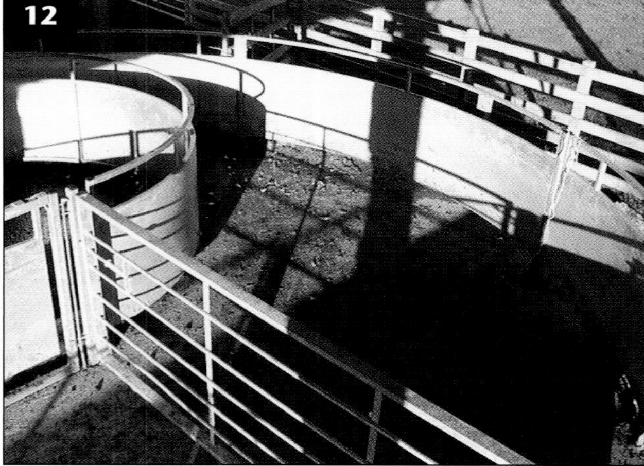

12 Smooth-sided funnel system into a handling race.

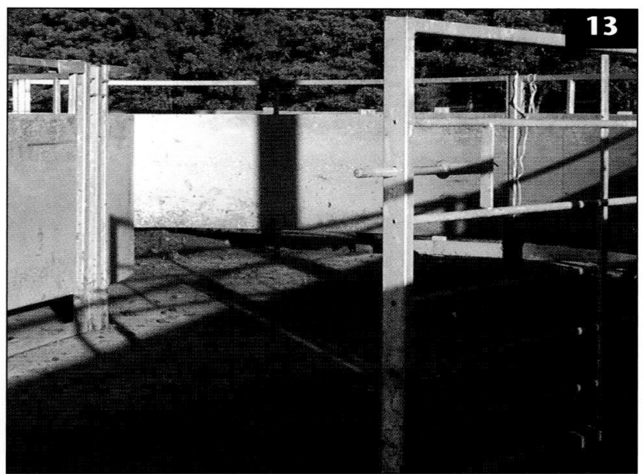

13 Solid partitions free of any sharp protrusions.

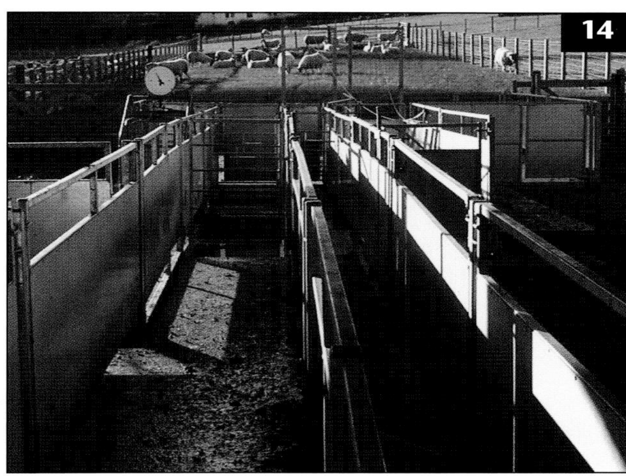

14 Exit via footbaths. The sheep take a 180° circuit.

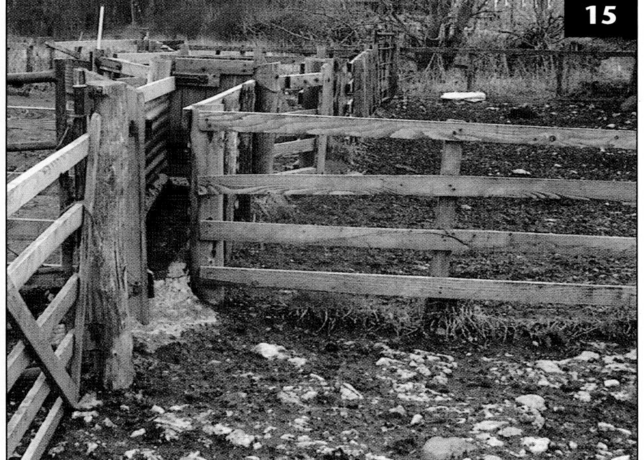

15 Inadequate flooring/surfaces that cannot be cleaned/disinfected between groups of sheep.

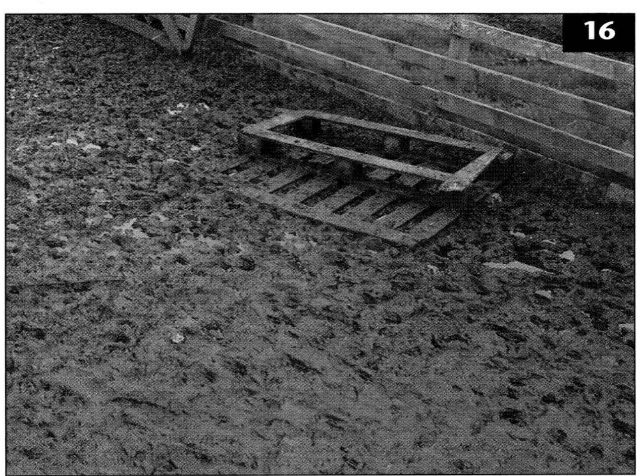

16 Unacceptable handling facilities. There is deep mud/faeces and a risk posed by a wooden pallet left lying around.

The pens must have smooth surfaces with no protruding hinges or latches (**13**) that could cause injury. Wooden handling pens all too frequently have protruding nails or broken wooden rails. Limb fractures are not uncommon when growing lambs are caught in poorly designed pens with wooden rail partitions (**15**) or when pallets, used as temporary gates, are left lying around (**16**).

The sheep should have a clear view of the exit from the footbath (**14**), as this will encourage movement through the facility. The plunge dipper is positioned alongside the footbath. The sheep will have become accustomed to this route during numerous exits from the handling pens (**14**). A larger footbath may be installed to allow sufficient area for sheep to stand in a zinc sulphate footbath for the recommended time.

MATING PERIOD

The mating period is generally timed so that lambing coincides with the start of rapid grass growth in the spring.

Targets

- All ewes should be mated during the first 17 days of the service period.
- Less than 5% of ewes should return to service.
- Rams should be removed after two oestrous cycles (five weeks in the UK), though this can vary in other countries. For example, in New Zealand sheep farmers usually put a terminal sire (mutton breed ram) out for a further cycle.
- No ewes should return for a third service (detected by vasectomized ram).
- At scanning time 98% (or greater) of ewes should be pregnant.
- Abortions should total less than 2%.
- Ninety-five per cent (or greater) of ewes should rear lamb(s) to weaning.

Selection of ewes for breeding

Ewes are usually culled from the breeding flock after six crops of lambs (voluntary culling) but this depends on geographical and husbandry practices. In addition, ewes with palpable mastitis lesions, poor dentition, chronic lameness and poor body condition are culled from the breeding flock (involuntary culling). The involuntary culling rate should be <5%; if it is higher, investigation is warranted and this is detailed later (see Chapter 5, Clinical problem 1, p. 134).

Body condition scoring

Body condition scoring is a subjective means of determining an individual ewe's fat reserves and, to a lesser degree, the amount of skeletal muscle. The amount of fat and muscle covering the transverse processes of the lumbar vertebrae is determined by palpation and graded subjectively from 1 (very thin/emaciated) up to 5 (obese) in 0.5 unit increments. The target body condition score (BCS) for lowland sheep during early pregnancy is 3–3.5, falling to around 2.5–3 during mid-gestation, with little further loss, but ewes with a multiple litter may lose a further 0.5–1 unit during the last six weeks of gestation.

Some farmers, particular in New Zealand, use the weight their sheep to decide if they are ready for mating (e.g. New Zealand Romney 55–60+ kg, Texel 60–70 kg).

Mating period

Lambing time is planned to coincide with the start of rapid grass growth in the spring. Sheep have a gestation length of approximately 147 days, so in the UK, for example, lowland flocks traditionally introduce rams (**17**) on November 5th in order to start lambing on April 1st.

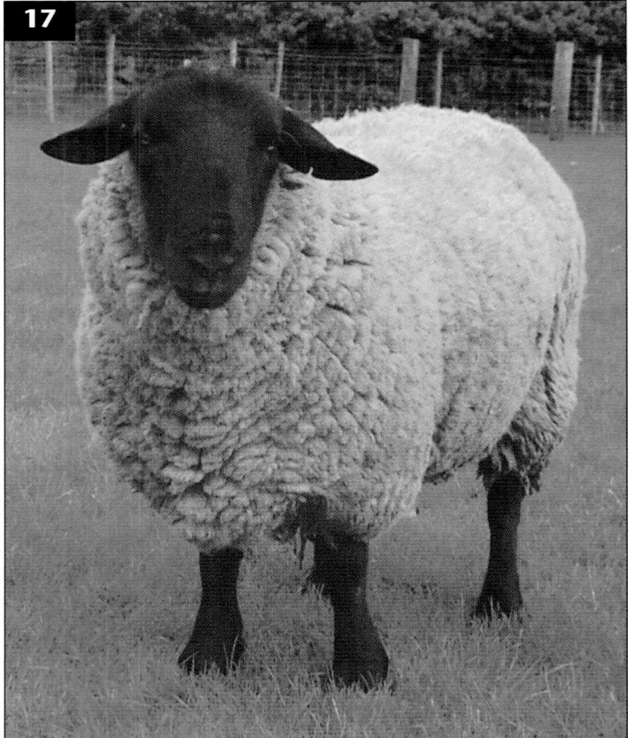

17 Suffolk ram in appropriate condition (body condition score 3.5).

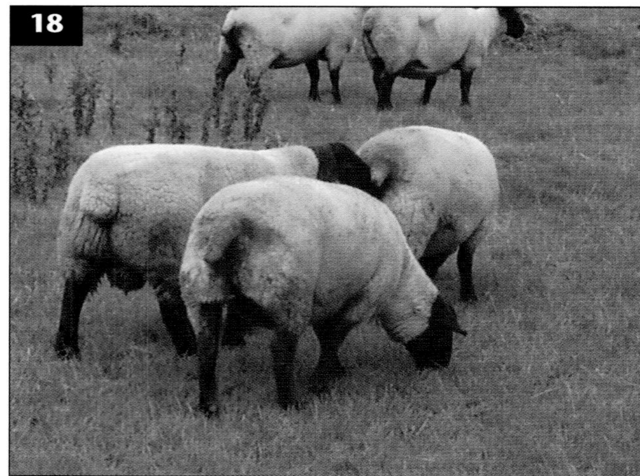

18 Keel paint markings indicate service. The ram is showing interest in this ewe, which has already been mated.

One ram is introduced to 30–50 ewes or, more commonly, three rams are added to a group of 100–120 ewes. Multiple matings of a ewe (**18**), often by different rams, increases the likelihood of conception and may also increase the ovulation rate and, ultimately, the litter size. The competition and constant search for oestrous females during the breeding season causes the rams to lose body condition rapidly and supplementary grain feeding (0.5–0.75 kg/day) is strongly advised to prevent excessive weight loss.

The oestrous cycle is 17 days and the rams are generally rotated after one cycle as an insurance policy in case one group of rams has poor fertility; therefore, ewes not pregnant to the first mating should conceive to the new group of rams.

Conception rate

The conception rate in mature sheep should be >90% and preferably >95%; therefore, the breeding season can be restricted to two oestrous cycles. Lower conception rates are almost invariably due to subfertile rams. Infertility in individual ewes is uncommon unless the ewe is emaciated or there is a history of previous dystocia. The fertility after caesarean section in ewes is very high and comparable to that of normal sheep.

FLUSHING EWES

In many sheep-producing countries, including the UK, the provision of improved nutrition to ewes by means of a good grass sward (**19**) for up to one month before mating and during the breeding season ('flushing') is a farming tradition on both lowland and upland farms. The object is to increase ovulation rates and embryo implantation rates, and this ultimately results in increased litter size. Nutritional manipulation might make physiological sense but there are real consequences of this management practice in hybrid flocks. Triplet-bearing ewes are more prone to OPT, vaginal prolapse, evisceration through a vaginal tear and rupture of the prepubic tendon. Mortality rates in excess of 40% have been reported for triplet lambs when their dams were underfed, compared with 7% in twin lambs born to well-fed dams. If ultrasound scanning data during mid-gestation (often 210% for lowland flocks) is compared with the weaning rate (often 155%), it is questionable whether sheep farmers really do need more lambs at lambing time and whether flushing is a sensible strategy. Such data should form the basis of any flock health scheme evaluation.

Reducing perinatal mortality from its present unacceptable rates (variably quoted as 15–25% in the UK, for example) is more important than producing even more weakly triplet lambs to ewes with insufficient milk on a farm where there is little skilled labour to deal with such highly susceptible neonates. On many farms artificial rearing of orphan lambs is a chore and these lambs are rarely well managed. Flushing may ensure improved ewe condition scores at mating but this can also be achieved by timely weaning and appropriate management thereafter.

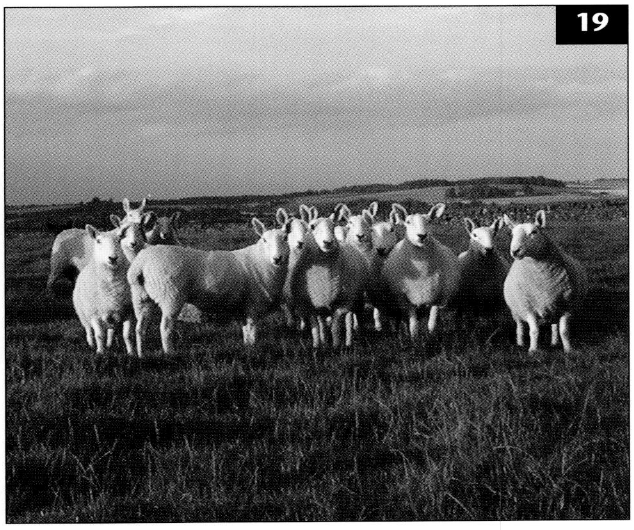

19

19 Scottish half-breed gimmers grazing good pasture prior to mating ('flushing').

PREGNANCY

Pregnancy can be divided into three stages:

- **First trimester:** implantation — weeks 2–7
- **Second trimester:** placental development — weeks 8–14
- **Third trimester:** fetal growth and development — weeks 15–21

Implantation

In many management systems pasture is reserved for the 5–6 week mating period and for one month or so thereafter. Dietary energy supply around the time of implantation, and during the first six weeks of gestation, is therefore adequate because sufficient autumn grass is still available.

Placental development

While the effect of ewe undernutrition during mid-trimester on poor placental development and, subsequently, reduced lamb birth weights (**20**) has been demonstrated under experimental conditions, it can prove difficult to be certain of such an influence in commercial flocks because many other factors affect lamb birth weights. Furthermore, placentas are never collected and weighed and their cotyledons counted and measured during farm investigations.

Weather and/or grazing conditions need to be severe for at least ten days during mid-gestation to impair placental development. However, reduced lamb birth weights can occur when placental development has been limited by competition in the uterus for caruncles, resulting in a reduced number of placentomes per fetus. This situation is not uncommonly encountered in multiple litters and where the birth of twins with disproportionate weights (e.g. 5.5 kg versus 3.5 kg) (lowland sheep breeds; **21**) probably indicates that three embryos implanted and underwent early fetal development but one fetus failed to develop further and was resorbed. The limited number of caruncles available to the remaining fetus in the ipsilateral horn results in poor growth and a much reduced birth weight compared to the co-twin, which developed without competition in the contralateral horn. While the placentomes can increase in size and blood flow, these compensatory mechanisms often fail to overcome their reduced number.

Real-time B-mode ultrasound scanning should be undertaken between 45 and 90 days of gestation to determine fetal number, thereby ensuring more accurate and selective concentrate feeding during the last six weeks of gestation when 75% of fetal growth occurs. The scanning process can be carried out easily and inexpensively, with up to 120 ewes scanned per hour.

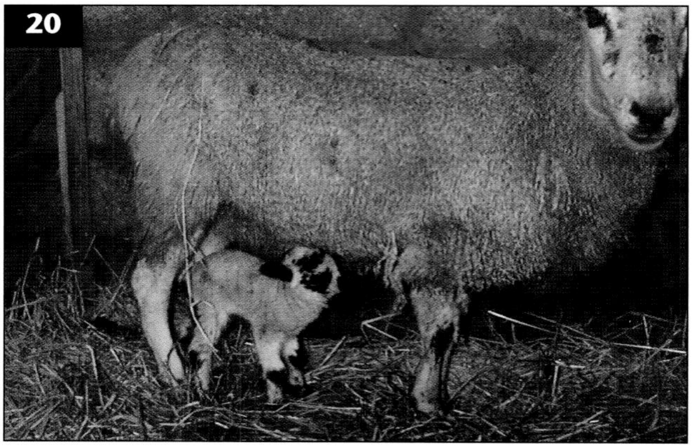

20 Chronic intra-uterine growth retardation as a consequence of poor placental development.

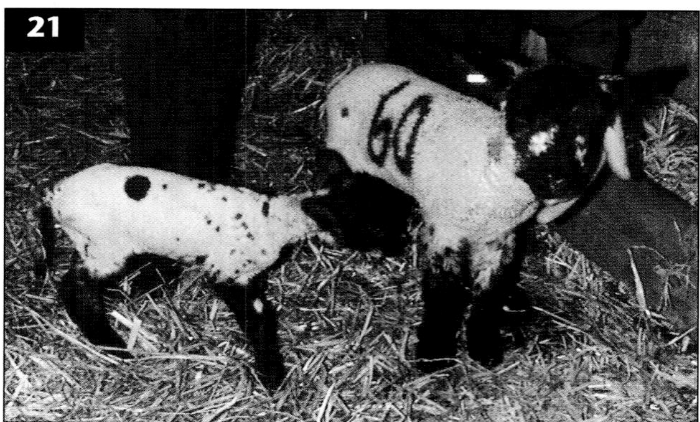

21 Marked difference in birth weights. The smaller lamb would have shared one uterine horn during early placental development but the other fetus has since been resorbed.

Fetal growth and development

Over the past 40 years perinatal lamb mortality has improved little in the majority of flocks worldwide. Many factors, including farm management, levels of flock supervision and infectious diseases, contribute to such losses. Correct lamb birth weight, together with good ewe body condition and adequate colostrum accumulation at lambing, remain fundamental to ensuring a good start for the lamb during the critical first 36 hours of life.

The importance and influence of adequate ewe energy supply during late gestation on lamb survival cannot be overemphasised. The direct influence of dam energy undernutrition during late gestation on reduced lamb birth weights and inadequate accumulation of colostrum in the udder was established almost 20 years ago by Russel[1]. Many studies have found significantly higher lamb perinatal mortality rates in the progeny of underfed ewes, with the effects greater in triplet than in twins lambs; singletons were largely unaffected by the dam's nutritional status (see Flushing ewes, p. 15). There are many excellent field studies, published in the 1980s, that have been largely overlooked, with unacceptable consequences in terms of lamb losses.

Dietary energy supply relative to metabolic demands can be accurately determined during late gestation by measuring the ewe's serum (or plasma) 3-OH butyrate concentration. Increased 3-OH butyrate concentrations (a ketone body) reflect inefficient fatty acid utilization caused by high glucose demand from the developing fetuses not being matched by dietary propionate or glucogenic amino acid supply. Experimental studies have determined an energy supply, reflected in the serum 3-OH butyrate concentration, that results in the birth of healthy lambs of normal birth weight and a dam with sufficient accumulation of colostrum in the udder. These factors combine to ensure the optimum start to the newborn lamb's life. The reader is directed to the excellent article written by Russell[1], which described the interpretation of the serum 3-OH butyrate concentration in relation to dam energy requirements. This article is the cornerstone of any sheep preventive medicine programme.

VETERINARY VISIT TO ASSESS LATE GESTATION EWE NUTRITION

Ewes due to lamb first should be body condition scored and blood sampled 4–6 weeks before the start of lambing (22), thereby allowing sufficient time to implement dietary changes. Primiparous sheep (ewe lambs and gimmers, approximately one year old and two years old, respectively) should not be sampled as they have significantly more singletons and may represent a skewed population. Thereafter, a random sample of 15–20 ewes should be sampled. If the flock has been scanned to determine fetal number, an equal number of twin- and triplet-bearing ewes should be sampled; there is little benefit in collecting samples from ewes with singletons other than to establish reference values. Sick ewes, thin ewes and those not representative of the flock must be investigated separately and not included as part of the nutrition assessment exercise.

Details of the diet (23–25), forage analyses (26) and future alterations should be noted. Feed allocations must be checked on weigh scales and the number of sheep per group accurately determined – approximations lead to unnecessary errors.

Australian and New Zealand farmers tend to use dry matter (DM) estimation of pasture to help control

22 Blood sampling ewes during the veterinary farm visit.

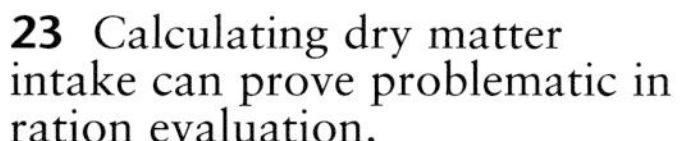

23 Calculating dry matter intake can prove problematic in ration evaluation.

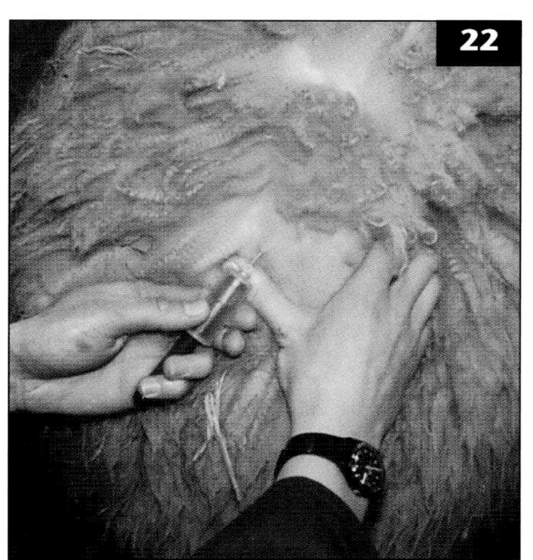

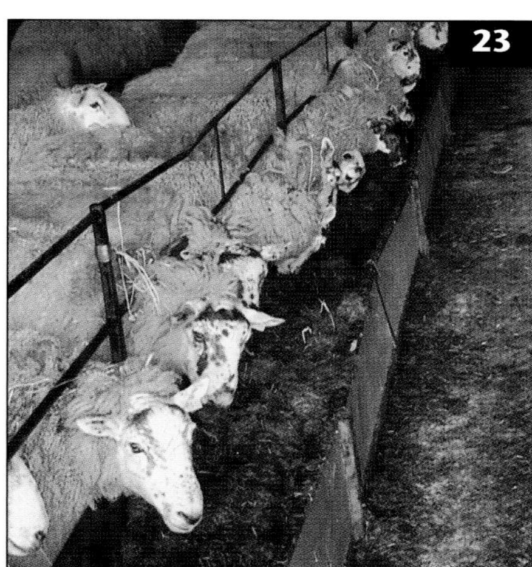

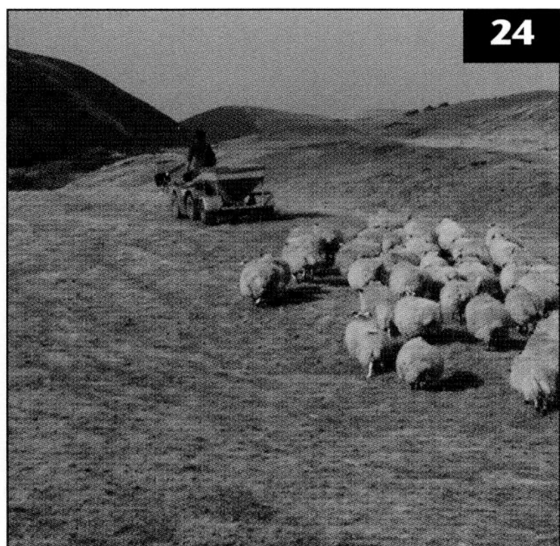

24 It is essential to measure concentrate allowance to all groups of sheep fed from one load.

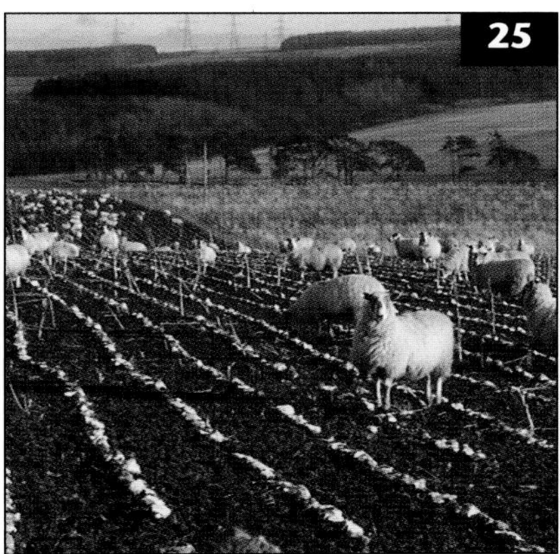

25 Estimating energy contribution from root crops proves very inaccurate.

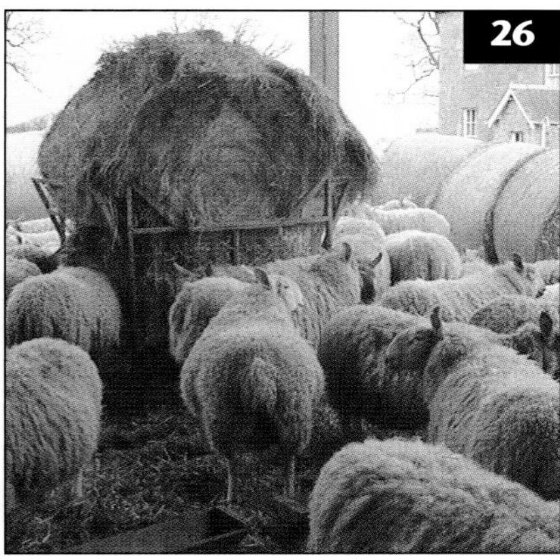

26 Hay intake can be variable between ewes with different fetal numbers.

ewe condition during pregnancy. Pasture with 1,000–2,000 kg DM per hectare is considered optimum, provided it is composed of high quality grasses.

Results and interpretation

A range of 3-OH butyrate concentrations is often encountered in a flock test, largely in relation to fetal number; therefore, a more reliable interpretation of results can be afforded those flocks where fetal number has been determined by prior ultrasound scanning.

The target mean 3-OH butyrate concentration is <1.0 mmol/l. Concentrations >1.6 mmol/l in individual ewes represent severe energy underfeeding, with the likelihood of OPT as pregnancy advances and fetal energy requirements increase unless dietary changes are implemented.

3-OH butyrate concentrations >3.0 mmol/l are consistent with a diagnosis of OPT. Ewes treated for hypocalcaemia may have high 3-OH butyrate concentrations due to inappetence over the previous 24 hours, but they respond to intravenous injection of calcium borogluconate alone without recourse to oral dextrose plus electrolyte solution etc.

Once the mean 3-OH butyrate concentration has been determined, any alteration in the ration can be made with reference to Russel[1] and the farmer advised immediately by telephone, and in writing, regarding future dietary or management changes (**27**).

For example, during a flock visit to determine nutritional management four weeks before lambing commenced, the mean serum 3-OH butyrate concentration of 10 ewes sampled at random is 1.5 mmol/l.

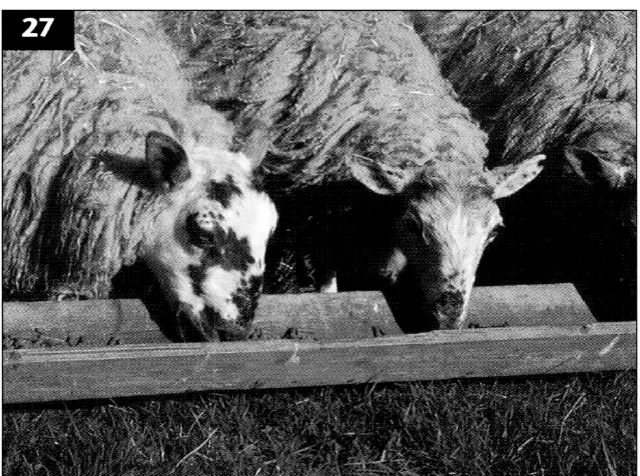

27 Energy shortfalls are quickly corrected by increasing concentrate allowance.

This underfeeding situation necessitates an extra 4 MJ ME/day (0.3 kg of concentrates) to return the ewes to a satisfactory level of energy supply (mean 3-OH butyrate concentration <1.0 mmol/l), with a further 2–6 MJ ME/day given for the last two weeks of pregnancy. The flock should be revisited and blood samples collected two weeks later to check on progress and further monitor any changes in ewe body condition scores.

Evaluation of protein status

Blood samples can also be analysed for blood urea nitrogen (BUN), which indicates short-term protein intake, and albumin, which reflects longer-term protein status. Care must be exercised with the interpretation of these parameters, as recent feeding can greatly influence BUN concentrations. Blood samples should be collected either before concentrate feeding or at least four hours later to avoid postprandial increases. Low BUN concentrations usually indicate a shortage of rumen degradable protein. Serum albumin concentrations fall during the last month of gestation as immunoglobulins are manufactured and accumulate in the udder; therefore, serum albumin concentrations in the region of 26–30 g/l are 'normal' during the last month of gestation. Plasma protein concentrations are often 10–20% higher than corresponding serum protein concentrations; therefore, it is essential to be aware of what samples were submitted to the laboratory before interpretation.

VACCINATION PROGRAMME

A recent survey in the UK showed that up to 16.4% of sheep farmers did not vaccinate their ewes against clostridial diseases. Farmers are advised to vaccinate their ewes against clostridial diseases four weeks before lambing. Ensuring that ewes are in good condition at vaccination time, and receiving an appropriate level of supplementation as determined by the blood samples collected, will guarantee a plentiful accumulation of protective antibodies in their colostrum at lambing time. It is vital that farmers are reminded of the importance of ensuring passive antibody transfer within the first few hours of the lamb's life.

If the flock has not experienced a problem with polyarthritis due to *Erysipelothrix rhusiopathiae* in previous years, such vaccination is not recommended. It is important that heavily pregnant ewes are not challenged with too many antigens at the same time. If there are few losses due to pasteurellosis in lambs less than one month old, consideration should be given to using a multivalent clostridial vaccine and not a vaccine containing the *Pasteurella* species components as well. If it is necessary to administer a *Pasteurella/Clostridia* vaccine and an erysipelas vaccine, separation of the two products by at least one week is recommended.

FOLLOW-UP VISIT DURING LAMBING TIME

A visit must be made during lambing time to discuss progress with the farmer and shepherd. Measurement (with a spring balance) and recording of lamb birth weights and ewe condition scores are essential to determine the success of the flock nutrition advice that has been given during late gestation. In highly productive flocks, particular attention must be paid to the triplet litters.

It is essential to determine any cost benefits from this exercise. Have reduced losses and greater lamb growth rates more than compensated for any increased feed bills? What are the improvements, if any, in terms of animal welfare? What improvements can be made for next year? Written reports should always be provided to remove any doubts over specific points and provide a record for future reference.

LAMBING FACILITIES

As an example, typical management practices during lambing time on farms in the UK are described. While much of this information may appear somewhat basic, it must be viewed against some harsh statistics. Neonatal lamb losses range from 15–25% and have not improved over the past four decades. Similarly, annual ewe mortality figures range from 5–7%, with the majority lost during the periparturient period. These shameful statistics emphasize the need for a fundamental review of management practices during lambing time and highlight the essential role of the practising veterinarian in client education.

Labour requirements

The single most important factor in ensuring a successful lambing period is adequate staffing. This is essential in providing 24-hour supervision of the flock during lambing time. During the first two weeks of lambing, when more than 85% of ewes should lamb (target of 95%), one person per 200 ewes is optimal (e.g. two regular experienced farm staff plus three 'students' working 12 hour shifts in a 1,000 ewe flock). The cost of additional casual labour is approximately 1% of the value of the ewe. Invariably, such labour is rarely available and basic tasks such as correct hygiene and feeding/watering sheep in individual lambing pens are overlooked. In almost all situations, prophylactic administration of oral antibiotic to newborn lambs is used instead of high hygiene standards to prevent watery mouth disease.

Lambing fields

Lambing fields are sometimes used during daylight hours. These are small, well-sheltered fields close to the farm, which allow regular inspection and access to feed stores and shelter. Ewes and their lambs are either confined in shelters in the field (**28**, **29**) or transported indoors.

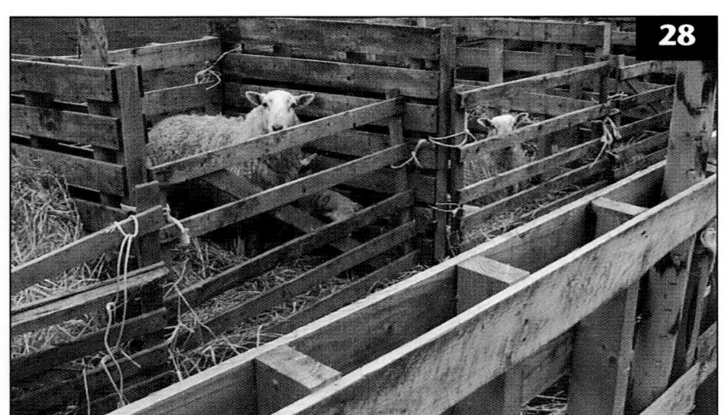

28 An outdoor pen exposed to the weather.

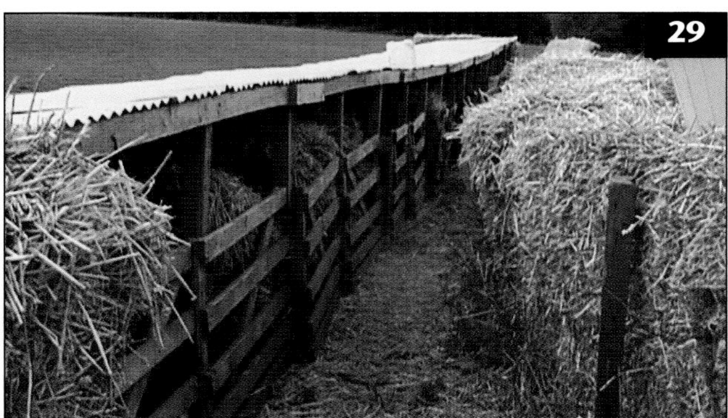

29 Roofed outdoor pens prove unpopular with staff during inclement weather.

Outdoor lambing pens involve a great deal of labour (**30**), and inspection of penned sheep, particularly during the hours of darkness, proves difficult. Outdoor pens are very difficult to clean because they have earth floors.

Traditional lambing fields have the advantage of reducing stocking density in the lambing shed during the day and, as a result, reducing the build-up of infection. During adverse weather the lambing paddocks become very wet and muddy, leading to problems of exposure and an increased incidence of umbilical infections in those lambs born outdoors (**31**).

Housing at night

Regardless of whether ewes are turned out into traditional sheltered lambing fields during the day, almost all flocks are housed during the hours of darkness. This allows continuous close supervision, prompt attention to any problems and penning of newborn lambs and their dam together in order to establish a strong maternal bond. However, such close confinement can cause many disease problems unless strict levels of hygiene are enforced. A wide range of facilities/buildings can be used during lambing to provide shelter (**32–34**).

Not all sheep farmers use covered lambing facilities. In New Zealand, for example, the vast majority of lambs are born unattended in the open air, in paddocks that are sheltered as far as possible from prevailing winds.

Housing

If there have been no previous problems on the farm with respiratory diseases such as sheep pulmonary adenomatosis or maedi, it is recommended that ewes are housed based on fetal number and their due lambing date (keel marks).

Pen dimensions

The critical dimensions of a sheep pen are that it should be three metres wide (**33**) with 450 mm trough space per ewe along one side, allowing 1.3 square metres of floor area per 60–75 kg ewe.

Bedding

The pens must be well bedded with barley straw (wheat straw does not last more than two days, especially with silage-fed ewes). It is essential that the pens are kept clean to prevent the development and spread of footrot and various other bacterial diseases at lambing time. Particular attention must be paid to water troughs to prevent overflowing and flooding of bedding material. Paraformaldehyde granules can be added to the bedding material daily in an attempt to limit bacterial multiplication.

Lighting

Good lighting in the building is essential, especially over the individual pens.

Ventilation

Ventilation of sheep sheds relies upon the natural stack effect. Air enters through the space boarding under the eaves and is drawn out through the central ridge gap in the roof. Ventilation problems can arise when buildings are sited too close together (**35**) or where the air can only enter at the front of the building (**36, 37**).

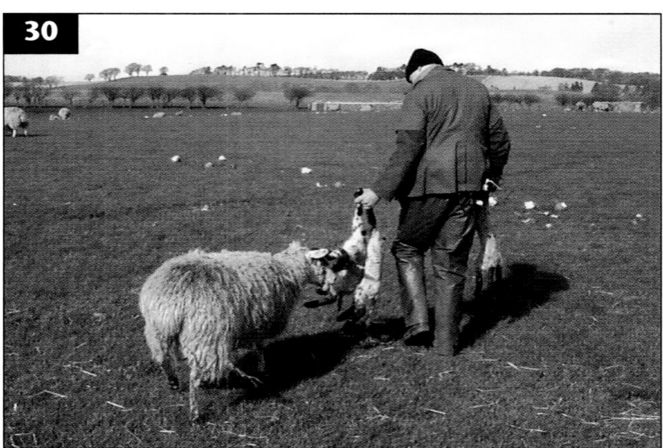

30 Carrying newborn lambs to an outdoor pen with confinement to ensure development of the maternal bond.

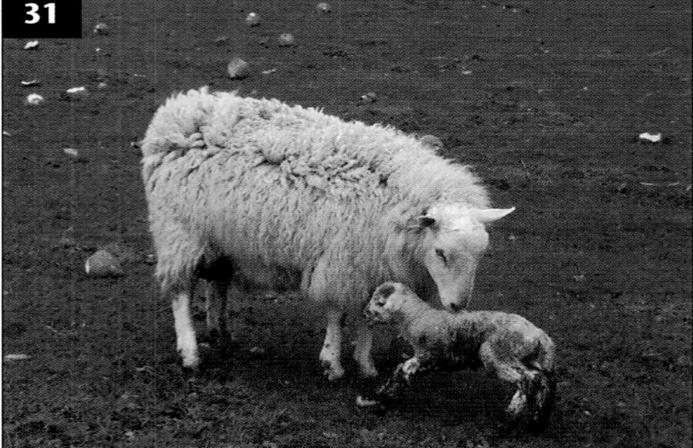

31 Outdoor lambing. There is soil contamination of the lamb, including the umbilicus.

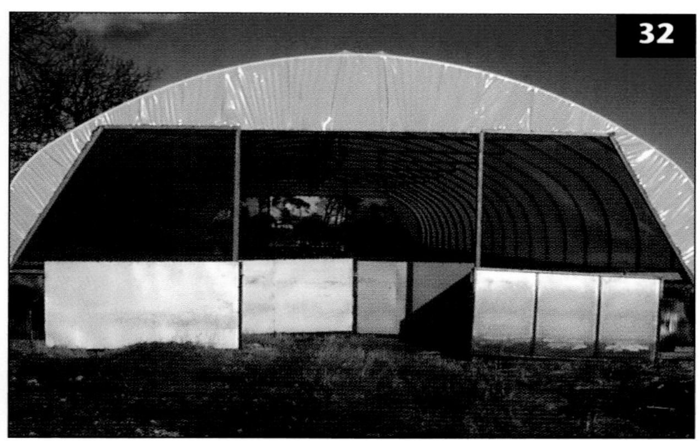

32 Polythene tunnel housing is cheap to erect.

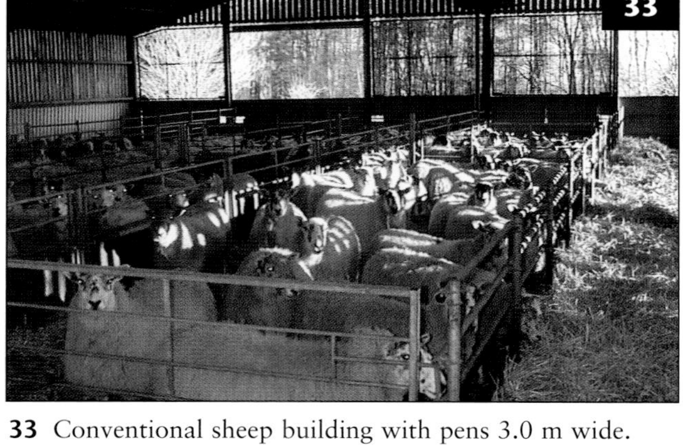

33 Conventional sheep building with pens 3.0 m wide.

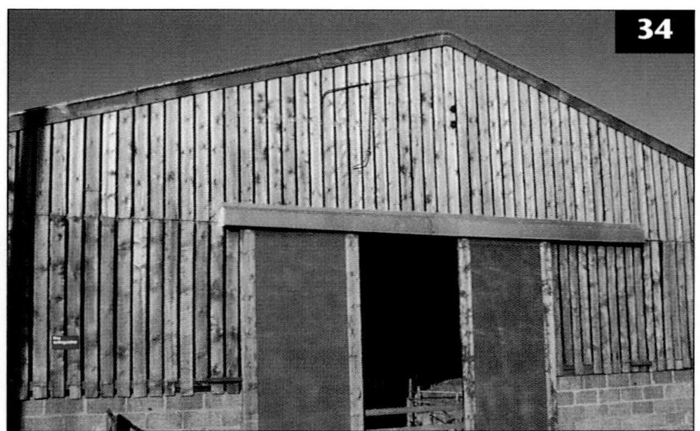

34 Sheep building with space boarding and central ridge gap.

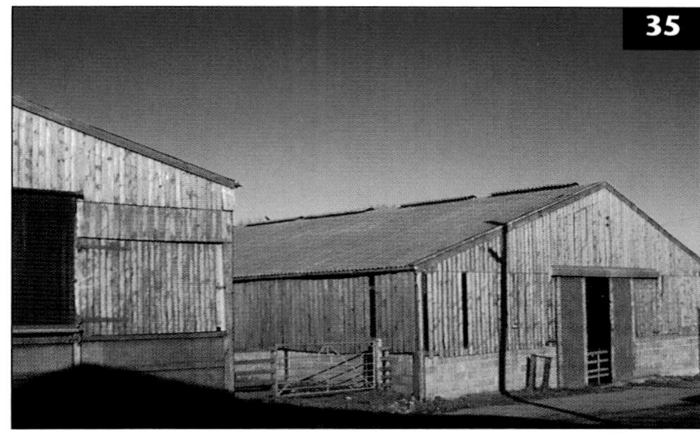

35 Sheep buildings too close together can adversely affect ventilation.

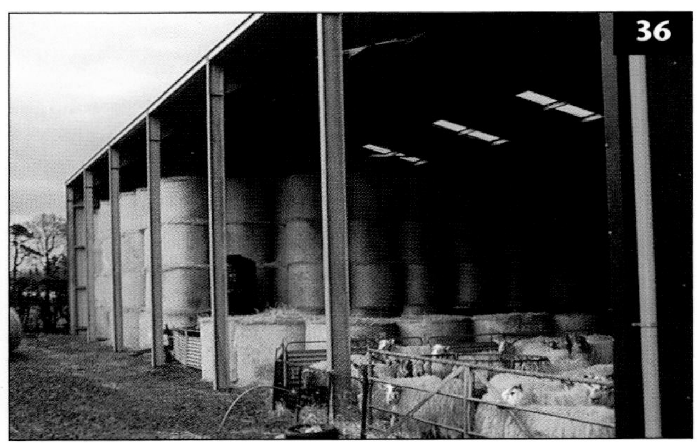

36 Multi-purpose farm building used as temporary sheep accommodation.

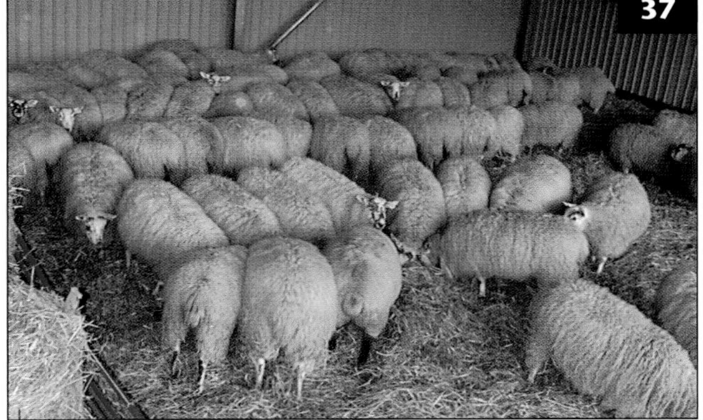

37 No pen divisions, leading to large group size in this multi-purpose farm building. Note the limited ventilation.

Individual pens

Individual pens must be well drained, be a minimum size of 1.5 m by 1.5 m, and have concrete floors with solid partitions. These pens should be cleaned out and disinfected between every ewe but this practice is rarely achieved on most commercial farms. Each pen must be provided with a water bucket and feed container. Six buckets cannot service 50 or more lactating ewes. Newly-lambed ewes will often drink more than ten litres of water after lambing. Placentas must be removed from the individual pens and put into plastic sacks for burning or burial.

During an intensive lambing period (up to 15% of ewes lambing in a 24-hour period), given the practice of fostering lambs and the likelihood of adverse weather conditions, one pen per five ewes is needed to avoid accommodation shortages. During adverse weather farmers rarely have sufficient housing and overcrowding can lead to problems with infectious bacterial diseases.

Use of multi-purpose buildings for housing sheep

Problems arise when attempting to adapt multi-purpose farm buildings to house sheep during late gestation and for the first few days after lambing. Straw sheds can be used to house sheep but problems can arise at feeding time when the building has not been subdivided.

MISMOTHERING

Mismothering is much more common in flocks where ewes are closely confined during lambing (**38–42**) compared with outdoor lambing (**43**).

ORPHAN LAMBS

Orphan lambs are generally small birth weight twin or triplet lambs removed because of poor dam milk yield. The majority of these lambs have failed to ingest sufficient colostrum and are therefore prone to a wide range of bacterial diseases during the neonatal period, including polyarthritis, enteric infections and respiratory disease. These lambs have often been hungry for a number of days before removal from the dam.

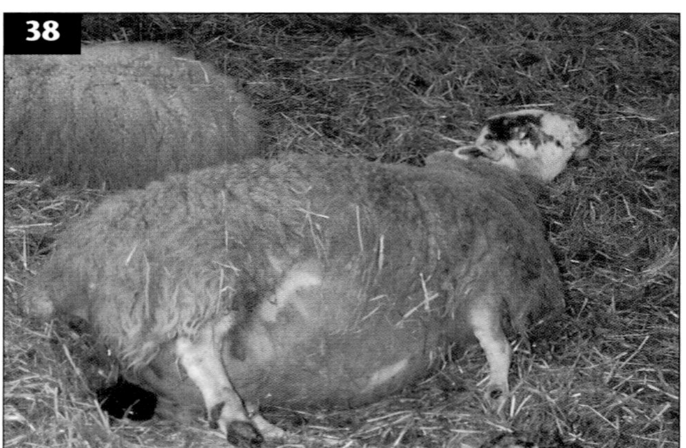

38 End of first stage labour. The close proximity of other sheep in this artificial confinement situation is alien to the ewe's natural instincts.

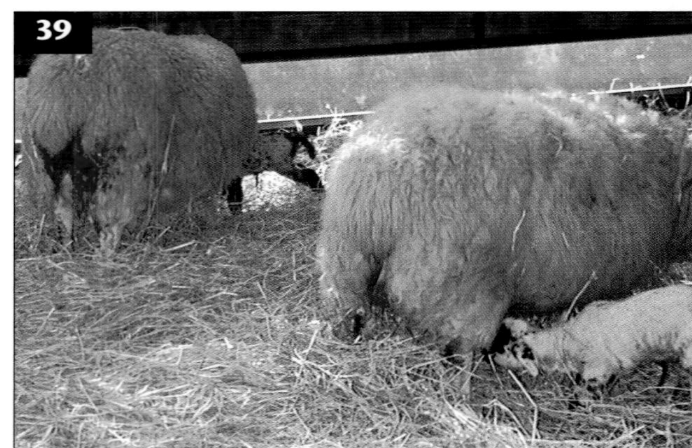

39 'Stealing' behaviour by the ewe on the right.

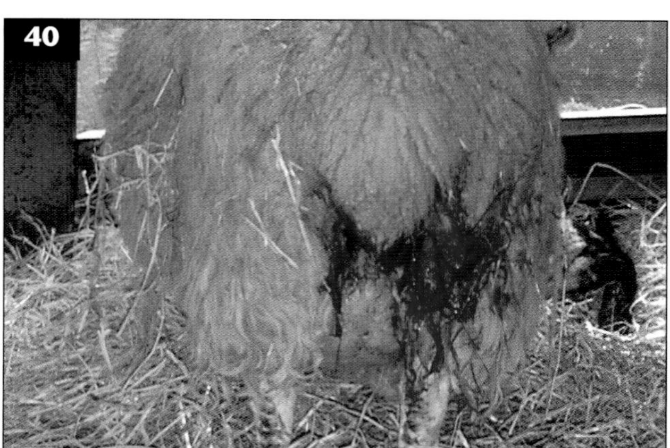

40 Blood and fetal fluids on the wool around the perineum of this newly lambed ewe.

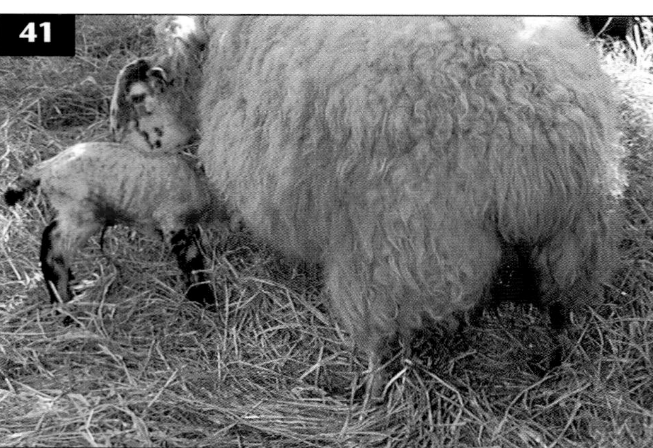

41 Absence of blood and fetal fluids on the wool around the perineum of this ewe, which has claimed a lamb from another ewe.

Rearing orphan lambs presents many problems. It has been recommended that 'surplus' lambs are removed from the ewe as early as possible because they learn to suck much more quickly from the milk bar than if left with their dam for two or three days. It could be reasoned that the smallest triplet of every litter should be removed within hours of birth, fed colostrum and either fostered immediately or reared artificially. The ewe and its two remaining lambs could then be turned out to pasture the following day.

Triplet lambs must not be viewed simply as 'spare lambs' to replace losses. If there is a surplus of lambs, a review of the flock nutrition prior to and during mating (flushing) should be undertaken.

Fostering of orphan lambs

Fostering triplet lambs on to ewes that have lost a lamb, whether stillborn or from other causes, is a routine management procedure undertaken on most farms in an attempt to maximize financial returns. In addition, lambs are also fostered on to ewes that produce a single lamb.

In general terms, 10% of ewes on lowland farms produce only one lamb, 65% produce two lambs and 25% produce three or more lambs; thus, there exists an abundance of lambs for fostering. No large scale survey has been undertaken to determine the number of attempted 'fosterings' in lowland flocks but it could be conservatively estimated at >10–15% and therefore warrants discussion. Furthermore, fostering is not as simple as would first appear and the long-term acceptance rate by the ewe is likely to be <60%. Numerous welfare concerns arise from the various methods employed to convince a ewe to accept another lamb. Veterinarians must be aware of these management procedures to enable them to advise their clients and, more importantly, ensure the health and welfare of these sheep.

Transfer of fetal fluids

Rubbing an orphan lamb in the fetal fluids (**44**) of the newborn single lamb before the ewe licks her own lamb is the most successful fostering method. Good acceptance rates are achieved when the foster lamb is as young as possible and preferably newborn. It has been suggested that the shepherd should gently insert a well-lubricated gloved hand into the ewe's posterior reproductive tract to simulate birth of another lamb but the practical use of this 'kidology' has not been scientifically proven.

If the foster lamb is more than a few hours old and its coat is dry, it should first be immersed in a bucket of warm water to aid transfer of fetal fluids

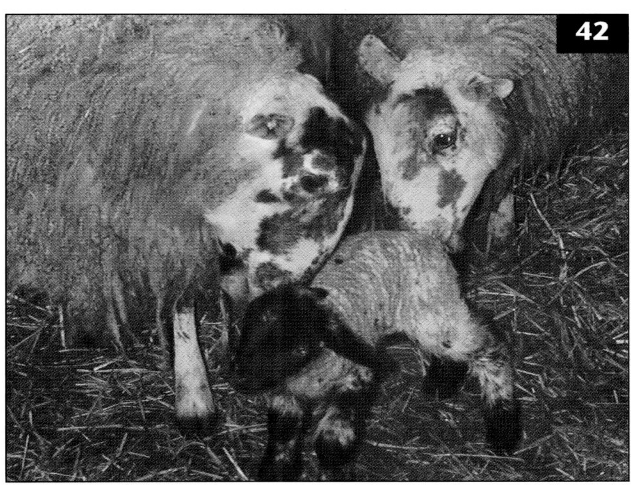

42 'Stealing' behaviour is common in ewes managed in close confinement.

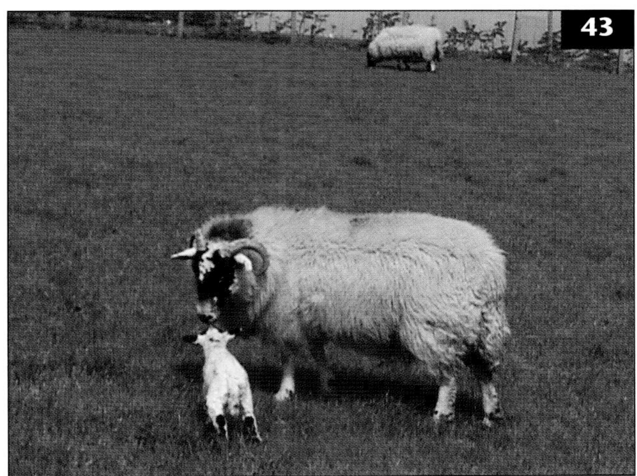

43 Lambing under natural conditions.

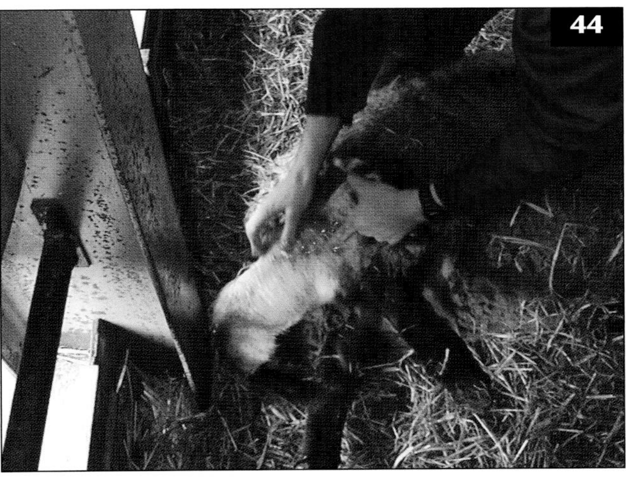

44 Transferring fetal fluids to the foster lamb immediately after delivery of a singleton.

and associated odours onto the wet fleece. Many shepherds will place only the foster lamb in the pen with the ewe for a period of time before introducing the ewe's own lamb. Time spent ensuring initial acceptance by the ewe is well worthwhile. Some shepherds may elect to castrate and tail dock the foster lamb using elastrator rings at this time to delay its normal active behaviour and teat searching, because the ewe is suspicious of a 'newborn' lamb that is already ambulatory (**45**).

A variation on the fostering method described above is to place both lambs in a hessian sack, which is then tied at the neck and placed in the pen with the ewe for one hour (**46**). This practice facilitates mixing of odours and increases the foster lamb acceptance rate when the lambs are introduced to the anxious ewe.

Disparity in size (**47**) of the new 'pair' of lambs frequently results (6–7 kg singleton and 3.5 kg triplet). The smaller foster triplet lamb may be unable to keep up with the much larger singleton when the litter is turned out to pasture, and careful supervision of fostered lambs is essential to achieve good results and ensure the welfare of the smaller lamb.

'Skinning' lambs

Fostering lambs with the aid of the dead lamb's skin (**48**) has mixed success depending on the age of the dead lamb and the age of the foster lamb. Unless both lambs are less than two days old, a period of time in various foster crates usually becomes necessary (see below).

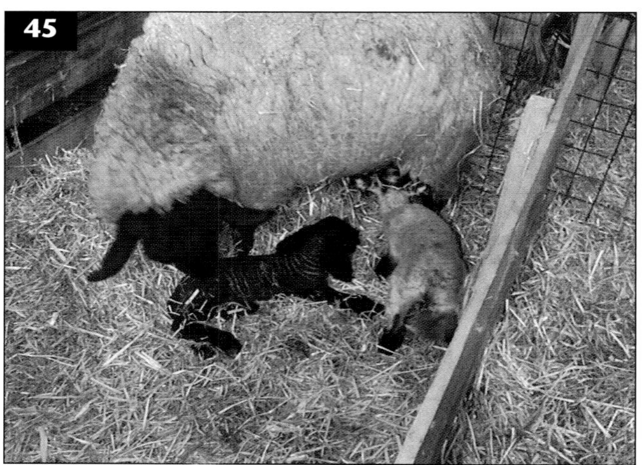

45 This day-old foster lamb is already sucking. The ewe will recognize this immediate ability to walk/suck as abnormal and may reject the foster lamb.

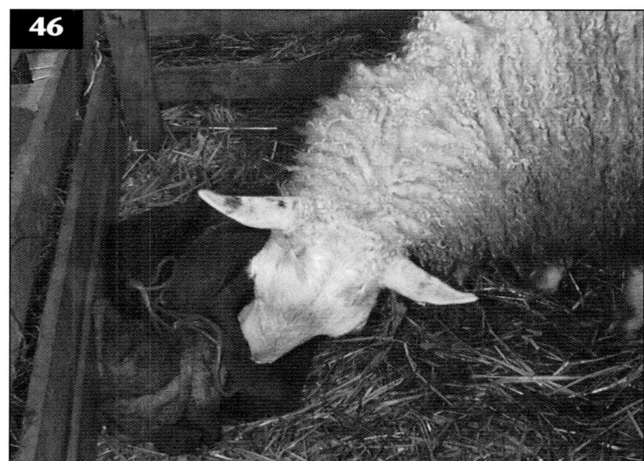

46 Both lambs have been placed in a hessian sack, which is then tied at the neck and put in the pen with the ewe for about one hour.

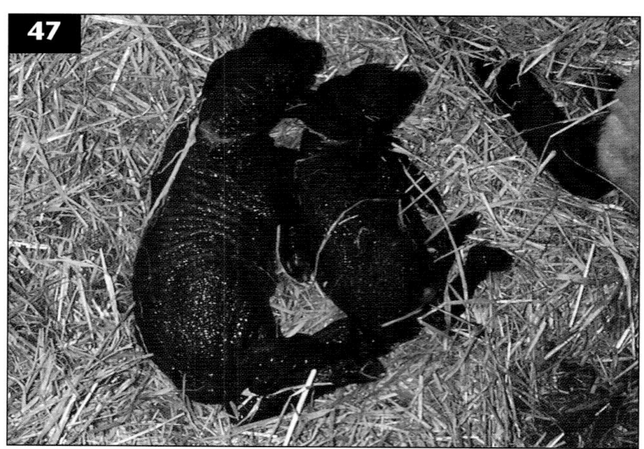

47 Fostering a triplet lamb results in marked disparity in live weight.

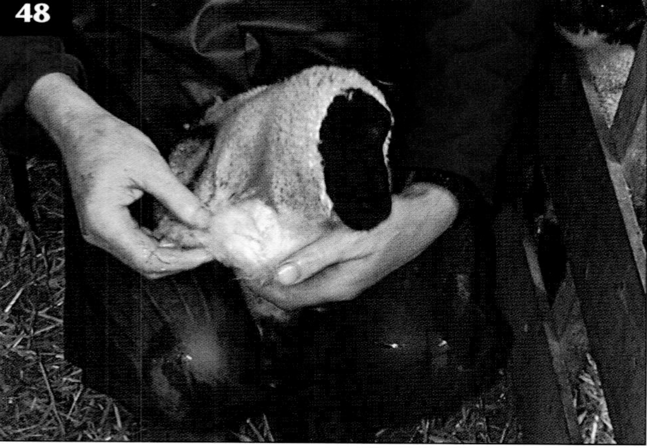

48 Transferring a dead lamb's skin on to a foster lamb.

Foster crates

There are many designs of foster crates (**49–52**), and none are satisfactory. Some are totally unacceptable (**53**). However, the welfare of the ewe could be greatly improved if more attention was exercised to ensure that clean water and good quality roughage was always available (**49**) and that concentrates were fed at least twice daily where the ewe could reach them. Inadequate ewe nutrition merely leads to poor milk production and poor long-term acceptance rates.

Rope halters

A rope halter provides limited freedom and improved comfort for the ewe provided it does not tighten across the bridge of the ewe's nose.

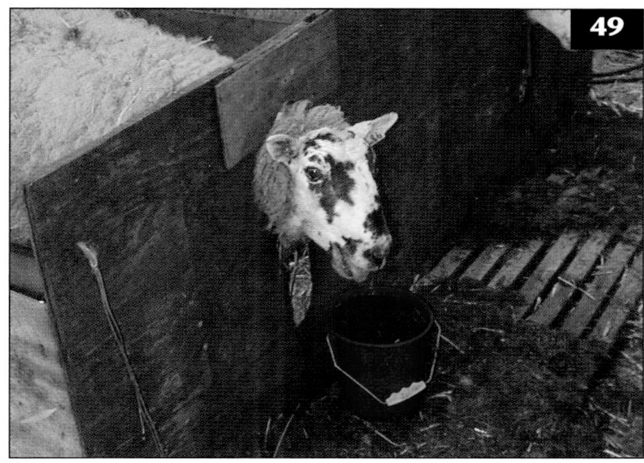

49 Foster crate showing water bucket and feed.

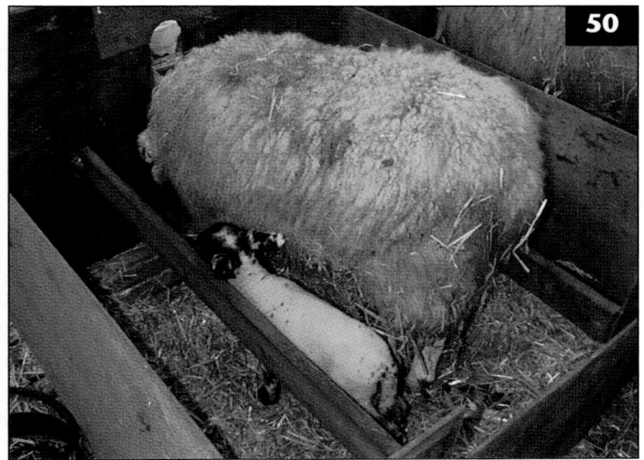

50 Rear view of foster crate.

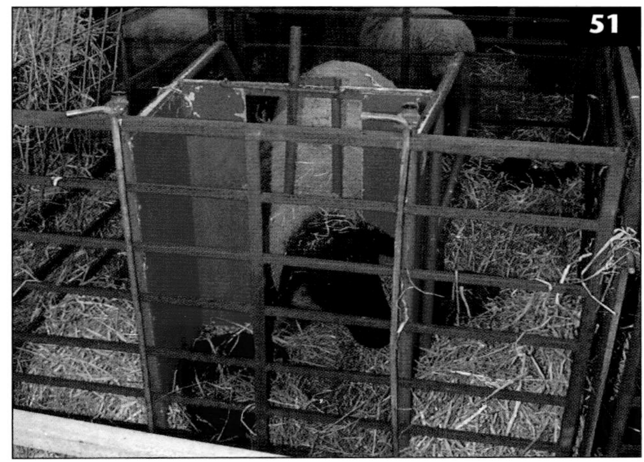

51 Another foster crate design.

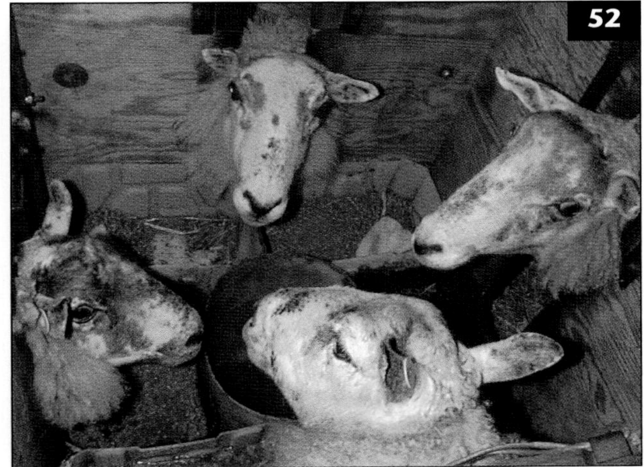

52 Foster crate for four ewes with advantage of central feed/water provision for all ewes.

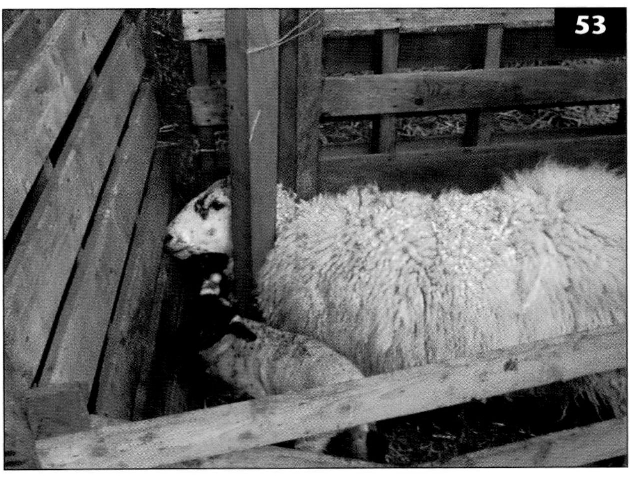

53 Inappropriate 'stocks' design used to restrain a ewe.

Halters should be made of soft rope and not a single strand of polypropylene baler twine (**54**). Occasionally, the rope is tied around the ewe's horns, which is unacceptable (**55**).

Rejection of foster lamb

The ewe and lambs must be carefully supervised to detect early rejection such as not letting the foster lamb suck, pushing the lamb away and vigorous head butting, which can cause severe chest trauma and even death of neglected lambs. The transfer of marker fluid used to identify lambs on to the ewe's forehead can often detect head-butted lambs.

Ewes can reject the orphan lamb at any stage but especially following turnout from a small pen to pasture. Ewes with foster lambs should be clearly marked and allocated to small paddocks for up to one week before rejoining the main flock.

ARTIFICIAL REARING OF ORPHAN LAMBS

Orphans lambs can be reared very successfully on artificial rearing systems using automatic milk dispensers. Such systems can produce excellent lamb growth rates and a low incidence of digestive disturbances (e.g. abomasal bloat and/or volvulus). Haphazard feeding of lambs from a bucket and teat system does not work. At weaning, at around five weeks old, these lambs are small, poorly fleshed and pot-bellied, and they remain so for many months (once a runt, always a runt). Unless farmers are prepared to devote time and resources to rearing orphan lambs, they should consider selling them within the first week of life.

Diseases of artificially reared orphan lambs

Enteric infections

Colibacillosis is common in orphan lambs due to overwhelming bacterial challenge caused by poor hygiene in the 'pet pen'. It can prove very difficult to maintain dry bedding in the pet pen; therefore, lambs must be transferred between disinfected pens on a regular 2–3-day rotation. A wooden slatted floor is essential to allow effective drainage and there must be ample dry barley straw bedding.

Improved pen hygiene, as detailed above, should also limit cryptosporidiosis. Coccidiosis is a major problem in orphan lambs because farmers are often not prepared to purchase medicated feed for only 20–30 lambs. Orphan lambs should be offered fresh lamb pencils containing decoquinate in clean troughs from two weeks old. While prevention of coccidiosis with diclazuril is effective, and cheaper, than in-feed decoquinate medication, it may prove difficult to determine the appropriate timing for prophylaxis.

Orphan lambs are frequently turned out in to small areas of grass around the farm buildings that are also used for sick ewes at lambing time; therefore, these 'paddocks' are often heavily infested with nematode larvae arising from the periparturient rise in egg output. Regular anthelmintic treatment of orphan

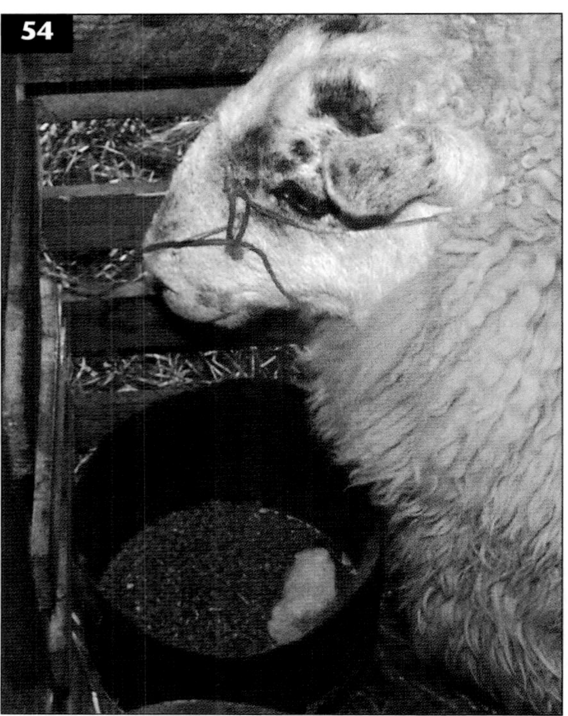

54 Ewe restrained by a halter fashioned from polypropylene twine.

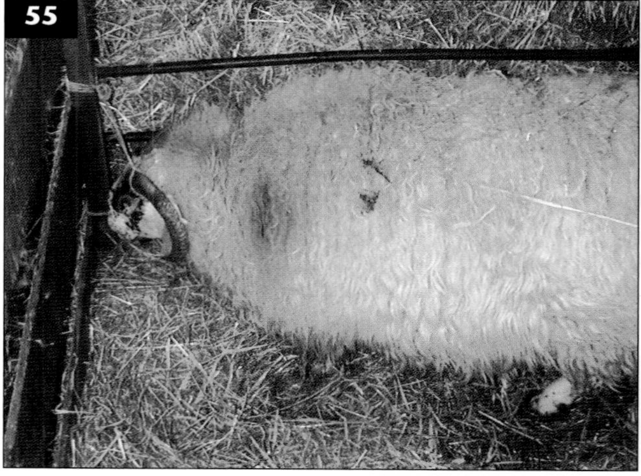

55 Ewe restrained by a rope tied around the base of her horns.

lambs at pasture is essential to prevent significant parasitic burdens but is often neglected. Orphan lambs should be fed concentrates throughout the grazing season to achieve satisfactory growth rates.

Skin infections
Contagious pustular dermatitis (CPD, orf) can spread very rapidly through a group of orphan lambs, causing large granulomatous lesions that impair sucking and eating. It not uncommon to find orphan lambs severely affected by orf, while all the naturally reared lambs appear unaffected or have only minor lesions. Affected lambs may act as a source of infection to the flock and should be kept in isolation.

Leakage of milk replacer from the teats onto the lamb's face during sucking can predispose to superficial skin infections, whether caused by *Staphylococcus aureus* (**56**) or *Dermatophilus congolensis*.

Respiratory tract infections
Respiratory tract infections, caused by a combination of parainfluenza 3 (PI3) infection, *Pasteurella* species and various pyogenic organisms, notably *Arcanobacterium pyogenes*, are especially common in orphan lambs (**57**, **58**).

Cutaneous myiasis
Blowfly strike is not uncommon in orphan lambs because they often have faecal staining of the tail and/or perineum. Orphan lambs often have not been tail docked because they missed that routine procedure at turnout to pasture with their dam when one day old.

Conclusion
The welfare of orphan lambs requires urgent review. There are no benefits to be gained from producing even more triplet lambs on lowland and upland farms, so why do veterinarians and agricultural advisers persist with the recommendation to flush ewes?

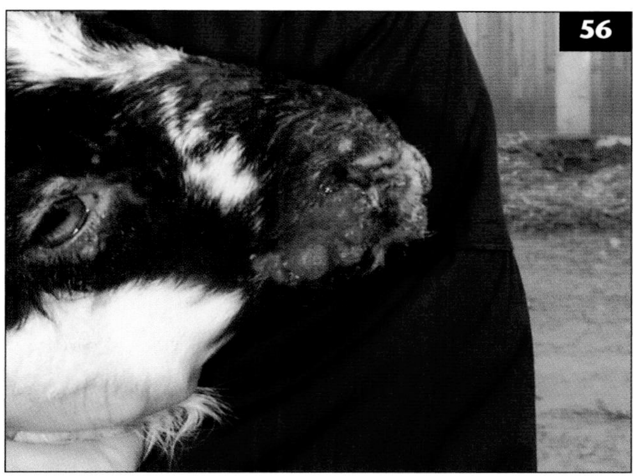

56 Staphylococcal dermatitis in an orphan lamb.

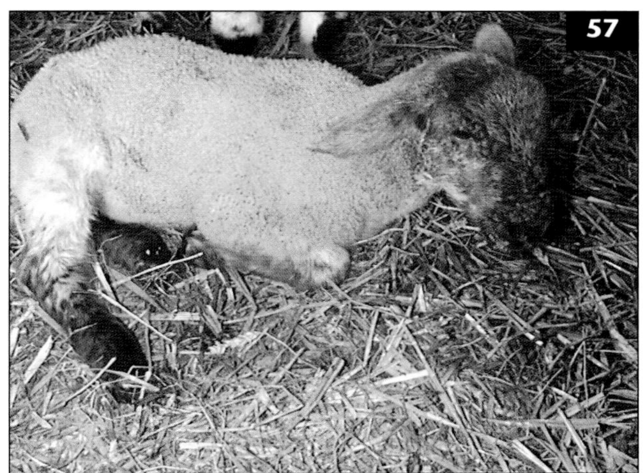

57 Foster lamb suffering from chronic suppurative pneumonia.

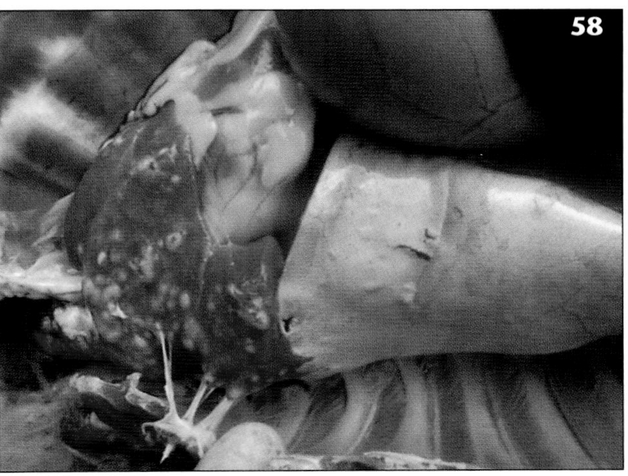

58 Postmortem illustration of chronic suppurative pneumonia.

CASTRATION AND TAIL DOCKING

Definition/overview
Castration and tail docking of young lambs is traditionally undertaken in many countries worldwide.

It is generally believed that tail docking prevents faecal contamination of the perineum, thereby reducing the likelihood of cutaneous myiasis; however, cutaneous myiasis affects mountain breeds in the UK (e.g. the Scottish Blackface), yet tradition dictates that they are not docked. It is unlikely that tail docking

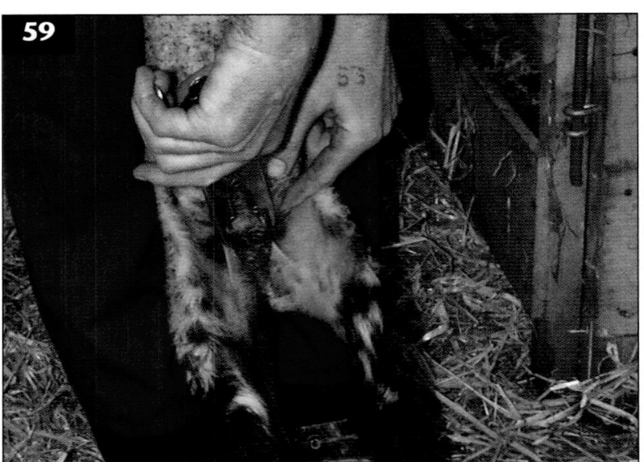

59 Applying an elastrator ring to the neck of the scrotum.

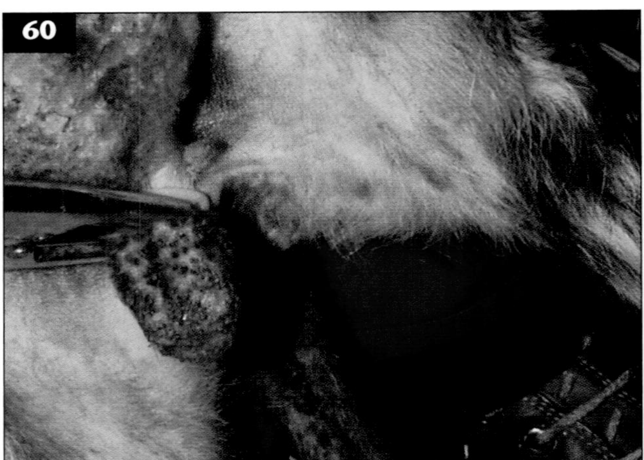

60 Elastrator ring applied to a scrotum containing both testicles. Note the ring is distal to the vestigial teats.

would be necessary if farmers practised good control of parasitic gastroenteritis and used pour-on preparations to control blowfly strike. Increasing concerns over zoonoses have dictated that sheep must have a clean fleece when presented at the slaughter plant. Docked sheep may be cleaner than sheep with tails but correct parasite control and a clean environment should limit most fleece contamination.

Castration is used to eliminate indiscriminate breeding but in many intensive management systems entire male lambs are sold for slaughter before they are sexually mature. An entire male lamb production system operates most effectively where lambs are intensively managed and marketed at no later than four months old. This system is typically found in the UK, where January lambing flocks produce lambs for the Easter market. Castrated lambs have the disadvantage that they grow more slowly and produce a fatter carcase than entire males.

However, on many farms an extended interval to slaughter, often up to one year old, greatly increases the likelihood of unwanted pregnancies in ewe lambs and in the ewe flock. Few farms have stock-proof fences, except for boundary fences, and this prevents segregation of the sexes.

In the UK elastrator rings can be used only during the first week of life (**59**, **60**). Castration with a knife or bloodless castrator (Burdizzo) can be performed without an anaesthetic in lambs up to three months old; tail docking can be performed in lambs up to two months old. Thereafter, an anaesthetic is required but it would be very uncommon for these procedures to be undertaken at such a late stage. The restrictions on the timing of these procedures are completely arbitrary and there exists considerable difference of opinion on this subject. In practice, castration and tail docking of six-week-old hill lambs is still commonly performed with rubber elastrator ring without anaesthetic (**61**, **62**).

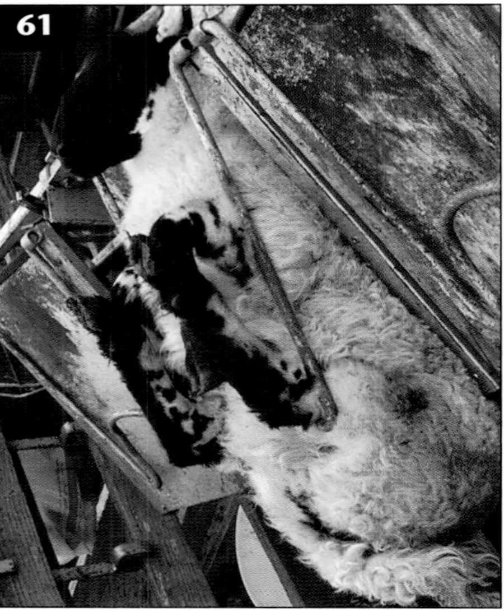

61 Restraining crate for older lambs. This lamb is more than six weeks old yet is castrated using an elastrator ring.

Elastrator rings

It is a legal requirement in the UK that sufficient tail remains to completely cover the anus and, in females, the vulva. The correct position for the elastrator ring is distal to (i.e. towards the tip of the tail) the two folds of skin that arise from either side of the anus and attach to the tail (caudal folds). Many ram breeders attempt to flout these regulations in the belief that a shorter tail makes the male rear quarters

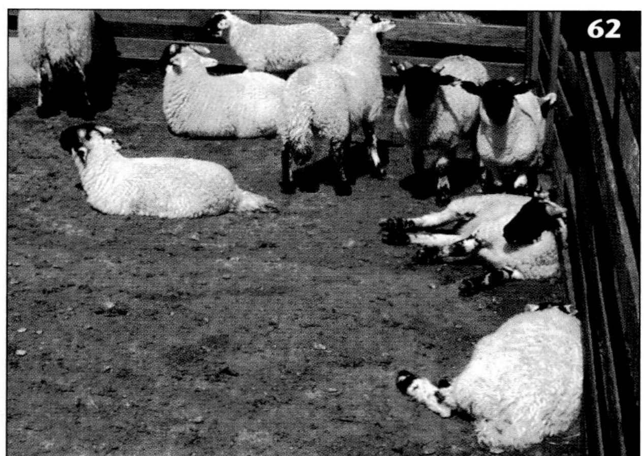

62 Abnormal active behaviours indicating acute pain minutes after elastrator ring application.

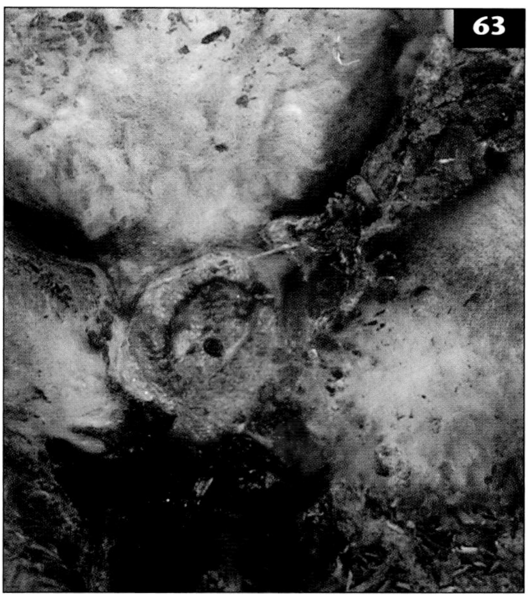

63 Granulating wound caused by application of an elastrator ring to a six-week-old lamb.

look more 'meaty'. In the USA, many Suffolk show sheep have no tail whatsoever.

Castration and tail docking using elastrator rings is most commonly undertaken when lambs are still confined in the lambing pens during their first day of life. One person can efficiently process up to 200 lambs per hour under such a management system. There is no evidence that the application of elastrator rings increases neonate mortality.

Local anaesthetic injection into the spermatic cord proximal to the elastrator ring blocks conduction of pain stimuli for up to two hours; however, this is not a practical method because of the time taken and the requirement of a second person to restrain the lamb adequately.

Economics

Elastrator rings cost very little; therefore, the economics of the procedure do not unduly concern farmers.

Welfare implications

Few farmers believe that castration and tail docking with elastrator rings are significant welfare issues. Farmers reason that ewe lambs show few pain responses and ram lambs appear to have recovered from their abnormal postures and rolling behaviour within 1–2 hours of the procedure. It is claimed that castration and tail docking with elastrator rings cause chronic inflammation, sepsis and pain until the necrotic areas detach from healthy tissue. This rarely occurs in lambs that are less than one week old when the elastrator rings are applied but it can present problems (**63**) when rings are applied illegally to older lambs.

Currently, there is no evidence to demonstrate that castration has a significant long-term effect on daily live weight gain. There is also no evidence that the superficial infection noted around the elastrator ring gives rise to a bacteraemia and focal infections (e.g. vertebral empyema, polyarthritis and endocarditis).

Castration and tail docking have attracted considerable research interest and there has been a trend to classify castration and tail docking of young lambs as mutilations.

SURGICAL CASTRATION AND TAIL DOCKING

Surgical castration and docking has no practical advantages over the elastrator ring method except that it can legally be performed without an anaesthetic for castration of lambs up to three months old and for tail docking of lambs up to two months old. There is a risk of herniation through the inguinal ring in older lambs, especially when the operator does not incise the vaginal tunic and applies traction to the vaginal tunic and spermatic cord (effectively a closed castration). This action damages the inguinal ring and increases the risk of herniation, which occurs within hours of castration. The herniated intestines become contaminated and traumatized and they may rupture. Affected lambs must be euthanased immediately for welfare reasons.

Infection leading to diffuse peritonitis and death is a major risk in open castration. This procedure must not be undertaken when lambs are wet. Older lambs often have diarrhoea with faecal staining of the perineum. It can prove very difficult to maintain any semblance of sterility when castrating large numbers of lambs.

BLOODLESS (BURDIZZO METHOD) CASTRATION

The bloodless castration method has the welfare advantage that the nerve supply to the testicles is destroyed. Rupture of the blood vessels in the spermatic cord results in testicular atrophy. The skin of the scrotum is not broken; therefore, there is no risk of peritonitis.

The procedure is time-consuming and it is not simple. Bloodless castration of day-old lambs takes 5–10 times longer than the elastrator ring method and necessitates two operators, one person to hold the lamb and the other to do the castration.

The major concern is that, unlike with calves, it is not possible to be certain that both spermatic cords have been sufficiently crushed to result in avascular necrosis of the testicles. Failure to crush the spermatic cord results in a potentially fertile male lamb and unwanted pregnancies should his masculinity not be detected before the autumn (breeding/mating season). In many lambs there is not sufficient length to the spermatic cord to permit a second attempt at crushing.

However, most observant shepherds will readily detect entire male lambs from about three months old. The older the lamb, the more noticeable the broader head, thicker neck and more aggressive behaviour. From six months old these entire male lambs show the flehmen response. In horned breeds, entire male lambs have much larger and thicker horns.

Much greater emphasis must be placed on the overall efficiency of rapid growth systems in lamb production rather than rely on improved seasonal prices, which dictate that many lambs are not slaughtered until 12 months old even though they have the genetic potential to reach their target weights by four months old.

HEALTH STATUS OF PURCHASED FLOCK REPLACEMENTS

All too frequently, selection of replacement females and stock rams is based more on traditions, prejudices and phenotype selection than on the general health status of the sheep and the flock of origin (if known). This policy is a great concern because of the alarming number of diseases that can be readily introduced and disseminated throughout a flock, with potentially disastrous financial consequences (**64**). For example, the on-going debacle with sheep scab in the UK, and the 2001 FMD epidemic, clearly illustrate how contagious disease can become widely disseminated throughout the national flock in the absence of effective control measures. Chlamydial abortion, caseous lymphadenitis, paratuberculosis, maedi-visna, sheep pulmonary adenomatosis (SPA) and anthelmintic-resistant nematodes have also become increasingly prevalent on sheep farms over the last decade in the UK. The lack of national disease control strategies reinforces the need for farm gate disease security with veterinary supervision.

The annual ewe mortality rate is around 5–7%, with many more ewes culled each year for poor condition/ill-thrift. The difference between the breeding stock replacement rate and the cull rate (number of ewe lambs and gimmers purchased compared with the number of ewes sold as culls) indicates the annual ewe mortality rate. Cull ewes can be further defined as those involuntary culls removed prematurely from the flock because of disease or poor condition, and those voluntary culls sold after a predetermined number of lambs crops (generally 4–6 crops). Comparison should also be made between the prices paid for replacements and those received for culls.

Unfortunately, few commercial flocks can achieve the ideal situation of establishing closed breeding flocks, and some introduced breeding replacements are needed in almost every flock. Almost without exception, two-crop ewes and older replacements pose significantly greater disease risks and, wherever possible, clean sheep (not previously bred) must be purchased. The most important contagious diseases that can be introduced through purchased flock replacements, using the UK as an example, in are shown in **Table 1**.

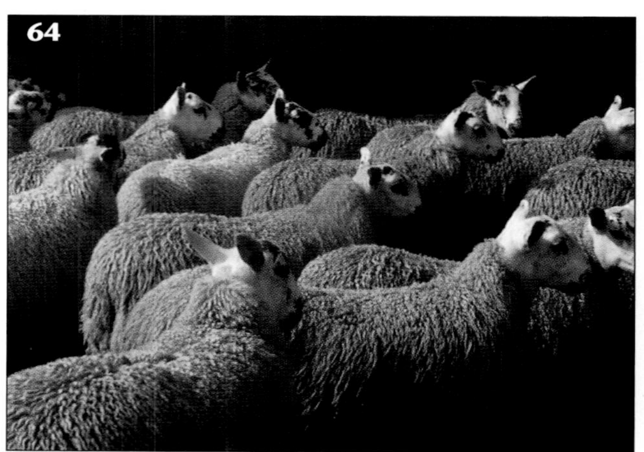

64 Purchased ewe lambs of uncertain health status.

Selection

Wherever possible, breeding replacements should be purchased from a flock of known health status but such information is rarely available or reliable. Many farmers will buy from a source whose stock has performed well in the past, and this makes a useful starting point.

Sheep health schemes that offer breeding stock for sale from flocks free of chlamydial abortion, and vaccinated against pasteurellosis and clostridial diseases, are to be applauded; however, the question remains whether these are the most important sheep diseases. For example, there are potential risks involved with establishing a totally naive flock with respect to chlamydial abortion when neighbouring farms are much less diligent; disease can be transmitted between farms with common borders. The availability of an effective chlamydial abortion vaccine questions whether a large financial premium is justified for breeding female replacements from supervised flocks.

General inspection of breeding stock at markets is largely worthless because of the subclinical nature of many diseases and the number of lots for sale. There may be no greater disease risk from purchasing gimmers (one to two year olds) than ewe lambs (less than one year old) because certain diseases are passed transplacentally (border disease), via the colostrum (maedi-visna) or during the nursing period (paratuberculosis, SPA).

Table 1 Diseases that can be introduced through purchased flock replacements in the UK.

- Maedi-visna
- Sheep pulmonary adenomatosis (jaagsiekte)
- Contagious pustular dermatitis (orf)
- Border disease
- Scrapie (homozygous genotype for shortened incubation period)
- Virulent footrot
- Ovine digital dermatitis
- Caseous lymphadenitis
- Paratuberculosis (Johne's disease)
- *Chlamydophila abortus* abortion (enzootic abortion of ewes)
- *Campylobacter fetus fetus*
- Various *Salmonella* species serotypes
- *Psoroptes ovis* (sheep scab, including pyrethroid-resistant strains)
- Pediculosis (lice)
- *Melophagus ovinus* (keds)
- Multiple anthelmintic-resistant nematode strains (*Haemonchus contortus* and *Teladosagia* species, in particular)
- *Fasciola hepatica* (liver fluke)

Routine inspections and treatments

The risks posed by anthelmintic-resistant nematode species and sheep scab must be fully recognized. On arrival on the farm all purchased sheep must be treated with an appropriate macrocyclic lactone preparation, and levamisole, and left in the handling pens overnight to prevent pasture contamination with nematode eggs. The sheep should then be turned on to contaminated pasture in case the nematodes have not all been eliminated and resistant strains are still present.

Careful inspection for ectoparasites is essential because macrocyclic lactone preparations do not kill lice and, under certain situations, plunge dipping may be an appropriate treatment option (**65, 66**).

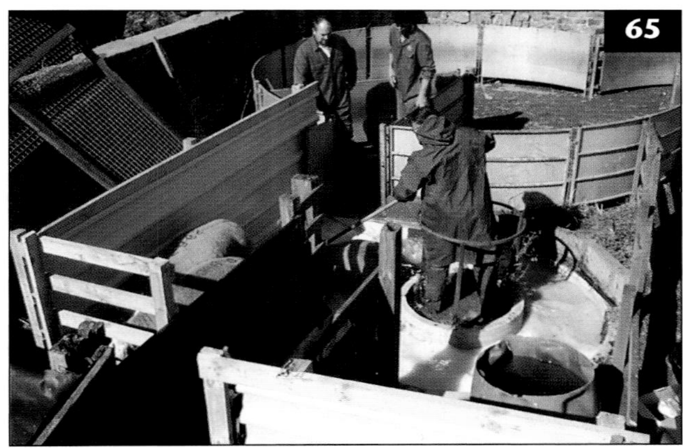

65 Plunge dipping to control external parasites.

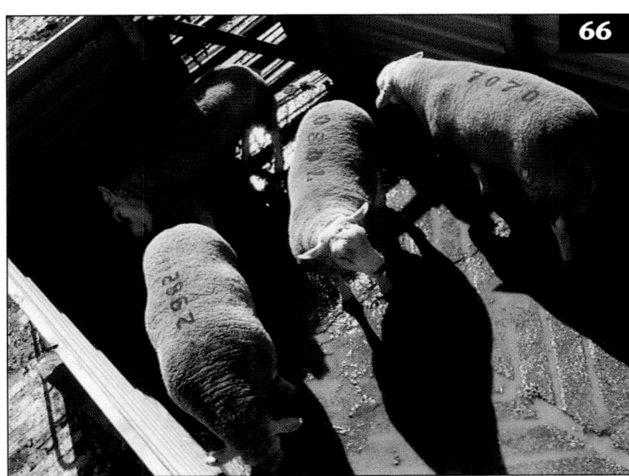

66 Purchased rams after being plunge dipped.

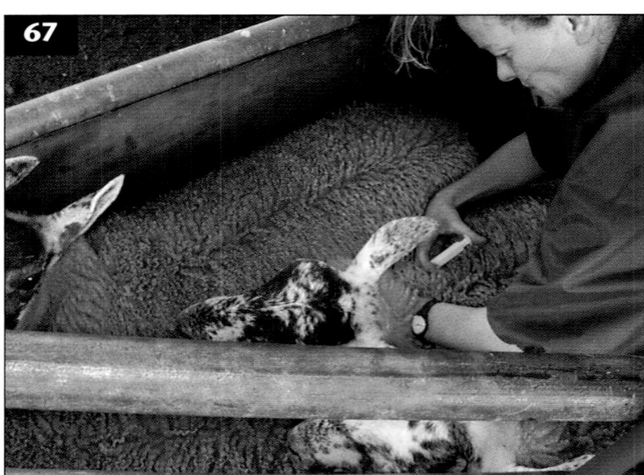

67 Clostridial disease vaccination.

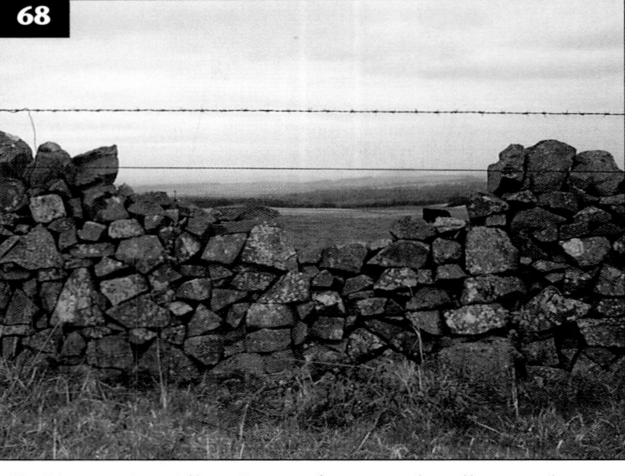

68 Biosecurity. All perimeter fences and walls must be maintained.

Routine foot bathing in zinc sulphate or formalin solution should be considered, especially if there are lame sheep in the batch. The sheep should be turned out to pasture the following day but contact with other sheep on the farm must be avoided for at least one month.

Vaccination against the clostridial diseases, toxoplasmosis and chlamydial abortion is strongly recommended for newly-introduced breeding replacements in lowland flocks (67). Vaccination against pasteurellosis will depend on the farm history.

Quarantine

All purchased sheep must be maintained in strict quarantine for at least one month after arrival on the farm (68).

Clinical examination cannot differentiate between the causes of thick-walled abscesses and discharging sinuses on the face and neck, and these lesions must be considered to be caseous lymphadenitis until proven otherwise.

Serological screening against maedi-visna virus infection is possible but seroconversion, detected by agar gel immunodiffusion, takes many months to develop and false-negative results have been obtained in sheep less than two years old, with serious financial consequences to the purchaser. The introduction of maedi-visna virus infected sheep may not result in overt disease for 8–10 years but, thereafter, considerable losses could be experienced.

There is no serological screening test presently available for SPA. Some control of spread of SPA can be achieved by maintaining sheep in age groups, especially during housed periods. Paratuberculosis has become a significant financial burden on some hill farms but the true prevalence has yet to be accurately determined. Flock screening for paratuberculosis is not a practical option.

During the quarantine period particular attention must be paid to any sick sheep, as such individual cases may be the forerunners of future flock problems. If doubts exist about the clinical diagnosis, individual sick sheep should be euthanased and a detailed postmortem examination undertaken at the local veterinary laboratory.

REFERENCE

1 Russel A (1985) Nutrition of the pregnant ewe. *In Practice* 7, 23–28.

3 Reproductive System

Part 1: Female Reproductive System

CLINICAL EXAMINATION OF THE FEMALE REPRODUCTIVE SYSTEM

Clinical examination of the female reproductive system in sheep can be divided into six stages of the reproductive cycle: failure to become pregnant during a restricted breeding period; embryonic loss/abortion; pregnancy diagnosis; vaginal/uterine prolapse; dystocia; metritis.

Failure to become pregnant during a restricted breeding period

Unlike cattle, sheep have a high fertility rate, with >90% of females of appropriate body weight and body condition score conceiving during one cycle of the normal breeding season to a fertile ram. This figure may be as high as 95% when about 40 ewes are managed with one fertile ram. Less than 2% of females should be non-pregnant after a restricted breeding period of only 35–42 days (two reproductive cycles). Investigation of a high barren rate in a group of ewes is detailed later (see Infectious causes of abortion, Toxoplasmosis p. 62, Border disease, p. 67).

Investigation of infertility is rarely undertaken in individual non-pedigree sheep. If non-pedigree sheep do not breed during their first season, they should be culled, as many fail to become pregnant the following season. Infertility in ewes is generally considered to arise from previous uterine infection and/or physical damage arising from dystocia, but there have been no detailed large-scale studies.

Investigation of infertility in a pedigree female should cover a history detailing previous breeding performance, including any dystocia, and a diary of service dates and ram(s) used. A complete physical examination must be undertaken, as infertility may be the result of disease in another organ system (e.g. chronic suppurative pneumonia) causing poor body condition. Investigation of the female reproductive tract is restricted to the external genitalia and percutaneous ultrasonography of the caudal abdomen using a 5 MHz sector scanner, although this will not reveal the normal involuted uterus, which is contained within the pelvic canal. Ultrasonography will only identify gross abnormalities such as pyometra when there are large fluid accumulations within the uterus.

More detailed examination of the uterus and ovaries could involve laparoscopy. Certain 'infertile' pedigree ewes undergo an embryo-flushing programme, with the laparoscopic examination undertaken at the time of surgical insemination or embryo collection if transcervical insemination is used. The cost of the flushing programme is relatively inexpensive, with embryos collected if no abnormalities are present; if there are abnormalities present preventing successful embryo collection, the only added cost is that of the flushing programme.

Embryonic loss/abortion

Embryo/fetal loss from non-infectious causes is considered to be very low in sheep. Detailed investigation is not generally undertaken unless the number of sheep returning to service after 30 days exceeds 2% (more commonly 5% in commercial situations). In many situations the rams are removed after a 35–42 day breeding period and embryo/fetal loss may not be detected until scanning time, which may be up to 90 days post service. Embryo/fetal loss may only become apparent when ewes are found to be barren at the end of the lambing period. Vasectomized rams can be returned to groups of breeding ewes after removal of the rams to identify returns to service.

Infectious causes of embryo loss and abortion are detailed later (see Infectious causes of abortion).

Pregnancy diagnosis

The percentage of non-pregnant sheep is generally around 2% after two breeding cycles. Pregnancy can be assumed following failure of the ewe to return to oestrus during the normal breeding period as determined by a ram or, outside the selected breeding period, by a vasectomized ram. Pregnancy can be confirmed from as early as 20–25 days post service using transrectal linear array B-mode ultrasound scanners but such information is of little practical application.

Determination of fetal number is commonly undertaken for management purposes. Greater than 95% accuracy can be achieved with transabdominal ultrasonography using a sector scanner between 45 and 90 days post service. These data are used for determining dietary energy allowances during late gestation in conjunction with 3-OH butyrate sampling (see

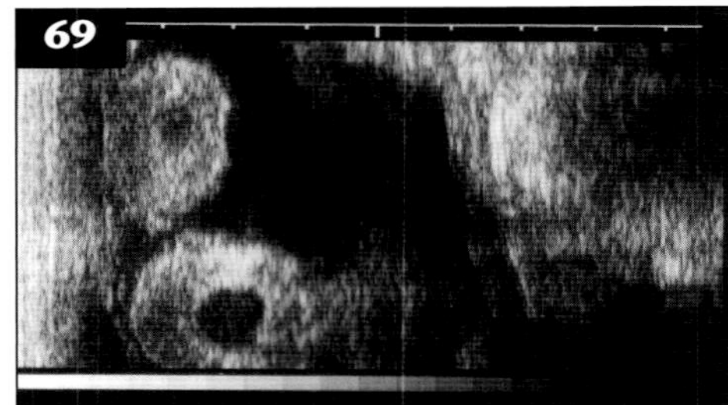

69 Advanced pregnancy. The classical 'doughnut rings' represent the placentomes.

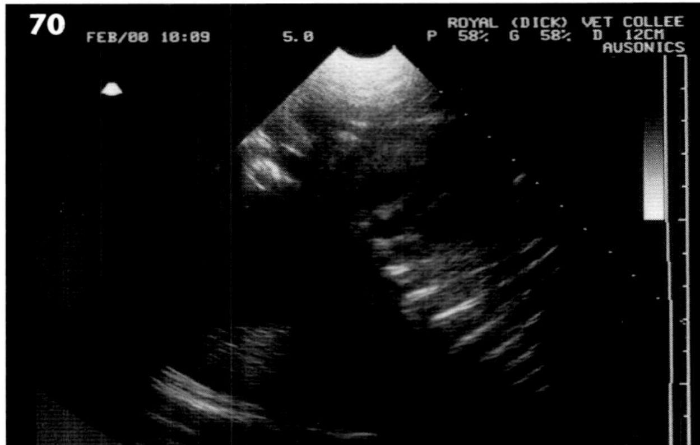

70 Retained fetus. The fetal ribcage is represented by broad parallel hyperechoic lines.

Chapter 2: Husbandry, p. 16). Litter size can be determined very quickly, with experienced operators scanning 80–120 sheep per hour. Determination of fetal number is much less accurate after day 90 of pregnancy.

Caruncles are readily identifiable from around day 45 of pregnancy, appearing as hyperechoic doughnut-shaped structures at the periphery of the anechoic fluid (**69**). The fetal skeleton is not always visualized during brief examinations and a positive diagnosis is based on imaging caruncles with adjacent anechoic fluid. During late pregnancy, fetal movement and/or fetal heartbeat can be determined to indicate a viable fetus (e.g. when examining a ewe with a vaginal prolapse or OPT). Ultrasonography may also be useful to determine the presence of a retained fetus following contraction of the cervix (**70**).

Vaginal/uterine prolapse

The investigation and treatment of vaginal and uterine prolapse is detailed later in this chapter (pp. 46–54). Ultrasound studies have demonstrated that the vaginal prolapse may contain either urinary bladder or uterine horn. These studies are very important because they highlight the risks of needle decompression to facilitate replacement. Indeed, having identified that the vaginal prolapse contains urinary bladder effectively instructs the clinician to elevate the prolapse after extradural injection and relieve the kink in the urethra and allow urine to drain.

The interval from parturition to uterine prolapse is very important; while uterine prolapse may occur spontaneously after prolonged second stage labour in a sheep with a singleton lamb, prolapse 12–48 hours after parturition indicates excessive manual interference of a dystocia, resulting in tenesmus that causes prolapse. In the latter group there is typically marked oedema, bruising and superficial infection of the posterior reproductive tract.

Dystocia

Normal parturition and the approach to dystocia cases are detailed below. This is an important area of veterinary work in many countries. The importance of a full clinical examination before attempting to correct the dystocia cannot be overemphasized, as uterine rupture and other iatrogenic traumas are not uncommon. The attendant farm staff must be informed of the origin of these traumas and instructed as to their prevention.

Metritis

A diagnosis of metritis is not simple in sheep and largely involves ruling out other common diseases. Manual vaginal examination for the presence of uterine discharges is not possible, and vaginoscopic examination is rarely undertaken. Percutaneous ultrasonography of the caudal abdomen using a 5 MHz sector scanner will identify the uterus for 2–3 days after parturition but interpretation of uterine diameter and fluid accumulations is problematic. There are no definitive data on the significance of bacteria isolated from vaginal swabs.

OBSTETRICS

Overview

Ewe deaths around lambing time in lowland flocks in the UK are quoted as 5–7%, with an estimated 70% of the deaths caused by dystocia. Similar figures are reported in many other countries with intensive lambing systems for meat breed sheep, although the development of easy-care sheep breeds lambing outdoors in Australia and New Zealand has greatly reduced the incidence of dystocia. The practice of lambing sheep indoors in the UK may itself lead to problems with the normal birth process but lambing outdoors may lead to problems of exposure and hypothermia in lambs.

There has been a disturbing trend in the UK over the past ten years towards fewer veterinary visits for ovine obstetrical problems. In a recent survey, which asked Welsh (UK) sheep farmers why they did not request veterinary assistance for dystocia cases, 33% of the respondents quoted excessive professional fees and 31% considered themselves as competent as their veterinarian in such matters.

The survey, which involved 183 sheep flocks comprising 89,000 sheep, revealed that 289 ewes with lambing difficulties that could not be corrected by farm staff received veterinary attention, with 104 cases being resolved by caesarean section.

In conclusion, economics are the critical factor in ovine obstetrics in the UK and in many other countries worldwide.

Easy-care lambing system

Many countries, such as New Zealand and Australia, have developed an 'easy-care' lambing system, though this has not been attempted in the UK. Under this system lambing takes place outdoors in carefully selected lambing paddocks that utilize natural shelter. Set stocking of paddocks is preferred to the daily group movement that occurs in drift lambing. A stocking rate of around 18 ewes per hectare has been recommended but this depends on grazing conditions and other factors. The easy-care lambing system allows supervision of lambing ewes without unnecessary disturbance. Ewes may spend up to six hours at the selected birth site before the start of first stage labour and they should not be disturbed during this period.

Selection of breeding stock should be based on the ability of ewes to rear at least one lamb. Rams should be selected from families that show strong maternal instincts. Conversely, ewes that have not reared a lamb should be culled.

Hygiene/antibiotic therapy approach to dystocia cases

In a survey of 90 UK sheep farms, 14 farmers always used water and approved surgical scrub prior to examination of lambing difficulties (**71**), 17 mostly did, 14 did on occasion, and the majority of shepherds (45 [50%]) never washed their hands (**72**). Arm-length disposable plastic gloves were always used on 29 farms (**73**), six farms used gloves for most lambings, eight farms used them occasionally, and the majority (52 [57%]) never used gloves. More than one third of the shepherds (32 [35%]) neither washed their hands nor used arm-length gloves before attempting correction of a difficult lambing.

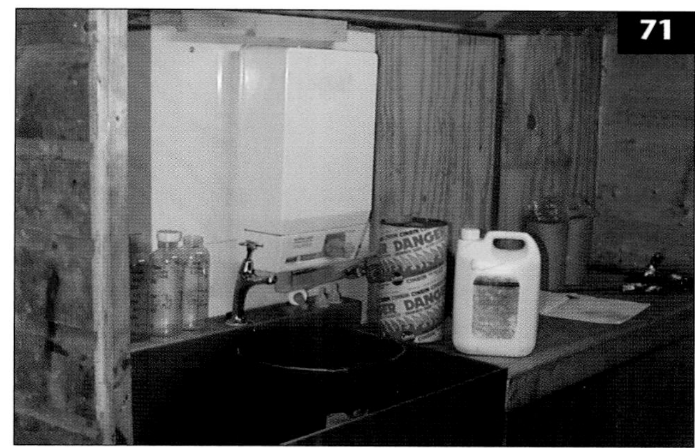

71 All lambing sheds must have hot water and washing facilities.

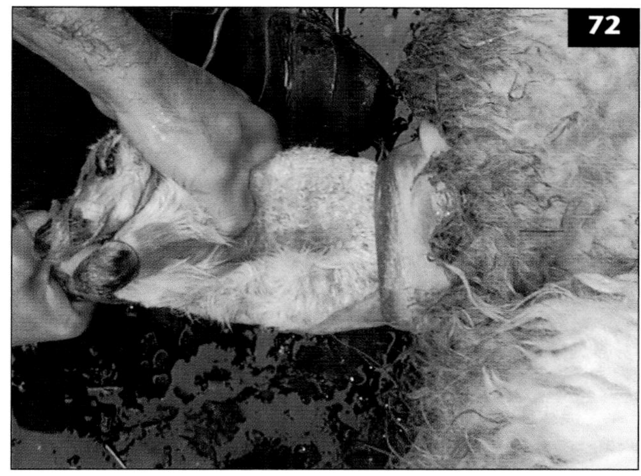

72 Inadequate hygiene precautions add to the risk of metritis and zoonotic infections.

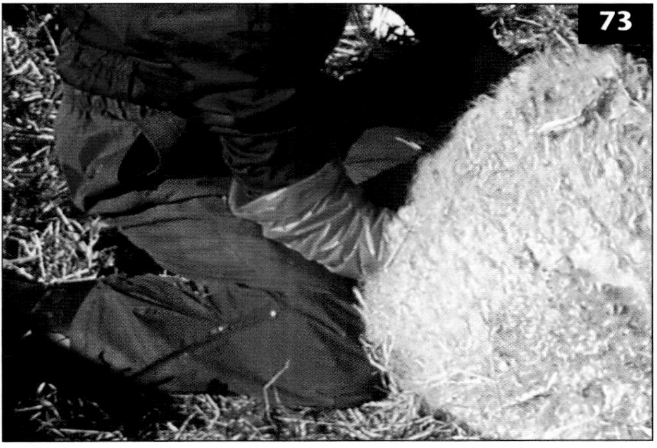

73 Arm-length disposable gloves must always be worn during dystocia correction; there are no excuses.

On 33 farms all assisted lambings received an antibiotic injection, while the majority of farmers (65%) treated only ewes that became sick some days after the assisted lambing (74). Sick ewes were treated with a single antibiotic injection on 47 farms (52%), a course of three consecutive days' antibiotic was given on eight farms (9%), and on seven farms the duration of therapy was based on response to treatment (8%). Penicillin was the antibiotic most commonly used by sheep farmers.

It is evident from these data that the basic hygiene approach to dystocia cases could be greatly improved on the majority of UK sheep farms by farmers washing their hands in approved scrub solution and using arm-length disposable gloves prior to correction of all dystocia cases (73–76). Arm-length disposable plastic gloves are cheap and easily carried within pockets; therefore, there can be no excuse for non-compliance with such basic hygiene, even under extensive management systems. With regard to infectious causes of abortion, such precautions should be a minimum standard to limit the risk of zoonotic infections.

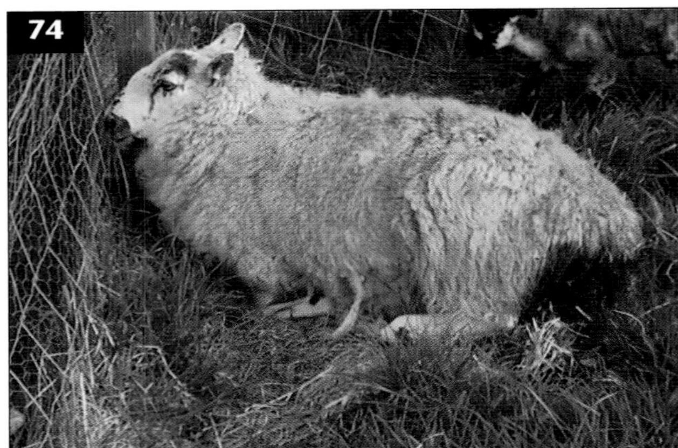

74 Metritis due to unhygienic and excessive unskilled interference during second stage labour.

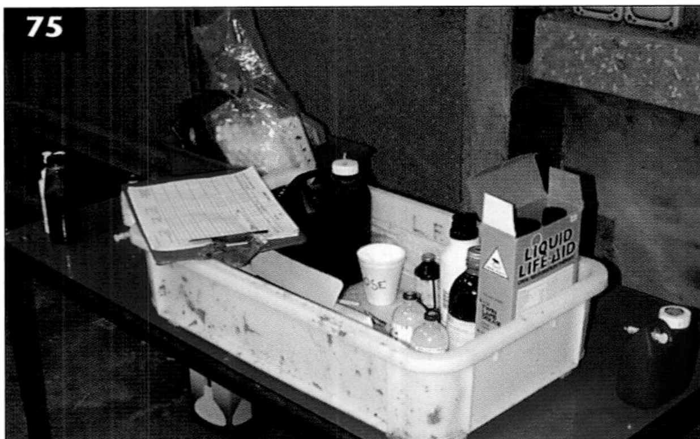

75 Exemplary tidiness, cleanliness, medicine records and recording forms.

Euthanasia

Euthanasia of ewes with dystocia is a recent development in the UK sheep industry and is based solely on economic considerations, because success rates exceeding 97% have been reported for caesarean sections undertaken in field situations.

Animal welfare implications

These data highlight important questions relating to the adoption of veterinary services on UK sheep farms and explain, in part, the 5–7% mortality rate of adult sheep, 70% of which die as a result of lambing difficulties.

There have been considerable advances in the provision of analgesia for ovine obstetrical conditions under field situations, with visible improvements in the animals' well-being. Such improved care and welfare of sheep can only be brought about by veterinary involvement in obstetrical problems. In the UK, for example, if a 50% reduction in the ewe periparturient mortality rate could be achieved by greater direct veterinary involvement in dystocia cases, this would save an estimated 500,000 ewes annually.

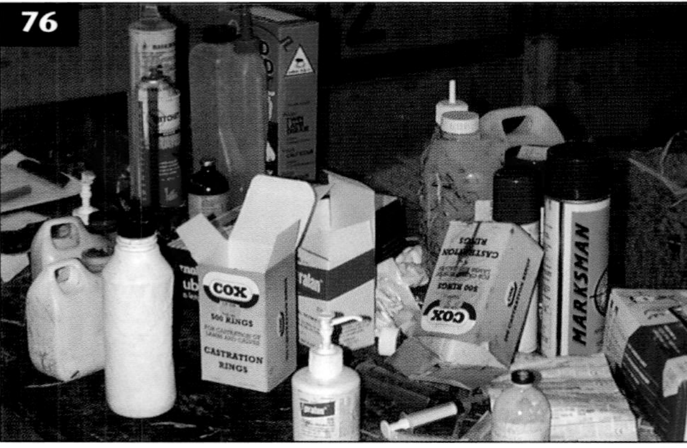

76 Disorganization in the lambing shed only adds to delays.

Definitions

- **Presentation.** Signifies the relationship between the long axis of the fetus and the maternal birth canal. It includes anterior or posterior longitudinal presentation and ventral or dorsal transverse presentation.
- **Position.** Indicates the surface of the maternal birth canal to which the fetal vertebral column is applied. It includes dorsal, ventral and right or left lateral position.

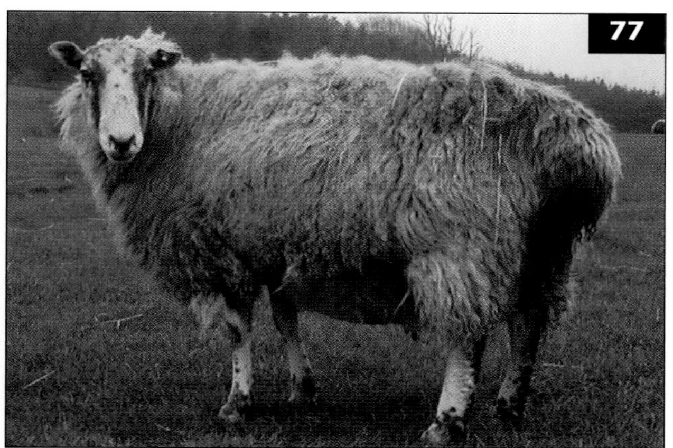

77 Early first stage labour. Ewes isolate from the flock wherever possible.

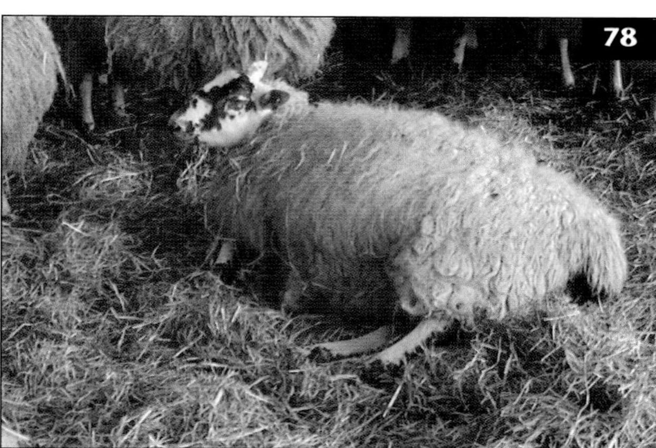

78 Early first stage labour.

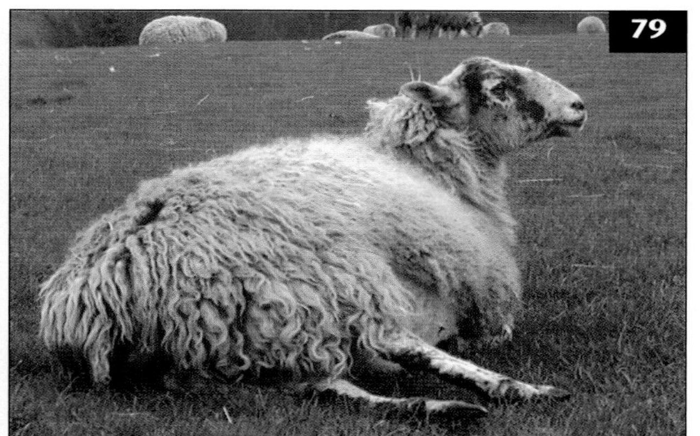

79 Early second stage labour. The allantochorion has appeared at the vulva.

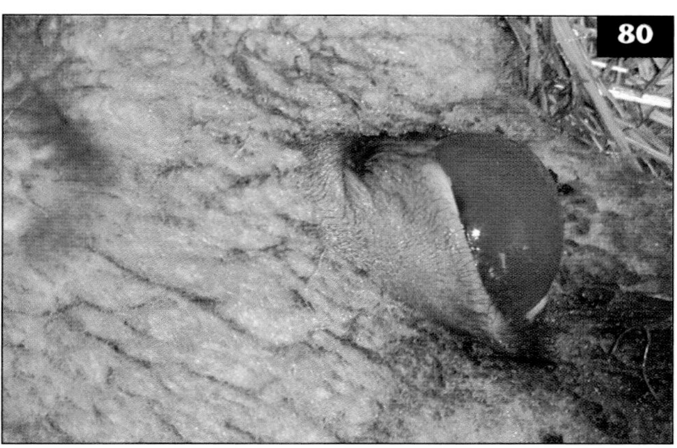

80 Appearance of the allantochorion at the vulva.

- **Posture.** Refers to the disposition of the moveable appendages of the fetus and involves flexion or extension of the cervical and limb joints (e.g. bilateral hock flexion posture).
- **Fetal oversize:**
  - Relative oversize: fetus normal dimensions, maternal pelvis too small.
  - Absolute oversize: fetus abnormally large, maternal pelvis normal.

Normal parturition in the ewe

The gestation period in ewes is 143–147 days. Imminent parturition can be detected by udder development, accumulation of colostrum and slackening of the sacroiliac ligaments. The birth process has three stages:

- **First stage labour.** First stage labour is represented by cervical dilation, which usually takes 3–6 hours but is more rapid in multiparous ewes. There are various behavioural changes, including the ewe not coming to the feed trough or leaving before other sheep in the group. The ewe seeks a sheltered area of the field (77) or corner of the barn (78) and will paw at the ground, frequently sniffing at this area, and alternately lying/standing (79). These periods of increased activity often occur at 15-minute intervals, with abdominal contractions lasting 15–30 seconds. A thick string of mucus is often observed hanging from the vulva. The bouts of straining then occur more frequently, usually every 2–3 minutes. This increased activity coincides with a change in fetal position, with extension of the forelimbs. At the end of first stage labour the cervix is fully dilated.
- **Second stage labour.** Second stage labouris represented by expulsion of the fetus(es), and typically takes about one hour. There is rupture of the allantochorion (80), accompanied by a rush

of fluid. The amnion and fetal parts are then engaged in the pelvic inlet (81). The amniotic sac appears at the vulva and frequently ruptures at this stage. Powerful reflex and voluntary contractions of abdominal muscle and diaphragm ('straining') serve to expel the fetus (82–85). However, the amniotic sac may not rupture until the ewe stands up after the lamb has been expelled. The delayed rupture of the amnion, referred to colloquially as the lamb being 'sheeted' or 'born with the skin over its nose', may result in death of the lamb due to asphyxiation. This scenario is not uncommon in multiple births, especially with later born lambs. In multigravid ewes the interval between lambs being born varies from 10–60 minutes; intervention should be considered after one hour.

- **Third stage labour.** Third stage labour is completed by expulsion of fetal membranes, which usually occurs within 2–3 hours of the end of second stage labour.

Veterinary approach to every lambing case

As a veterinarian it is essential to assess the patient in detail before attempting to correct any dystocia. Distant assessment of the ewe will frequently give an indication of prolonged dystocia (86). Lateral recumbency (87, 88) with frequent abdominal straining and vocalization may result from engagement of the lamb within the pelvis or from excessive manual interference, leading to trauma of the posterior reproductive tract (89). Bruxism (teeth grinding) and an elevated respiratory rate with an abdominal component (panting) may indicate more serious concerns such as uterine rupture.

Attempted delivery by an unskilled shepherd frequently results in oedema, reddening and bruising of the vulval labiae (90). There may be evidence of vaginal bleeding on the tail and perineum (89), especially on the lower side if the ewe was recumbent. The ewe's mucous membranes must be checked for evidence of pallor.

81 Second stage labour.

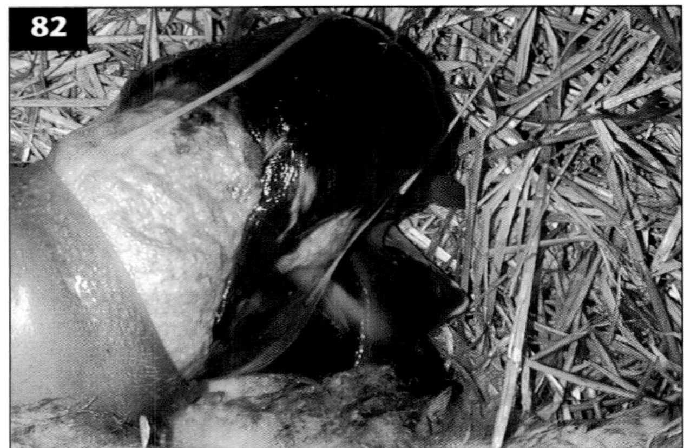

82 Delivery of lamb in anterior presentation.

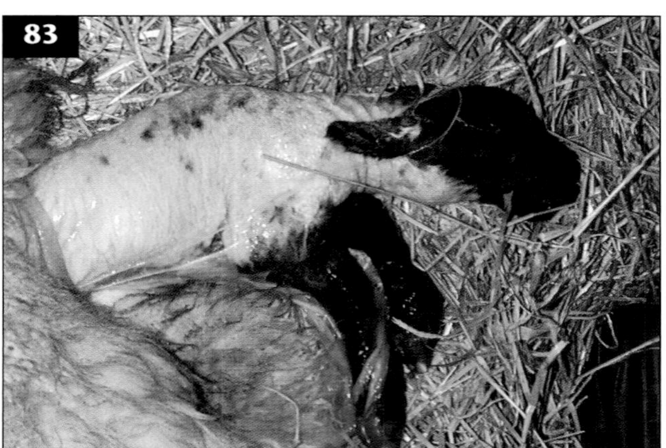

83 Delivery of lamb in anterior presentation.

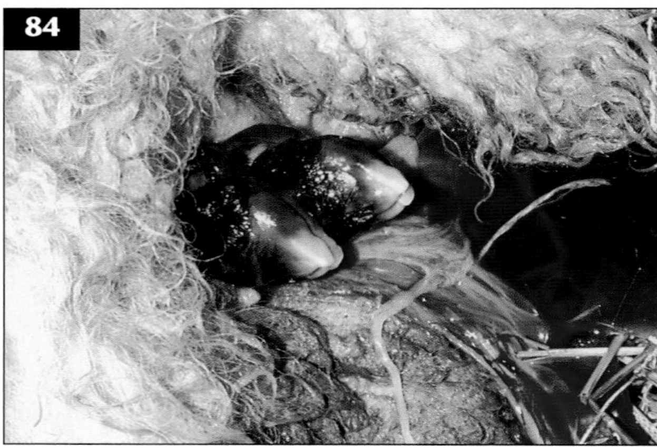

84 Appearance of lamb in posterior presentation.

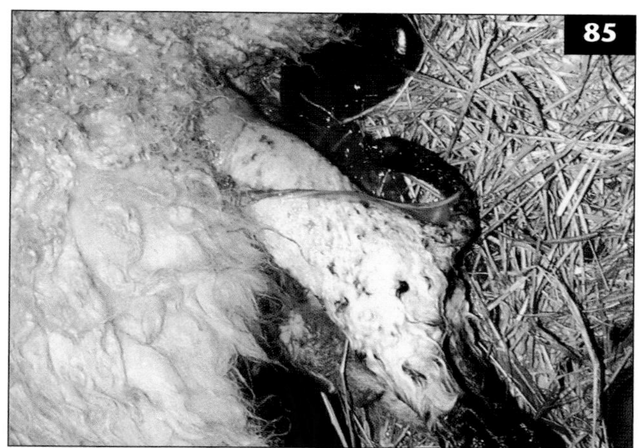

85 Delivery of lamb in posterior presentation.

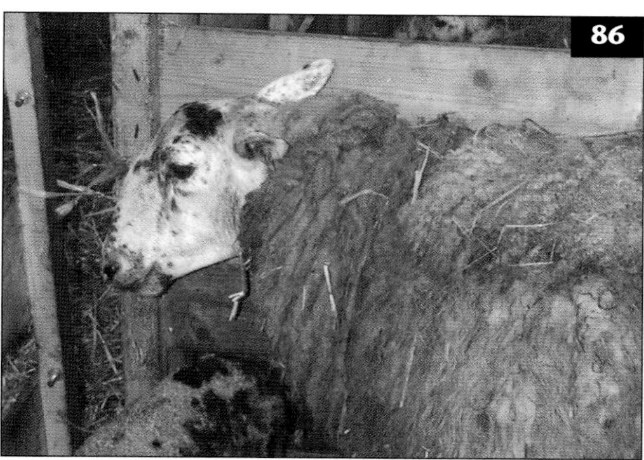

86 Dull, depressed ewe. A full clinical examination is essential before progressing to examination of the dystocia.

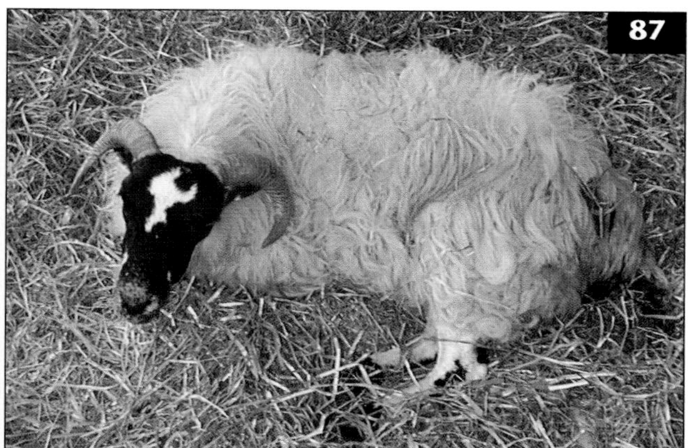

87 Sick ewe presented in second stage labour showing tenesmus.

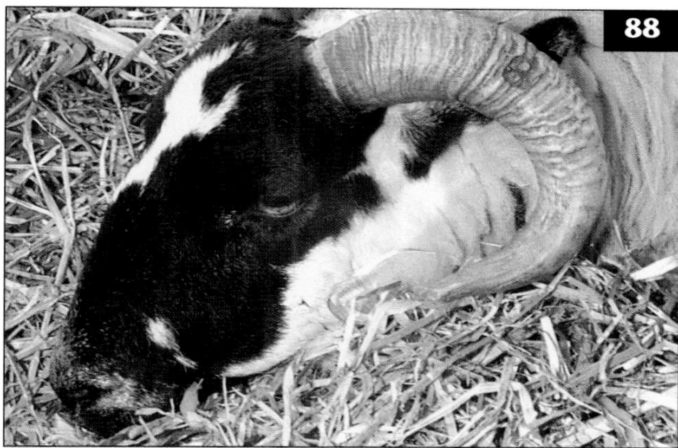

88 Closer examination reveals toxic mucous membranes.

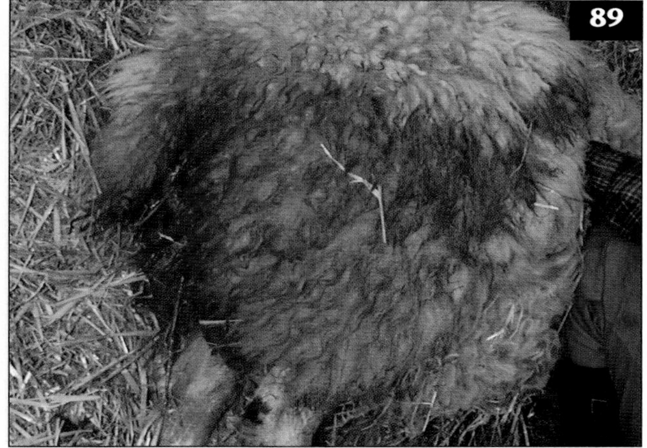

89 This degree of haemorrhage suggests serious trauma to the posterior reproductive tract. The client should always be forewarned about any veterinary concerns.

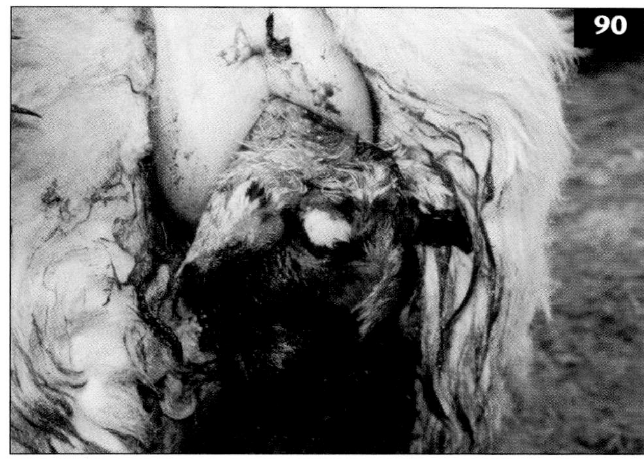

90 Attempted delivery causing trauma to the vagina, with considerable oedema, reddening and bruising of the vulval labiae.

The presence of a fetid yellow-brown vulval discharge indicates the presence of autolytic lambs *in utero*. It is important to discuss any concerns with the client before attempting correction of the dystocia.

Caudal analgesia

Caudal analgesia is essential for all corrections/manipulations undertaken by a veterinarian. This involves injection of 2% lidocaine solution (0.5 mg/kg) at the sacrococcygeal site (caudal block). Blockage of the ewe's reflex abdominal contractions greatly assists corrections/manipulations of dystocia cases and has obvious animal welfare benefits.

Reliance on strength by the shepherd to repel the fetus is unacceptable. Likewise, having an assistant raise the ewe by its hindlimbs or using a pulley system is totally unacceptable as this merely transfers the full weight of the rumen, gravid uterus and other abdominal viscera on to the ewe's diaphragm. Tension on the broad ligaments may also cause pain.

The reader is directed to Chapter 15 (Anaesthesia, p. 315) for a detailed approach to extradural analgesia in dystocia cases.

Hygiene

Hygiene is very important and is frequently overlooked by shepherds in their haste to correct a dystocia. Shepherds must use arm-length disposable gloves during the correction of all dystocia cases. The shepherd should use his free hand to hold the ewe's tail clear of the vulva. Ideally, an assistant restraining the sheep should do this but such help is rarely available. The vulva is then washed with a diluted surgical scrub solution. Obstetrical gel is then applied liberally to the hand of the shepherd's gloved arm; the fingers of the hand are forced together at their tips to form a cone-shape, and then gently introduced into the vagina. Careful examination is essential, not only for welfare reasons, but because the likelihood of infection of the posterior reproductive tract is greatly increased by trauma.

DYSTOCIA

INCOMPLETE CERVICAL DILATION

(*Syn*: ringwomb)

Definition/overview

The true incidence of ringwomb is difficult to determine because in most situations the onset of first stage labour has not been noted by the farmer, especially in overcrowded, housed flocks and in extensive pasture-managed systems. It is probable that some dystocia cases are classified as ringwomb but merely represent overzealous interference during early first stage labour. A working definition of ringwomb could be 'the presence of an incompletely dilated cervix more than six hours after first appearance of the fetal membranes (allantochorion) at the vulva'.

Aetiology

Some authors refer to cervical trauma during previous births but ringwomb has been described in primiparous sheep.

Clinical presentation

Fetal membranes can be seen at the vulva for six or more hours, with an incompletely dilated cervix detected on digital examination of the posterior reproductive tract. Typically, the external cervical os is only 3–5 cm in diameter, allowing passage of only two or three fingers.

Differential diagnoses

- Disturbed early first stage labour before complete cervical dilation.
- Uterine torsion.
- Incomplete cervical dilation associated with a lamb in posterior or transverse presentation.

Diagnosis

Diagnosis is based on digital examination of the reproductive tract and failure of the cervix to dilate under digital pressure applied for 10–15 minutes. The cervix feels approximately 1 cm thick and has obvious corrugations.

Treatment

Digital pressure applied for 5–15 minutes will gradually dilate the cervix in some cases but these cases may well represent those ewes disturbed during early first stage labour. If the cervix feels 2–3 mm thick and with no obvious corrugations at first presentation, then it will probably dilate under digital pressure.

If no progress has been made in 10–15 minutes, continued manual interference will simply lead to contamination of the fetal extremities, posterior reproductive tract and uterus, with an attendant risk of contamination of the peritoneal cavity when the lamb is delivered during the corrective caesarean section. Trauma to the posterior reproductive tract frequently results in reflex abdominal contractions, which may complicate the caesarean section, although this complication is resolved following routine extradural injection given by the veterinarian. Various smooth muscle relaxants have been used in sheep with ringwomb but there is no compelling evidence that they are effective.

Prevention/control measures

Too early/too frequent human interference may delay normal progression of first stage labour by inhibiting the ewe's normal behavioural patterns. Shepherds should be encouraged to leave sheep undisturbed for four hours after the appearance of a mucus string or allantochorion at the vulva, especially in primiparous animals. However, frequent bouts of powerful abdominal contractions occurring more frequently than every five minutes or so must be investigated because of the likelihood of fetal malposture.

Economics

Failure to deliver the lamb(s) *per vaginam* in cases of ringwomb requires veterinary assistance. Correction of dystocia at a veterinary surgery could cost 10–25% of the value of the ewe and a further 20–35% if a caesarean section is necessary. A visit charge could add a further 15–25%.

Welfare implications

Excessive unskilled interference in cases of ringwomb results in trauma to the posterior reproductive tract. Trauma may cause continued straining after the end of second stage labour and uterine prolapse. Unhygienic conditions and failure to wash hands and use disposable arm-length gloves increase the risk of metritis.

UTERINE TORSION

Uterine torsion is very uncommon in the ewe. Correction is usually made following delivery of the lamb(s) by caesarean section. The author has encountered only one case of uterine torsion in a ewe in 25 years of clinical practice. However, in some countries uterine torsion is considered a relatively common cause of dystocia presented to veterinarians.

UTERINE INERTIA

Primary uterine inertia occurs infrequently in the ewe. Unlike cattle, hypocalcaemia is very uncommon around the time of parturition in sheep.

RUPTURE OF THE PREPUBIC TENDON

Rupture of the prepubic tendon on the left side occurs in older multigravid ewes during the last 2–3 weeks of pregnancy. A large, 30 cm diameter swelling appears immediately cranial to the pubis (**91**). There may be extensive ventral oedema and the skin may touch the ground. Rupture of the ventral body wall results in an altered position of the uterus in relation to the pelvic inlet, and human assistance with delivery is frequently necessary because the lambs are not correctly presented (**92**). The ewe should be euthanased for welfare reasons following delivery of the lambs.

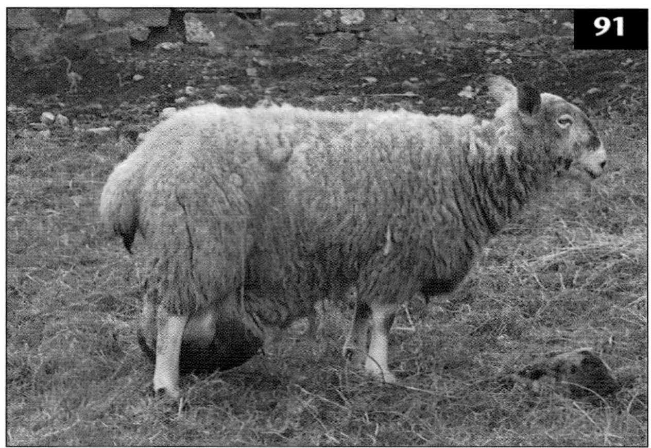

91 Rupture of the prepubic tendon.

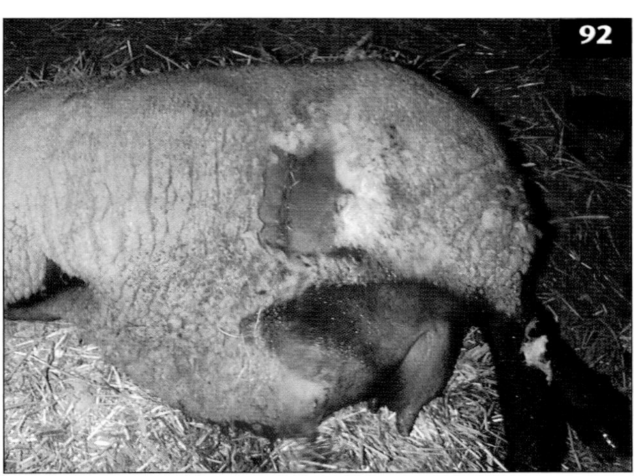

92 Ewe with rupture of the prepubic tendon with lambs delivered by caesarean section.

FETAL DYSTOCIA

Overview

Presentation and postural abnormalities are very common in sheep; however, they are generally simple to correct provided such dystocias are identified early during second stage labour. Congenital abnormalities, while usually rare on individual farms, are not uncommonly presented to the veterinary practitioner because of the large number of sheep within the practice area.

Anterior presentation

When a lamb is presented in anterior presentation (head and both forelimbs presented normally), it is often born after 5–10 minutes' vigorous abdominal straining.

In the case of a large single lamb, the forelimbs protrude as far as the feet while the muzzle and tongue only become visible when the ewe strains. If no progress is made within 30 minutes, the ewe should be gently restrained in lateral recumbency and patient assistance given. If both forefeet are present at the vulva and the muzzle can be touched, each forelimb should be extended in turn. One forefoot is held between the thumb and forefinger and steady traction is applied when the ewe strains. Such traction should extend the elbow and the forelimb will protrude to the carpus (knee). A sudden 'clunk' sensation is often appreciated when the elbow is extended. The other forelimb is extended in the same manner. Slight traction on both forelimbs should cause the head to protrude from the vulva. At this stage the poll of the head is grasped and slow, steady traction applied to the poll and both forelimbs. The lamb should be delivered in a downward arc without undue force over 10–30 seconds. Note that the traction is applied in an arc and the lamb is pulled 'down and around' and not 'straight out'.

The lamb should be left for a few minutes with the umbilical vessels still intact. The newborn lamb should not instantly be snatched away and placed at the ewe's head. It may take up to 30 seconds before the lamb takes its first deep breath but this is normal. There are no indications for swinging the lamb around by its hindlimbs – any fluid that appears at the mouth or nostrils during swinging originates from the lamb's stomach, not from its lungs. After delivery of one lamb it is usual to ballot the abdomen gently, which readily reveals whether there is another lamb(s) *in utero*. Opinion is divided on whether to deliver the second lamb or to leave well alone. Unnecessary interference in unhygienic conditions only increases the likelihood of uterine infection (metritis). It is reasoned, however, that the second lamb may be born in the intact amnion ('skin over its nose', 'sheeted') and therefore all remaining lambs should be delivered at this time to avoid such risks. However, this event is relatively uncommon, although it is more likely in triplet and larger litters, where a small lamb can be born and the amnion not be broken.

Time should be taken to observe a ewe that lambs unaided. She will always lie for 1–2 minutes before regaining her feet and licking her lamb. Parturition is a feat of great physical exertion and the ewe should not be expected to leap instantly to her feet as soon as the first lamb is born.

Head and only one forelimb presented

In this situation the retained forelimb lies alongside the lamb's chest (**93**) and must be brought forward (**94**) before any traction is applied to the lamb (**95**). Correction of this malposture involves flexing the shoulder, elbow and carpal joints, then carefully extending the carpus and elbow joints in that order, which presents the foot at the pelvic inlet. Gentle traction applied to both forelimbs should result in delivery of the lamb within 30–60 seconds.

Some shepherds will attempt to deliver a lamb with only one foot presented at the vulva, after checking that the other foot is not within the pelvic canal (this implies that the other limb lies alongside the lamb's chest). This practice will usually be successful if the

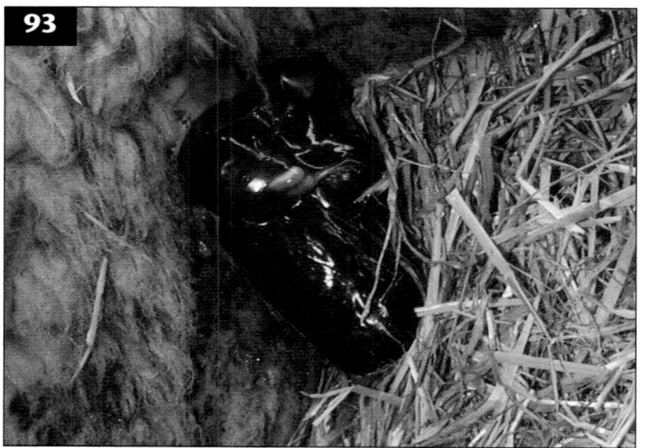

93 Anterior presentation with unilateral shoulder flexion. There is early detection of postural abnormality in this case.

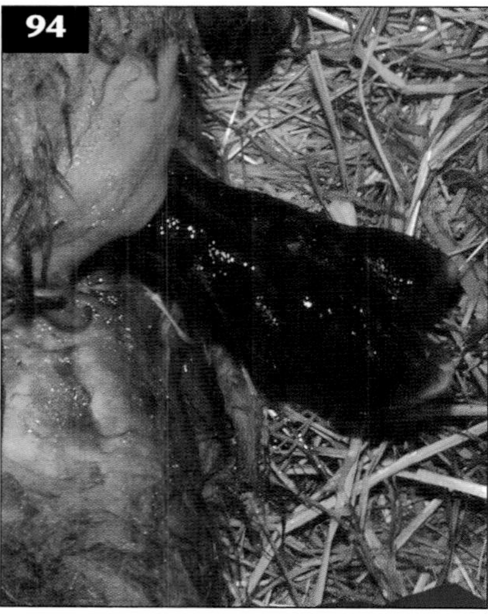

94 Extension of shoulder flexion.

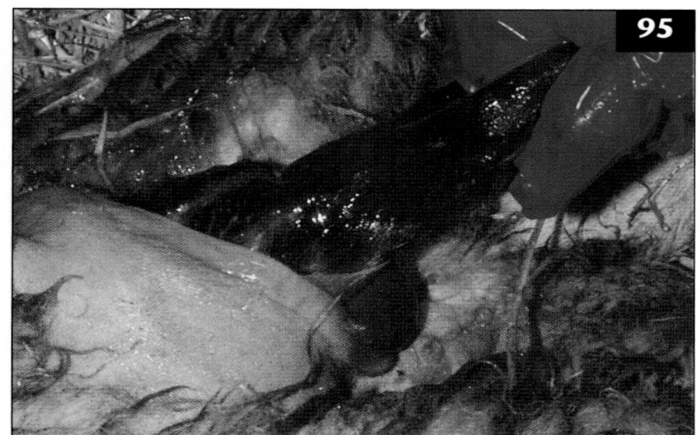

95 Steady traction to deliver lamb. Plastic arm-length gloves are being worn.

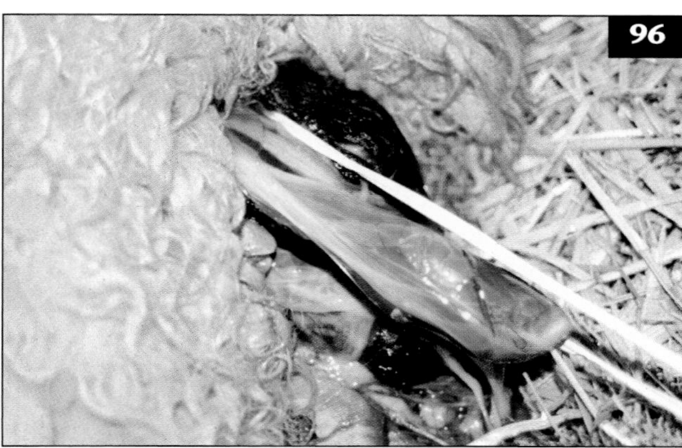

96 Use of snare rope to assist delivery of a lamb in anterior presentation.

lamb is a twin (see mark on ewe if previously scanned for litter size) but must never be undertaken if the lamb is a singleton.

Bilateral shoulder flexion (hung lamb)

The head is presented through the vulva but both forelimbs are retained alongside the chest. Correction of this malposture involves gentle repulsion of the head into the vagina, flexing the shoulder, elbow and carpal joints of one forelimb, and then carefully extending the carpus (knee) and elbow joints in that order, which presents the foot at the pelvic inlet. These manipulations are then repeated for the other forelimb. Repulsion of the lamb's head is greatly facilitated after sacrococcygeal extradural lidocaine injection, which blocks the reflex abdominal contractions of the ewe. The traditional method of repelling a lamb is to ask an assistant to suspend the ewe by its hindlimbs and then force the lamb back against the ewe's strong abdominal contractions. This procedure causes considerable distress to the ewe because the weight of the pregnant uterus, rumen and other abdominal viscera is forced against the diaphragm. The risk of trauma to the uterus and vagina is greatly increased if the lamb is forced back into the body of the uterus against such powerful opposition. Some clinicians apply a wire snare rope around the lamb's poll before gentle repulsion of the head into the vagina. The snare is helpful for applying traction (**96**) once the forelimbs have been successfully extended.

The lamb's head and tongue may remain swollen for a few hours and it is prudent to stomach tube these lambs to ensure that they receive sufficient colostrum before six hours old, if not sooner.

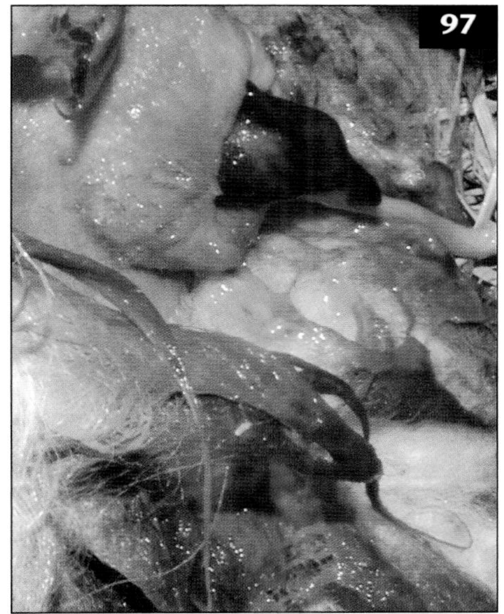

97 Posterior presentation with bilateral hip flexion. Only the tail is presented at the vulva.

Posterior presentation

First stage labour proceeds normally but there is much reduced straining during second stage labour because the lamb does not become fully engaged within the ewe's pelvis, which stimulates the powerful reflex abdominal contractions. The shepherd examines the ewe because it has made no progress since being noticed in first stage labour 2–6 hours previously. Digital examination of the vagina reveals the lamb's hooves facing the roof of the vagina (not the floor) and the hocks can be felt by progressing forward. Sometimes the tail can be felt (**97**).

Trauma to the rib cage at the costochondral junctions is common in large lambs (especially singletons) delivered in posterior presentation (**98, 99**). Fractures of the ribcage can severely impair respiratory function and may cause death. It has been suggested that lambs that sustain rib fractures during delivery are more prone to respiratory disease. Excessive traction of lambs in posterior presentation can also cause rupture of the liver and rapid death (**100**) in breeds such as the North Country Cheviot and Texel that have a relatively short sternum, thus exposing the liver to potential trauma.

In most situations a twin lamb in posterior presentation can be delivered without trauma by using steady traction. If one twin is in posterior presentation, it is very likely that the other twin will also be in posterior presentation; therefore, this is one situation where it may be prudent to check the presentation of a second lamb immediately after delivery of the first lamb.

Posterior presentation with bilateral hip extension (breech presentation)

Signs of second stage labour (e.g. powerful abdominal straining) are not observed when the lamb is in breech presentation because the lamb does not enter the maternal pelvis; instead the lamb's pelvis/tailhead becomes lodged at the pelvic inlet. Occasionally, the lamb's tail may protrude for 2–3 cm through the ewe's vulva (**97**).

Diligent shepherds will detect breech presentation by recognizing the signs of first stage labour and realizing that the ewe has not progressed to second stage labour. Sometimes these dystocia cases are not recognized until 24–48 hours after the lambs have died and the ewe has become sick. The lambs rapidly become emphysematous (**101, 102**), and this may result in the death of the ewe in neglected cases.

Correction of a breech presentation involves extending the hips while the hindlimb joints (stifle, hock and fetlock) are fully flexed. In this manner a breech presentation is first converted to a posterior presentation and then the lamb is delivered as described above. Singleton lambs are rarely presented as a breech delivery.

Correction of the breech presentation is facilitated by gently repelling the lamb into the body of the uterus. Great care must be taken during extension of the hip joints, especially if the uterus is clamped down around the lamb. It is not uncommon for an unskilled person to rupture the uterus during these manipulations, and veterinary assistance must

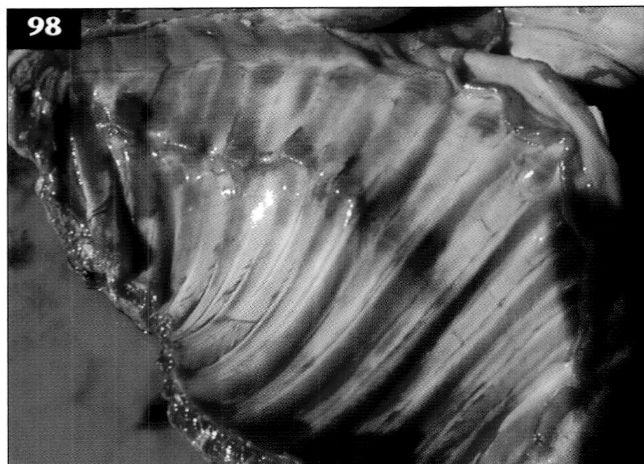

98 Multiple rib fractures at the costochondral junction after posterior delivery. This traumatic delivery led to death of the lamb at around 36 hours old.

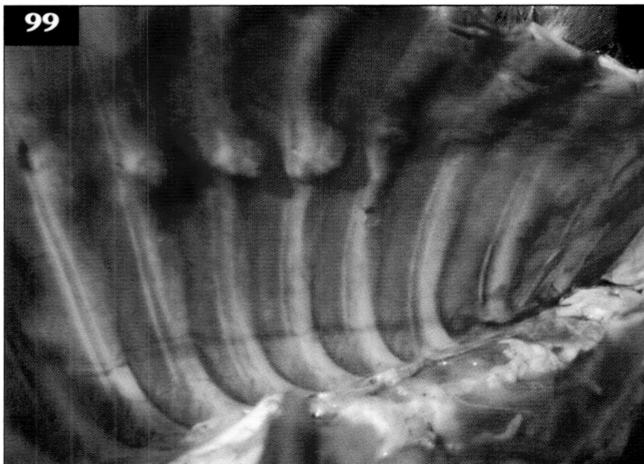

99 Healed rib fractures at the costochondral junction in a yearling sheep.

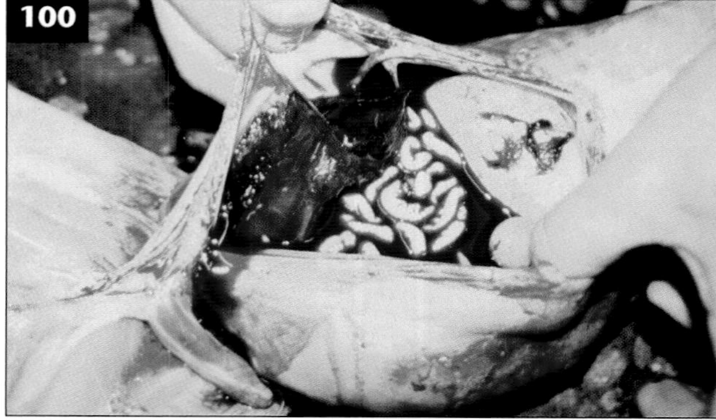

100 Ruptured liver with massive intra-abdominal haemorrhage.

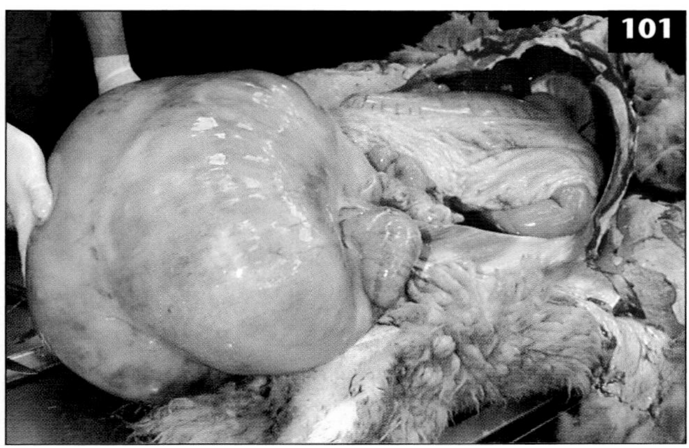

101 Necropsy reveals devitalized uterine wall and emphysematous lambs *in utero*.

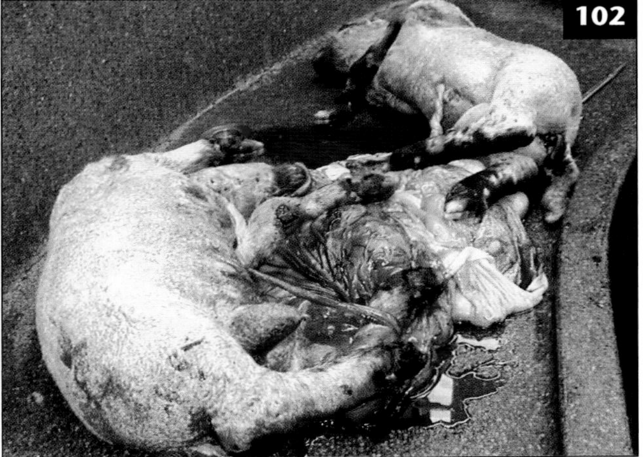

102 Emphysematous lambs at necropsy of a ewe.

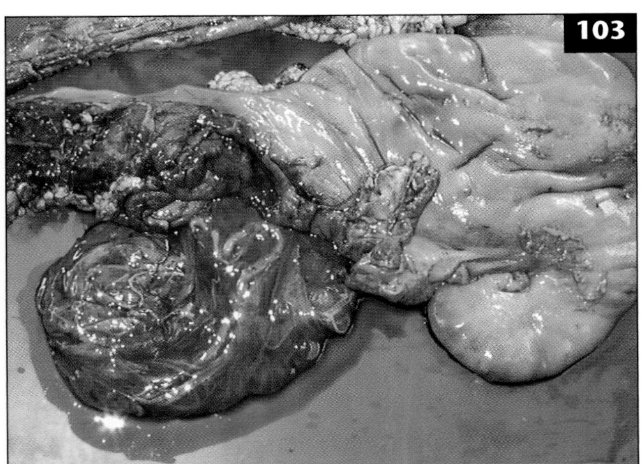

103 Ruptured uterus identified at necropsy.

be called if there is any doubt regarding correction of the presentation. Extradural lidocaine injection facilitates the various manipulations during correction of a breech posture by blocking the powerful abdominal contractions.

Prolonged second stage labour

Ewes that appear to have stopped straining after two or more hours should be examined. Reasons for cessation of abdominal straining include fatigue, a lamb in either posterior presentation or posterior presentation with bilateral hip extension (breech presentation), simultaneous presentation of two lambs, the ewe being continually disturbed, or other reasons.

Simultaneous presentation of two lambs

There are many possible combinations of heads and feet/limbs when two lambs are presented simultaneously. It is necessary to identify which forelimb corresponds to which head by tracing from the foot to the shoulder, and then on to the neck and head. Once both forelimbs and head have been correctly identified, one lamb is gently repelled as traction is applied to the other. Only gentle traction should be necessary to deliver a twin lamb in this situation; if little progress is being made, it is essential to check that the correct anatomy has been selected.

Lateral deviation of head

The lamb is often dead when there is lateral deviation of the head. Both feet are presented in the pelvis. The forelimbs and neck are gently repelled and a wire head snare is placed behind the lamb's ears and around the poll. The head is then drawn into the pelvic inlet just after the forefeet enter the pelvis. Plenty of lubrication is needed if the lamb is dead and its fleece is dry.

Rupture of the uterus

Excessive manual interference can cause rupture of the uterus, with subsequent shock, acute septic peritonitis and death of the ewe (**103**). This unfortunate event is more common where lambs are presented in breech posture and/or where excessive unskilled force has been used. The ewe presents in shock, with fast, shallow abdominal breathing and a rapid pulse. There is frequently odontoprisis (bruxism). Abdominal straining, with arterial blood at the vulva, may be seen. In these cases, signs of excessive manual interference should be obvious and an explorative laparotomy/caesarean section is the only treatment.

Retained fetus

Very occasionally a ewe presents with a retained full-term fetus some months after the end of the lambing period (**104**). Why the fetus did not become autolytic and result in toxaemia and eventually death of the ewe within days of fetal death cannot easily be explained. Attempted delivery of the fetus by caesarean section can prove difficult, if not impossible, due to fibrous adhesions between the uterus and the abdominal viscera (**105**). Leakage of purulent material (**106**) into the abdominal cavity during surgery almost inevitably results in septic peritonitis. The grossly thickened uterine wall (**106**) was identified during an attempted caesarean section.

VAGINAL PROLAPSE

Definition/overview

The diameter of a vaginal prolapse varies from approximately 8 cm (**107**) up to 20 cm (**108, 109**), especially if the prolapse contains urinary bladder (**110**) or uterine horn(s), or both of these structures. Prepartum vaginal prolapse occurs in mature ewes during the last month of gestation, with a 0–15% flock incidence. A recent UK survey revealed a 1% incidence of vaginal prolapse – this represents 160,000–200,000 sheep out of a national flock of 16–20 million. Only 10.5% of these ewes received veterinary attention. Other surveys have generally reported an overall incidence of around 1%; however, the high mortality

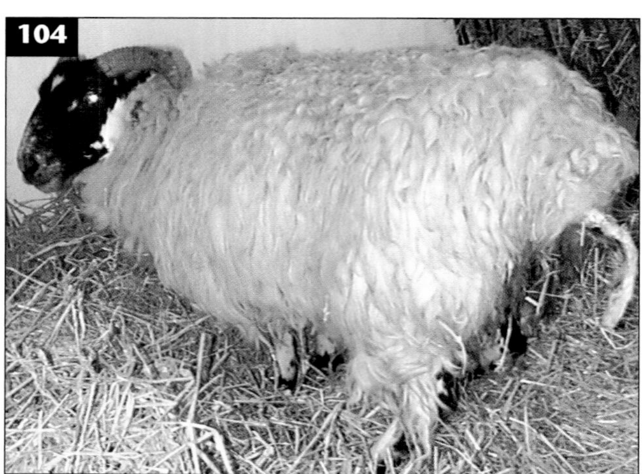

104 Gimmer presenting with a retained fetus two months after the end of the lambing period.

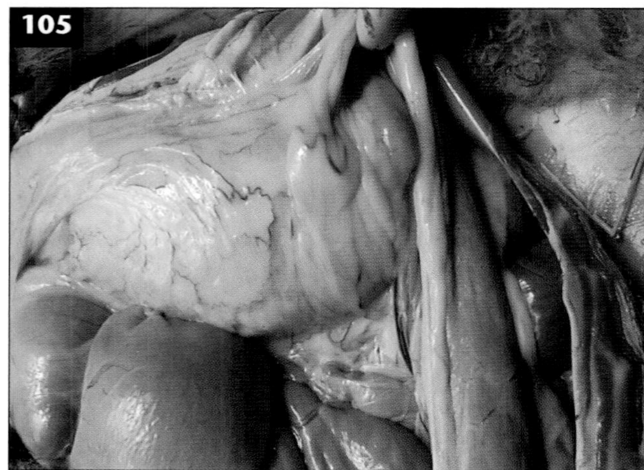

105 Fibrous adhesions between uterus and omentum and grossly thickened uterine wall first recognized during attempted caesarean section.

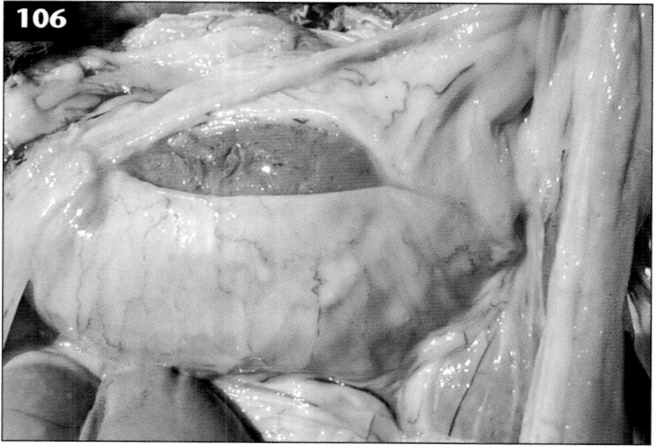

106 Grossly thickened uterine wall associated with an autolytic fetus.

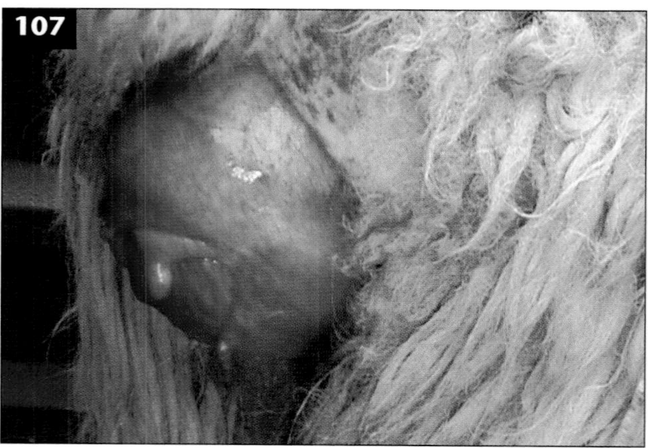

107 Early vaginal prolapse.

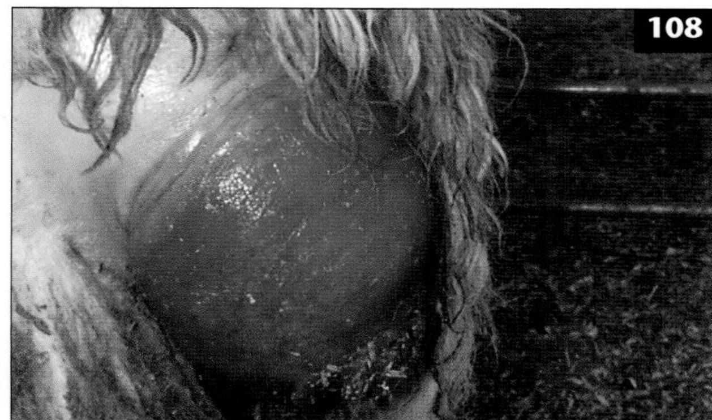
108 Contaminated vaginal prolapse.

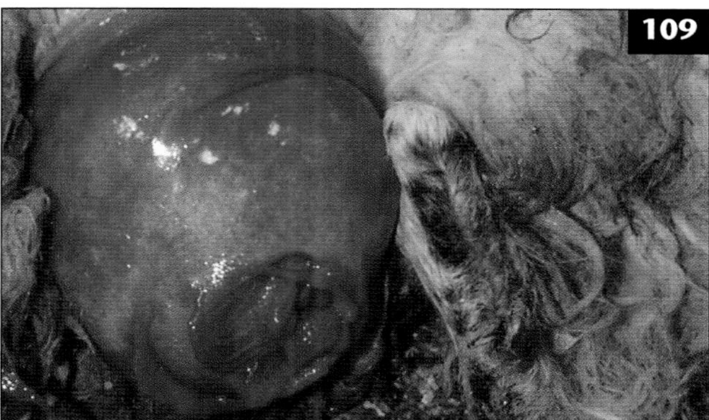
109 Cleaning of the prolapsed tissues.

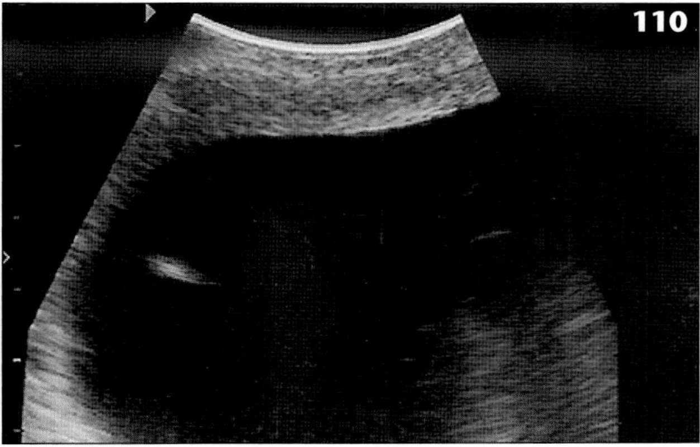
110 Ultrasonogram of a vaginal prolapse containing urinary bladder represented by the large uniform anechoic area.

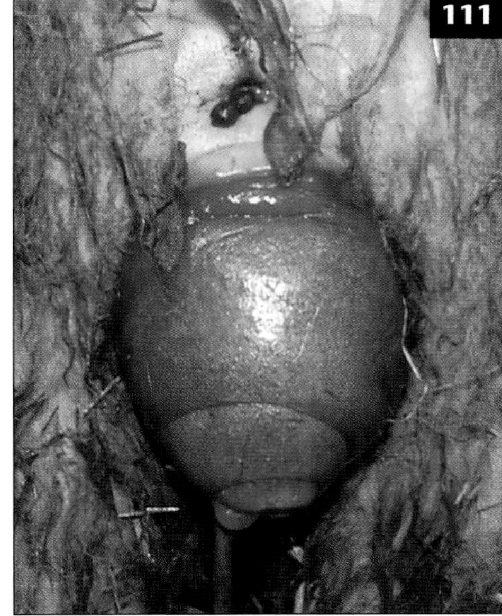
111 Vaginal prolapse in a ewe in first stage labour. The allanto-chorion can be seen.

rate, increased incidence of dystocia (**111**) and recurrence of prolapse in 40–55% of ewes during later pregnancies result in significant production losses and raise serious animal welfare problems.

Aetiology

Many factors have been implicated in the aetiology of vaginal prolapse including: excess body condition (BCS 3.5 and above); multigravid uterus; high-fibre diets, particularly those containing root crops; limited exercise in housed ewes; lameness leading to prolonged periods in sternal recumbency; steep fields; and subclinical hypocalcaemia. Short-docked tails have been implicated in vaginal prolapse but the condition also occurs in mountain breeds with undocked tails.

Clinical presentation

Extra care is needed when checking ewes with undocked tails and long fleeces as vaginal prolapse is easily overlooked. In extensively managed systems, vaginal prolapse may not be noted for some days, with resultant gross contamination (**112**), vascular compromise of prolapsed tissues and superficial bacterial infection.

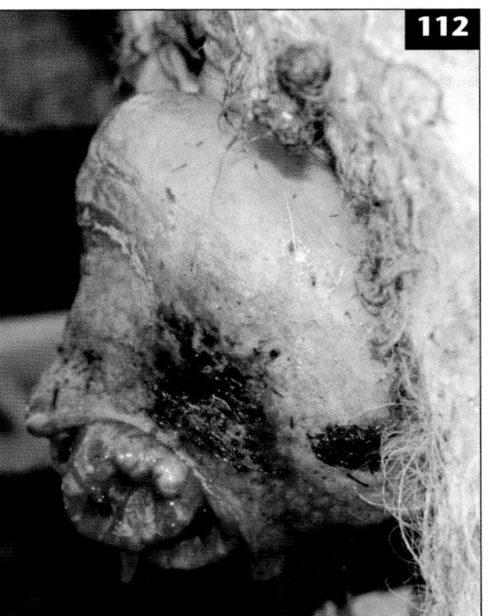
112 Vaginal prolapse contaminated with faeces.

Ewes with vaginal prolapse may show many behavioural signs consistent with first stage labour, including isolation from the remainder of the flock, failure to come forward for concentrate feeding and periods spent in lateral recumbency with repeated, short-duration, forceful abdominal contractions and associated vocalization. Frequent attempts to urinate, with no urine voided, are often noted when the ewe raises herself. Neither cervical mucus plug nor fetal membranes are visible at the vulva; instead a red spherical prolapse measuring 8–20 cm is present.

The duration of prolapse directly affects the degree of contamination with faeces, bedding material and soil, and this compromises the integrity of the vaginal mucosa. The vaginal wall quickly becomes oedematous and turgid, greatly increasing the risk of rupture during manual replacement, especially if this procedure is attempted without effective caudal analgesia. The vaginal prolapse may become damaged when the ewe is transported to the farm or confined in a pen while awaiting veterinary attention.

A full clinical examination of ewes with vaginal prolapse must be undertaken as clinical signs indicating toxaemia (inappetence, reduced ruminal contractions, raised pulse and congested mucous membranes) may be consistent with fetal death, associated metritis and impending abortion. Particular attention should be paid to the cervix and the nature of any discharges. The accumulation of colostrum in the udder may give some approximation of the due lambing date.

If there is doubt regarding the viability of the fetus(es) after the vaginal prolapse has been replaced, fetal movement can be reliably demonstrated in near-term sheep using a transabdominal real-time B-mode ultrasound machine with a 5 MHz sector transducer. Fetal heartbeats can prove more difficult to detect in near-term fetuses even after searching for five minutes. It must be remembered that ultrasonographic findings only indicate the presence of one or more live fetuses at the time of examination; fetal death may occur subsequent to the examination. If no fetal movement is detected after five minutes, it is highly probable that the fetuses are dead and very close supervision of the ewe is essential to detect signs of impending abortion. However, it is unlikely that consecutive daily ultrasound examinations to monitor pregnancy would be undertaken except for valuable pedigree ewes.

Diagnosis

Diagnosis is easily confirmed on clinical inspection. The contents of the vaginal prolapse can be readily determined using real-time B-mode ultrasonography with a 5 MHz transducer and either linear array or sector scanners. The vaginal prolapse may contain dorsal vaginal wall, urinary bladder, uterine horn(s), or both urinary bladder and uterine horn(s). Urinary bladder is readily identified as a markedly hypoechoic (black) area on the sonogram, usually >10 cm in diameter and compressed dorsoventrally (**110**). A fold in the bladder wall, which presents as a hyperechoic (white) line, can often be visualized in the ventral one-third of the hypoechoic area.

Sections through the tips of uterine horn(s) have been visualized ultrasonographically; they appear as round hypoechoic structures measuring 3–5 cm in diameter. Uterine horn containing fetal membranes has been visualized in vaginal prolapses that also contained urinary bladder. Fetal skeleton has been visualized within the pelvis of ewes with vaginal prolapse by directing the ultrasound beam cranially from the vulva.

Differential diagnoses

- Rectal prolapse.
- Eversion of the bladder.
- Evisceration of intestines through a tear in the dorsal vaginal wall.
- Impending parturition.

Treatment

Attempts at replacement and retention of vaginal prolapses by farmers are totally unacceptable because the techniques used cause unnecessary suffering (**113–116**).

Effective caudal analgesia is essential before replacement of a vaginal prolapse is attempted. Emptying of the bladder can be readily achieved in the standing ewe by raising the prolapse relative to the vulva, thereby reducing the fold in the neck of the bladder, at which point urine flows from the urethral orifice.

It is essential to determine the contents of the vaginal prolapse if needle decompression of a suspected fluid-filled viscus is attempted before replacement. Puncture of the allantochorion would greatly increase the risk of introducing infection and thus cause subsequent abortion. Furthermore, puncture of a major blood vessel may occur if uterine horn is contained within the prolapsed tissues.

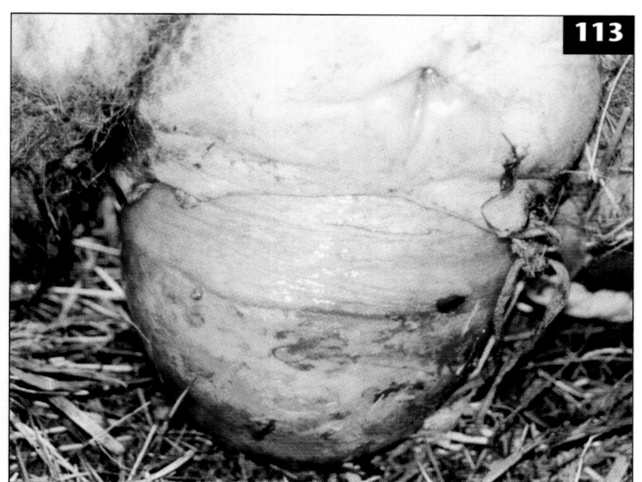

113 Totally inappropriate suture for retention of a vaginal prolapse. Polypropylene baler twine has been used. This situation has caused unnecessary suffering.

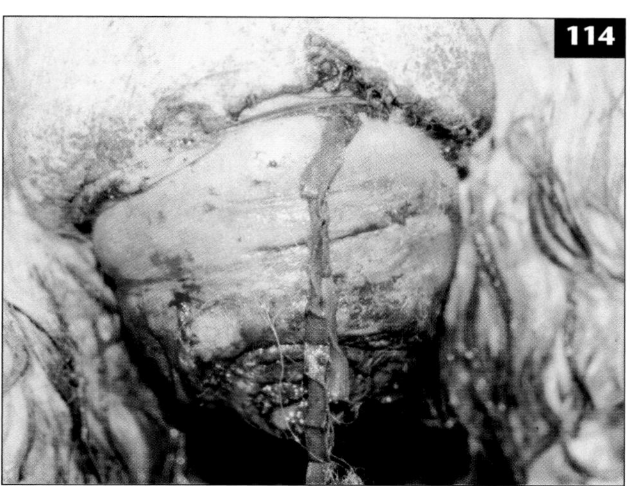

114 Totally unacceptable management of a vaginal prolapse.

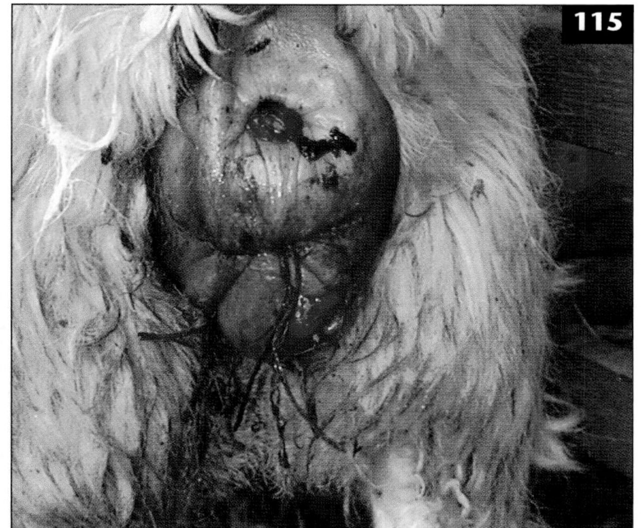

115 Use of polypropylene baler twine to retain a vaginal prolapse. This situation has caused unnecessary suffering: note the extensive oedema. The photograph was taken after extradural injection, which blocked the tenesmus that had caused the rectal prolapse.

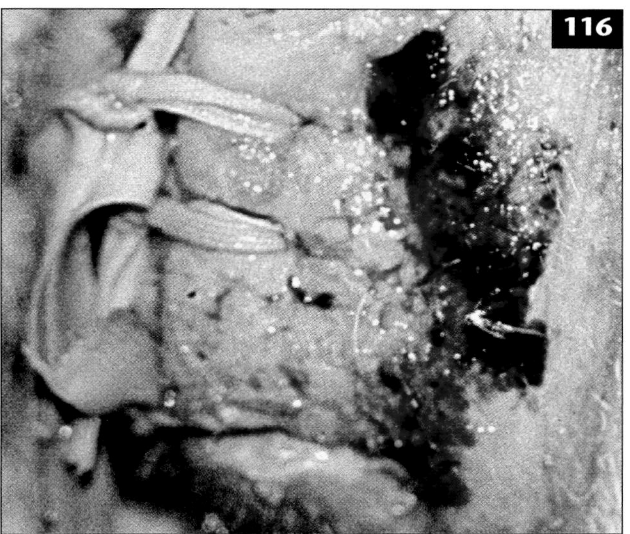

116 Totally unacceptable attempt at a retention suture. There is vulval tearing and diphtheresis.

The ten-minute interval between extradural injection and prolapse replacement affords the veterinarian time to remove gross contamination from the mucosal surface of prolapsed tissues using warm dilute antiseptic solution. The vaginal prolapse should be replaced with the ewe standing; in fact, the vaginal prolapse will frequently return to the normal position within five minutes once caudal analgesia has commenced and tenesmus has ceased. There is no indication whatsoever to suspend the ewe by its hindlimbs.

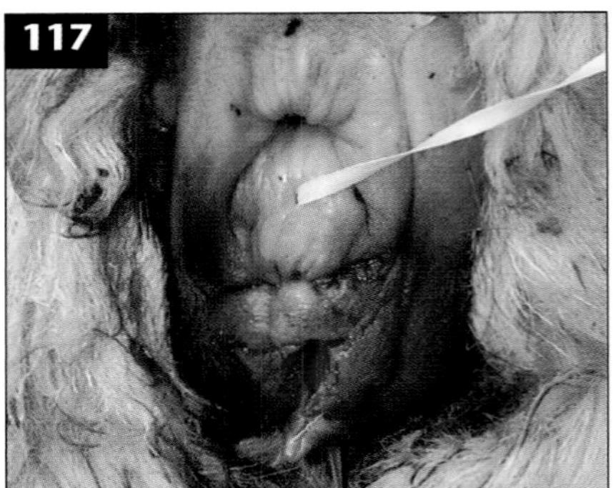

117 Insertion of a Buhner suture of 5mm umbilical tape to the ewe in **115**.

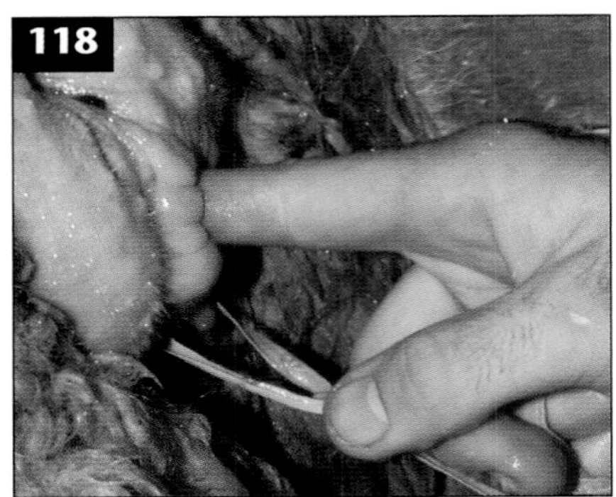

118 Tightening a Buhner suture to 'one finger' diameter.

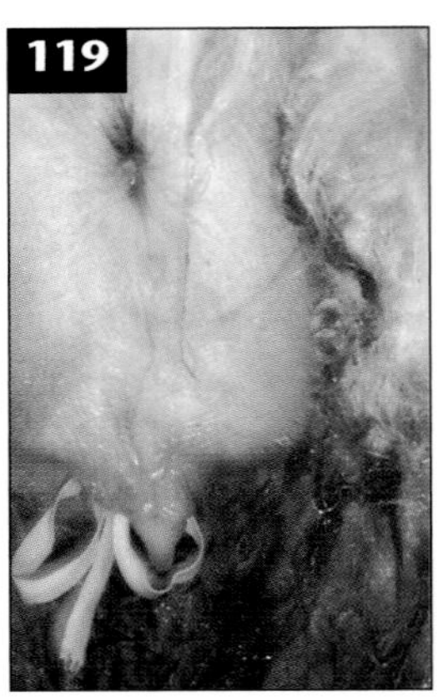

119 A Buhner suture of 5 mm umbilical tape. Compare with **116**.

There are several methods of retention of the vaginal prolapse after it has been after replaced:

- **Buhner suture.** A modified Buhner suture of 5 mm nylon tape is placed in the perivulvar subcutaneous tissue 1.0 cm from the labia (**117**) and tightened to allow an opening of 1.5 cm diameter (**118, 119**). Procaine penicillin (44,000 iu/kg) should be injected intramuscularly once daily for 3–5 consecutive days. The ewe is clearly marked and the shepherd instructed to observe her closely for signs of impending parturition. The modified Buhner suture can easily be untied to allow examination of the posterior reproductive tract for signs of first stage labour. Oedema surrounding the vulva often follows placement of a Buhner suture but this rarely causes significant problems and no specific treatment is necessary except for monitoring to check that the ewe can urinate freely.

  Sutures that penetrate the vaginal mucosa (e.g. single interrupted or mattress sutures) must be avoided as urine scalding of vaginal mucosa around the suture material, in conjunction with secondary bacterial infection, forms large diphtheritic areas (**116**), which cause considerable discomfort and tenesmus. Furthermore, single interrupted and mattress sutures must be removed to permit digital examination of the posterior reproductive tract during periods of suspected first stage labour, and they cannot easily be retied.

  Hindlimb paresis occasionally results 10–15 minutes after extradural injection of combined lidocaine and xylazine solution and may persist for up to 36 hours. The shepherd must be warned of this possibility in advance and affected sheep should be confined to well-bedded pens until ambulatory. Fresh food and clean water must be placed within easy reach of recumbent sheep. Recumbent ewes must be observed regularly for signs of first stage labour and this will involve raising the tail and examination of the vulva for the presence of fetal membranes.

  All ewes with retention sutures for vaginal prolapse must be clearly identified and staff notified that there could be problems at lambing with this group of sheep. Permanent ewe identification is essential to ensure culling before the next breeding season.

  In some countries there are no analgesic agents licensed for use in sheep (e.g. the UK); however, non-steroidal anti-inflammatory drugs (NSAIDs) have been shown clinically to be helpful in the treatment of painful lesions in sheep (e.g. lameness and following dystocia), and this should support their use after replacement of vaginal prolapse. When using such drugs a standard 35-day meat withdrawal period is recommended. Daily monitoring of ewes after replacement of vaginal prolapse under combined xylazine and lidocaine extradural injection revealed that tenesmus was significantly reduced for up to 36 hours. Conversely, when only local infiltration of the vulva was used, 75% of ewes with prepartum vaginal prolapse experienced straining.
- **Plastic retention devices.** Plastic retention devices are shaped so that the central loop (**120**) is placed within the vagina and then held within the pelvic canal by two side arms tightly tied to the fleece of the flanks (**121**). These devices can cause considerable discomfort, with irritation and secondary infection of the vaginal mucosa resulting in frequent tenesmus and even re-prolapse (**122**).
- **Harnesses or trusses.** Harnesses and trusses (**123**) are useful in situations where the prolapse is detected early and there is little superficial trauma/contamination. However, these devices may prove difficult to fit and they can give rise to pressure sores if too tight and not inspected regularly. Faecal staining of the perineum and detection of first stage labour can become problematic when harnesses or trusses are used.

Shepherds often use plastic retention devices, harnesses and trusses because they think (mistakenly) that there is no need for veterinary attendance of vagi- nal prolapse cases. However, as there is no caudal analgesia, the cycle of prolapse/trauma/superficial infection/tenesmus continues, and may even be aggravated by poorly fitted retention devices. It remains an unfortunate fact of farm animal practice that many shepherds do not want to seek veterinary attention, so they only present vaginal prolapse cases that they have failed to control by their own efforts.

In most ewes tenesmus is not observed after replacement of a vaginal prolapse and, under these circumstances, it is recommended that the Buhner suture is untied and slackened after an interval of 3–4 days. If re-prolapse occurs, it will be quickly detected due to the increased group supervision, and the tissues can be cleaned and replaced and the suture tightened and re-tied.

In most situations the retention suture(s) are not untied by the shepherd until signs of first stage labour – including separation from the remainder of the group, inappetence, frequent getting up and lying down, sniffing at the ground, and abdominal straining with fetal membranes present at the vulva – have been observed (**124**). If the cervix is already fully dilated, and first stage labour has been completed, a lamb may be forcefully expelled as soon as the retention suture has been slackened. Unfortunately, if the ewe has not been closely supervised, the forceful abdominal and myometrial contractions may force the lamb(s) through the vaginal wall before the suture has been slackened, causing perineal laceration.

120 Plastic spatula for retention of a vaginal prolapse.

121 Plastic spatula inserted into the vagina, with the wings tied to the fleece of the ewe's flanks.

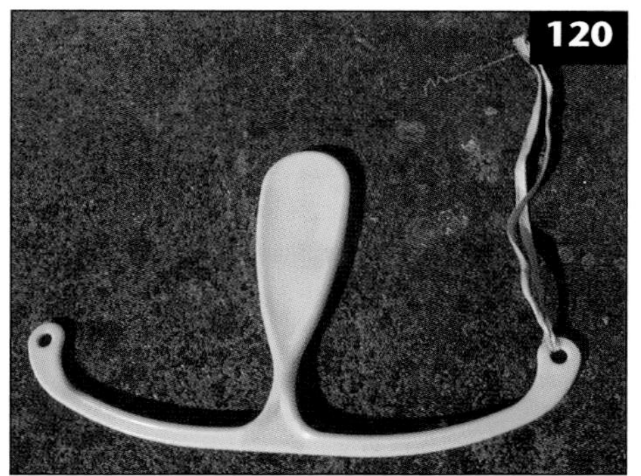

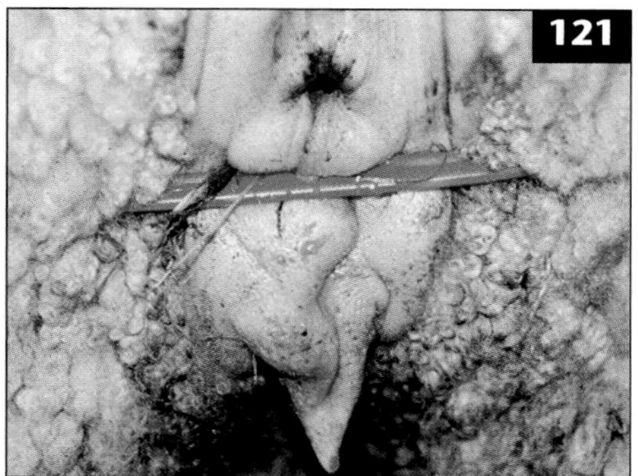

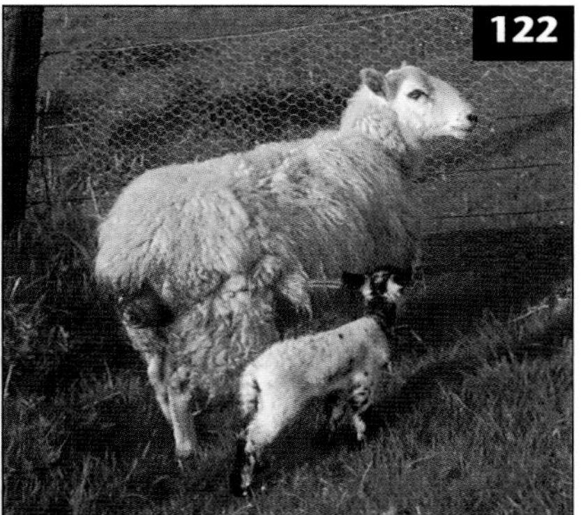

122 Neglected vaginal prolapse that has recurred post partum. This situation is unacceptable.

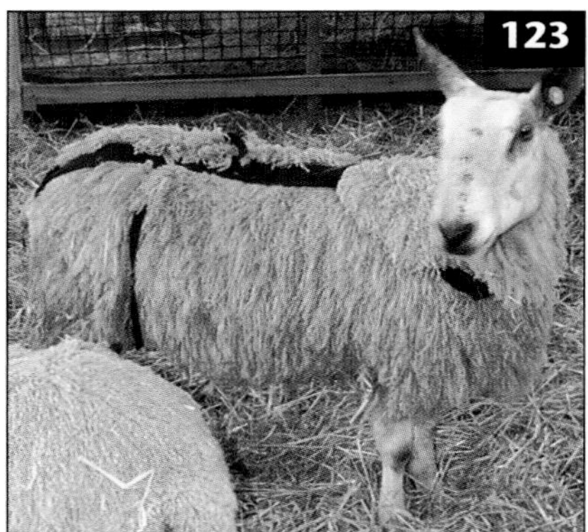

123 Use of a harness to retain a vaginal prolapse.

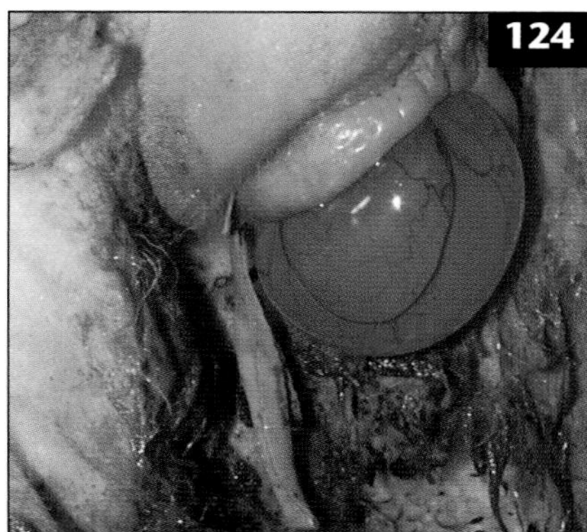

124 End of first stage labour with a Buhner suture still in place. This situation could result in birth of the lamb(s) through a perineal tear if forceful tenesmus occurs.

Complications of vaginal prolapse

Abortion. Abortion may occur 24–48 hours after replacement of the vaginal prolapse. It is not known whether this event is a consequence of trauma to the feto – placental unit during prolapse or to other factors. Ewes must be confined and carefully supervised after replacement of a prolapse for signs of impending abortion.

Incomplete cervical dilation. Considerable trauma, superficial infection and oedema of the vaginal prolapse at the time of replacement may result in incomplete cervical dilation during first stage labour. Typically, the fetal membranes are presented through the external cervical os and vulva.

Digital pressure over 5–10 minutes may result in partial cervical dilation in ewes that present with incomplete cervical dilation associated with prior vaginal prolapse; however, trauma to an inadequately dilated cervix during delivery of the lambs results in tenesmus post partum, and uterine prolapse is not an uncommon sequela. Prolonged manual interference during attempted delivery of the lambs also greatly increases the risk of metritis, and affected ewes often fail to nurse their lambs.

Performing a caesarean section when presented with a ewe with incomplete cervical dilation and a history of vaginal prolapse that has usually been replaced by the shepherd without due care has numerous advantages. These include a much improved prognosis for both ewe and lambs and greatly improved animal welfare. Sadly, the cost of a caesarean section becomes the deciding factor in the management of these cases. However, even under less than optimal farm operating conditions, and prior attempts at delivery of lambs by numerous farm staff, the success rate of caesarean section is >97%.

Prevention/control measures

Great care must be exercised when transporting sheep with a vaginal prolapse due to the friable nature of the oedematous and congested mucous membranes. Wherever possible the veterinarian should visit the farm to deal with such cases. Cases that cannot be successfully managed using either harnesses or plastic retainers should be sutured using a Buhner pattern.

Economics

The farm visit comprises the major component of the veterinary fee (**Table 2**) but lacerations to the friable vaginal wall caused during transport can prove very difficult to repair and the welfare aspects of such transport may be difficult to support on economic grounds alone. If it is necessary to transport a ewe with a vaginal prolapse to the surgery, the prolapse should be covered with a towel soaked in warm water to prevent further trauma and desic-cation.

If a caesarean section is performed in addition to replacement of the vaginal prolapse, the total invoice for veterinary services may well exceed the commercial value of the sheep. However, if a caesarian section is required, it must be performed for the welfare of the ewe and lamb(s).

UTERINE PROLAPSE

Definition/overview

In a survey of over 89,000 sheep, 93 cases of uterine prolapse (0.1% of ewes at risk) were reported. Only 41 of the ewes were presented to a veterinarian, with a success rate of 75.6%. The other 52 ewes were treated by the farmer, with a mortality rate of 45.3%.

Aetiology

Uterine prolapse results from powerful abdominal straining. It may occur either immediately after delivery of the (last) lamb (**125, 126**) or after an interval of 12–48 hours (**127, 128**). In the first instance, prolapse usually results as a consequence of prolonged second stage labour culminating in the delivery of a large singleton lamb. Uterine prolapse occurring after an interval of 12–48 hours generally results from tenesmus caused by pain arising from infection and swelling of the posterior reproductive tract, which has developed consequent to excessive and unskilled interference by the shepherd during delivery of the lamb(s).

Clinical presentation

The everted uterus is readily identifiable by its large size (up to 40 cm long and 25 cm in diameter and extending from the vulva to below the level of the

Table 2 Typical cost of vaginal prolapse replacement by a veterinarian. (Current UK conditions. All figures as percentages of the value of the ewe.)

Item	%
• Value of breeding ewe with twin lambs at foot	100%
• Visit farm	15–25%
• Replace vaginal prolapse	10%
• Drugs (xylazine, lidocaine, penicillin)	2%
• Total	25–35%

hocks) and prominent caruncles (**125, 126**). The fetal membranes may still be attached to the caruncles.

Differential diagnoses

- Vaginal prolapse.
- Eversion of the bladder.
- Evisceration of intestines through a tear in the dorsal vaginal wall.

Treatment

Unless the uterus is replaced correctly and fully inverted to its normal position within the abdomen, the ewe will continue to strain, causing considerable distress and suffering, and re-prolapse. For welfare reasons uterine prolapse must only be replaced by a veterinarian using extradural anaesthesia (see Chapter 15: Caudal injection technique, p. 316); this makes return of the uterus into the abdominal cavity relatively simple.

If the uterus is not completely inverted, partial eversion may occur, with the tip of the uterus retained within the vagina by the retention suture. This situation causes vigorous straining; therefore, any discomfort shown by a ewe after replacement of a uterine prolapse must be carefully investigated and veterinary assistance sought.

Antibiotics, either procaine penicillin or oxytetracycline, should be administered intramuscularly daily for 3–5 consecutive days to limit bacterial infection of the traumatized tissues.

The ewe's milk yield will be reduced for a number of days and her lambs will require supplementary feeding. Unlike vaginal prolapse, it is unusual for a ewe to prolapse its uterus the following year; therefore, there is no indication to cull such ewes prematurely.

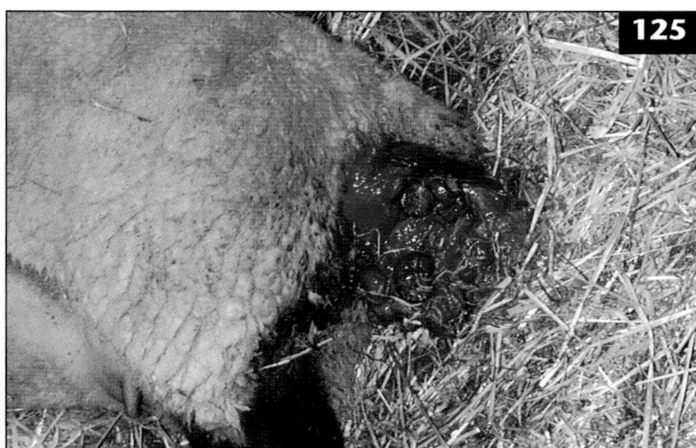

125 Uterine prolapse immediately after delivery of the lamb. Congested caruncles are seen with attached placenta.

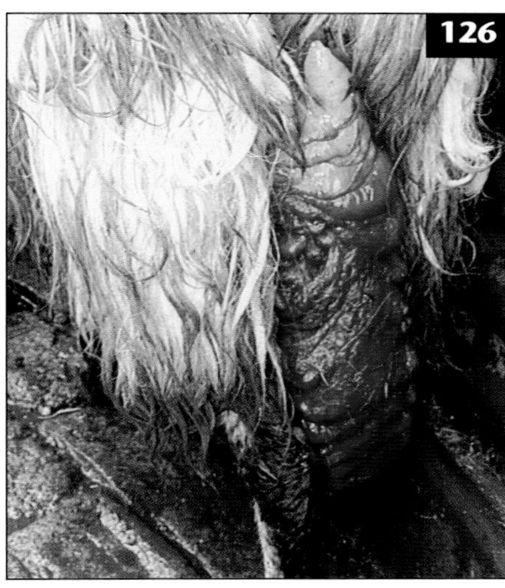

126 Turgid uterine prolapse of approximately 4–6 hours' duration.

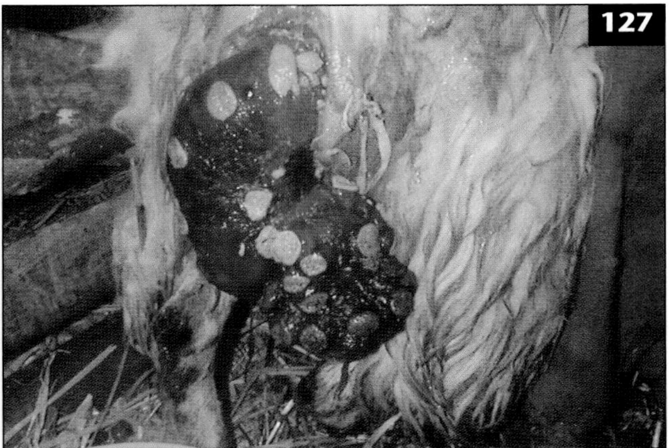

127 Attempted uterine prolapse replacement by the farmer: note the remnant of the mattress suture. Persistent tenesmus resulted in recurrence after 36 hours. The caruncles are necrotic.

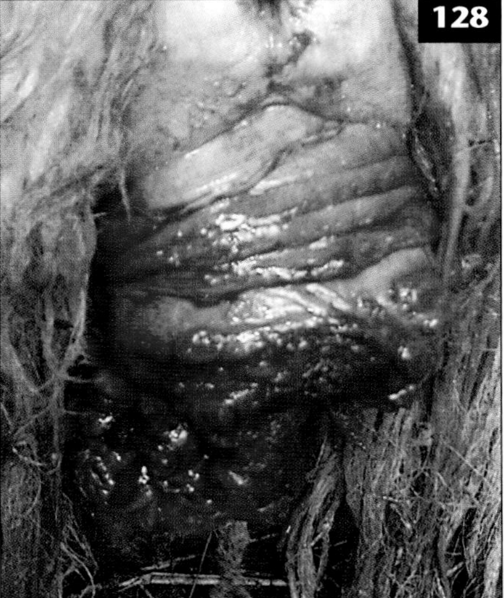

128 Uterine prolapse associated with a prepartum vaginal prolapse. The vaginal wall is oedematous.

Prevention/control measures

While it may prove difficult to prevent sporadic uterine prolapse following delivery of a large singleton lamb, uterine prolapse after protracted unskilled interference can be avoided by timely correction of the dystocia by a veterinarian.

Economics

Replacement of a uterine prolapse under extradural analgesia at the veterinary surgery could cost 20–25% of the value of the ewe. Correct replacement of the everted uterine horn should prevent recurrence and there should be a rapid return to normal appetite/lactation. While the ewe may not rear two lambs, she should have sufficient milk for one lamb.

Welfare implications

Replacement of a uterine prolapse is an act of veterinary surgery and not a procedure that someone with no training should ever attempt. Attempted replacement of a uterine prolapse simply by suspending the ewe by its hindlimbs is both unacceptable and unnecessary. The veterinary profession must cooperate more effectively with farmers to resolve this issue. Education is essential to inform farmers and their staff what can be achieved using appropriate extradural analgesia.

EVISCERATION THROUGH A VAGINAL TEAR

Evisceration of intestines, caecum and omentum through a tear in the dorsal vaginal wall occurs spontaneously in heavily pregnant ewes during the last month of gestation (**129**). There is usually no history of prior vaginal prolapse or tenesmus. The incidence may reach 2–5% in some housed flocks for no obvious reason, as management factors have not changed from previous years. Excess body condition, triplet pregnancy and high-fibre diets are thought to be risk factors but the precise mechanism is unknown.

There is no treatment and affected ewes must be destroyed immediately for welfare reasons. If the ewe is due to lamb within three days, she could be shot and an emergency caesarean section undertaken to salvage the lambs; however, this procedure is rarely successful. Furthermore, when evisceration occurs during late gestation in flocks lambing over a concentrated period, there are no ewes to accept such weakly foster lambs.

RECTAL PROLAPSE

In most situations rectal prolapse occurs in ewes that show tenesmus caused by a vaginal prolapse. The rectal wall extends for 2–3 cm (**130**). Provision of effective caudal analgesia to block tenesmus will allow the rectal prolapse to return to its normal position (see Chapter 15: Caudal analgesia, p. 316). If the rectal prolapse does not return, it should be retained by a purse string suture of 5 mm umbilical tape placed subcutaneously around the anus and tightened to reduce the internal diameter to approximately 1.5 cm. However, this procedure should be considered carefully, as it may prove difficult to judge if the ewe is still able to defecate easily yet retain the previously prolapsed rectal tissue.

Very occasionally, continued tenesmus after vaginal prolapse replacement may cause rectal prolapse (**131**). On rare occasions the rectal prolapse may extend to more than 10 cm and, under these circumstances, the prolapsed rectum should be amputated under caudal analgesia.

In the USA rectal prolapse presents as a problem in overconditioned show lambs with very short-docked, or absent, tails. It is a legal requirement in the UK that sufficient tail must be left to cover the anus of male lambs and the vulva of female lambs, including the caudal skin folds. Notwithstanding such anatomical differences, rectal prolapse has been effectively treated after caudal extradural injection of xylazine and lidocaine and placement of a Buhner suture of 5 mm umbilical tape. There is no justification for percutaneous injection of irritant substances around the serosal surface of the rectum in order to produce intrapelvic inflammation and adhesion formation.

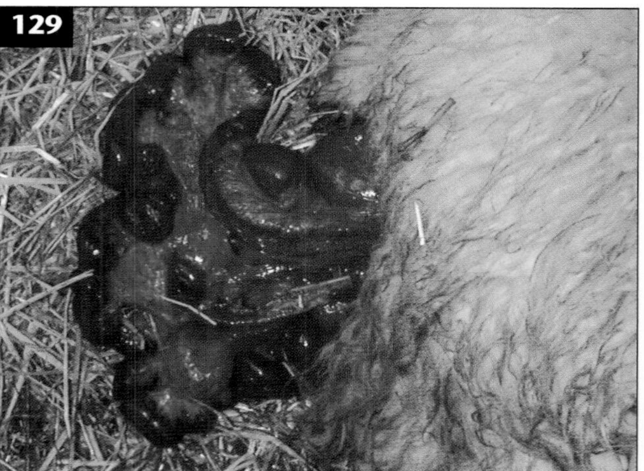

129 Evisceration through a vaginal tear.

An alternative regimen for inhibition of tenesmus is to produce temporary damage to the cauda equina by caudal extradural injection of isopropyl alcohol. Accurate dose calculation and injection technique is required to block tenesmus but not compromise the lumbosacral outflow to the hindlimbs; this can cause prolonged posterior paralysis and its consequences. There are no published studies describing sacrococcygeal isopropyl alcohol injection in sheep but there is no indication for such a regimen when timely veterinary management employing extradural injection of lidocaine and xylazine can prove successful, even in advanced cases. Where necessary, it is recommended that the extradural injection of lidocaine and xylazine is repeated after 36–48 hours in problem cases.

CAESAREAN SECTION

Caesarean section to correct dystocia has been performed routinely and with excellent success rates in general veterinary practice. Emphasis on sheep meat production and carcase conformation within Europe has resulted in the development of breed characteristics that directly increase the likelihood of absolute fetal oversize. Sire selection is still based on phenotype, with no attention given to the possibility of dystocia. However, in many countries worldwide careful selection of sheep for ease of lambing under pastoral management systems, such as practised in NewZealand and Australia, have greatly reduced the dystocia rate so that caesarean section is rarely necessary. In addition, other factors such as cost and proximity to veterinary services preclude surgery on sheep of low financial value.

The most common conditions necessitating delivery of lamb(s) by caesarean section are relative fetal oversize, particularly in the immature primiparous animal (one year old) with a singleton fetus, incomplete cervical dilation, absolute fetal oversize in the Texel, Beltex and Suffolk breeds, and vaginal prolapse. The incidence of caesarean section is often high in ewes that have been treated for prolapsed vagina, because gross oedema and trauma of the vagina, in association with incomplete cervical dilation, prevent normal delivery of the lambs.

Analgesia

(see also Chapter 15: Anaesthesia)

There are three options:

- Analgesia of the left flank can be achieved using local line infiltration of the incision site with approximately 5 mg/kg of 2% lidocaine solution.
- Xylazine (0.07 mg/kg) injected into the extradural space at the sacrococcygeal site affords analgesia of the flank approximately 30 minutes after injection.
- Excellent analgesia of the flank for caesarean section can be achieved after lumbosacral extradural injection of 4 mg/kg of 2% lidocaine solution.

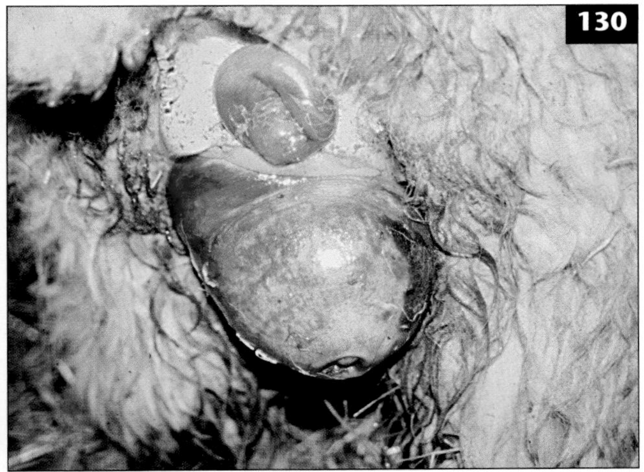

130 Concurrent rectal and vaginal prolapses.

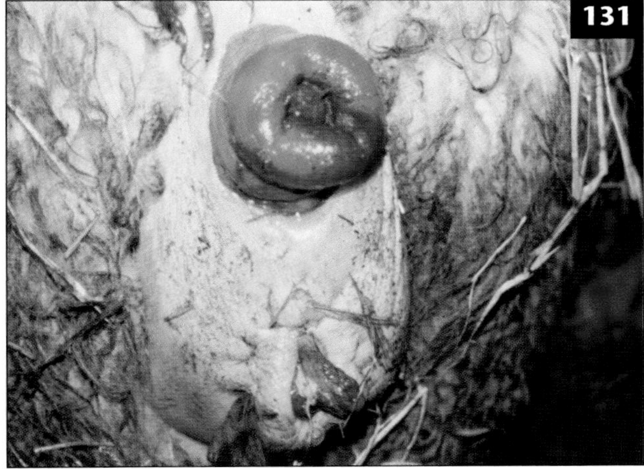

131 Rectal prolapse caused by persistent tenesmus after inappropriate retention method for a vaginal prolapse.

Surgery

The ewe is positioned in right lateral recumbency. A large area of the left flank is shaved; under no circumstances should the wool be plucked from the skin. A plastic disposable drape is fenestrated and held in position with towel clips (**132**).

Surgery is performed through a left flank incision midway between the last rib and the wing of the ilium, commencing 10 cm below the level of the transverse processes of the lumbar vertebrae. A 15 cm incision is made through the skin, subcutaneous fat (**133**), external abdominal oblique muscle (**134**) and internal abdominal oblique muscle. The transversus muscle and closely adherent peritoneum are grasped with forceps and raised. A small nick is made with scissors and extended as necessary (**135**). Care is necessary at this stage to avoid puncturing any underlying viscus, especially if the ewe is bloated or shows tenesmus.

Care is necessary when exteriorizing the gravid uterine horn (**136**) because of its thin wall and friable nature. In a multigravid uterus the left horn is always chosen (**137**). The abdominal wound can be packed with sterile gauze swabs prior to the incision being made in the greater curvature of the uterus in an attempt to prevent leakage of uterine fluids into the abdomen, but this is not usually necessary. Using

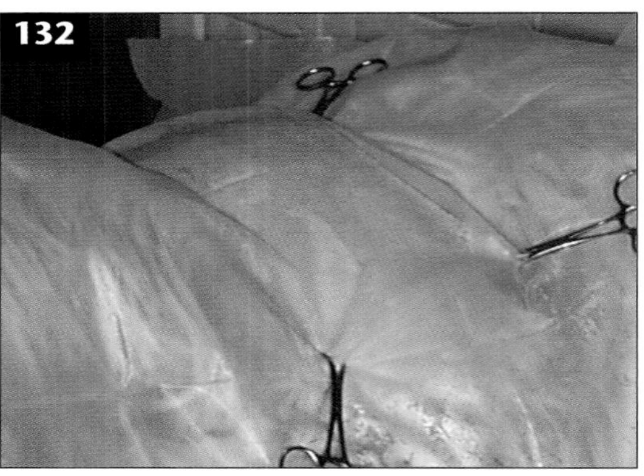

132 Left flank shaved, prepared and draped for surgery.

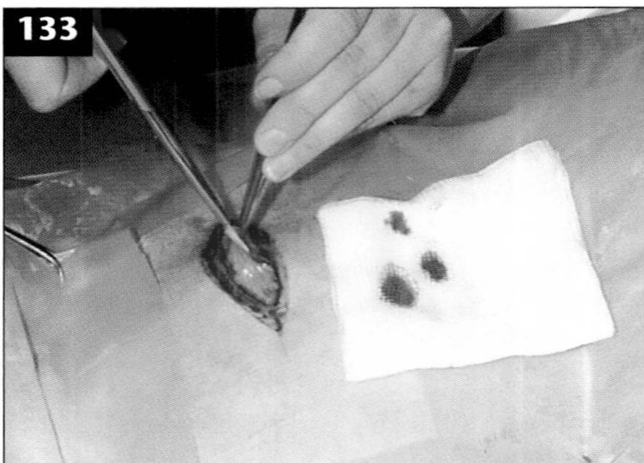

133 Incision through the subcutaneous fat.

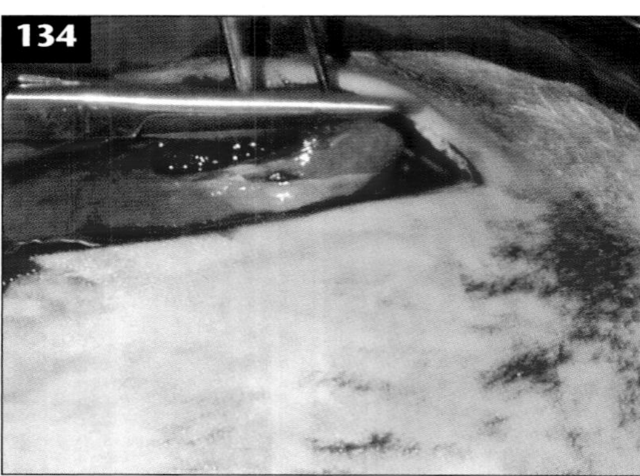

134 Incision through the external abdominal oblique muscle.

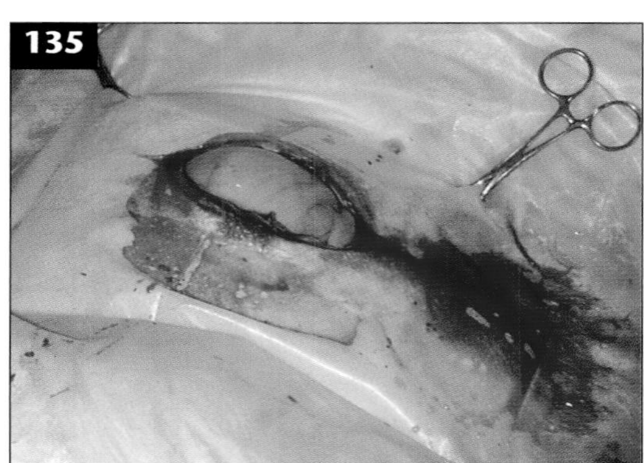

135 Abdominal incision completed: appearance of the dorsal sac of the rumen.

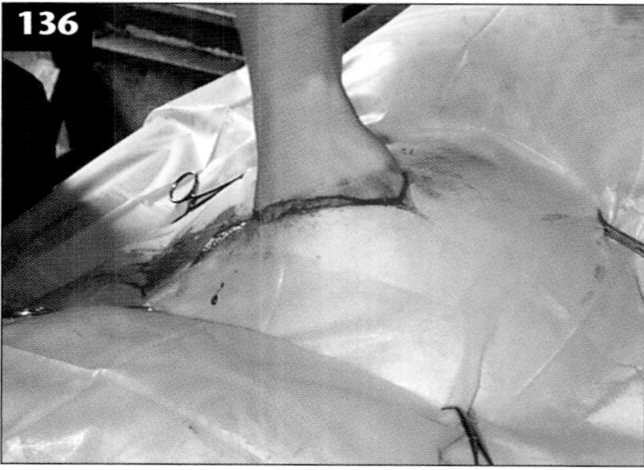

136 Entry into the abdominal cavity.

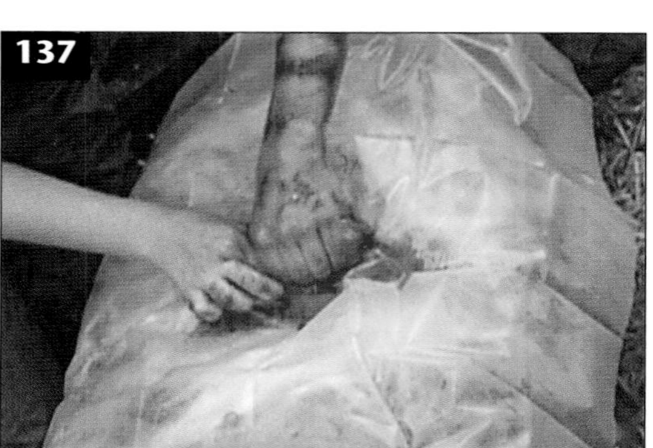

137 Exteriorization of the left uterine horn.

scissors an incision is made, starting 6–8 cm from the tip of the uterine horn (at the level of the lamb's hind fetlock joints in those lambs in anterior presentation) and extending towards the cervix as necessary (**138**). The uterine incision is normally extended to just over the lamb's hock. Because of the oedematous and friable nature of the uterus, considerable difficulty may be encountered when manipulating and attempting to exteriorize part of the uterine horn when emphysematous lambs are present *in utero*. When the lamb in the left uterine horn is presented in anterior presentation, it will be delivered hindlimbs first (**139**). If present, the lamb(s) in anterior presentation in the right uterine horn is delivered head first (**140**).

The uterine incision is closed with an inversion suture pattern of 7 metric chromic catgut, or equivalent, suture material (**141, 142**). The suture line is

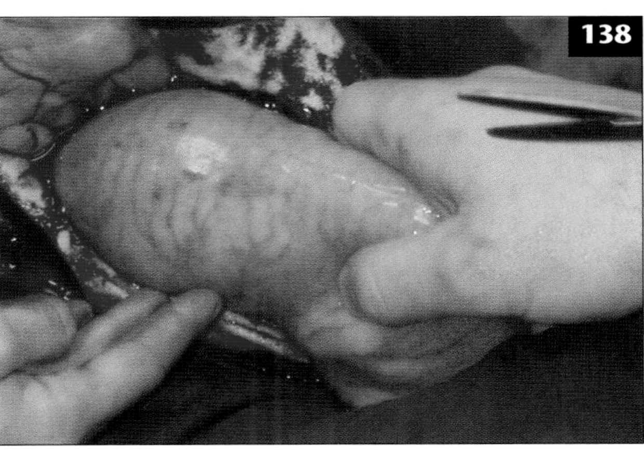

138 Preparing to incise along the greater curvature of the uterus from the lamb's fetlock to just proximal to the hock joint (lamb in posterior presentation). The pattern of blood vessels can be seen.

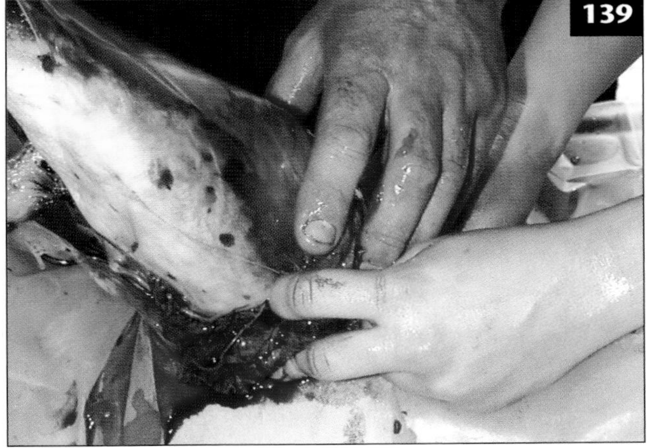

139 Delivery of a lamb from the left uterine horn when in normal anterior presentation.

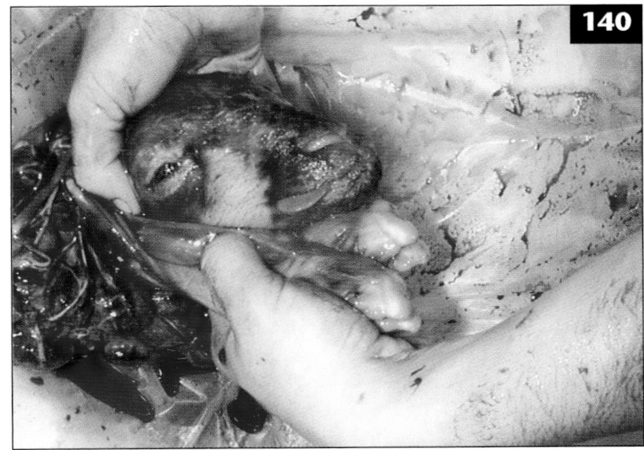

140 Same operation as in **139**. Delivery of a lamb from the right uterine horn. The lamb was in normal anterior presentation, hence delivered head first.

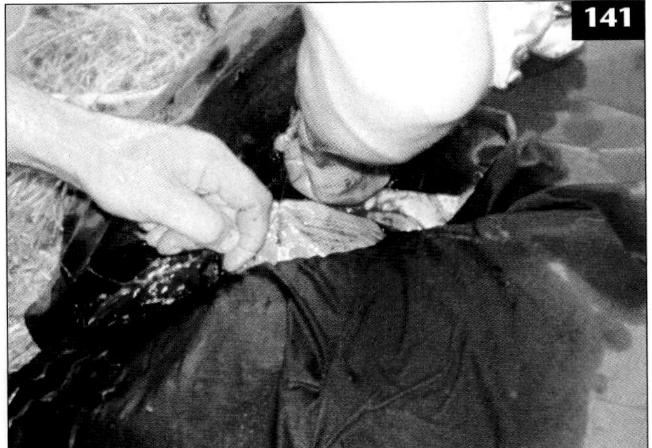

141 Repair of uterine closure using inversion suture pattern. The left uterine horn is resting on a surgical drape.

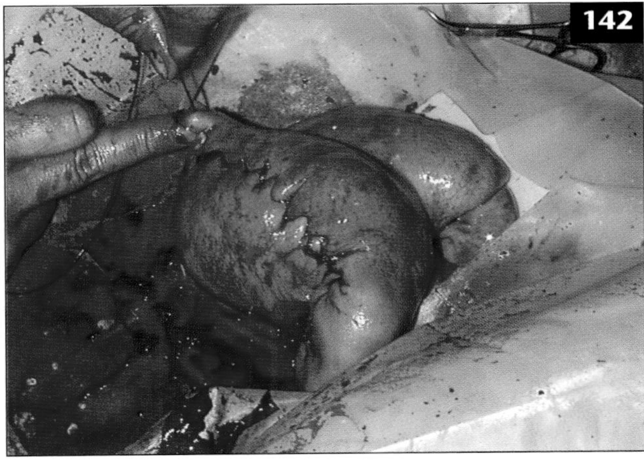

142 Uterine closure.

checked carefully for leakage of uterine contents. The peritoneum and transverse abdominal muscles are closed with a continuous suture of 7 metric chromic catgut. The internal and external abdominal oblique muscle layers are then closed with a continuous suture of 7 metric chromic catgut. The skin incision is closed with interrupted horizontal mattress sutures of 6 metric monofilament nylon or similar.

Supportive therapy

Procaine penicillin (44,000 iu/kg i/m) should be administered before surgery commences and then for three consecutive days postoperatively. Ewes should also be given flunixin (2.2 mg/kg i/v) before surgery. In toxaemic sheep, where costs permit, supportive therapy could include up to three litres of isotonic saline (50 ml/kg/hour) administered intravenously during surgery.

Application of ultrasonographic examination in sheep presenting with obstetrical problems

Ultrasonographic examination at full-term can prove very helpful when transabdominal ballotment suggests the presence of a fetus *in utero* after delivery of a lamb(s) some 12–48 hours previously, but contraction of the cervix prevents manual examination of the uterine lumen. Ewes are scanned in the standing position using a 5 MHz sector scanner immediately cranial to the udder where the skin is free of wool and only requires application of ultrasound gel to obtain good contact.

Metritis

Definition/overview

Metritis commonly affects ewes after unhygienic manual interference to correct fetal malpresentation/malposture, after delivery of dead lambs and following infectious causes of abortion. Metritis is also common following replacement of uterine prolapse.

Aetiology

Illness follows bacterial entry and multiplication within the uterus, with production of toxins that are absorbed across the damaged endometrium. A recent survey revealed that more than one third of shepherds neither washed their hands nor used arm-length disposable plastic gloves before attempting correction of a difficult lambing. The likelihood of metritis is increased if the lambs are dead and further increased if the lambs are autolytic. Unlike cattle, metritis in ewes is not commonly associated with retained fetal membranes.

Clinical presentation

A ewe with metritis shows little interest in her lamb(s) and spends long periods in sternal recumbency (**143**). The ewe is depressed (**144**) and inappetent, and has a poor milk yield as evidenced by hungry lambs who attempt to suck whenever the ewe stands. Often a lamb has been 'fostered-on' to replace a dead lamb, and its gaunt appearance may be masked by the covering dead lamb's skin. The ewe's rectal temperature is often only marginally elevated (40°C). The mucous membranes are congested. There are reduced/absent ruminal sounds

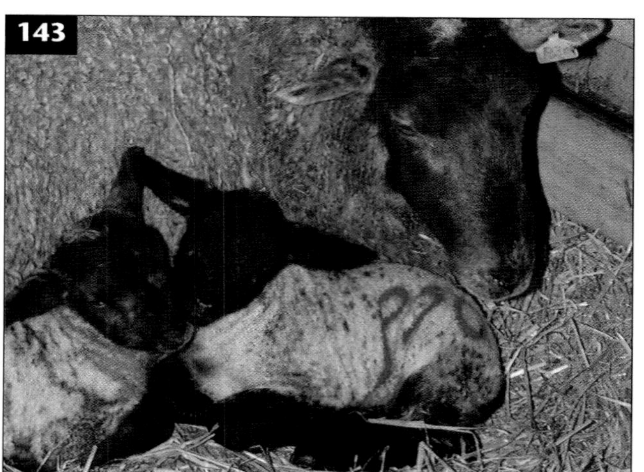

143 Sick ewe with metritis. The ewe has little interest in its offspring and the lambs are hungry. (See also **147**.)

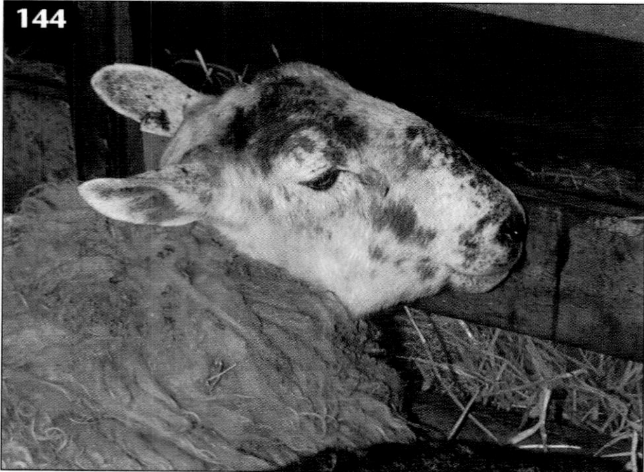

144 Sick ewe with metritis.

and the sublumbar fossae may be sunken, reflecting reduced rumen fill. The vulva is usually swollen and oedematous as a result of manual interference during second stage labour, with evidence of a red/brown fetid discharge on the wool of the tail and perineum (**145**). The vulval discharge may appear more purulent with an increasing postpartum interval. The posterior reproductive tract can be examined digitally but not the cervix or uterus. Digital examination frequently provokes forceful straining and vocalization. Abdominal ballotment fails to detect evidence of a retained fetus.

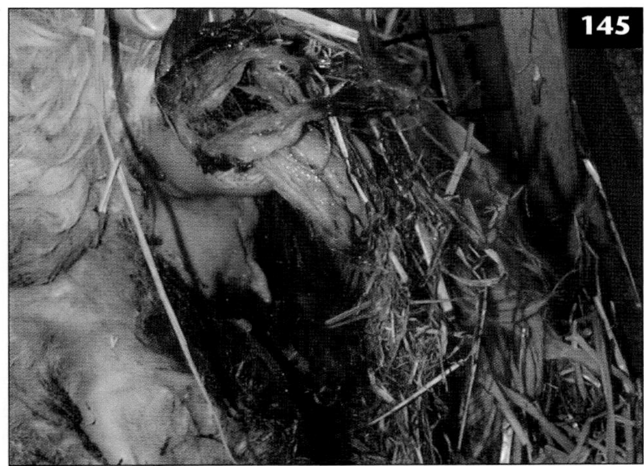

145 Purulent vaginal discharge staining a ewe's tail.

Differential diagnoses

Differential diagnoses to consider for inappetent recumbent ewes could include:

- Ruptured uterus if considerable difficulty encountered during delivery of fetus.
- Retained fetus.
- Acidosis if ewe overfed concentrates post lambing.
- Peritonitis.
- Mastitis.
- Hypocalcaemia.

Diagnosis

It can prove difficult to be certain that the cause of illness is metritis, because the uterus cannot be examined in detail and vulval discharge is present on the tail and perineum of many postpartum ewes (**146**). A provisional diagnosis of metritis is based on a history of dystocia, clinical findings and exclusion of other diseases of the postpartum ewe.

Treatment

The common agents causing abortion in sheep are sensitive to a wide range of commonly used antibiotics. Typically, there is dramatic improvement in the sheep's demeanour and appetite within 12 hours of intravenous injection of oxytetracycline and dexamethasone (**147**). The inclusion of dexamethasone in the treatment regimen achieves a more rapid response than antibiotic injection alone. Other antibiotics (e.g. procaine penicillin) can also be administered. There is no risk from septicaemia as a consequence of corticosteroid injection and the author has used this treatment protocol with

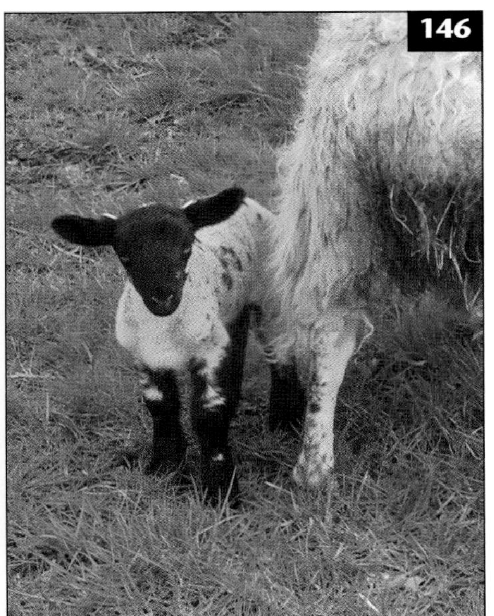

146 A scant purulent vaginal discharge staining the tail is common in many healthy postpartum ewes.

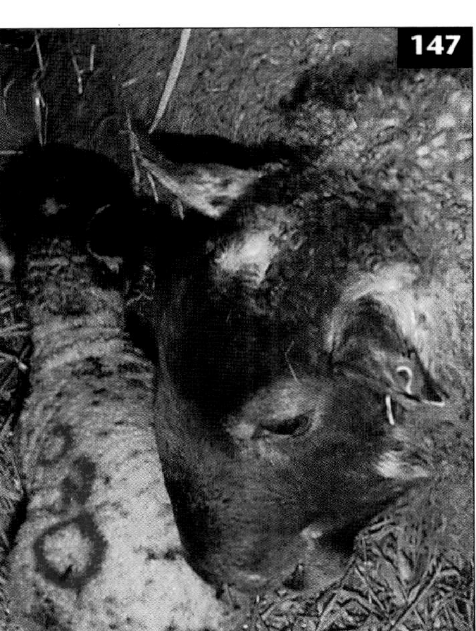

147 Ewe in **143** 12 hours after treatment. She is showing maternal instincts and the lamb is happy.

excellent results for many years. Deterioration in the clinical presentation in a small percentage of metritis cases results from developing septic peritonitis associated with a uterine tear, rather than treatment failure, but few such deaths are subjected to postmortem examination.

Prevention/control measures

Almost without exception, farmers' attitudes to overall hygiene standards during dystocia correction could be greatly improved, thereby avoiding many of the problems encountered after such interference. Often there is no hand-wash basin in the lambing shed. Farmers should wash their hands in an approved surgical scrub solution and they must use arm-length disposable gloves prior to correction of all dystocia cases. Arm-length disposable plastic gloves are cheap and easily carried within pockets; there is no excuse for non-compliance with such basic hygiene precautions even under extensive flock management systems. With infectious causes of abortion, these precautions should be seen as a minimum standard to limit the risk of zoonotic infections such as *Salmonella*, *Campylobacter* and *Chlamydophila* species. In multigravid litters, delivering all the lambs, not just the lamb in malpresentation/malposture, greatly increases the likelihood of introducing infection deep into the uterus.

Economics

Death of hungry lambs may result if they are turned outdoors during adverse weather. In some cases it may prove necessary to remove one or both lambs and cross-foster them or rear them on milk replacer. Death of the ewe is very uncommon but the check in lamb growth during the critical first few days of life is not recovered over the next few weeks to months, with a consequent extended period to market.

Welfare implications

Metritis in ewes results in poor milk production and hungry lambs, which may die if not given supplementary milk.

ABORTION

Overview

Infectious causes of abortion are most common after day 120 of pregnancy. While sporadic losses are variably attributed to overcrowding, competition during feeding (**148**), handling procedures or movement, an abortion rate in excess of 2% is suggestive of an infectious aetiology and laboratory investigation is strongly recommended. A standard set of samples will allow laboratory identification of the abortifacient agent(s) in most situations. Farmers must isolate all suspect aborted sheep and remove all aborted material. The zoonotic potential of many abortifacient agents must be stressed to anyone attending sheep. Appropriate hygiene precautions must also extend to the household, where infection could arise from contaminated clothing and footwear.

Sample collection

The minimum requirements for laboratory submissions for abortion investigation include the fetus(es) or fetal stomach content, a piece of placenta and a maternal serum sample. Instructions regarding safe packaging of pathological material can be obtained from the veterinary laboratory. While the first submission may identify a recognized abortifacient agent, it is important to collect aborted material throughout the outbreak, as more than one agent may be present within the flock and such knowledge is essential when formulating treatment, control and prevention strategies.

CHLAMYDIAL ABORTION (*Syns*: enzootic abortion of ewes [EAE], *Chlamydophila abortus* infection)

Definition/overview

Chlamydial (*Chlamydophila abortus*) abortion is a major cause of abortion and ewe and lamb deaths in many countries, with the exception of Australia and New Zealand, and it is the main cause of ovine abortion in the UK. Pregnant women are at serious risk from *C. abortus* infection, because the organism is able to colonize the human placenta, causing abortion, stillbirth and maternal illness.

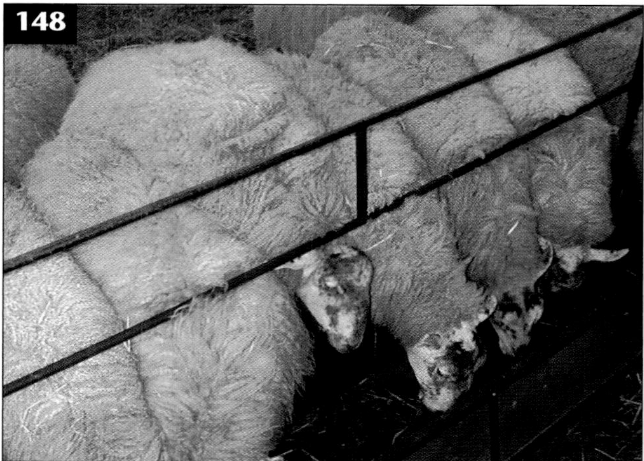

148 Abortion caused by overcrowding, competition during feeding, handling procedures and movement are uncommon.

Aetiology

Disease is transmitted by the oral route following exposure of susceptible females to high levels of infected uterine discharges/aborted material. Such exposure and transmission is greatly increased when sheep are intensively managed during late gestation and during the lambing period. Infection does not result in clinical signs unless the ewe is more than six weeks from the due lambing date, infection remaining latent until the subsequent pregnancy.

Colonization of the placenta takes places from about day 90 of gestation, coinciding with rapid fetal growth. Rapid bacterial multiplication takes place within the placentome, with a resultant inflammatory response and infection and reaction spreading to the intercotyledonary areas of the chorion. Impaired nutrient transfer across diseased placentomes results in fetal debility. Abortion may be triggered by reduced progesterone synthesis by damaged chorionic epithelial cells and altered concentrations of oestradiol and prostaglandin.

Live lambs born to infected ewes, and lambs fostered on to aborted ewes, may acquire infection during the neonatal period and develop placental infection and/or abort if bred during their first year.

The role of venereal transmission of *C. abortus* is generally assumed to be uncommon but may occur in certain situations.

Clinical presentation

Infection typically results in the abortion/birth of fresh dead and/or weakly lambs during the last three weeks of gestation. The ewe is not sick and may only be identified by a red/brown vulval discharge staining the wool of the tail/perineum (**149**), and a drawn-up abdomen (**150**) compared with a ewe at a similar stage in gestation (**151**). Aborted lambs have a sparse short coat and a distended abdomen due to accumulation of fluid within the abdominal cavity. Live lambs rarely survive more than a few hours despite supportive care. Retention of fetal membranes may lead to metritis and a sick ewe.

Differential diagnoses

Other causes of abortion including:

- *Salmonella* species serotypes.
- *Campylobacter fetus intestinalis.*
- *Listeria monocytogenes.*
- *Pasteurella* species.
- Toxoplasmosis.

Diagnosis

A provisional diagnosis is based on abortion of fresh lambs during the last three weeks of gestation and an associated necrotic placentitis; the ewe is not sick. Chlamydial abortion is confirmed following demonstration of large numbers of elementary bodies in placental smears stained by the modified

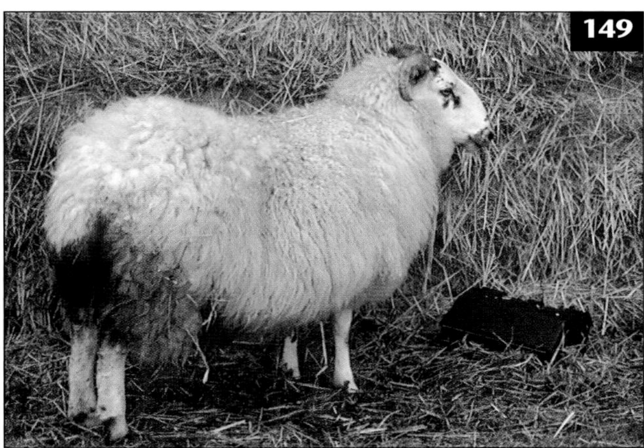

149 Aborted ewe with a bloody vulval discharge and sunken right flank.

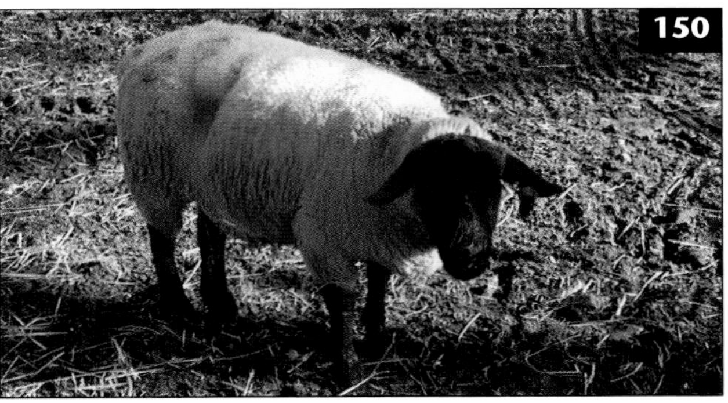

150 Aborted ewe. The right flank is sunken. Compare with **151**.

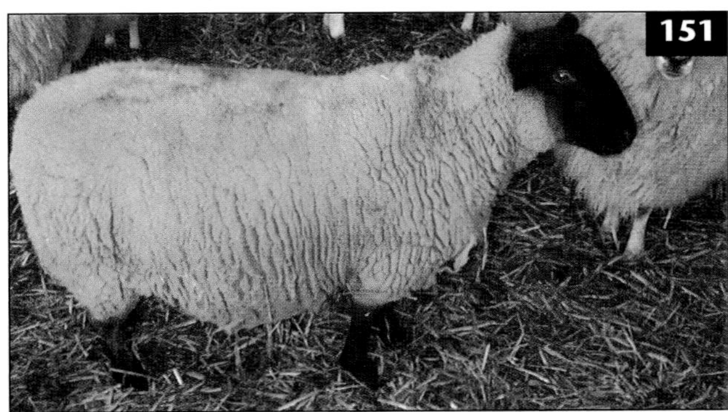

151 Ewe at same stage of pregnancy as the ewe in **150**. Compare the distended right flank with the ewe in **150**.

Ziehl-Neelsen (ZN) method. Serology involves a complement fixation test (CFT) but this might not distinguish between recent field infection and vaccination and is therefore undertaken in conjunction with placental examination. It is important to continue to submit abortion material throughout an outbreak in case more than one abortifacient agent is involved, as this may impact upon future control strategies.

Treatment

With abortions typically occurring in the last 3–4 weeks of gestation, prompt action is necessary if any benefit is to be gained from antibiotic therapy. Metaphylactic long-acting oxytetracycline injection (20 mg/kg) may reduce the number of abortions from *C. abortus* infection but cannot reverse placental damage. As a result, lambs are carried closer to term but they are weakly at birth with consequent high mortality. From a practical standpoint, while such antibiotic metaphylaxis may not save the litter of infected sheep, it allows healthy lambs to be fostered on to ewes that abort much closer to term and consequently have reasonable udder development and sufficient milk to nurse a single lamb.

Prevention/control measures

In common with all infectious causes of abortion, aborted ewes must be isolated and aborted material and infected bedding removed and destroyed. Ewes that give birth to dead/weakly full-term lambs should also be isolated. Lambs fostered on to aborted ewes should not be retained for future breeding.

Freedom from *C. abortus* infection is best achieved by maintaining a closed clean flock with strict biosecurity, although there have been situations where infected material has been transmitted between neighbouring farms by birds and foxes.

Various accreditation schemes operate in some countries. These offer breeding female replacements from flocks declared free of *C. abortus* infection. Accredited status is achieved by a serological survey of a statistically representative sample of the whole flock, and all aborted and barren ewes. Careful consideration must be given to establishing a clean but susceptible flock when the health status of neighbouring flocks cannot be guaranteed.

Purchase of *C. abortus*-infected carrier sheep presents the greatest risk to a clean flock, with infection transmitted following abortion. Infection of susceptible sheep, typically occurring following direct contact with aborted material or uterine discharges, can lead to an abortion storm the following year, with up to 30% of ewes aborting. Once infection becomes endemic in a flock, losses are largely confined to one-crop ewes that acquired infection at their first lambing, and this may give an annual abortion rate of 5–10% thereafter.

Ewes that have aborted or given birth to weakly lambs as a consequence of *C. abortus* are solidly immune and will maintain a normal pregnancy subsequently. In view of the possible venereal transmission from carrier ewes to clean ewes, it would be prudent to maintain the former as a distinct group at mating time.

Vaccination offers an excellent means of control for farms buying breeding replacements from non-accredited sources and in those flocks with an endemic *C. abortus* problem. In the UK, for example, there is a choice of either inactivated or live *C. abortus* vaccines, with administration before the start of the mating period. Vaccination of sheep already infected with *C. abortus* will not prevent all abortions but may reduce the incidence. It is recommended that vaccination should be repeated after three years.

Economics

Vaccination against *C. abortus* is expensive. In many commercial situations revaccination is not performed (with no appreciable loss of immunity), so the cost can be divided over three years (i.e. the productive lifespan of the average non-pedigree ewe). Even then the cost is approximately 3–5 times the cost of annual clostridial vaccination; however, this must be viewed against the cost of purchasing replacements. Female breeding replacements generally command a premium, though this can be very variable. The 'gold standard' is to purchase accredited stock and vaccinate them against *C. abortus*.

Welfare implications

Welfare concerns arise from the loss of weakly lambs and the confinement of ewes during fostering procedures.

TOXOPLASMOSIS

Definition/overview

Toxoplasma gondii infection during pregnancy can result in embryo/early fetal loss, fetal death and abortion/mummification, and birth of weakly lambs. *T. gondii* has a worldwide distribution and is the second most common cause of ovine abortion in the UK. Together with *Campylobacter* species infection, *T. gondii* infection is the most common cause of abortion in New Zealand. Toxoplasmosis is a zoonosis with a seroprevalence 30% in some human populations, although clinical illness is rare. People with an immunosuppressive illness are at most risk of illness. Infection of susceptible women during pregnancy can result in infection of the fetus.

Aetiology

Toxoplasmosis results from infection of susceptible sheep with the protozoon parasite *T. gondii*. The sexual cycle takes place in cats, while the asexual cycle can occur in a range of species, including sheep.

Clinical presentation

Infection during early pregnancy may manifest as embryo/early fetal loss, with an increased number of returns to service after irregular extended periods. As the ram is often removed after a breeding period as short as 5–6 weeks, these returns to service are not noted unless a vasectomized ram is present with the ewes. Embryo/early fetal loss is then manifest as an increased barren rate, often >8–10%; a 4% rate is acceptable and 2% is the target after a six-week breeding period. Often the highest number of barren sheep is within the youngest age group.

T. gondii infection during mid-pregnancy results in abortion or production of weakly live lambs near term, often with a small mummified fetus. The mummified fetus has a dark brown leathery appearance and a crown-rump length of approximately 8–10 cm (**152**).

Differential diagnoses

- The irregular and extended interval of return to oestrus suggests that ram infertility is unlikely to be the cause of a high barren rate. Other common abortifacient agents cause abortion during the last trimester and do not cause infertility in this manner.
- The birth of a normal lamb and a small mummified fetus is highly suggestive of toxoplasmosis but other causes of abortion should also be considered (e.g. *C. abortus*, *Salmonella* species serotypes, *Campylobacter fetus intestinalis*, *Listeria monocytogenes*, *Pasteurella* species, border disease).

Diagnosis

Serological testing merely indicates past infection; therefore, a single positive titre is not diagnostic for embryo/fetal death caused by toxoplasmosis.

It may prove difficult to establish a definitive role for toxoplasmosis in an increased barren rate in a group of sheep. Blood should be collected from 6–10 barren ewes and their serological titres compared with those from an equal number of pregnant sheep; the former group should show higher titres and a higher seroprevalence when the cause is toxoplasmosis. However, the pregnant ewes may have encountered infection just prior to mating or during late pregnancy and therefore have high titres themselves.

Toxoplasma-induced abortion is confirmed following histopathological examination of placentas and a high serology titre. The cotyledons appear dark red, with numerous white foci that become more visible under pressure from a microscope slide; the remainder of the placenta is unaffected. Antibody may also be present in the fetal fluids.

Antibody can also be detected in pre-colostral blood samples from newborn lambs but such samples are difficult to acquire during a single farm visit.

Treatment

While effective treatment has been reported with a combination of pyrimethamine and sulphadimidine, this is unlikely to have practical application because the timing of infection has passed before evidence of barren or aborting ewes appears. Rather than treatment, efforts are directed at prevention through vaccination.

Prevention/control measures

Feed should be stored in vermin-proof facilities to prevent contamination by cats and other vermin. Oocyst excretion is much greater in young cats and those with debilitating viral infections such as feline leukaemia virus and feline infectious peritonitis. Maintaining a healthy adult cat population by an appropriate vaccination and neutering policy, and controlling the feral cat population, should limit

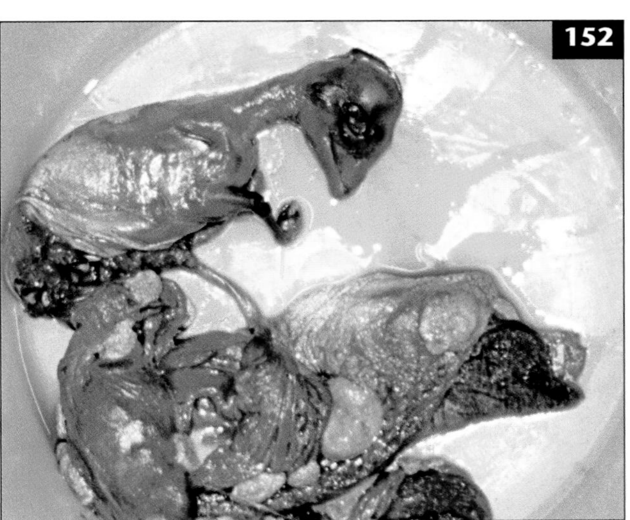

152 Mummified fetus with the dark brown leathery appearance caused by toxoplasmosis.

active excretion and contamination on the farm; however, prevention of toxoplasmosis is more readily and effectively achieved by vaccination of breeding replacement sheep. In common with all infectious causes of abortion, all aborted material must be collected and disposed of in an appropriate manner.

Vaccination using a live attenuated vaccine is available in many countries (e.g. New Zealand) and provides excellent immunity to natural infection; it is administered at least three weeks before the breeding season. Care should be taken when administering the vaccine; detailed safety instructions are provided by the manufacturer.

In-feed medication from mid-gestation with the commonly used coccidiostat decoquinate (2 mg/kg body weight daily) has been shown significantly to reduce perinatal lamb losses from toxoplasmosis, but this is rarely practicable under farm situations and proves more expensive than vaccination when fed throughout every pregnancy, as challenge and immunity cannot be guaranteed during the first pregnancy. Monensin sodium (fed at 15 mg/kg per head daily) has also been shown to be effective but this is no longer licensed for sheep in many countries.

Economics
The vaccine is expensive but, as a single vaccination effectively provides lifelong immunity, the cost can be divided over the sheep's productive life.

Welfare implications
Abortion and the birth of weakly lambs can be prevented by timely vaccination, which is cost-effective under all production systems.

SALMONELLA ABORTUS OVIS ABORTION

Definition/overview
Salmonella abortus ovis is a sheep-adapted serotype and is a major cause of abortion and neonatal lamb deaths in many countries worldwide. *S. abortus ovis* is not a zoonosis.

Aetiology
S. abortus ovis is introduced into a clean flock by apparently healthy carrier sheep, with bacterial shedding greater after stressful events. Subsequent bacteraemia leads to invasion of the pregnant uterus in susceptible ewes and fetal death with abortion or birth of full-term lambs depending on gestational age. Abortion rates may exceed 50%, with ewe deaths in susceptible flocks encountering infection for the first time. Thereafter, females pregnant for the first time and purchased susceptible sheep are most at risk.

Clinical presentation
The major clinical presentation is abortion during the last trimester, which may not be detected. However, metritis following abortion is common and this may lead to septicaemia and death.

Infection close to term leads to stillbirths and increased lamb losses during the neonatal period, some of which show respiratory disease.

Differential diagnoses
Differential diagnoses include other causes of abortion, especially other *Salmonella* species serotypes.

Diagnosis
Fetal stomach contents provide the best material for bacterial culture but vaginal swabs can be taken for up to one week after abortion.

Treatment
By the time the cause of abortion has been identified, infection is widespread throughout the group and metaphylactic antibiotic injection is unlikely to be economically justifiable. Metaphylactic long-acting oxytetracycline injection (20 mg/kg) may reduce the number of deaths from metritis following abortion during an outbreak of *S. abortus ovis*. Most *Salmonella* species serotypes causing abortion in sheep remain sensitive to a wide range of commonly used antibiotics; most diagnostic laboratories routinely provide antibiotic sensitivity of bacterial isolates.

Prevention/control measures
Prevention is best achieved by maintenance of a high health status closed flock; where this is not possible, purchased sheep must be kept segregated until after lambing.

While mixing non-pregnant breeding replacement stock with aborted ewes may confer lifelong protection against *S. abortus ovis*, this practice will also disseminate all other abortion agents present within the flock and is not without risk. Vaccines are available in certain countries against *S. abortus ovis*. The choice of which vaccine to use will depend on the published literature relating to those available vaccines and knowledge of individual flock situations.

Economics
In endemic areas, vaccination is likely to prove necessary where a closed flock status cannot be assured. Introduction of *S. abortus ovis* into a susceptible flock could prove financially disastrous.

Welfare implications

Prompt identification and antibiotic treatment of sick ewes and lambs should limit any welfare implications of this disease.

OTHER *SALMONELLA* SPECIES SEROTYPES

Definition/overview

Numerous *Salmonella* species serotypes have been associated with abortion and death of pregnant ewes worldwide. Whilst the number of flocks affected is small, losses within a flock can be substantial.

Aetiology

In addition to *S. abortus ovis* described previously, a number of *Salmonella* species serotypes, including *S. montevideo*, *S. dublin* and *S. typhimurium,* have been associated with abortion and death in pregnant ewes. Other serotypes cause disease in different parts of the world. Of considerable concern in New Zealand at present is the recent appearance of *S. brandenburg* as a cause of abortion and ewe deaths. *S. brandeburg* is a zoonosis and human cases have been recorded.

Frequently, the interval between infection and abortion means that the source is not identified with certainty. Wild birds have been incriminated in the transmission of certain serotypes, particularly *S. montevideo*. Cattle are frequently carriers of *S. dublin* but show no clinical signs. Cattle, especially calves, and human sewage are common sources of *S. typhimurium*.

Clinical presentation

Abortion is the main presenting feature with *S. montevideo*. Affected sheep are dull and depressed and may be found standing isolated from the flock, often next to their aborted fetus(es). The abdomen is drawn up in ewes that have aborted, which contrasts with the normal distended appearance of late gestation. Abdominal ballotment fails to detect evidence of any fetuses. There is a fetid red/brown fluid vaginal discharge. The udder is poorly developed and there is no accumulated colostrum in the glands.

Sheep affected with *S. typhimurium* may simply be found dead, with autolytic lambs that have not been aborted *in utero*. Profuse dysentery is often observed in other sheep with *S. typhimurium*. These ewes are very depressed (**153**) and are often heard tooth-grinding.

The rectal temperature is elevated to 41.0°C. The mucous membranes are congested. Affected ewes rapidly develop severe metritis following abortion and deaths are not uncommon. The clinical picture of *S. dublin* infection is similar to that of *S. typhimurium* infection.

Differential diagnoses

Other causes of abortion including:

- *Chlamydophila abortus*.
- *Campylobacter fetus intestinalis*.
- *Listeria monocytogenes*.
- *Pasteurella* species.

Diagnosis

Fetal stomach contents provide the best material for diagnostic purposes. Where aborted fetuses are not available or have been scavenged, vaginal and rectal swabs from the ewe should be submitted to the laboratory. Blood samples can be collected for chlamydial and *T. gondii* serology but they are not useful for *Salmonella* species. A provisional diagnosis of salmonellosis can often be given after 24 hours' culture.

Treatment

Sick ewes should be treated with intravenous oxytetracycline, NSAIDs and oral fluids administered by orogastric tube, but the prognosis for ewes with autolytic, often emphysematous lambs, is hopeless unless these lambs can be delivered. Death of the ewe may occur 5–7 days after delivery of rotten lambs because the devitalized uterine wall ruptures, followed by development of a peracute septic peritonitis with rapid toxin uptake via the peritoneum.

All aborted sheep must be isolated and not mixed with other sheep for at least six weeks.

Prevention/control measures

There are many potential sources of salmonellae in a group of sheep, including contaminated feedstuffs and watercourses, sewage effluent overflow, other farm stock

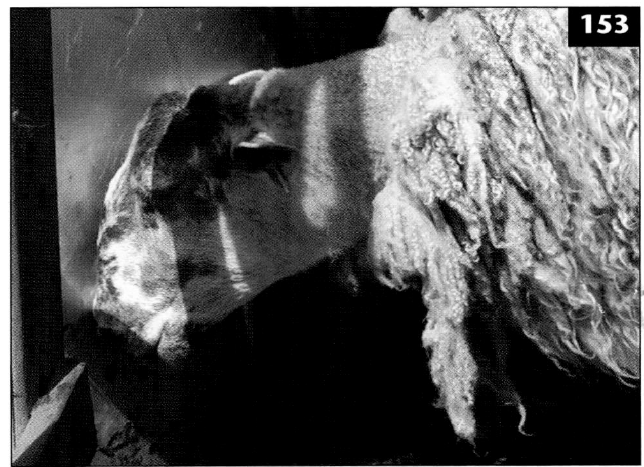

153 Sick ewe after abortion due to *Salmonella typhimurium*.

and carrion. All feed must be stored in vermin-proof bins but this is not implemented on many farms. Wherever possible, water should be supplied from a mains supply and ponds and surface water fenced off. If possible, pregnant sheep should be managed separately from cattle.

The farmer must be advised regarding the zoonotic risk from suspected/confirmed salmonellosis and told to adopt strict personal hygiene when handling sick sheep. If infection occurs in one group of sheep, then that field must be visited last at feeding times. Feeding troughs must be turned over and moved at least ten metres across the field immediately after each feed to limit the risk of transmission by birds to others groups of sheep. Many farmers now feed cubes on a clean area of pasture each day to reduce the risk of birds contaminating the area around feed troughs.

Metaphylactic long-acting oxytetracycline injections (20 mg/kg) may reduce the number of abortions during an outbreak of salmonellosis in sheep, although there are few split-flock data to demonstrate any economic advantages of this strategy.

Economics
The economic consequences of *Salmonella* species abortion can be devastating, with ewe losses as high as 10–20%. Unfortunately, infection is widespread throughout the group by the time abortions/deaths are identified and confirmed. In most situations ewe mortality must be reduced by around 3% for metaphylactic long-acting oxytetracycline injections to be cost effective.

Welfare implications
Prompt identification and antibiotic treatment of sick ewes should limit any welfare implications. Ewes should be euthanased for welfare reasons when autolytic lambs cannot be delivered *per vaginam*.

CAMPYLOBACTERIOSIS

Definition/overview
Campylobacteriosis is a common cause of abortion where sheep are managed intensively, leading to heavy contamination and unhygienic environments during late gestation. *Campylobacter* species infection is one of the most common causative agents of abortion in New Zealand.

Aetiology
Campylobacter fetus subspecies *fetus* (*intestinalis*) and *C. jejuni* are the species involved. Infection is by the faeco-oral route, largely following introduction of carrier sheep into the flock, although wild birds have been shown to carry infection.

Clinical presentation
The common presentation is abortion during late gestation, although some lambs are carried to full term, are born weakly and succumb during the neonatal period.

Differential diagnoses
Other infectious causes of abortion including:
- *Salmonella* species serotypes.
- *Chlamydophila abortus*.
- *Listeria monocytogenes*.
- *Pasteurella* species.

Diagnosis
Diagnosis is confirmed following culture of fetal stomach contents.

Treatment
All aborted ewes must be isolated immediately and the main flock moved to other accommodation/pasture whenever possible. Treatment options are limited because infection has already spread rapidly through the group by the time the first abortions are recognized. There appears to be no economic advantage if metaphylactic antibiotic injection is given.

Prevention/control measures
Sheep should be managed in clean environments and not subjected to unhygienic conditions, especially during late gestation. Particular attention should be paid to the feeding troughs/areas. Purchased sheep must be managed as a separate group until after lambing.

Following infection, ewes are immune to further challenge and should not abort. While mixing non-pregnant breeding replacement stock with aborted ewes could confer lifelong protection against campylobacteriosis, this practice could also disseminate other abortion agents present within the flock (e.g. *Chlamydophila abortus*), with potentially disastrous consequences. A vaccine against campylobacteriosis is available in many countries (e.g. New Zealand) and used routinely in some flocks.

Economics
Losses from campylobacteriosis can be high in many countries; however, vaccination confers affordable protection.

Welfare implications
Apart from abortion, there are no major welfare implications arising from campylobacteriosis.

Border disease (*Syn*: hairy shaker disease)

Definition/overview

Border disease has a worldwide distribution. It is one of the less commonly diagnosed causes of abortion but this may not reflect its true impact upon flock reproductive performance. Losses from congenital infection are difficult to quantify because a high barren rate may be mistakenly attributed to other causes, and hairy shaker lambs may not present in a group of neonatal lambs infected with border disease, which has a high mortality rate.

Aetiology

Border disease is caused by a pestivirus serologically related to bovine virus diarrhoea (BVD), with cross-infection between cattle and sheep.

Clinical presentation

Exposure of healthy lambs and adult sheep to border disease virus causes nil or only mild signs of disease. Clinical signs are only seen following infection of susceptible pregnant ewes.

Infection during early pregnancy can cause fetal death and resorption, with no outward signs other than an extended interval to return to service and/or an increased barren rate at scanning or lambing time.

Infection from mid-gestation onwards results in abortion. Infection later in gestation results in the birth at full term of small weakly lambs that succumb during the neonatal period to adverse physical factors and/or infectious disease. It is possible that such mortality is overlooked amongst other perinatal lambs losses, which frequently exceed 20% in many flocks. Congenitally infected lambs show symptoms ranging from few clinical signs up to classical cerebellar disease, skeletal abnormalities and coat changes.

Many lambs with cerebellar hypoplasia are unable to stand or maintain sternal recumbency. They may present with seizure activity progressing to opisthotonus. Less severely affected lambs show fine muscle tremors over the head and ears, which are exacerbated when the lamb is excited or stimulated, typically when the lamb is assisted to feed, resulting in forceful jerking movements of the head. Coat changes are often difficult to appreciate in many breeds and it is important to examine some normal lambs for comparison before diagnosing a 'classical' hairy shaker lamb on coat change alone. It is reported that affected lambs have a hairy rough fleece due to proliferation of longer guard hairs, most noticeably over the neck and back. Skeletal abnormalities include shortened long bones, which are of narrower diameter than normal. There may be evidence of hypertensive hydrocephalus, with doming of the head, and brachygnathia.

While most lambs infected *in utero* die during the first few days of life from a combination of physical factors and infectious disease, some lambs survive but have a poor growth rate and remain susceptible to other diseases, while others survive as apparently normal but persistently infected sheep. It is this latter group that provides a source of virus for susceptible pregnant sheep.

Differential diagnoses

- The irregular and extended intervals of return to oestrus suggests that ram infertility is unlikely to be the cause of a high barren rate.
- Toxoplasmosis would be an important differential diagnosis.
- Swayback (see Chapter 7: Swayback, p. 170) must be distinguished from newborn lambs with border disease presenting with opisthotonus.
- Bacterial meningoencephalitis rarely affects lambs less than ten days old.
- Septicaemia is usually accompanied by depression progressing to stupor and death within 24 hours.
- Polioencephalomalacia does not occur in lambs less than four months old.
- There are many causes of weakly lambs with low birth weights and the reader is directed to the section on perinatal mortality (see Chapter 4: Perinatal lamb mortality p. 83).

Diagnosis

A provisional diagnosis of border disease can be reliably based on the clinical examination of a significant number of hairy shaker lambs; other congenital neurological disorders are more usually sporadic in nature and tend not to occur as an outbreak. The diagnosis is confirmed following demonstration of border disease virus in either blood samples from affected lambs before they suck colostrum or in tissues from fresh dead lambs submitted to the laboratory.

Treatment

There is no treatment for border disease other than supportive therapy. Hairy shaker lambs have a very poor prognosis and should be euthanased for welfare reasons.

Prevention/control measures

There are no practical preventive strategies for border disease in non-pedigree flocks that do not have the disease, because screening is cost prohibitive. Blood sampling to identify all antibody-negative, virus-positive purchased sheep is not economically realistic in non-pedigree flocks. The cost could represent approximately 10% of the purchase price of the sheep.

Infection can be introduced into a susceptible flock by apparently healthy rams or breeding replacements. Screening could be undertaken if only rams are introduced into an otherwise closed flock.

Virus is readily transmitted from persistently infected BVD cattle and therefore it is essential to keep sheep separate from cattle during the breeding season and the first half of pregnancy. BVD virus is widespread in the cattle population, with 1% of young stock/growing cattle estimated to be persistently infected in the UK.

Once border disease is identified within a group of lambs, none of the lambs in that cohort should be kept within the breeding flock unless screened and found to be seropositive. This is likely to prove cost prohibitive in most non-pedigree flocks.

At present there is no border disease vaccine available in the UK but a killed adjuvant vaccine is available in some countries. Natural vaccination can be attempted in endemically infected flocks, whereby females to be retained for future breeding are deliberately mixed with persistently infected border disease sheep at least three months before the start of the breeding season. Close confinement (i.e. essentially housing these sheep) for at least three weeks is necessary to ensure exposure to virus. This policy is by no means guaranteed and carries the risk of spread of other infectious agents, including abortifacient agents, if aborted ewes are mixed with susceptible replacements without first establishing the cause of abortion.

Economics

The true economic impact of border disease after introduction into a susceptible flock is likely to be considerable in terms of increased barren rate, hairy shaker lambs and increased neonatal losses, but there are few data available. In endemically infected flocks, border disease losses could be easily overlooked in the general poor performance and high losses of the many non-pedigree flocks that have little veterinary supervision.

Welfare implications

Increased perinatal mortality due to physical factors and infectious disease has obvious welfare implications.

BRUCELLA MELITENSIS

Definition/overview

Brucella melitensis is a sporadic cause of ovine abortion in some Mediterranean and Middle Eastern countries. It is absent from Australia, New Zealand, the USA and much of Europe.

Aetiology

B. melitensis, and much less commonly *B. abortus*, can cause abortion in sheep. Infection of susceptible pregnant sheep may result in abortion, with excretion of the organism for many months. The mammary gland is frequently colonized, with resultant poor milk production. Sheep milk is a potential source of human infection.

Clinical presentation

Abortion close to term occurs in a percentage of susceptible ewes infected during pregnancy. Rams may occasionally develop orchitis.

Differential diagnoses

Other causes of abortion including:

- *Chlamydophila abortus*.
- *Salmonella* species serotypes.
- *Campylobacter fetus intestinalis*.
- *Listeria monocytogenes*.
- *Pasteurella* species.
- Border disease.

Diagnosis

Diagnosis is based on bacteriology of aborted fetuses and placentas, and serological testing of aborted ewes.

Treatment

The intracellular nature of this organism renders it largely refractory to antibiotic therapy.

Prevention/control measures

Infection is transmitted to susceptible flocks by infected carrier animals and by the products of abortion transferred between neighbouring flocks by scavenging wildlife. General approaches to biosecurity and maintenance of a closed flock strategy should prevent infection gaining entry. Strict hygiene, appropriate isolation of all aborted ewes and disposal of all aborted material will limit the spread of infection during the lambing period. *Brucella* organisms can be present in vaginal discharges for up to two months post abortion.

In many countries control is attempted by identification and culling of infected sheep, often in combination with a vaccination policy during the early stages of such schemes. Vaccination never affords complete protection and persistently infected vaccinated sheep can continue to disseminate infection.

Welfare implications

Apart from abortion, there are no major welfare implications arising from brucellosis.

OTHER CONDITIONS OF PREGNANT EWES

PERIVULVAL OEDEMA

Definition/overview

Perivulval oedema is seen sporadically in multiparous ewes.

Aetiology

Incomplete farm records prevent scrutiny of past breeding history to see if there is a possible link with previous vaginal prolapse and the use of a Buhner suture. The localized nature of the oedema and absence of systemic signs suggest impairment of lymphatic drainage from the perineum. Localized oedema of the vulva can occur after insertion of a Buhner suture to retain a vaginal prolapse but the extent of the oedema is not as pronounced (**154**).

Clinical presentation

Affected ewes are bright and alert and have a normal appetite. Shepherds rarely report the associated tenesmus as observed with vaginal prolapse. The udder is very pendulous and there is considerable oedema of the subcutaneous tissue overlying the mammary tissue and teats. The perineum is extremely oedematous, extending up to 6–8 cm deep and giving the overlying skin a translucent appearance. The shepherd's descriptive term of 'baboon bum' is surprisingly apposite.

Differential diagnoses

Cellulitis following puncture wound and blackleg can readily be distinguished from perivulval oedema on clinical examination.

Diagnosis

Diagnosis is based on clinical examination and the presence of extensive pitting oedema.

Treatment

There is a risk that birth of lambs through the swollen and oedematous posterior reproductive tract could cause tearing of the vaginal mucosa. The perineal oedema will be considerably reduced 24 hours later if the ewe is injected intramuscularly with 3 mg of dexamethasone (**154**).

Prevention/control measures

Perivulval oedema occurs sporadically with no obvious cause; therefore, there are no practical control measures. Dexamethasone produces a good response and does not cause abortion at normal dose rates.

Economics

Perivulval oedema does not represent a major economic concern.

Welfare implications

Timely recognition and corticosteroid therapy will produce a good response, thereby addressing any welfare concerns.

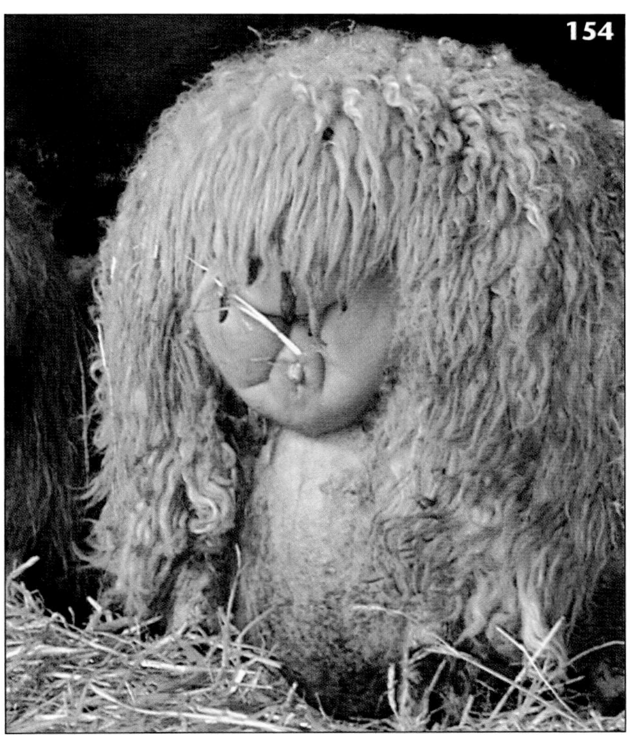

154 Extensive perivulval and udder oedema ('baboon bum').

CLINICAL PROBLEM 1

A Suffolk ewe is presented that has had an assisted lambing only minutes earlier. Tenesmus after delivery of the lamb has caused uterine prolapse (**155**).

How should this case be dealt with?

Treatment/management

A combined sacrococcygeal extradural injection of 2% lidocaine (0.5–0.6 mg/kg) and xylazine (0.07 mg/kg) (2 ml and 0.25 ml, respectively, for an 80 kg ewe) greatly facilitates replacement. The area over the tailhead is clipped and swabbed with diluted povidone iodine solution. The first intercoccygeal space is identified by digital palpation during slight vertical movement of the tail, and a 25 mm 20 gauge needle is directed at 20° to the tail, which is held horizontally. The correct position of the needle is determined by the lack of resistance to injection.

After waiting 5–10 minutes after the injection, the prolapse is replaced with the ewe in lateral recumbency, starting at the cervical end and gently working towards the uterine tips. Suspending the ewe by its hindlimbs is not necessary.

A perivulval Buhner suture of 5 mm umbilical tape is inserted to prevent re-prolapse. It is important not to penetrate the vaginal mucosa when inserting the suture. The Buhner suture should not be necessary if the uterus is correctly replaced. However, if the posterior reproductive tract is oedematous, this could provoke tenesmus despite the extradural injection.

The ewe should be injected with procaine penicillin to counter any bacterial infection of the uterus during prolapse. Non-steroidal anti-inflammatory drugs, such as ketoprofen or flunixin meglumine, can also be given for their analgesic properties but they are not licensed for use in sheep. Extradural xylazine injection provides analgesia for up to 36 hours after sacrococcygeal injection.

The total veterinary professional fee (mostly the cost of the visit) will be about 25–30% of the value of the ewe. Caudal extradural lidocaine injection is an inexpensive and safe procedure with obvious animal welfare benefits. Hindlimb ataxia caused by slight overdosage of lidocaine could cause practical husbandry problems arising from lambs being unable to find the udder and suck colostrum but this situation can be overcome by careful supervision.

CLINICAL PROBLEM 2

A 'difficult lambing' occurs in a pedigree Suffolk ewe. The lamb is presented with unilateral shoulder flexion. The ewe was noted in first stage labour four hours earlier. The farmer has attempted to deliver the lamb for ten minutes but has been unable to extend the second forelimb into the pelvis (**156**) due to the ewe's forceful contractions.

How should this case be approached?

Action

Gentle repulsion of the lamb is greatly facilitated after sacrococcygeal extradural lidocaine injection, which blocks the reflex abdominal straining of the ewe.

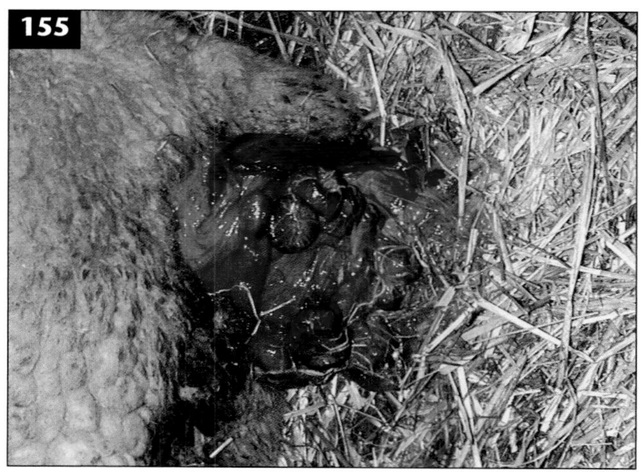

155 Uterine prolapse.

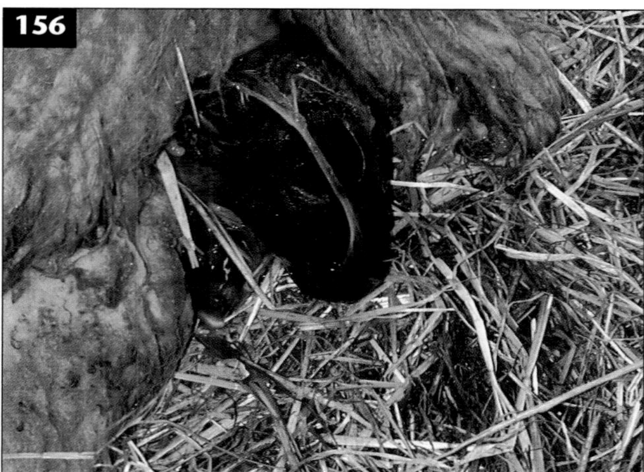

156 A pedigree Suffolk ewe with a lamb presented with unilateral shoulder flexion.

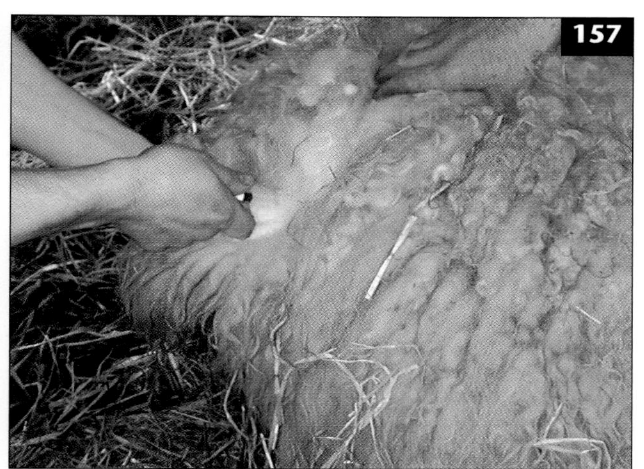

157 Sacrococcygeal extradural injection of 2% lignocaine.

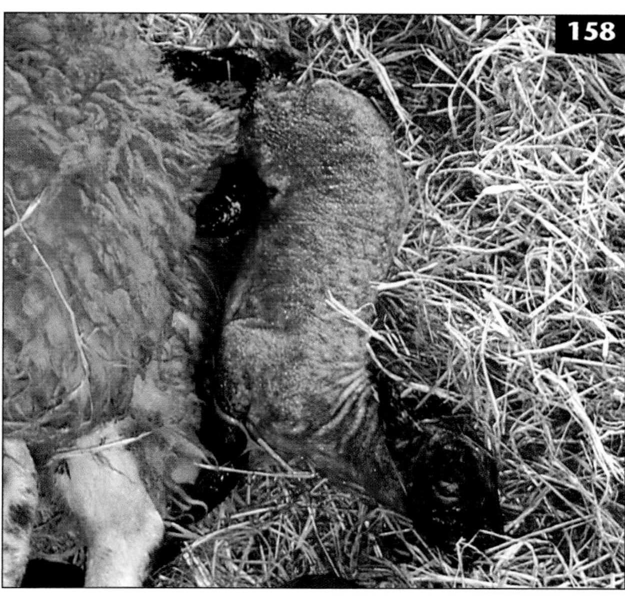

158 Meconium staining of the lamb associated with extended second stage labour.

This technique greatly improves ewe welfare as well as rendering the various manipulations much easier to perform. Two ml of 2% lidocaine is injected at the sacrococcygeal site (**157**).

The more traditional means of repelling a lamb during correction of a dystocia is to enlist the help of an assistant who suspends the ewe by the hindlimbs while the lamb is forced back against the ewe's strong abdominal contractions. This procedure causes considerable distress to the ewe because the pregnant uterus, rumen and other abdominal viscera are forced against the diaphragm. The risk of trauma to the uterus and vagina is greatly increased if the lamb is forced back into the body of the uterus against such powerful opposition.

Correction of the malposture

Correction of this malposture involves gentle repulsion of the lamb's extended forelimb and the head. Repulsion of the head well into the pelvis, and possibly just into the body of the uterus, allows the joints of the other forelimb to be first fully flexed until the foot is firmly grasped, then extended as the foot is gently drawn into the maternal pelvis. A wire snare can be passed behind the lamb's poll to a level below the ears before gentle repulsion. The forelimbs are extended such that the fetlock joints are level with the entrance into the maternal pelvis. The lamb's head is drawn into the pelvic inlet using the wire snare. Each forelimb is extended in turn so that both fetlocks joints are level with the vulva. The lamb's muzzle should appear at the vulva. Each forelimb is now extended so that the carpal joints appear at the vulva. Gentle traction using the head snare (if necessary) and both forelimbs effects delivery of the lamb. There is meconium staining of the lamb (**158**) but no arterial blood contamination of the lamb's fleece, which would indicate trauma to the ewe's posterior reproductive tract.

Follow-up

The ewe showed mild hindlimb paresis for two hours after the extradural injection but this did not interfere with maternal bonding. The lamb received 50 ml/kg of colostrum stripped off the ewe and given by stomach tube immediately, and its umbilicus was immersed in strong veterinary iodine BP. The ewe was treated with procaine penicillin (44,000 iu/kg i/m for 3 consecutive days).

Part 2: Male Reproductive System

MANAGEMENT OF RAMS

While the breeding period may only extend to five or six weeks on many intensive sheep farming enterprises, effective management of rams necessitates year round attention. Routine vaccination and anthelmintic treatment (**159**) is equally important for the rams as for the ewes. Foot care is essential to maintain ram soundness (**160, 161**). Lameness can have a marked adverse affect on the ram's willingness to follow ewes (**162, 163**) and serve all the oestrous ones. Lame rams must be replaced immediately and the source of the lameness identified and corrected.

Rams must be in good body condition (**164**) prior to the mating period, ideally BCS of 3.5; this may necessitate a prior period of concentrate feeding. Supplementary feeding is critical during the mating period, when many rams may lose considerable body condition (up to two units on the five-point scale). Debility following such weight loss may render rams more prone to respiratory disease and other infections.

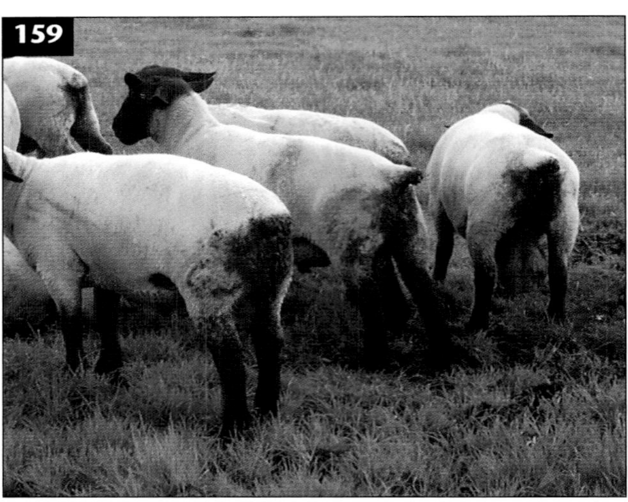

159 Poor internal parasite control in a group of stud rams.

IDENTIFICATION OF MATED EWES

Raddles/harnesses

Raddles are frequently applied to rams (**165**) to determine service dates and, following colour change, indicate returns to service. Knowledge of the service date and absence of return to service enables prediction of the lambing date, so that ewes can be fed

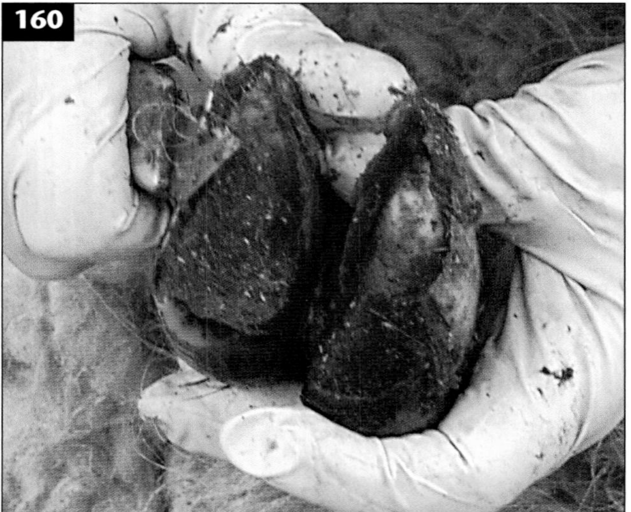

160 Year-round foot care is essential in rams.

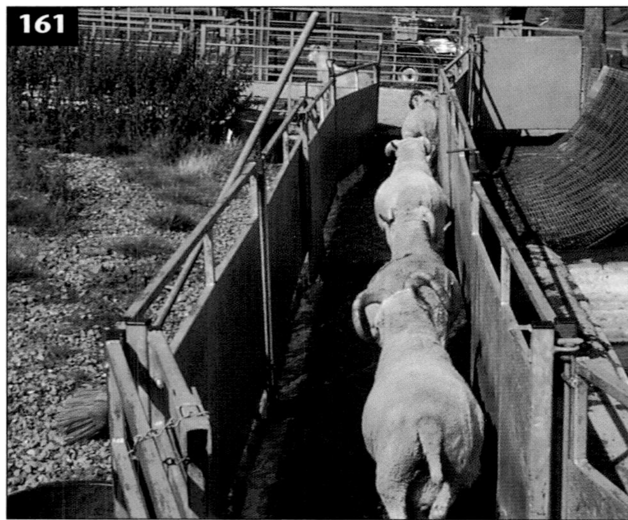

161 Regular foot bathing is an integral component of ram management.

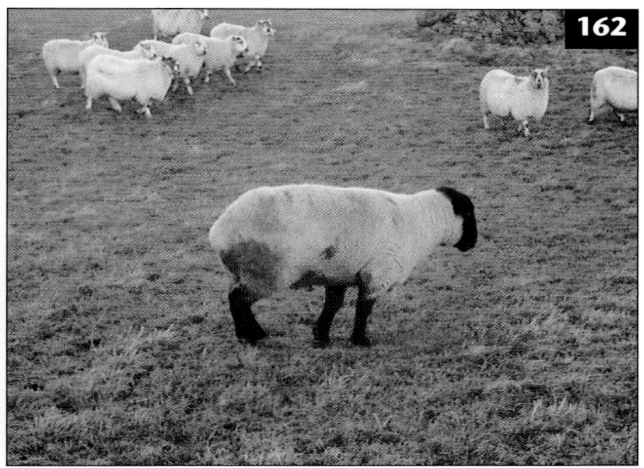

162 Severely lame (10/10) ram separated from ewes.

more precisely during late pregnancy. Many sheep farms do not have sufficient space to house the whole flock, so ewes are housed based on the lambing date indicated by the keel mark. In many countries, sheep are set-stocked in paddocks depending upon the expected lambing date.

Ill-fitted ram keel harnesses and blocks often cause large brisket sores (**166**), which heal very slowly, if at all, and raise serious welfare concerns. Correct fitting of the harness is essential to avoid these sores and extra padding, usually carpet underlay material or similar, should be placed under the harness. The harnesses should be checked daily. Harnesses that are fitted too tightly around the axillary region may damage the brachial plexus and manifest as radial nerve paralysis.

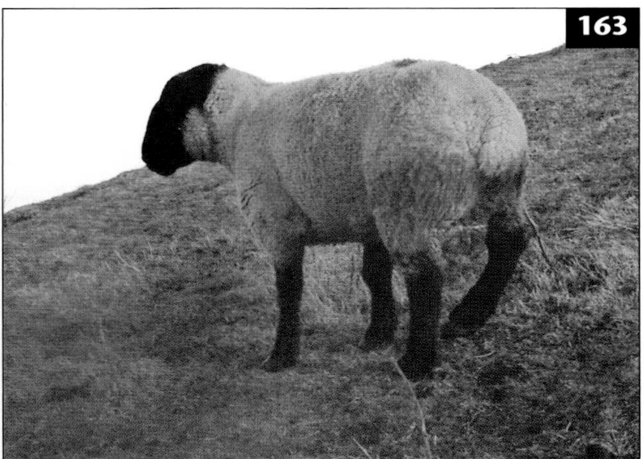

163 Same ram as in **162** ten days later. Note the ram is still 10/10 lame and isolated from ewes.

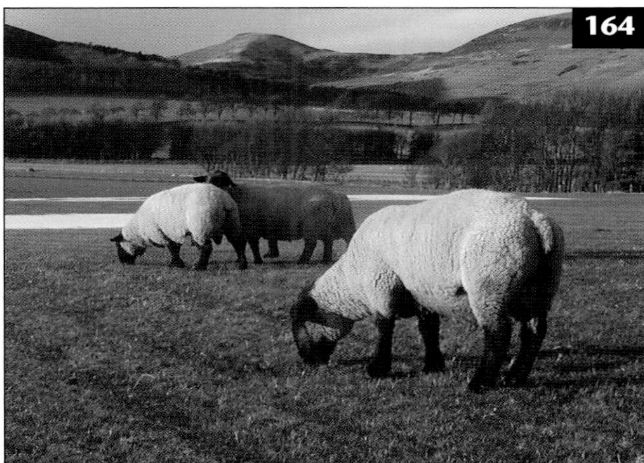

164 Suffolk rams in good body condition prior to the mating period.

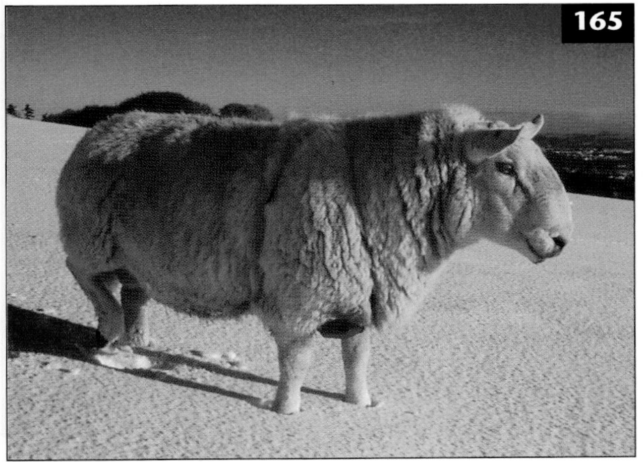

165 Raddle applied to a Cheviot ram.

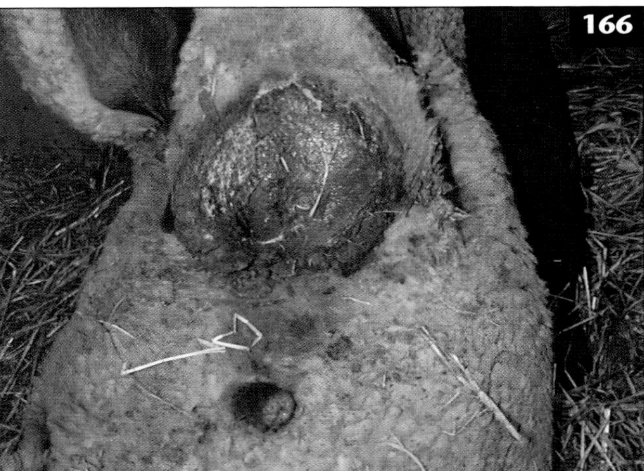

166 Large brisket sore from a poorly-fitted raddle.

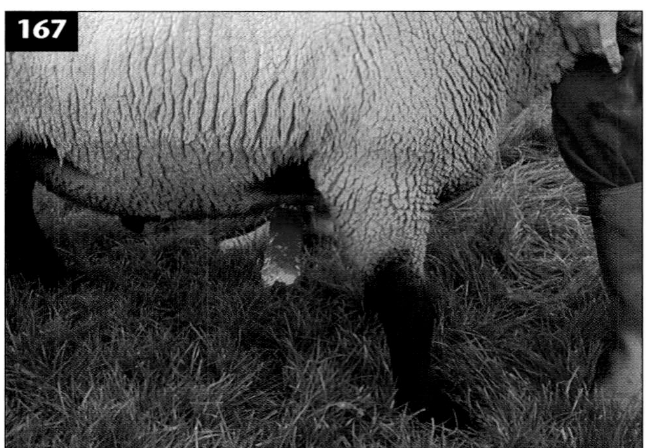

167 Keel paint applied to the fleece immediately in front of the prepuce.

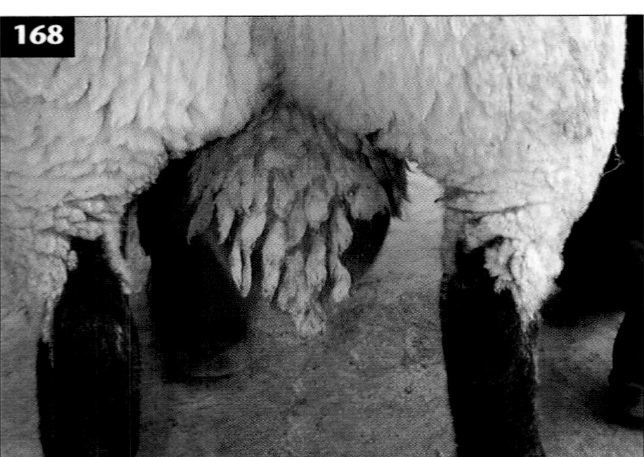

168 Wool on the scrotum is common in many breeds and does not appear adversely to affect fertility.

Keel paint

Some shepherds prefer to use keel paint instead of harnesses or raddles. The paint is applied to the fleece immediately in front of the prepuce (**167**) or on the brisket. Keel paint must be replenished daily and this can be achieved when the rams are fed concentrates. Keel paint has a number of advantages and should be used wherever possible in preference to raddles. Firstly, there is no risk of brisket sores developing from a poorly fitted harness. Secondly, in order to mark the ewe the ram must fully mount her; sometimes a harness can mark the ewe if the ram simply rests his chin on the ewe's hindquarters.

BREEDING SOUNDNESS EXAMINATION IN RAMS

Physical evaluation at the sale ring

Ram selection at auction sale is a lottery; therefore, farmers must undertake a basic physical examination of their possible purchases in order to reduce the likelihood of selecting an infertile ram. Farmers must be constantly reminded that sale price is not a guarantee of a ram's fertility.

Maximum scrotal circumference has a particularly high heritability coefficient and pedigree breeders must be alerted to this fact. Taking of scrotal measurements should be seriously considered before purchase of a stud ram. Progressive sheep breeders have made considerable progress in flock fertility management by selecting rams with maximal scrotal circumference rather than rams with 'presence', a bold head, heavy bones and large ears.

Using a tape measure, farmers should measure the maximum scrotal circumference of all potential ram purchases, looking for values above 36 cm for shearlings and 32 cm for ram lambs. This simple measurement allows a large number of potential ram purchases to be examined prior to commencement of the sale. Rams with measurements below these threshold values must be rejected. The presence of wool on the scrotum (**168**), unless excessive, does not influence testicular function.

Symmetry of the testicles and free movement in the scrotal sac can be readily determined. Consistency of the testicles and/or epididymes should be evaluated by an experienced veterinarian and not performed by farmers prior to the appearance of the ram in the sale ring. Ultrasonographic examination of palpable scrotal abnormalities by the veterinarian can provide much useful information (**169, 170**).

Semen evaluation

There has been a gradual change in the recommended practice for ram breeding soundness assessment over the past 15–20 years. During the 1980s it was standard practice to collect semen from all rams on the farm prior to commencement of the breeding season. However this practice has been replaced by collection of semen only from rams that have a palpable scrotal abnormality.

Despite numerous disadvantages with regard to assessment of rams' libido, occasional collection of an unrepresentative poor sample and animal welfare concerns, electroejaculation remains the most convenient method for checking individual suspect rams for breeding soundness on commercial farms. However, for many insurance claims, companies insist on examination of a semen sample(s) collected from an artificial vagina. Quantity and nature of samples

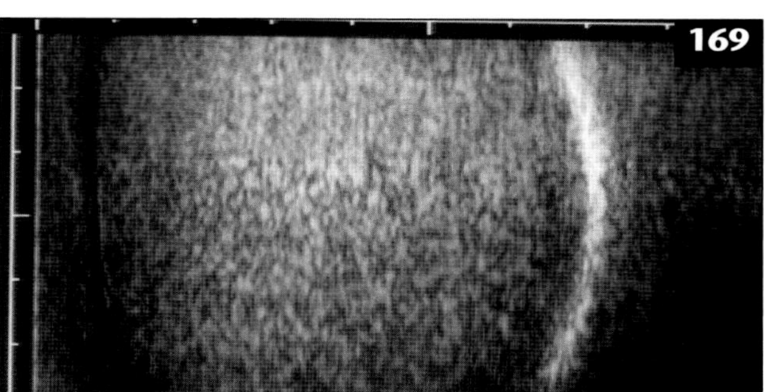
169 Ultrasonogram of a normal testicle. Note the normal 7 cm diameter and uniform echogenic pattern.

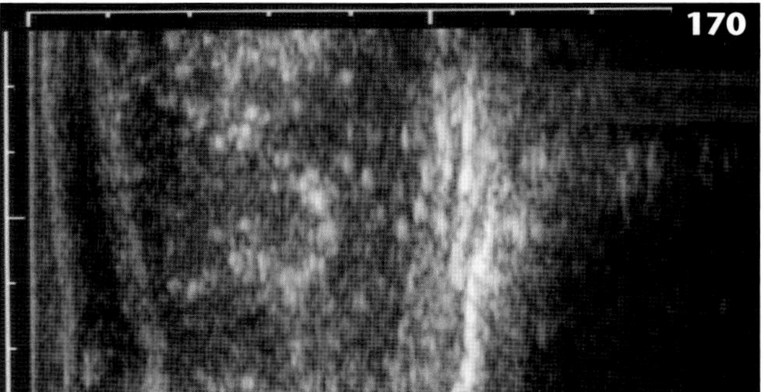
170 Ultrasonogram of an atrophied testicle. Note the 5 cm diameter and irregular echogenic pattern with multiple hyperechoic (white) dots in a more hypoechoic (dark) background.

collected by electroejaculation using certain probes such as the Ruakura probe, which has two circular electrodes at the tip, are often too variable to be useful parameters. Much more reliable results have been demonstrated using a probe with longitudinal electrodes[1] (Lane Manufacture, Denver, USA).

Routine semen examination should include evaluation of progressive sperm motility, the presence of white cells in the ejaculate and sperm morphology. Progressive motility is a more accurate assessment of forward sperm motion than the swirling action observed when an undiluted semen sample is examined under ×10 magnification. The presence of large numbers of white cells, which can be observed in the ejaculate after the sample has been prepared and examined for progressive motility, alerts the veterinarian to the presence of an inflammatory lesion involving the urinogenital system. Most veterinarians do not routinely perform such examinations; they prefer to observe movement of an undiluted semen sample only. Sperm morphology is an integral part of all semen examinations.

Examination for the presence of white cells in the ejaculate has the disadvantage that the ejaculate must be collected from the vermiform appendage without cellular contamination from the prepuce; therefore, the penis must be extruded and held extended during the collection process.

Method for semen sample collection

The ram is positioned in lateral recumbency and the penis extruded by extending the sigmoid flexure. A gauze swab is wrapped around the penis proximal to the glans to prevent retraction into the prepuce. A warmed 7 ml plastic collection tube is held over the glans penis. A probe is introduced into the rectum to a pre-determined length just caudal to the pubic symphysis. The handle of the probe is gently raised, positioning the stimulatory electrodes along the probe adjacent to the accessory sex glands. The ram is stimulated for four seconds, then the probe is switched off for four seconds. If the Ruakura-type probe is used, stimulation often causes vocalization and sudden muscular spasm, with resultant arching of the back and extension of the hindlimbs. Rigid extension of one hindlimb during stimulation indicates that the tip of the probe is not positioned in the midline but has moved toward the side of the extended hindlimb. With the electric current switched off, the probe is slowly moved to massage the accessory sex glands.

The ram will ejaculate during massage of the accessory sex glands, when the probe is switched off. A colourless/pale yellow watery sample of 0.5 ml probably represents pre-ejaculatory fluid. A semen sample (thick creamy white, 0.7–2.0 ml) will be collected after the next cycle of electric stimulation/accessory sex gland massage. This sequence can be repeated for a maximum of three stimulations. If no sample is collected, the ram should be released and a further attempt made later.

Examination of semen samples

Progressive motility and white blood cells

One drop of semen is transferred to the centre of a warmed (approximately 37°C) slide. A small amount of semen is then collected on the corner of a cover slip and transferred to five drops of warm phosphate buffered saline (PBS). After mixing, the cover slip is placed on top of the now-diluted semen sample and examined under dark ground microscopy (×100). Vigorous forward motility of individual sperm can be readily identified in normal semen samples. White cells, whose presence is grossly abnormal, appear as round transparent cells somewhat smaller than the sperm heads.

Sperm morphology

Five drops of nigrosin/eosin stain is now added to the drop of semen in the centre of the slide and thoroughly mixed. A thin smear is then made by picking up a small amount of semen sample/stain on the corner of a microscope slide and pushing this slide at a shallow angle along the original slide.

To save time the nigrosin/eosin stained smear can be made before examining the PBS-diluted semen sample for progressive motility and white cells. By the time that examination has been performed (30–60 seconds) the stained smear will be dry and ready for examination under oil immersion (×400). Drying is expedited when a warm microscope stage is used.

Interpretation of results

Forward motility of 60% or more spermatozoa is expected in normal semen samples. It is important always to be aware that cold shock can dramatically reduce both swirling movement observed in undiluted ejaculates and in samples diluted in PBS to examine progressive motility. Urine contamination of the ejaculate will also adversely affect sperm motility but this should be readily recognized by the yellow tinge to the increased volume of diluted sample collected and an ammoniacal smell.

The presence of white cells is a significant finding and indicates inflammation of the urinogenital system. In rams, epididymitis caused by either *Brucella ovis* or *Histophilus ovis* is the most common cause of such inflammatory changes. In countries with endemic *B. ovis* infection, such as the USA, detection of white cells in the ejaculate, in addition to a high percentage of detached sperm heads, may be the first indication of infection in previously uninfected flocks. Inflammatory changes in semen often occur before serological evidence of *B. ovis* infection.

Sperm abnormalities

Spermatozoan abnormalities are recorded as either primary or secondary. Primary abnormalities involve the head and acrosome and are associated with serious testicular conditions. Tail abnormalities are often associated with less severe problems and disease of the epididymis. Sperm abnormalities should not total more than 30% of the spermatozoa examined.

Welfare considerations

Recent studies in New Zealand have indicated that electroejaculation may be no more 'stressful' for rams than routine procedures such as shearing and handling for anthelmintic drenching. However, such fertility examinations should be limited to those rams where there is either a history of infertility or a palpable scrotal abnormality that cannot be conclusively defined during ultrasonographic examination.

EPIDIDYMITIS

Definition/overview

Epididymitis caused by *B. ovis* and *Actinobacillus seminis/H. ovis* is a major cause of ram infertility in many countries, including the USA, Australia and New Zealand, where control measures are in operation for *B. ovis*. The condition causes reduced fertility in affected rams. While the clinical signs are similar despite the bacterial cause, implications and control measures differ considerably. Many other countries remain free of *B. ovis* infection, including much of Europe.

Aetiology

B. ovis can enter the body via various mucous membranes, including the vagina, rectum, conjunctivae and nasal passages, localizing in the epididymis and accessory sex glands in addition to other organs. Transmission has been described from infected and non-infected rams serving the same ewe but it occurs more commonly from sodomy. Significant pathological changes are largely confined to the epididymis (**171**). Infection of the ewe very rarely results in subsequent abortion under field conditions.

Epididymitis caused by *A. seminis/H. ovis*, a group of organisms also referred to as gram-negative pleomorphic organisms, most commonly affects ram lambs and shearlings. In infected flocks, *A. seminis/ H. ovis* can be cultured from the prepuce/distal urethra in almost all rams lambs. Contamination of the prepuce may be acquired from the environment or during homosexual activity in pubertal ram lambs. Such homosexual behaviour is not uncommon even in mature rams. Infection may also be transmitted by different rams mating the same ewe. It has been postulated that retrograde travel of the organism from the prepuce results in infection of the accessory sex glands and epididymis(es). Hormonal changes which effect puberty may facilitate retrograde migration of the organism from the prepuce and explain the age prevalence of males most commonly affected.

Clinical presentation

Lesions caused by *B. ovis* generally involve the tail of the epididymis (**171, 172**) and may develop rapidly to form large palpable granulomas, which progress to abscesses (**173–175**). The scrotum is grossly enlarged, with the affected side up to three times the normal size in severe cases (**173**). If the lesion is unilateral, the contralateral testicle is atrophied but freely moveable

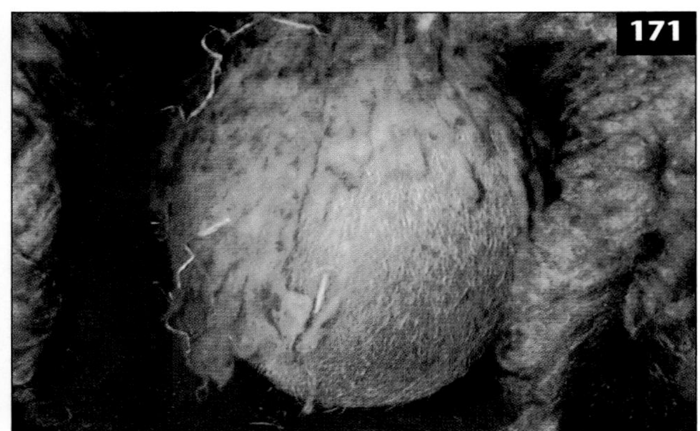

171 Marked unilateral scrotal swelling (right side) in a ram with epididymitis.

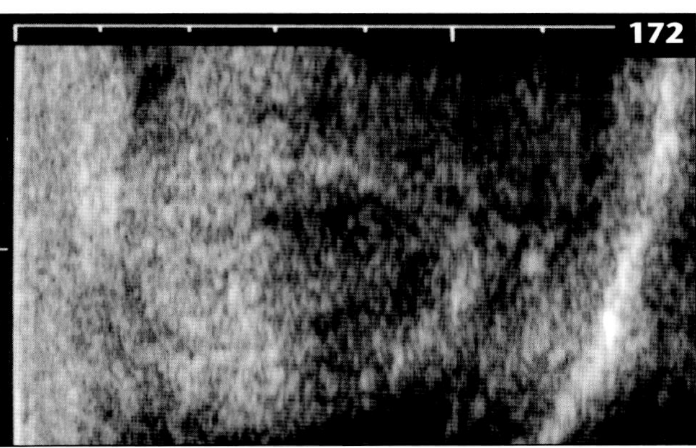

172 Ultrasonogram (5 MHz linear scanner) of the tail of the epididymis. There is an encapsulated abscess, which appears as an anechoic (black) area containing multiple hyperechoic (white) dots surrounded by a hyperchoic capsule.

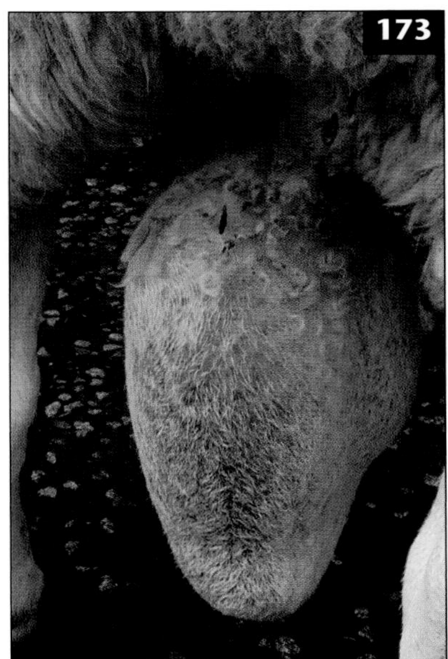

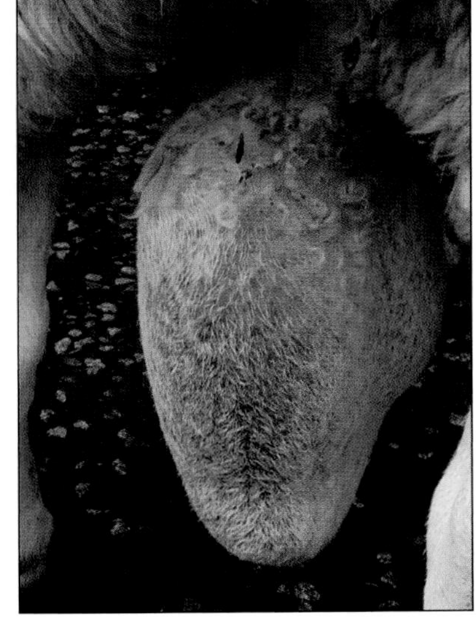

173 Border Leicester ram with epididymitis involving the tail, body and head of the left epididymis causing considerable scrotal swelling. There is atrophy of the right testicle.

174 Ultrasonogram of the proximal portion of the tail of the epididymis. There are well-encapsulated abscesses visible.

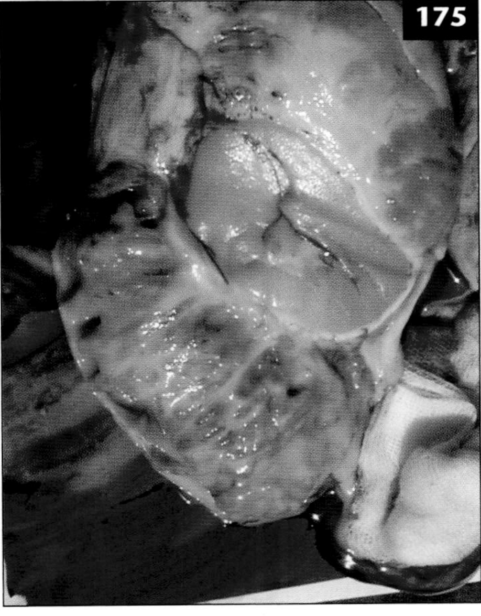

175 Necropsy specimen of the ram in **173** and **174** revealing severe epididymitis.

within the scrotum. Irrespective of a distal lesion, palpation reveals a normal spermatic cord and neck of the scrotum. The testicle and epididymis cannot readily be differentiated on palpation as the contents are firm and adherent to the scrotal skin, thus preventing free movement. There may be one or more discharging sinuses along the ventral border of the swelling.

Acute disease caused by *A. seminis/H. ovis* has not been reported in the UK, although reports in New Zealand have described anorexia and marked lameness progressing to recumbency.

Lesions caused by *A. seminis/H.ovis* more commonly affect the head of the epididymis (**176–179**). In this Suffolk ram the larger abscess in the head of the left testicle (**176**) is not associated with ipsilateral testicular atrophy (**177**); rather it is the right testicle that has atrophied (**179**).

Differential diagnoses

Differential diagnoses of scrotal swelling caused by epididymitis include:

- Inguinal hernia with omentum extending through the inguinal ring.
- Accumulation of ascitic fluid.
- Oedema of the scrotal skin.
- Haematoma.
- Orchitis.
- Varicocele.
- Spermatocele.
- Puncture wound causing cellulitis.

Diagnosis

It is rarely possible to differentiate between orchitis and epididymitis by palpation alone. Ultrasonographic examination of the scrotum in standing sheep using a 5 MHz linear scanner connected to a real-time B-mode ultrasound machine provides the most valuable information regarding location of the lesions. If necessary, ultrasonographic examination of normal rams can be undertaken first to establish normal measurements and sonographic appearance before progressing to those rams with scrotal swelling(s).

Sequential examination of the pampiniform plexus, testicle and tail of the epididymis is undertaken as the transducer head is moved distally over the lateral aspect of each spermatic cord, testicle and epididymis. The pampiniform plexus reveals a matrix of hyperechoic (bright white) lines throughout the conical anechoic area. The normal testicle appears as a uniform hypoechoic area (**169**) with a hyperechoic mediastinum clearly visible. The tail of the epididymis is distinct from the testicle and considerably smaller in diameter (2–3 cm compared with 6–7 cm) and with a distinct capsule. It may prove difficult to obtain

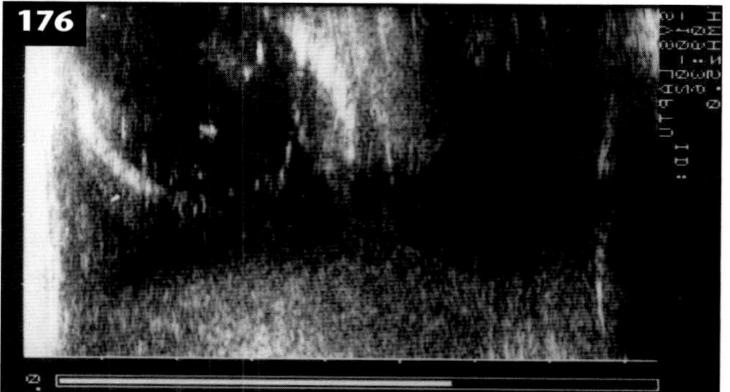

176 The head of the left epididymis of a ram revealing a 4 cm diameter well-encapsulated abscess.

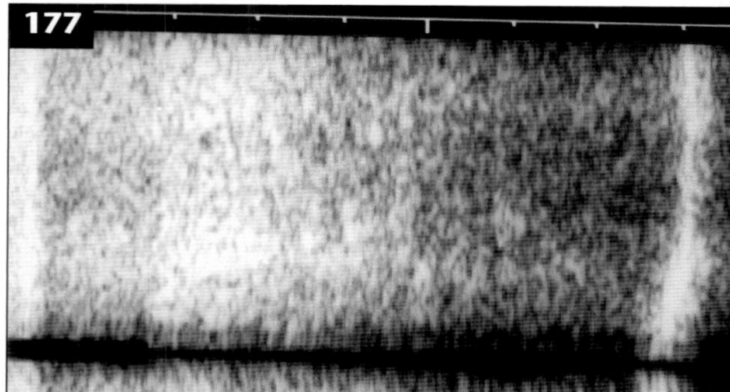

177 The left testicle has a normal ultrasonographic appearance and a normal 8 cm diameter.

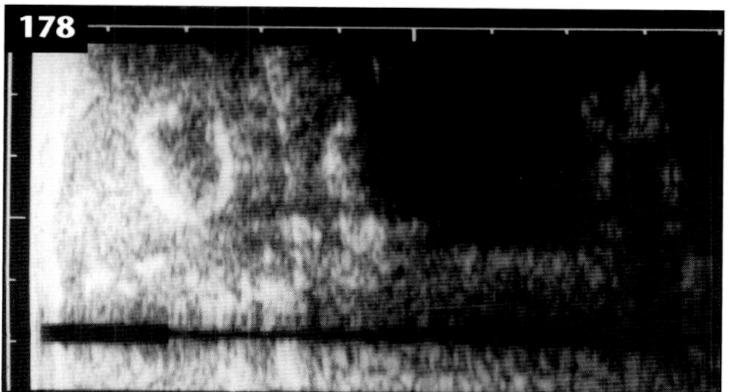

178 The head of the right epididymis revealing a 2 cm diameter well-encapsulated abscess.

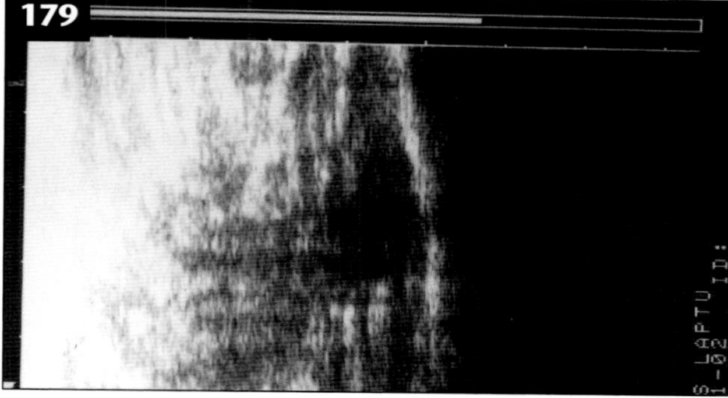

179 The right testicle. There is atrophy of the testicle. It has a 5 cm diameter. Compare with **177**.

good contact between the linear probe head and the small diameter tail of the epididymis.

Ultrasonographic examination in rams with epididymitis reveals a normal pampiniform plexus. The swollen scrotal contents frequently appear as multiple, 1–5 cm diameter anechoic areas containing many bright spots (**172**) surrounded by broad hyperechoic lines (fibrous capsule) extending up to 1 cm in thickness, typical of thick-walled abscesses. The abscesses generally involve the tail of the epididymis (**174**) but may extend to involve the body and head of the epididymis (**176, 178**), respectively. The testicle is embedded within this fibrous tissue reaction, is much reduced in size, appears more hypoechoic than normal and contains numerous hyperechoic spots consistent with testicular atrophy. In sheep with unilateral epididymitis the contralateral testicle is much smaller than normal and appears more hypoechoic.

In countries with endemic *B. ovis* infection, detection of large numbers of white cells in the ejaculate, in addition to an increased percentage of detached sperm heads, typically >20% but often much higher, may be the first indication of infection in previously uninfected flocks. Inflammatory changes in semen often occur before serological evidence of *B. ovis* infection. Similar semen changes are found in *A. seminis/H. ovis* infections. Semen collection should not be attempted in rams with palpable swellings that can readily be differentiated during ultrasound examination.

Culture of the semen will confirm the cause of epididymitis. Seroconversion to *B. ovis* may occur some time after changes in the semen and palpable scrotal swellings. Serological testing is based on the ELISA test. There are at present no serological tests for *A. seminis/H. ovis* epididymitis.

Treatment

In cases of unilateral *A. seminis/H. ovis* epididymitis the owner may request hemicastration with the expectation that regeneration of the other testicle will occur over a 3–6 month period. Such surgery is generally ill-advised because the extensive adhesions between the inflamed (and abscessed) epididymis and the tunica vaginalis render castration problematic.

Prevention/control measures

Finding large numbers of white cells and a high percentage of dead sperm with detached heads in the ejaculate during a pre-breeding ram soundness examination is significant and indicates marked inflammation of the testicle and/or epididymis. In rams, epididymitis caused by either *B. ovis* or *A. seminis/H. ovis* is the most common cause of such inflammatory reaction and such changes in the ejaculate can be detected months before palpable enlargement of the epididymis. Antibiotic treatment can be attempted during these early stages but the best advice is to cull affected rams from the flock.

In countries with endemic *B. ovis* infection, regular serological testing and culling of positive rams will eradicate the problem. Replacement rams should be purchased from accredited flocks. If the seroprevalence is high, replacement of all rams will be the quickest method of eradicating *B. ovis* infection.

There are no recognized control measures for *A. seminis/H. ovis* epididymitis in pedigree flocks producing ram lambs and shearlings. Improved environmental hygiene may limit contamination. Rams lambs often congregate on bare earth, which rapidly becomes contaminated; therefore, access to such areas should be prevented. Regular rotation through small paddocks may reduce the level of environmental exposure. Dividing the ram lambs into small groups may limit the spread of infection. Irrigation of the prepuce with dilute chlorhexidine solution at regular intervals as the ram lambs reach puberty has been recommended. This procedure is cheap and access to the prepuce can be achieved using a foot turning crate. Administration of parenteral antibiotics to ram lambs as they reach puberty has not proven successful but long-term inclusion of antibiotics in feed has proved beneficial. The different results achieved by these antibiotic regimens may be related to the duration of medication. These potential control measures are not exclusive and there may be good reason to adopt most, or all, of them.

Economics

Epididymitis caused by *A. seminis/H. ovis* is not a major concern to the commercial farmer purchasing rams for cross-breeding purposes, where the disease is recognized sporadically and affected rams are promptly culled. Epididymitis is most problematic in pedigree flocks selling high priced ram lambs and shearlings, where spread may occur during the pubertal period, thus rendering rams unfit for sale.

In countries with endemic *B. ovis* infection the economic effects resulting from an increased barren ewe rate, a reduced lambing percentage and an extended lambing period are considerable. Farmers must be encouraged to purchase accredited stock and maintain a *B. ovis*-free flock.

Welfare implications

Rams with palpable scrotal lesions should be culled. Hemicastration is ill-advised in rams with unilateral epididymal lesions.

VASECTOMY

Overview

Vasectomized rams are widely used to induce ovulation and synchronize oestrus in ewes before the introduction of fertile rams, thereby compacting the lambing period, optimizing seasonal labour and reducing the consequences of disease build up as the lambing season progresses.

It is common practice to introduce the vasectomized ram for one week starting two weeks before the breeding season. This management practice will generally induce ovulation in ram-responsive ewes within 2–3 days, with normal behavioural oestrus around 17 days later (i.e. around six days after the introduction of fertile rams). The prior introduction of vasectomized rams should guarantee that the vast majority of ewes are mated during a ten-day period, with a subsequently compacted lambing period. Before advising a client about using vasectomized rams, it is essential that the veterinarian check that there are sufficient fertile rams to cope with such a compacted breeding period (approximately one ram per 30 ewes) and that there is sufficient labour to cope with the challenges of a concentrated lambing period.

Vasectomy is more easily performed in shearlings than in either six-month-old lambs or subfertile mature rams. Crossbred sheep (e.g. Suffolk × Greyface) grow to live weights in excess of 100 kg and often become aggressive and unmanageable in later years; therefore, where available, it is better to vasectomize yearling Suffolk rams that have failed to make the grade for sale as breeding stock. However, with increasing awareness of biosecurity, it would be prudent to vasectomize home-bred stock in order to reduce the number of sheep introduced onto the farm.

Analgesia

A full description of the various analgesia options available for vasectomy can be found in Chapter 15 (p. 315).

Surgical technique

The ram is positioned on its hindquarters (**180**). An incision is made in the skin over the spermatic cord at the level of the accessory teats. The spermatic cord is exteriorized following blunt dissection and the vas deferens localized medially within the spermatic cord between the thumb and index finger (**181**). The tunic is nicked with the scalpel blade point (**182**) and a 6 cm length of vas deferens freed from connective tissue (**183**). The vas deferens is ligated twice and the 5 cm section between the sutures removed and submitted for histological examination. During closure the ligated ends of the vas deferens are incorporated in different fascial planes to further reduce the possibility of re-canalization. The skin incision is closed with interrupted mattress sutures and the procedure repeated for the other side. Sperm granulomas (**184**) may develop over a period of several years but do not affect the sexual behaviour of the vasectomized ram.

Some veterinarians prefer to hemicastrate rams rather than remove sections of both vasa deferentes because these rams are much more readily identifiable should a ram ever lose its ear tag and become the subject of a legal dispute.

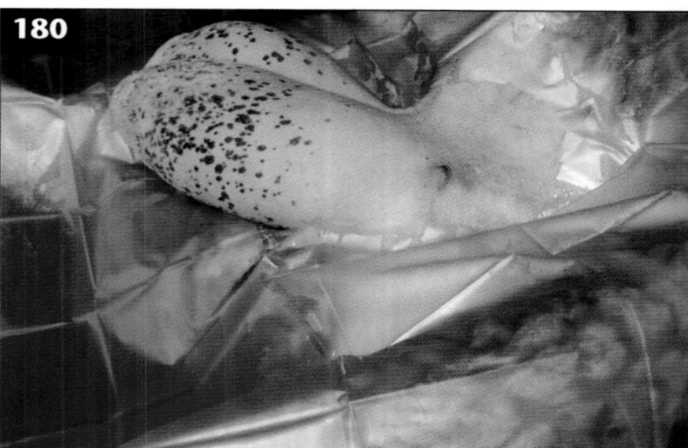

180 Preparation for vasectomy.

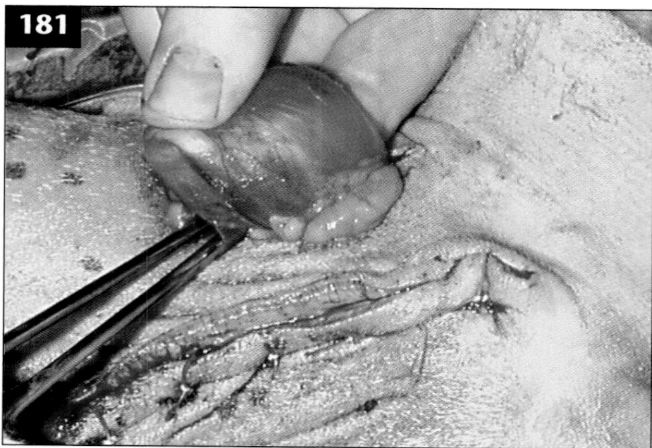

181 Isolation of the vas deferens at the axial (medial) margin of the spermatic cord.

Economic considerations/litigation

Occasionally, costly mistakes occur whereby pregnancies result from the use of 'vasectomized' rams, whether caused by errors at surgery or re-canalization of one vas deferens. Effective analgesia greatly facilitates surgery and therefore may reduce the likelihood of such mistakes. Dual identification of all vasectomized rams and storage of vasa deferentes is very important in case of litigation. While some surgeons prefer to submit samples for histological examination, this can prove costly. Experienced surgeons prefer to store specimens in formol saline and submit such specimens should a dispute arise. Electroejaculation of the 'vasectomized' ram would also be a vital part of any such investigation.

CLINICAL PROBLEM

A yearling Suffolk ram is presented with a two-week history of unilateral scrotal swelling and a discharging sinus from the ventral pole (**185**).

Clinical examination

The ram is bright and alert and was at the feed trough this morning. The rectal temperature is 40.0°C. The left side of the scrotum is markedly swollen (**185**). There is no evidence of any hernia and the spermatic cord is normal. There is no palpable distinction between the testicle and the epididymis. The contents of the left scrotal sac are hot, swollen and painful, and firmly adherent to the vaginal tunic. There is a

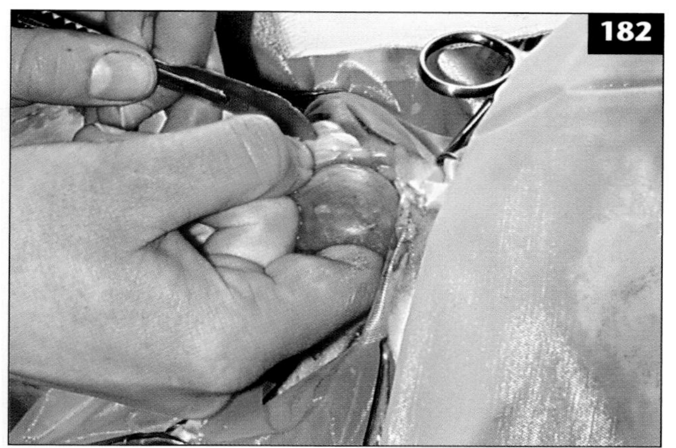

182 Incision over the isolated vas deferens.

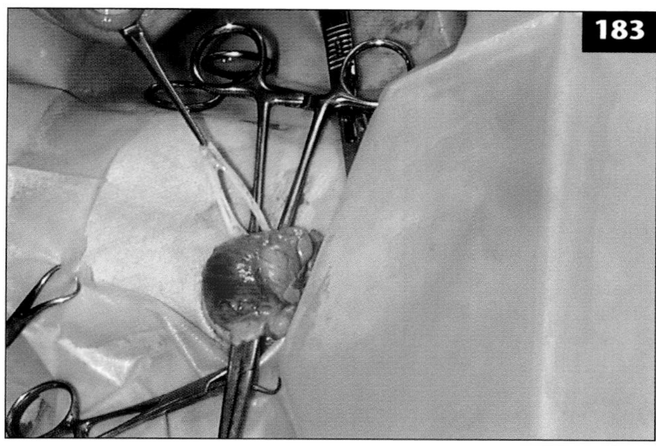

183 Exteriorization of the vas deferens.

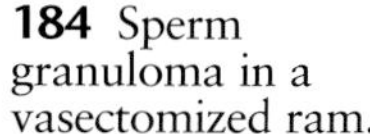
184 Sperm granuloma in a vasectomized ram.

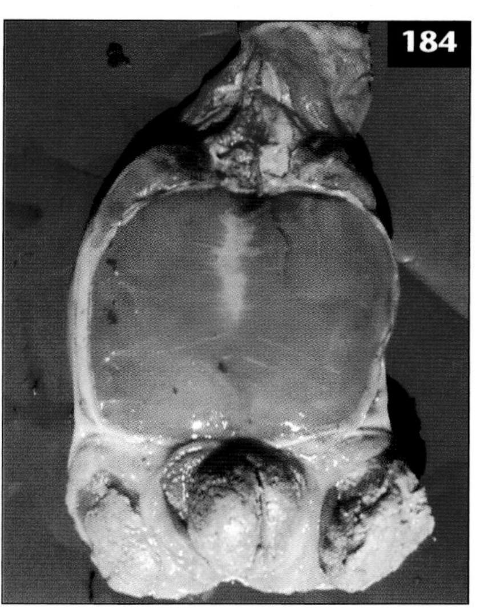

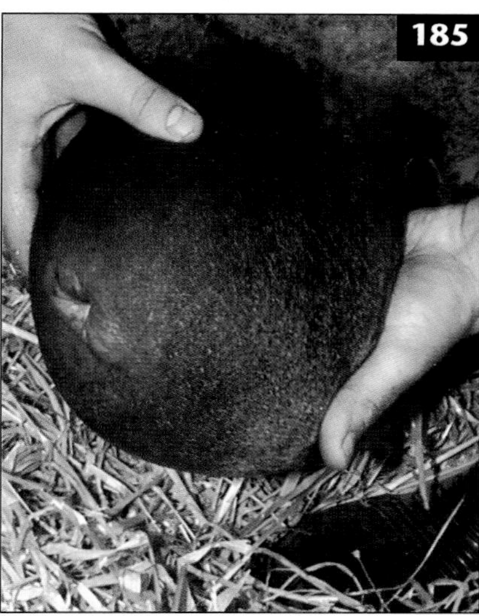

185 Left side of the scrotum is markedly swollen.

discharging sinus on the ventral pole. The right testicle and epididymis are smaller and softer than normal but freely moveable within the scrotum. No other abnormalities are noted on clinical examination.

What conditions should be considered?
What further tests could be undertaken?

Differential diagnoses

- Epididymitis caused by *A. seminis/H. ovis* or *B. ovis*.
- Orchitis.
- Haematoma.
- Scrotal hernia (discounted during the clinical examination).
- Cellulitis following puncture wound of the scrotum.

Further tests

- Ultrasonography.
- Bacteriology from discharging sinus.
- Semen evaluation.

Diagnosis

The clinical presentation of this ram was typical of epididymitis involving the tail of the epididymis but possibly extending to involve the body and head.

Ultrasound examination using a 5 MHz linear scanner revealed a 4 cm diameter abscess; anechoic (black) area containing multiple hyperechoic gas echoes (white spots) on the left hand side of the sonogram (**186**). The furthermost wall (right-hand side) of the capsule is clearly visible as a broad hyperechoic (white) band resulting from acoustic enhancement of sound waves travelling through the fluid medium of the abscess.

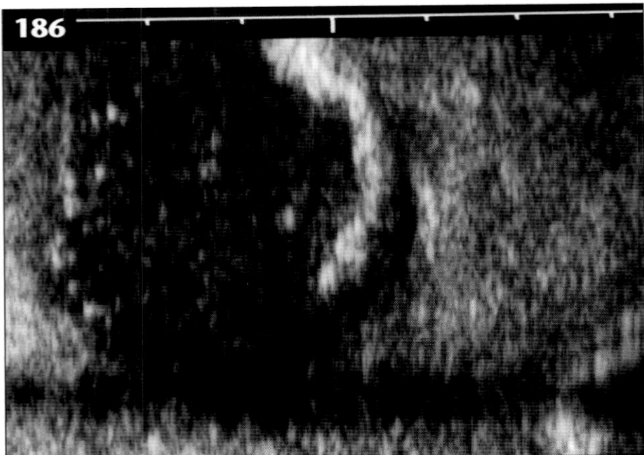

186 A 4 cm diameter abscess; note the anechoic (black) area containing multiple hyperechoic gas echoes.

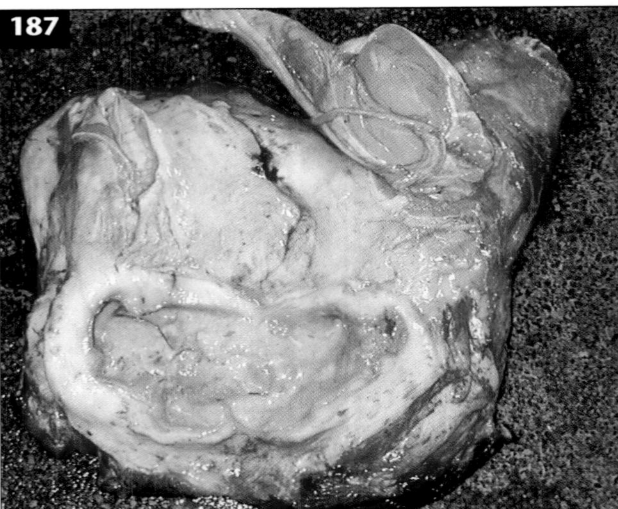

187 Diagnosis of epididymitis confirmed at necropsy.

Treatment

Treatment would have no effect on this condition and the ram lamb was destroyed for welfare reasons.

Postmortem examination

The diagnosis of epididymitis was confirmed at necropsy (**187**). Bacteriology yielded *Fusobacterium necrophorum*, which may have overgrown other organisms.

Further information and control

The occurrence of inflammatory lesions of the male urinogential tract caused by bacterial infections is much less common in UK flocks than in other countries worldwide because *B. ovis* has not been reported in the UK. However, infections caused by *H. ovis* do occur in the UK. The isolation of *Fusobacterium necrophorum* in this case of epididymitis is unusual.

REFERENCE

1 Kimberling CV (1988) Diseases of rams. In *Diseases of Sheep*, 3rd edn. (eds R Jensen and BL Swift) Lea and Febiger, Philadelphia, pp. 3–19.

4 Neonatal Lamb Diseases

PERINATAL LAMB MORTALITY

Definition/overview

Perinatal lamb mortality in the majority of UK flocks ranges from 15–25%, which represents 3–7 million dead lambs annually. Perinatal lamb mortality in New Zealand overall is approximately 15–20%. In some situations the major loss is due to dystocia and on some farms lamb mortality figures are as low as 5–10%. New Zealand farmers have worked hard on this problem and easy care lambing and better husbandry (nutrition) have played a big part in improving the national lambing data in that country. In the USA, lamb mortality reports consistently demonstrate a pattern of perinatal losses ranging from 10–35% of the annual lamb crop.

In well-managed flocks (**188**), which vaccinate against toxoplasmosis and enzootic abortion (or EAE-accredited flock) and lamb indoors (or outdoors during good weather), the target perinatal lamb mortality figure should be <7%, with 5% readily achievable. The importance of the lambing shed environment cannot be overemphasized (**189–193**). Poor hygiene standards (**190**) increase the prevalence of watery mouth disease, infectious polyarthritis and omphalophlebitis. Individual

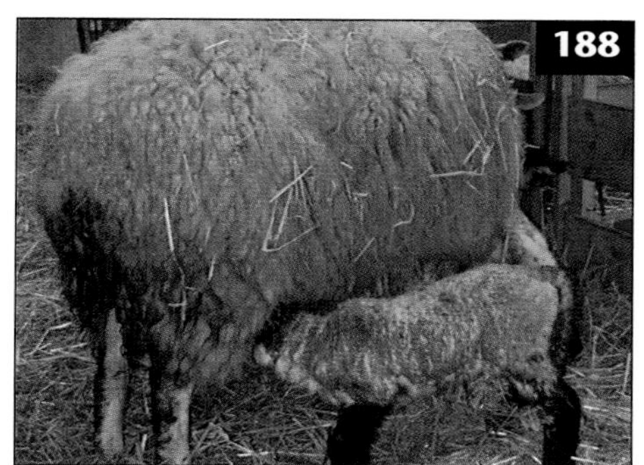

188 A normal litter.

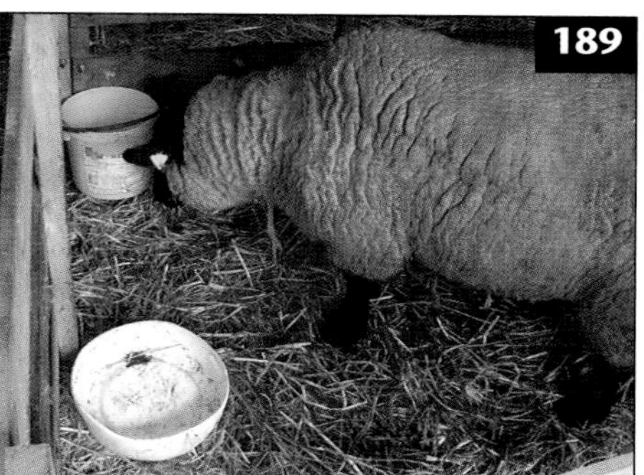

189 Poor management. Dirty pen with neither food or water for the ewe.

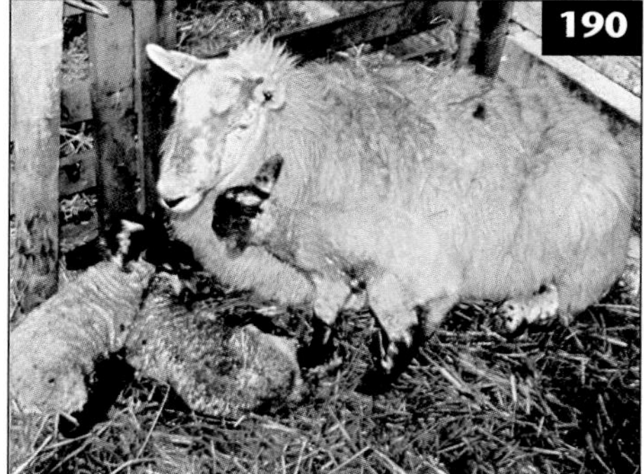

190 Triplet lambs born into a very dirty environment. The lambs are still wet and the ewe shows no interest. Without prompt action all three lambs could be dead within 36 hours.

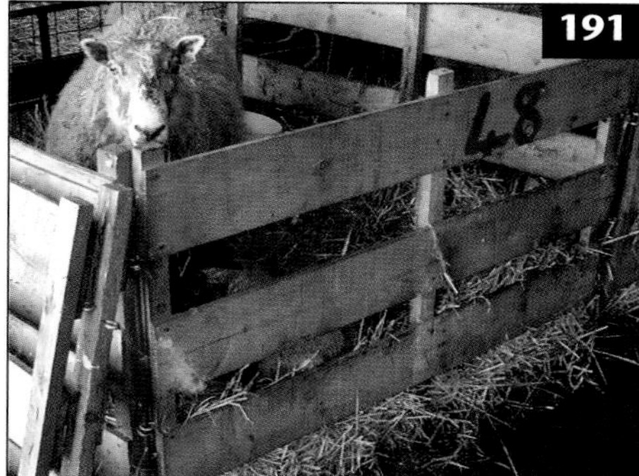

191 Build-up of dirty straw bedding in individual pens affords the ideal environment for bacterial multiplication.

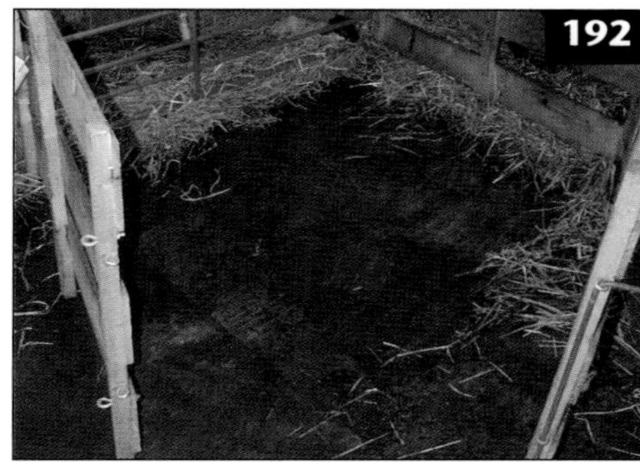

192 Pen should be left to dry before using again.

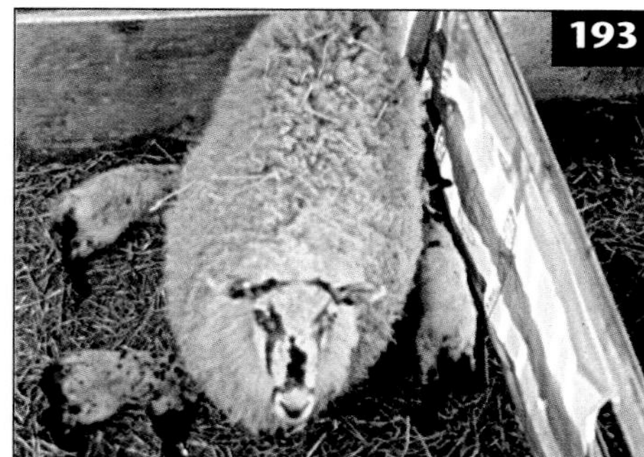

193 Clean, dry pen with concrete floor. Compare with **190.**

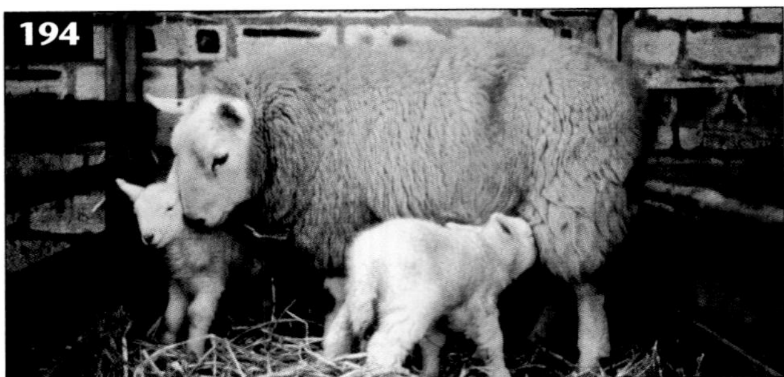

194 Individual pen too small, which could result in overlying.

pens must be large enough (1.3 m × 1.3 m minimum) to prevent overlying by the ewe (**194**).

Aetiology

While many factors, including farm management, levels of flock supervision and infectious diseases, contribute to high levels of perinatal lamb mortality, lamb birth weight, together with colostrum accumulation in the ewe's udder at lambing, remains fundamental to ensuring a good start for the lamb during the critical first 36 hours of life. Perinatal lamb mortality is an area where veterinary advice can have a major impact in terms of flock production and profitability and, importantly, welfare of the flock.

Clinical presentation

Lamb birth weights

In UK lowland flocks, for example, approximately 15%, 65% and 20% of ewes produce single, twins and triplets, respectively. Breed, parity and nutrition at tupping time (flushing) influence these lambing statistics.

Optimum lamb birth weights using a Suffolk or other terminal meat breed sire crossed on to a F1 hybrid female (e.g. Greyface or Scottish Halfbred) are:

- Single – 5.5–7.0 kg.
- Twins – 5.0–6.0 kg.
- Triplets – greater than 4.0 kg.

The live weight measurements for the hybrid ewes listed above range from 60–85 kg.

Recording birth weights

Lamb birth weight changes little within the first 24 hours of life; therefore, all lambs born within the previous 24 hours can be weighed to provide a representative population sample during on-farm investigations. Lamb birth weights >1.0 kg lighter than those quoted above are strongly suggestive of chronic ewe undernutrition during late gestation. Ewe body condition scores must also be checked, with low values being consistent with poor energy supply.

Hill breeds (e.g. the Scottish Blackface in the UK – live weight range of 45–65 kg) will have birth weights 1–1.5 kg lighter than those stated above, and it is best to establish target values for particular breeds by visiting farms with excellent production figures and measuring lamb birth weights there.

Ewe body condition score

Ewe body condition scores are low (2.0 or less) when late gestation nutrition has been inadequate for more than two weeks. Where the flock is managed as one group, low body condition scores are most noticeable in multigravid ewes, especially those ewes with three or more lambs *in utero*. In prolific flocks it is good practice to manage pregnant ewes based on fetal number determined by ultrasonography. Where feeding of the whole flock started on the same date, later born lambs typically have heavier birth weights due to a longer period of dam supplementary feeding.

Flock problems such as chronic parasitism, particularly fasciolosis, can lead to low body condition in a large percentage of ewes but this problem is exacerbated by fetal load.

Hungry lambs within the first 24 hours of life

Hungry lambs appear dull and lethargic (**195**) and spend a lot of time lying in sheltered areas. After the normal enthusiastic teat-searching behaviour immediately after birth, these lambs make only pathetic attempts to suck (**196**). They quickly become gaunt and have a 'hunched up' appearance, with all four limbs held on the same spot (**197**). If neglected, the condition may progress to coma and death. This may take 2–3 days, during which time these lambs should be detected by the shepherd and fed accordingly. Coma and death occurs more rapidly in starved lambs exposed to severe weather conditions. In many situations, lambs that have failed to ingest sufficient colostrum, which contains protective immunoglobulins, succumb to infectious diseases such as watery mouth disease or septicaemia.

Lamb starvation after 24 hours

Starvation after 24 hours (**198**) results from dam rejection, often after fostering a lamb; poor dam milk supply, which can be caused by mastitis, poor dam nutrition or infectious disease; and misadventure after turnout. Hungry lambs often try to suck other ewes, especially while the ewes are at the feed trough. Hungry lambs may even attempt to eat concentrates. Diarrhoea is frequently encountered in such hungry lambs.

After 24–36 hours starvation the condition may progress to coma and eventual death but close supervision of newly lambed ewes turned out into well-sheltered paddocks should prevent this neglect; however, losses may still occur during adverse weather or in triplet litters.

Differential diagnoses

Weakly lambs

There are many causes of weakly lambs at birth, including the infectious causes of abortion listed below:

- Toxoplasmosis.
- Border disease.
- *Chlamydophila abortus.*
- *Salmonella* species serotypes.
- *Campylobacter fetus intestinalis.*
- *Listeria monocytogenes.*
- *Pasteurella* species.

Lack of colostrum

Lack of colostrum accumulation within the udder can arise from:

- Mastitis.
- Chronic debilitating disease such as paratuberculosis.
- Maedi-visna virus.

Diagnosis

Birth injuries

There is considerable debate as to the relative importance of dystocia, and in particular intrapartum hypoxaemia, as a contributing factor to neonatal losses. The relative importance of dystocia as a cause of neonatal deaths varies between countries, and this reflects on the breed, management system and level of supervision. For example, an extensive survey in New Zealand involving 23,000 lambs suggested that dystocia was the main cause of death, with 74% of lambs showing evidence of trauma, while a survey in the UK reported only 0.5% deaths due to dystocia.

It is important to define what is meant by dystocia in this respect. Postural abnormalities are very common in multigravid sheep and may affect 10–25% of all births in UK lowland flocks. Diligent staff should readily detect such problems within 30 minutes so that they can be promptly corrected and the lambs delivered with minimal traction. These lambs require close supervision but no more than any other litter.

Lambing problems that require more than 10–15 minutes assistance may comprise another group altogether. A typical example might be anterior presentation with either unilateral or bilateral shoulder flexion. Such lambs may present with considerable oedema of the head due to reduced venous return when the head is lodged within the maternal pelvis. In

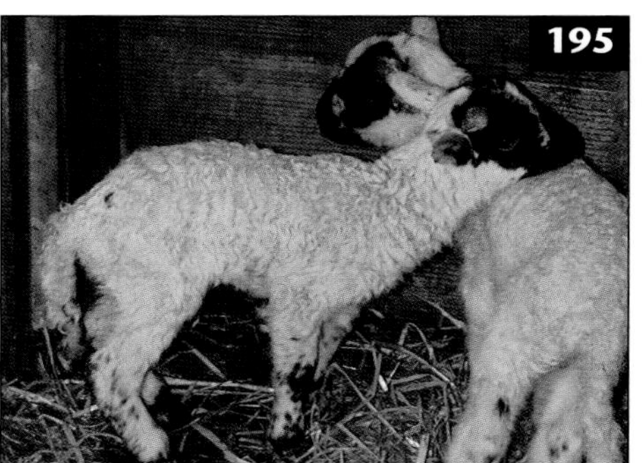
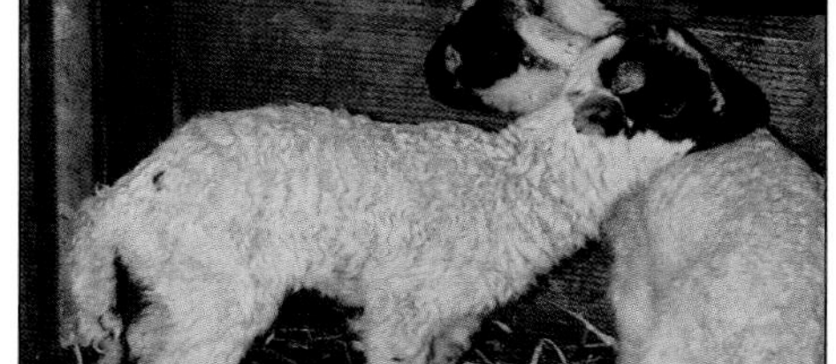

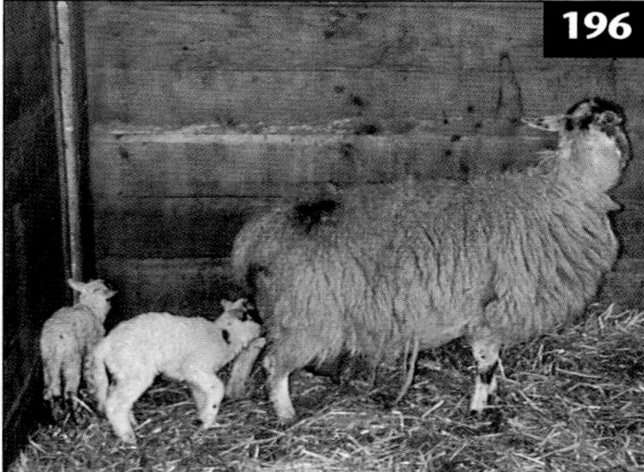

195 Newborn lambs, which have not sucked colostrum.

196 Newborn lambs, which have not sucked colostrum. There are pathetic attempts at searching for a teat.

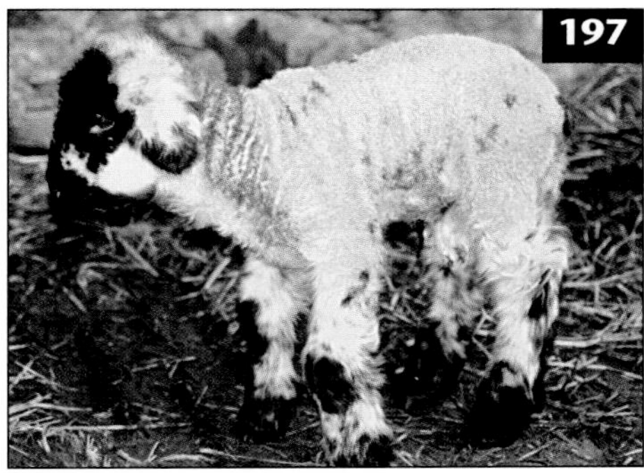

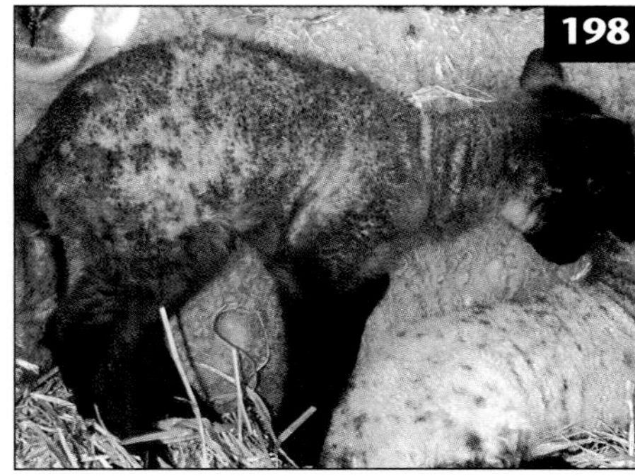

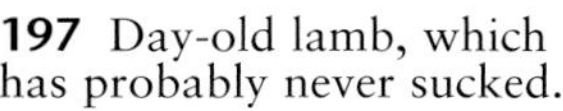

197 Day-old lamb, which has probably never sucked.

198 Very hungry two-day-old lamb.

these cases it is possible to envisage that intracranial haemorrhage may occur. However, practical experience indicates that with appropriate supervision these lambs have a normal survival rate.

Meconium staining of the fleece
It has been suggested that meconium staining of the fleece is an indication of a stressful birth and that such lambs are less able to adapt quickly to extra-uterine life, although there are few supporting data. While lambs with meconium staining of the fleece may warrant special attention, in particular ensuring early colostrum ingestion, there are no convincing data that show they have a significantly higher mortality rate.

Weakly lambs at birth
The investigation of infectious causes of abortion is detailed in Chapter 3, Part 1 (Abortion, p. 60). Investigation of dam dietary energy supply with respect to lamb birth weight and perinatal mortality is based on serum 3-OH butyrate determination during late gestation (see Chapter 2: Late gestation nutrition, p. 17).

Determination of passive antibody transfer

Transabdominal palpation of the abomasum
Colostrum in the lamb's abomasum immediately caudal to the costal arch can readily be detected by gentle transabdominal palpation. This can be undertaken in the standing lamb (**199**) or with the lamb held up by its forelimbs (**200**).

The gastrointestinal tract of the newborn lamb is relatively empty and it should be easy to detect whether the lamb has ingested up to 500 ml of colostrum (more than 10% of its body weight). Abdominal distension does occur in watery mouth disease but affected lambs are usually 24 hours old. This distension should not be confused with colostrum ingestion by lambs within the first few hours of life.

Ultrasonographic determination of abomasal diameter
Ultrasonographic examination of the abomasum of neonatal lambs will show immediately whether lambs have sucked or not and may highlight an area for more detailed examination whilst the veterinarian is still on the farm. The abomasal diameter of newborn lambs before sucking is approximately 3.0 cm (range 2–4 cm) compared with 8 cm (range 7–10 cm) recorded for lambs that have sucked normally.

Determination of plasma protein concentration
During investigation of perinatal lamb mortality, venous blood samples should be collected into lithium heparin vacutainers from 10–20 randomly selected day-old lambs. Samples are then spun down in a microhaematocrit centrifuge and plasma protein concentration determined using a hand-held refractometer. The plasma protein concentration for lambs that have not sucked sufficient colostrum is <45 g/l, compared with >65.0 g/l for lambs that have sucked adequate colostrum within the first 12–18 hours after birth. Such tests are accurate, inexpensive and very informative when the data are used in conjunction with transabdominal palpation of the abomasum and ultrasonographic determination of abomasal diameter.

Treatment

Ensuring the lamb's best start in life
There are three critically important events that must happen to ensure that newborn lambs have the best chance of survival:

- Lambs must be born into a clean environment to an attentive dam with a good colostrum supply.
- The lamb must ingest sufficient colostrum (200 ml/kg) during the first 24 hours of life and 50 ml/kg within the first 1 hours, if not sooner.

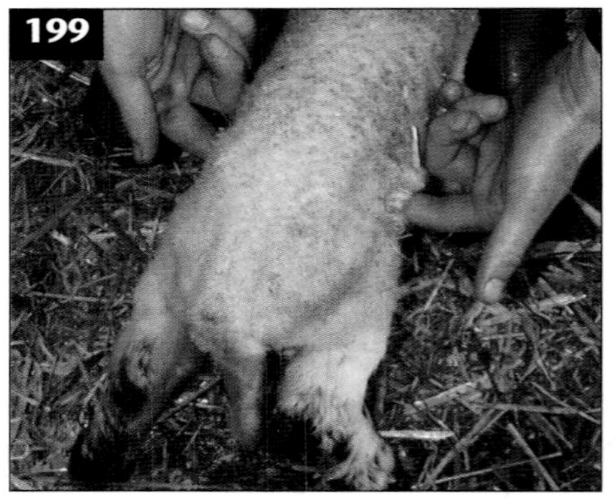

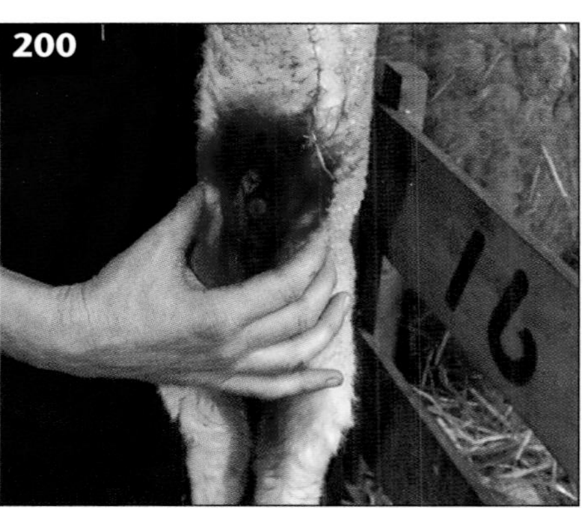

199 Palpation of the abomasum extending beyond the costal arch.

200 Palpation of the abomasum dropped below the costal arch.

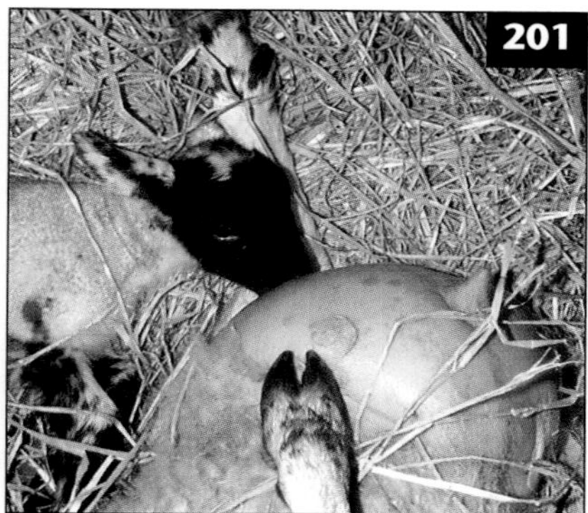

201 Ensuring colostrum intake during the first two hours of life.

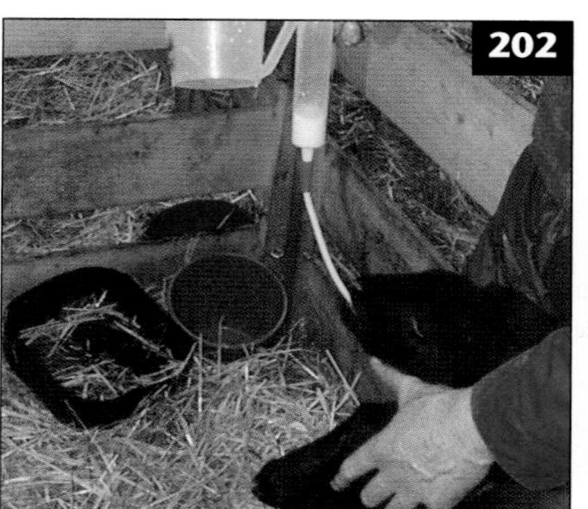

202 Feeding colostrum by oesophageal tube.

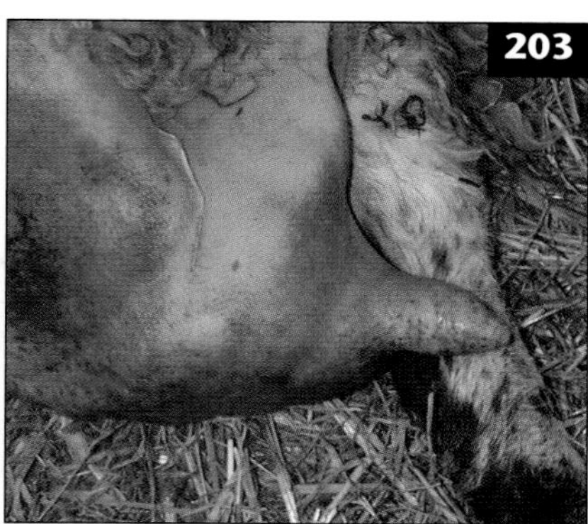

203 Twin lambs sucking only the right teat, leading to distension of the left gland.

- The navel must be fully immersed in strong veterinary iodine BP within the first 15 minutes of life, and this procedure repeated at least once 2–4 hours later.

Ensuring colostrum ingestion

If the lamb has not sucked colostrum, then some assistance is necessary and various methods are employed:

- The ewe is restrained and the teat put gently into the lamb's mouth at the same time as some colostrum is gently expressed on to the lamb's tongue to encourage sucking.
- The ewe is sat on to her hindquarters and the lamb is laid on its side. The teat is then put into the lamb's mouth at the same time as some colostrum is gently expressed on to the lamb's tongue to encourage sucking (**201**).
- The lamb is encouraged to suck colostrum stripped from either the dam or another ewe, or bovine colostrum, from a bottle and teat.
- Colostrum stripped from the either the dam or another ewe, or bovine colostrum, is administered via a stomach tube (**202**). Ovine colostrum is very viscous and it may prove necessary to dilute the colostrum with warm water so that it will easily flow through the stomach tube. Alternatively, a 50–60 ml syringe can be filled then discharged through the stomach tube.

Teat-searching behaviour

Newborn lambs should be able to stand and search for the teat within 15 minutes of birth. Healthy lambs nuzzle their way along the ventral abdomen until they find the udder and teat. When sucking, lambs adopt a characteristic posture, with rapid tail movements, and the ewe invariably starts chewing her cud. A slurping sound can often be heard when the lambs are sucking vigorously and this can last 2–3 minutes. Provided the lambs are actively searching for the teat, the ewe and lambs should be left undisturbed. In many pastoral systems, disturbance of lambing ewes may affect maternal bonding and lead to increased lamb losses through abandonment, particularly in breeds with poor mothering instincts such as the Merino.

Udder problems

Many shepherds gently express a small amount of colostrum from each teat when the ewe is penned in order to remove the small waxy plug that has sealed the teat and check that there is no mastitis. Occasionally, twin lambs may only suck from one gland, leading to considerable distension of the other gland and teat (**203**).

Colostrum is uniformly thick and viscous with a yellow/white colour. Infection of the udder causes the mammary secretions to alter; mastitic milk is often straw-coloured, watery and contains white/yellow clots. The normal udder is firm but not hard, and should feel neither hot nor painful. Mastitis often results in swelling of the gland, with accumulation of subcutaneous and interstitial fluid, which will pit under pressure (oedema). Examination of a mastitic quarter may elicit a pain response from the ewe. The mammary gland becomes hot and painful and the ewe appears lame.

Mismothering

Mismothering occurs more commonly in housed sheep where there are high stocking densities; ewes are unable to isolate themselves from the remainder of the flock during first stage labour. It is interesting to note that a ewe that is attempting to 'steal' or 'pinch' another ewe's lambs is always the more possessive sheep.

Treatment of comatose lambs

The treatment of comatose lambs is divided into two age groups; those less than six hours old and those more than six hours old.

Treatment of comatose lambs less than six hours old

Coma should not arise in lambs less than six hours old unless the lambing flock has been neglected during adverse weather. This situation occurs most commonly when ewes lamb outdoors (**204**) during severe weather conditions, and in hill flocks that lamb outdoors and where there is no supervision during the hours of darkness.

The lamb is placed in a warming box with the thermostat set at 45°C. Colostrum should be stomach tubed at a rate of 50 ml/kg once the lamb has been warmed and it can maintain sternal recumbency. If there is insufficient ewe colostrum, it is possible to use cow colostrum pooled in advance from more than four dairy cows previously vaccinated with a multicomponent sheep clostridial vaccine preparation three, six and ten weeks prior to calving.

The true incidence of cow colostrum-induced anaemia is very low indeed and many more lambs die of starvation than anaemia. The possible occurrence of cow colostrum-induced anaemia is greatly reduced if pooled cow colostrum is fed. Laboratory checks for anaemia factor have a low specificity and are not generally undertaken.

Artificial milk replacers should not be used for the first colostrum feed but they can be used after the first feed to save colostrum stores. Electrolyte solutions contain very little energy (as little as 15% of daily requirements) and should be used for treating neonatal diarrhoea only.

Treatment of comatose lambs more than six hours old

Coma in lambs more than six hours old is a reflection of poor flock supervision, because it takes one to two days' starvation before a lamb finally exhausts all of its body reserves of glycogen/glucose precursors and brown fat. These metabolic crises can be corrected by intraperitoneal injection of 25 ml of 20% glucose solution, followed by placing the lamb in a warming box with the thermostat set at 45°C. The injection should be administered before the lamb is placed in the warming box. The lamb must be checked regularly if the box does not have a thermostat to prevent overheating.

The warm 20% glucose (dextrose) solution is made up by adding 12 ml of recently boiled water from the kettle to an equal volume of 40% glucose solution, which is available commercially from the farmer's veterinarian.

To give an intraperitoneal injection the lamb is first suspended vertically by the forelimbs. A 19 gauge, 25 mm long needle is introduced through the body wall 2–3 cm to the side of, and 2–3 cm caudal to, the navel. The point of the needle is directed towards the lamb's tail head. Once the needle has been introduced up to the hub, the solution is injected slowly into the body cavity. It is important not to attempt injection into the peritoneal cavity of lambs with watery mouth disease, as the needle point will usually puncture the very thin wall of the hugely distended abomasum, resulting in leakage of abomasal contents and the potential for peritonitis.

The recovery of hypothermic and hypoglycaemic lambs is dramatic within 30–60 minutes but such neglect should not have occurred in the first instance.

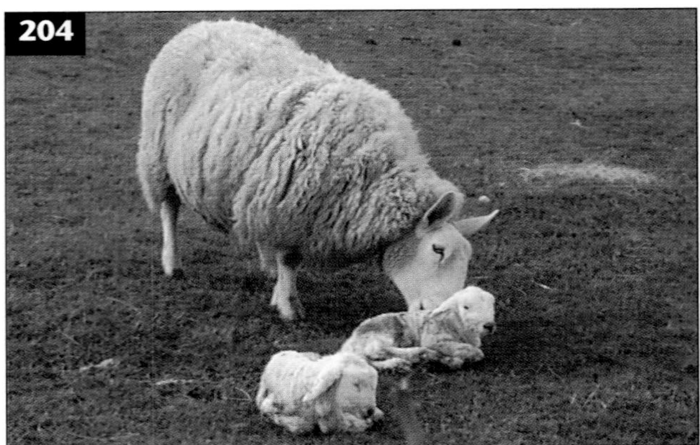

204 Newborn lambs born outdoors are prone to exposure during adverse weather conditions.

Prevention/control measures

Veterinary monitoring and adjustment of late pregnancy ewe nutrition could have a major impact on perinatal lamb survival and prevention of disease by ensuring adequate colostrum accumulation in the ewe's udder. Such advice, incorporated into a veterinary health plan for sheep flocks, could achieve increased financial returns (**Table 3**) and produce significant improvements in sheep welfare.

The data in **Table 3** represent a flock with moderate energy underfeeding that would require four MJ/head/day over the last six weeks of gestation to return 3-OH butyrate concentrations to target values[1]. This increase in dietary energy supply necessitates an extra 10.5 tonnes of feed (energy value 12 MJ/kg as fed), and this represents the major cost in the total expenditure.

The improved flock nutrition will prevent five ewes (0.5% of the ewes at risk) developing OPT. These ewes would have reared eight lambs (1.6 lambs per ewe) for sale as stores. In addition, an extra 90 lambs will be

Table 3 Simplified costings (2005 figures) for implementation of a veterinary flock plan targeting late gestation ewe nutrition in a 1,000 ewe lowland flock (all values in UK pounds).

• Visit to farm	£25
• Biochemical analyses (15 ewes)	£60–100
• Extra feed (0.25 kg/ewe/day for 42 days)	£1,050
• **Total costs for 1,000 ewe flock**	**£1,175**
Increased production:	
• 5 ewes (previously died of OPT)	£450
• 8 lambs (progeny of 5 ewes listed above)	£240
Reduction in perinatal mortality (15–10%):	
• 90 extra lambs reared	£2,700
• Reduced neonatal infections	£1,080
Increased income	**£4,670**
Profit (income less expenditure)	**£3,495**

weaned because the perinatal lamb mortality has been reduced by 5% due to ewes lambing with adequate colostrum accumulations, thereby preventing bacteraemia in their progeny following passive antibody transfer. Increased lamb birth weight is inversely correlated to perinatal mortality. As well as reducing mortality due to the increased lamb birth weight and improved immunoglobulin status, such changes also reduce focal bacterial infections such as polyarthritis, meningitis, omphalophlebitis and hypopyon, which were estimated to cause a 2% wastage in the 1,800 lambs born alive.

Turnout of ewes and lambs to pasture

Ewes and their 1–2-day-old lambs should be turned out in groups of 8–12 ewes in small 0.5 hectare paddocks, which have shelter provided on all sides. Ewes can be drawn to the sheltered areas by placing the feed troughs, root crops and hayracks in those areas. The lambs (and ewes?) are numbered to allow mothering-up at regular intervals, and especially just before dusk. After 2–3 days the ewes and lambs are walked into larger fields with more sheep.

WATERY MOUTH DISEASE

Definition/overview

Watery mouth disease is a colloquial expression used to describe a collection of clinical signs in neonatal lambs. This includes lethargy, unwillingness to search for the teat and suck, profuse salivation, increasing abdominal distension and retained meconium. The disease process is essentially one of endotoxaemia.

Aetiology

The condition is caused by colonization of the small intestine by *Escherichia coli*, with rapid multiplication followed by bacterial death and release of endotoxin from the cell wall. Initial contamination of the gastrointestinal tract results from a high environmental bacterial challenge in the dirty wet conditions of the lambing shed and pens. Colonization of the gut and rapid bacterial proliferation is facilitated by inadequate and/or delayed colostrum ingestion, especially in small, weakly triplet lambs.

Clinical presentation

Watery mouth disease is commonly encountered in twins but especially in triplet lambs aged 24–36 hours kept in unhygienic conditions. Affected lambs are dull, lethargic, depressed and reluctant to suck. They frequently lie in the corner of the pen and show little interest in sucking when encouraged to stand. They rarely stretch themselves when they stand. Within 2–6 hours there is profuse salivation, a wet lower jaw (205)

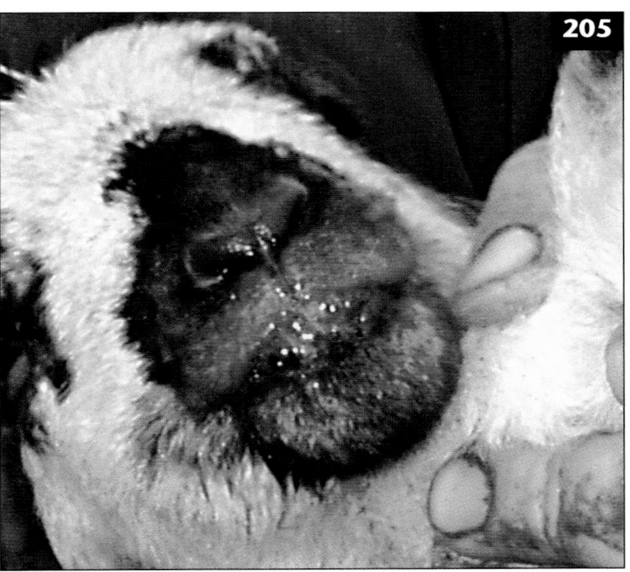

205 A 36-hour-old lamb with watery mouth disease. Note the wet lower jaw and excess salivation.

and increasing abdominal distension (**206**), even though the lamb has not been sucking. There is profound muscle weakness and the lamb is unable to stand (**207**). Scour is only a feature in the latter stages of disease in some lambs. Most lambs have retained meconium, which may be relieved after treatment (**206**) with a soapy water enema (washing-up liquid and warm water). The condition can quickly progress to coma and death.

Differential diagnoses

- Starvation/hypothermia/hypoglycaemia.
- Septicaemia.
- Intrapartum injury.
- Injury post partum, such as chest trauma.
- Toxoplasmosis.
- Border disease.

Diagnosis

Biochemistry reveals low plasma glucose concentration but elevated lactate and BUN concentrations consistent with endotoxaemia. Haematology reveals a leucopenia.

Necropsy reveals a grossly distended abomasum, which contains mucin, gas and unclotted milk. Care must be taken when interpreting these findings because the lamb may have been stomach tubed during the agonal stages of disease. The intestines are gas-filled; there may be meconium in the rectum. Bacteriological culture from liver, lungs, kidneys and heart blood often reveals evidence of agonal septicaemia.

Treatment

Soapy water enemas and mild laxatives/purgatives promote gut activity and expulsion of meconium during the early stages. (Metaclopramide administered orally is also effective but is too expensive for use in commercial flocks). These actions, in addition to supportive oral fluid therapy, are often effective in treating mild cases of watery mouth disease.

Oral antibiotics are effective during the early phase of the disease; an aminoglycoside such as neomycin or spectinomycin is probably the drug of choice because it maintains high concentrations within the gut. It is not unusual to find that a different antibiotic such as amoxicillin or apramycin may be needed towards the end of the lambing period, presumably due to selection for resistant strains of bacteria, although such epidemiology is seldom investigated in practice. Fluoroquinolone antibiotics such as enrofloxacin should be held in reserve and used only when all other measures and antibiotic treatments have failed.

Up to 40% of advanced clinical cases of watery mouth disease are bacteraemic; therefore, aminoglycoside antibiotics should not be used because they are not absorbed from the gut. These lambs are often treated with intramuscular amoxicillin.

Despite abomasal distension in lambs with watery mouth disease, oral electrolyte therapy (50 ml/kg q6h) is essential. Based on the endotoxic cause, administration of flunixin meglumine intravenously should be helpful but its use in farm situations is poorly documented. Intravenous fluid therapy, whether with isotonic or hypertonic saline, has not been documented. There is no evidence that lambs with endotoxaemia are acidotic and intravenous bicarbonate administration may be contraindicated.

Prevention/control measures

Problems with watery mouth disease are almost invariably encountered in housed flocks towards the end of the lambing period because of a build up of infection. Attempts must be made to improve hygiene standards in the lambing shed. Wherever possible the remaining pregnant ewes should be moved to another building or, weather permitting, turned out to pasture. Whilst not the primary factor in the disease process, it is still important to ensure adequate passive antibody transfer.

The single most effective means of controlling endotoxaemia in neonatal lambs in commercial sheep units is the administration of an oral antibiotic preparation within the first 15 minutes after birth

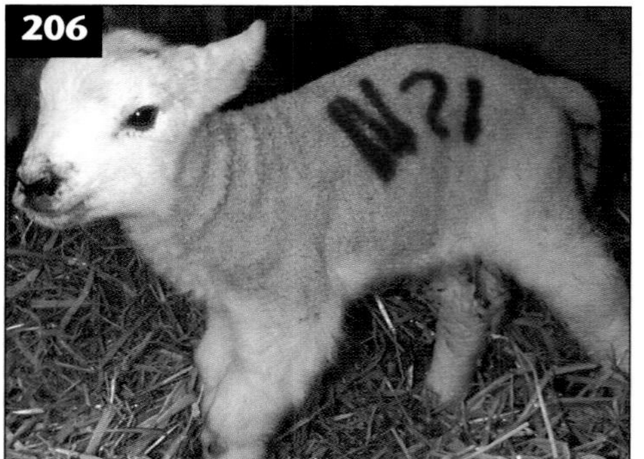

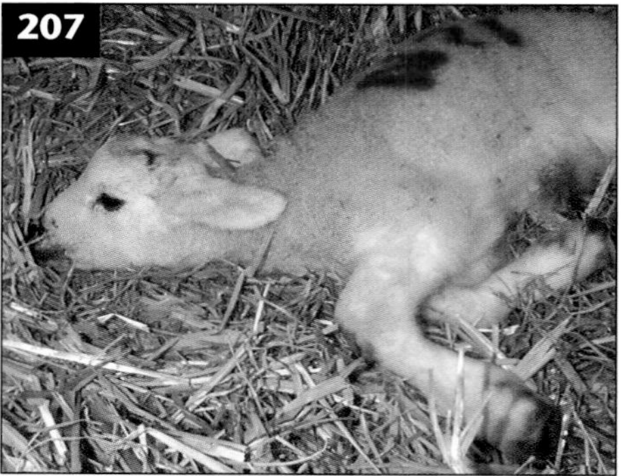

206 Depression with mild abdominal distension in a two-day-old lamb with watery mouth disease. The meconium (present on the tail and hindquarters) has been expelled after enema treatment by the farmer.

207 The lamb in **206** three hours later. There is marked abdominal distension and weakness.

(**208**); this limits bacterial colonization of the gut. On most farms it should be possible to delay the prophylactic use of oral antibiotics in lambs until the second half of the lambing period.

Control measures for neonatal infections should include:

- Abundant clean, dry straw bedding.
- Use of paraformaldehyde powder on straw bedding.
- Cleaning and disinfection of individual pens between lambing ewes.
- Collection and disposal of placentas.
- Ensuring that lambs suck colostrum as soon as possible following birth.

The role of probiotics in the prevention of watery mouth disease is uncertain, although competition between the live cultures of *Lactobacillus* species and *Streptococcus faecium* in the probiotic culture may limit proliferation of *E. coli* serotypes and other potentially pathogenic bacteria. The definitive probiotics control study is still awaited.

There are anecdotal reports that oral flunixin is effective in preventing watery mouth disease but substantive on-farm controlled studies are lacking.

Economics

There are no precise figures quantifying losses caused by watery mouth disease, because the bacteraemia that frequently accompanies the latter stages of this disease may be manifest subsequently as polyarthritis and lung and liver abscessation some days to weeks later. Assuming one quarter of perinatal lamb losses result from watery mouth disease, this approximates to 100 lambs in a 1,000 ewe lowland flock, which represents a significant loss of income to the sheep farmer. Therefore, reducing perinatal lamb mortality is key to increasing flock profitability.

The administration of an oral antibiotic preparation to every lamb within the first 15 minutes after birth costs approximately 0.2–0.5% of the anticipated market value of the lamb.

Welfare implications

Watery mouth disease is a major welfare concern because of the associated high mortality rate.

E. coli ENTERITIS

Definition/overview

Disease caused by enterotoxigenic strains of *E. coli* is relatively uncommon in sheep flocks.

Aetiology

Outbreaks of neonatal diarrhoea in lambs caused by enterotoxigenic strains of *E. coli* (e.g. K99 and F41 serotypes) are uncommon but may affect lambs less than four days old. There is rapid spread of disease in situations where lambs are crowded together (**209**).

Enterotoxigenic strains of *E. coli* possess two important properties: firstly fimbriae, which attach the bacterium to the enterocytes lining the gut; and secondly the production of an enterotoxin that interferes with normal water and electrolye transport mechanisms, causing net secretion and loss that leads to rapid dehydration.

Clinical presentation

Clinical signs include profuse yellow diarrhoea, with obvious staining of the tail and perineum (**210**), rapid dehydration, weakness and death within 24 hours of onset of signs. There is rapid dehydration resulting from secretion of water and electrolytes into the gastrointestinal tract, which becomes distended with fluid.

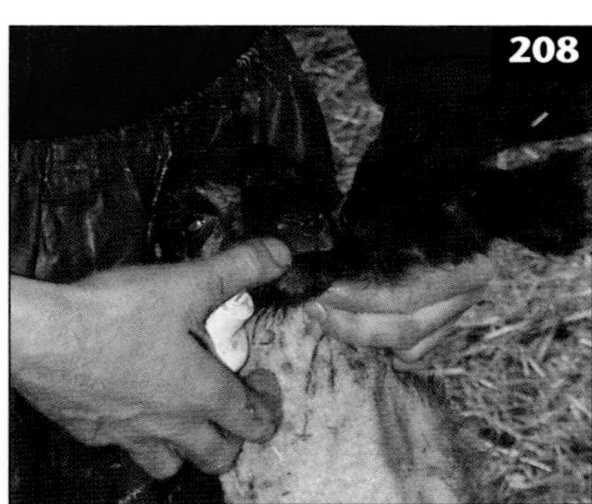

208 Administration of an oral antibiotic preparation within the first 15 minutes after birth. The lamb's fleece is still wet.

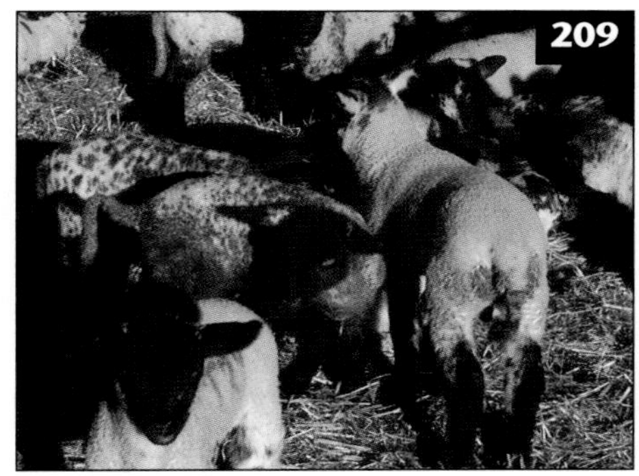

209 An outbreak of enteritis in a group of housed lambs. The stocking density is high.

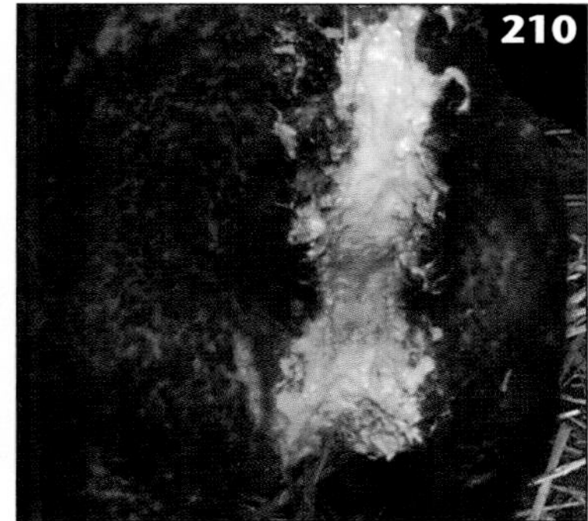

210 Profuse diarrhoea in a 36-hour-old lamb.

Differential diagnoses

- Watery mouth disease.
- Other *E. coli* infections.
- Cryptosporidiosis.
- Septicaemia.
- Salmonellosis.
- Lamb dysentery.

Diagnosis

Diagnosis requires faecal culture and serotyping for K99 and F41 fimbrial antigens.

Treatment

Affected lambs and their mothers should be isolated but this is rarely practical due to the high morbidity rate in the flock. Oral electrolyte therapy (50 ml/kg q6h) is essential for dehydrated lambs but this regimen presents considerable practical difficulties due to the large numbers of lambs affected.

Enterotoxigenic strains of *E. coli*, including K99 and F41 serotypes, are generally sensitive to the commonly used oral antibiotics such as neomycin or spectinomycin. They do not invade the gut wall and affected lambs do not develop a bacteraemia; therefore, systemic antibiotics are not necessary.

Prevention/control measures

Flocks with a history of infection with enterotoxigenic strains of *E. coli* (K99 and F41 serotypes) should be vaccinated eight and four weeks prior to the expected lambing date with multivalent vaccines containing these serotypes. However, such infections rarely become endemic on sheep farms and the infection may not appear in following years even if no action is taken. A compromise situation may be to vaccinate all introduced breeding stock and carefully monitor the disease situation.

Economics

Infection with enterotoxigenic strains of *E. coli* can cause considerable losses in young lambs, although figures will vary depending on the amount of supportive care provided.

Welfare implications

While infections with enterotoxigenic strains of *E. coli* only occur sporadically, they represent a major welfare concern because of the associated high mortality rate.

SALMONELLA SPECIES INFECTIONS

Definition/overview

Salmonellae serotypes are only a problem in young lambs if there is an obvious source of infection, either from an existing abortion problem in the ewes or infection gained from cattle or pasture contamination via sewage effluent.

Aetiology

There are many *Salmonella* species serotypes that can cause disease in lambs of all ages, particularly in young lambs when they are intensively managed and densely stocked:

- *S. typhimurium* can cause abortion in ewes and lead to further environmental contamination.
- *S. typhimurium* and *S. dublin* infections can be acquired from cattle by direct contact with aborted material or faeces, with the development of severe clinical signs.
- *S. typhimurium* and other serotypes can be contracted from sewage effluent.
- While *S. montevideo* is a common cause of abortion, neonatal enteritis is not a feature of this infection.

Clinical presentation

There is a wide range of clinical signs following infection, ranging from sudden death without premonitory signs to symptomless carrier sheep. The clinical signs are most severe in lambs less than one week old.

In young lambs there is rapid onset of dysentery, rapid dehydration, toxaemia, agonal septicaemia and death. Affected lambs appear gaunt and show signs of abdominal pain with frequent tenesmus. Initially, the rectal temperature may be raised but it becomes subnormal as the severity of signs increases. Dysentery is a feature of the disease in older lambs, when the faeces are malodorous and may contain mucosal casts and large blood clots.

Differential diagnoses

- Depending on age and management, coccidiosis is an important differential diagnosis of diarrhoea, tenesmus and passage of some blood clots, although toxaemia and sudden death are uncommon.
- Lamb dysentery should also be considered in lambs that have received no specific protective immunoglobulin for whatever reason.
- Nematodirosis can cause sudden death in lambs grazing infested pasture, while others in the group show signs of profuse diarrhoea.
- Causes of sudden death include pasteurellosis and other septicaemic conditions.

Diagnosis

The provisional diagnosis is based on clinical signs and elimination of other possible causes. Confirmation requires bacteriological isolation from faecal samples and viscera of septicaemic cases.

Treatment

While many exotic *Salmonella* species serotypes remain sensitive to most antibiotics, problems may arise with strains of *S. typhimurium*. Antibiotic selection can be directed by sensitivity testing in the latter group.

Prevention/control measures

It should be standard farm management that livestock do not have access to slurry storage areas. Overflow from septic tanks must be dealt with immediately. Sheep should not be co-grazed with cattle that have endemic salmonellosis. Feed storage areas must be vermin proof to prevent faecal contamination. Feeding areas must be changed daily to prevent environmental contamination by vermin and birds.

Economics

Salmonellosis is not a major economic problem in young lambs.

Welfare implications

Welfare concerns are addressed by prompt treatment. Recumbent sheep with dysentery should be euthanased.

OMPHALOPHLEBITIS (UMBILICAL INFECTION)

Definition/overview

Omphalophlebitis is common in young lambs (**211**) born in unsanitary conditions where there is inadequate navel treatment (**212, 213**). It is more common during inclement weather and in male lambs, presumably because urination delays desiccation of the umbilicus and removes some of the topical astringent/antibiotic applied by the shepherd, thus making bacterial invasion more likely.

Umbilical infections may remain localized and develop into a discrete abscess involving the body wall or they may extend to peritonitis, urachal infection and liver abscessation.

Aetiology

The consequences of nil or incorrect navel dressing include ascending infection to involve the body cavity, liver and urachus, and possibly more generalized infection involving the joints, meninges, lungs, kidneys and endocardium. Umbilical infection with *Fusobacterium necrophorum* and subsequent haematogenous spread to the liver causes the specific condition of hepatic necrobacillosis.

Clinical presentation

Septic peritonitis

The clinical signs vary with the extent and nature of the peritonitis. Lambs that develop septic peritonitis appear very dull and weak within the first week of life. They stand with their back arched and their head held lowered (**214**) and they spend long periods lying

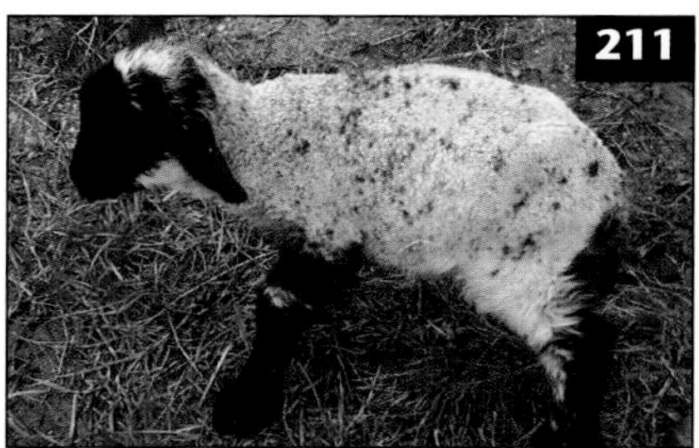

211 Depressed and lethargic four-day-old lamb suffering from omphalophlebitis and associated peritonitis. The lamb has a roached back stance and a painful expression.

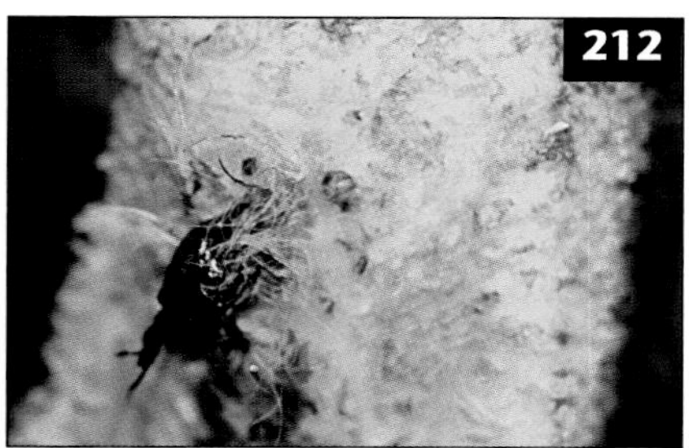

212 Totally inadequate navel dressing. There is umbilical swelling.

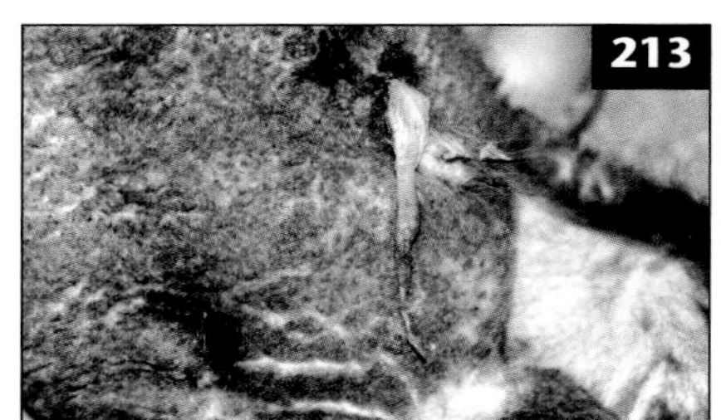

213 Totally inadequate navel dressing. The umbilicus is wet and there is abdominal distension due to peritoneal exudate.

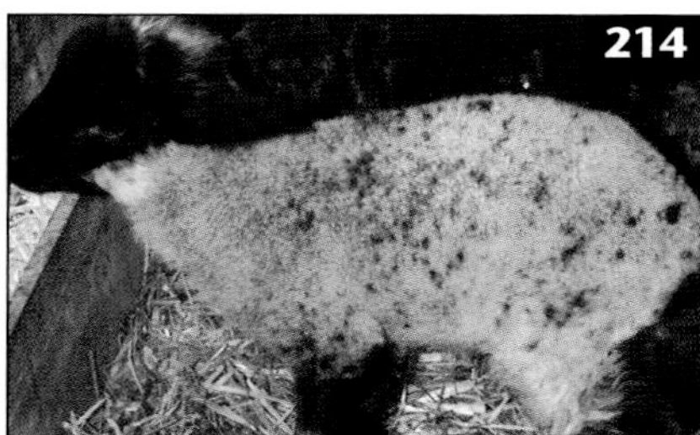

214 Depressed four-day-old lamb suffering from omphalophlebitis and associated peritonitis. The lamb has a painful expression.

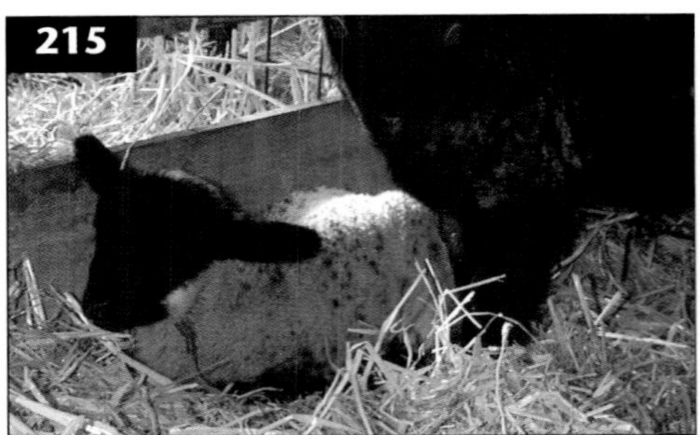

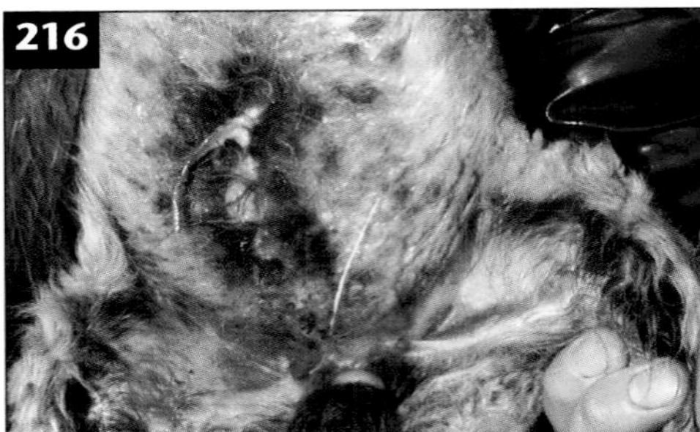

215 The attitude of the lamb in **214** is quite different to that of its healthy co-twin shown here.

216 Six-day-old lamb suffering from omphalophlebitis and associated peritonitis. The umbilicus is wet and there is abdominal distension.

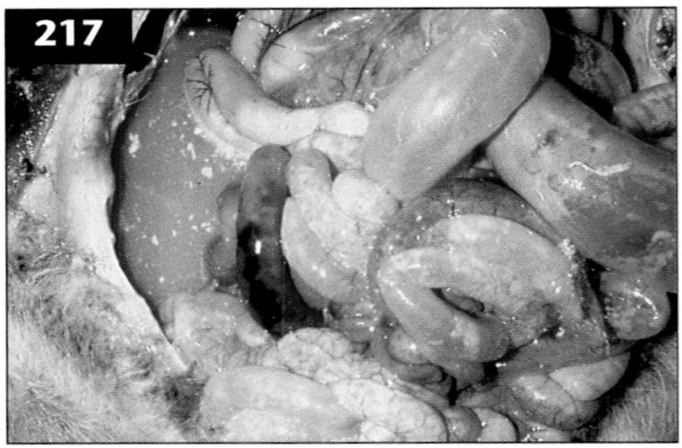

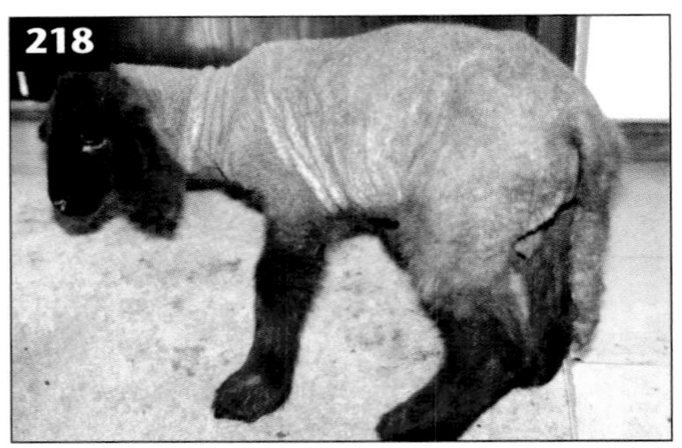

217 The lamb in **216** showing diffuse suppurative peritonitis arising from the umbilical infection.

218 Three-week-old lamb suffering from hepatic necrobacillosis.

in the corner of the pen (**215**). The rectal temperature may be subnormal. There is rapid loss of body condition and a prominent ribcage and bony prominences. This contrasts markedly with the well-muscled contours of the healthy co-twin (**215**). These lambs do not suck but there is increasing exudation in the peritoneal cavity, which causes moderate distension (**216**), contrasts with the lamb's gaunt appearance and expression. The abdomen may contain up to 200 ml of turbid fluid, with large fibrin clots that may develop to pus following cellular infiltration and bacterial multiplication (**217**). Affected lambs rapidly become dehydrated and die within a few days of clinical signs first appearing.

Localized fibrinous peritonitis

Peritoneal lesions may often be restricted to a small number of fibrin tags, which adhere readily to intestine and may loop around intestine, causing stricture and/or occlusion. This presentation is not uncommon when infection has extended along the urachus. These lambs present with a distended abomasum and small intestine proximal to the constriction and often show signs of mild colic, which may be mistaken for abomasal bloat. An overenthusiastic shepherd who continues to administer fluids by orogastric tube because the lamb is not sucking may exacerbate the abdominal distension. The important clinical feature in this condition is the absence of faeces over the preceding few days but such information is rarely available to the clinician.

Hepatic necrobacillosis

The clinical presentation of hepatic necrobacillosis depends on the number, site and size of the liver lesions. Abscesses involving the liver capsule, which stimulate localized peritonitis with adhesion formation to adjacent small intestine, are more important than deeper-seated lesions.

Typically, affected lambs are first noted from 10–14 days old, when they appear dull and depressed and are in much poorer condition than their co-twin. They have an empty, gaunt appearance and are too easily caught in the field. Many affected lambs may not follow the ewe and co-twin and they are found sheltering behind walls and hedgerows. Affected lambs stand with an arched back and all four limbs drawn together (**218**). In some lambs the liver can be palpated extending beyond the costal arch, and digital pressure caudal to the xiphisternum may elicit a painful response. Affected lambs are much more prone to predation than healthy lambs.

Differential diagnoses

Septic peritonitis

- Enteric infections.
- Abomasal bloat/torsion.
- Atresia coli.

Localized fibrinous peritonitis

- Watery mouth disease.
- Pyloric outflow obstruction (e.g. wool ball).
- Abomasal bloat/torsion.
- Atresia coli.

Hepatic necrobacillosis
- Starvation.
- Pneumonia.
- Polyarthritis.
- Coccidiosis.
- Nephrosis.

Diagnosis
Septic peritonitis
Abdominocentesis of turbid fluid with a high protein concentration and large numbers of degenerative white cells confirms the clinical diagnosis of septic peritonitis. Direct smears stained with Gram's stain may identify clumps of bacteria. Care must be taken not to penetrate the abomasum during abdominocentesis; therefore, this should be undertaken only after ultrasonographic demonstration of excess peritoneal fluid.

Localized fibrinous peritonitis
Diagnosis of gut stricture caused by fibrin tags is not simple. Ultrasonography typically reveals a grossly distended abomasum with little or no fluid within the intestines. It may be possible to visualize fibrin tags within excess peritoneal fluid but large accumulations are uncommon; therefore, abdominocentesis would not usually be undertaken.

Hepatic necrobacillosis
Diagnosis of hepatic necrobacillosis is based on clinical signs and the presence of anterior abdominal pain. Ultrasonography reveals the presence of liver abscess(es) and focal adhesions. Normal blood urea nitrogen concentration allows nephrosis to be excluded from the list of differential diagnoses. The diagnosis is confirmed at necropsy (**219**) when affected lambs are euthanased for welfare reasons.

Treatment
Treatment of septic peritonitis is hopeless and lambs should be euthanased as soon as the diagnosis is established. Prompt recognition and antibiotic treatment of hepatic necrobacillosis may arrest growth of the infective lesions; thereafter, liver regeneration may restore health. However, this is largely supposition and the extent to which the liver regenerates in hepatic necrobacillosis remains unknown.

Prevention/control measures
The umbilicus (navel) must be fully immersed in strong veterinary iodine BP (**220–222**) within the first 15 minutes of life. This must be repeated at least 2–4 hours later. Antibiotic aerosol sprays are much inferior to strong veterinary iodine BP for dressing navels and are much more expensive. All umbilical infections are a direct consequence of the farmer's neglect of sound husbandry practices.

Economics
Failure to adopt sound management practices with respect to hygiene standards and routine navel dressings can lead to considerable lamb mortality.

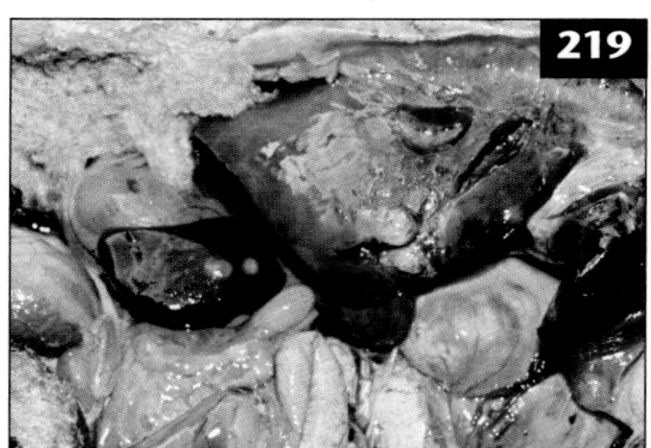

219 Necropsy findings of abscessation in the liver and associated peritonitis.

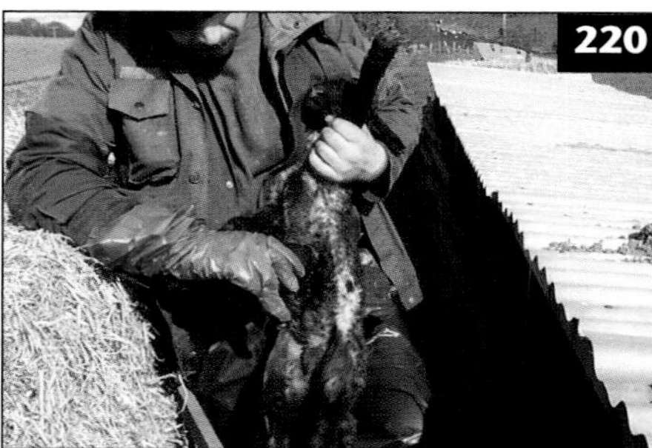

220 Correct navel dressing in the field.

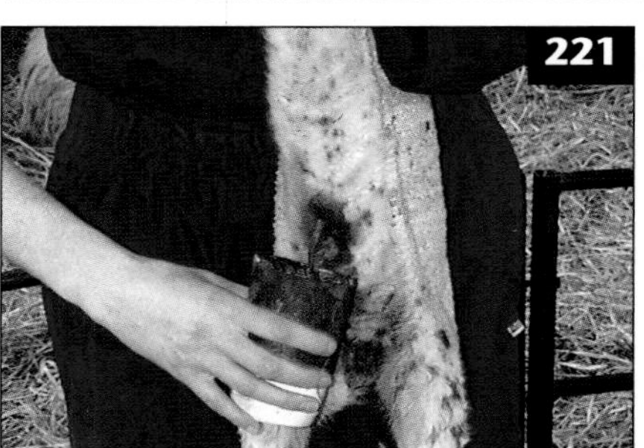

221 Complete immersion of the umbilicus in strong iodine solution.

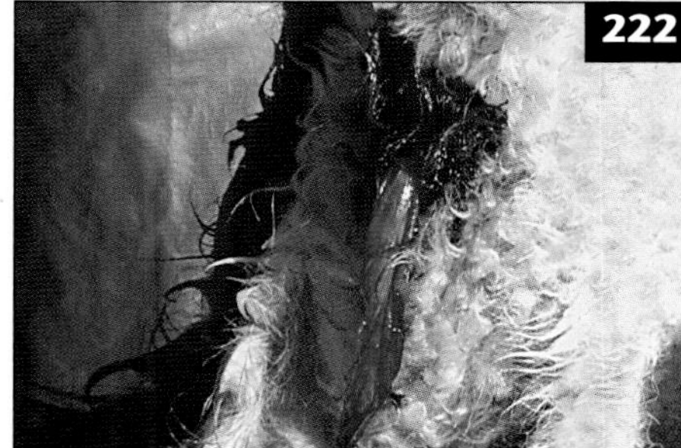

222 Correct application of strong iodine solution.

Welfare implications

Lambs with peritonitis appear gaunt and in obvious pain. Liver abscessation leads to debility and eventual death. This suffering is all the more poignant because it can be readily prevented.

POSTMORTEM EXAMINATION OF NEONATAL LOSSES

Postmortem examination of a representative number of neonatal deaths provides a great deal of useful information regarding lamb starvation and other causes of neonatal losses. The examinations can be undertaken very quickly on the farm and can highlight the cause(s) of death and allow control and prevention measures to be adopted. It is vitally important that a representative sample of lambs is necropsied; this is best achieved by examining all the lambs that have died one or two days previous to the veterinary visit, depending on the number. Care should be exercised if the visit is preceded by adverse weather conditions or other potentially unique events, as this could distort the data collected. This is overcome by undertaking necropsies on serial batches of lambs.

Lamb identified by farmer

Litter size, dam parity, dystocia, any illness and/or treatment and the age at death should be noted. Losses from starvation/exposure are greater in twins and triplets and this is associated with lower birth weight. Losses caused by dystocia are highest in primiparous females, especially if lambed as yearlings.

Lamb weight

Depending on the breed and live weight of the ewe, lambs <3.5 kg are more prone to starvation/exposure, while lambs with birth weights >5.5–6 kg are more likely to have caused dystocia.

Gross inspection

The presence of blood staining of the fleece and subcutaneous oedema of the head and hindlimbs may indicate dystocia. A dark yellow/brown discoloration of the whole fleece indicates meconium staining, which may reflect prolonged second stage labour/dystocia.

A tapered end to the umbilicus indicates prepartum death; a square end indicates death soon after parturition; and a dry shrivelled cord indicates death after 12 hours or more, although this appearance is influenced by iodine or other topical treatment. A blood clot within the umbilical vessels indicates that death occurred after first stage labour.

Necropsy

The lamb is positioned in dorsal recumbency and incisions are made between the chest wall and the scapulae. The strip of skin left covering the sternum is reflected toward the pubis and removed, taking care not to enter the abdominal cavity. An incision can be made into each hip joint to aid stabilization but is not necessary. The skin should also be removed from the ventral neck region and extended to the jaw to allow examination of the thyroid glands. Dead lambs have often had their skin removed for fostering purposes. This affords ready examination of the hindlimb extremities for signs of oedema caused by dystocia.

The abdominal wall is tented and an incision made immediately caudal to the sternum and extended caudally to the pubis with scissors, thus avoiding puncturing any viscus. The sternum is then removed by cutting through the costochondral junctions using a knife. (**NB**: A scalpel blade will suffice but it may snap.) The size and contents of the abomasum should be noted. The abomasum of well-fed lambs contains numerous large milk clots up to 2–3 cm in diameter, as well as milk. The presence of unclotted milk suggests feeding immediately prior to death. There should be evidence of chyle in the intestinal lymphatics. The presence of meconium should be noted.

The abomasum and intestines are then lifted out of the abdomen to allow inspection of the kidneys and the perirenal fat deposits. In normal lambs the kidneys are embedded in 5–10 mm of fat and are not visible (**223**). Exhaustion of fat reserves in starved neonatal lambs can occur within days, and the kidneys will be clearly visible. Fat reserves are also mobilized from the epicardial groove. Haemorrhage into the abdomen,

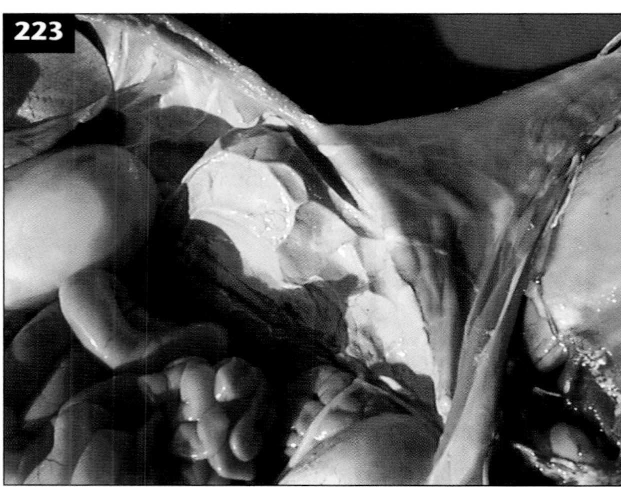

223 Necropsy revealing adequate perirenal fat.

with formation of large blood clots, is uncommon but may result from liver lobe rupture.

Full expansion and aeration of the lungs can be checked by immersion in water: aerated lung floats, unexpanded lung sinks. The pericardium is incised to check for excess fluid and mobilization of epicardial fat.

Removal of the brain and spinal cord is rarely undertaken during on-farm investigations of perinatal lamb mortality. Intrapartum injury to the CNS during dystocia is reported to result in subdural, subarachnoid and extradural haemorrhages, with a prevalence of 21% in lambs that died compared with 1.4% in a control group. However, other signs of dystocia such as peripheral oedema and haemorrhages in the thymus, pleurae, and epicardium are more easily observed during on-farm investigations.

STARVATION/EXPOSURE

Deaths due to starvation/exposure occur 1–3 days after birth. They are much more common in multiple births and in litters of ewes in poor condition with intercurrent illness such as mastitis or metritis.

Exposure

Losses occur within the first day of life, typically within the first 6–8 hours where there is poor supervision. During adverse weather conditions (e.g. winter storms, cold driving winds and snow) lambs can die of exposure, although there will be few lesions detected at necropsy. The lambs may not have risen, walked or sucked, and they are often found in the morning, where they were born, in lateral recumbency. All the lambs in a litter may be found dead. There are fewer losses of singletons. The lamb's coat may still be covered with fetal fluids. Necropsy findings may reveal peripheral oedema, absence of colostrum and depletion of fat reserves.

Starvation

If a lamb has died of starvation, there is an absence of milk clots and milk in the abomasum and no evidence of chyle in the intestinal lymphatics. The kidneys are clearly visible and fat reserves are also mobilized from the epicardial groove. There is loss of mesenteric fat. The liver may be smaller and less friable than normal.

CLINICAL PROBLEM 1

A six-day-old Suffolk-cross lamb presented in much poorer condition than its co-twin (224). The lamb was dull and weak, and stood with its head held lowered.

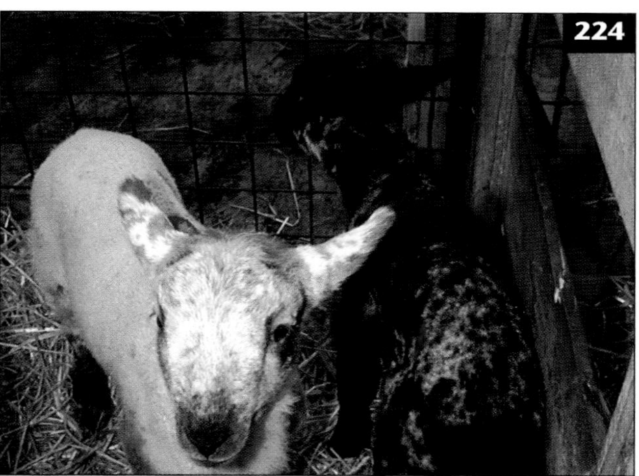

224 Suffolk-cross lamb presented in much poorer condition than its co-twin.

The rectal temperature was subnormal (38.0°C). The heart rate was 90 bpm. The mucous membranes appeared congested. The respiratory rate was increased to 40 breaths per minute. No abnormal sounds were heard on auscultation of the chest. The umbilicus was wet. Careful abdominal palpation over the umbilicus and caudal to the xiphisternum elicited a painful response. There was no evidence of diarrhoea. The ewe showed no evidence of mastitis to account for the lamb's poor condition.

What conditions should be considered in the differential diagnosis list?
What is the provisional diagnosis and how could this be confirmed?

Differential diagnosis list

- Localized peritonitis following umbilical infection.
- Hepatic necrobacillosis.
- Starvation.
- Viral pneumonia with secondary bacterial infection.
- Polyarthritis.
- Wool balls (trichobezoars).
- Nephrosis.

Provisional diagnosis

Hepatic necrobacillosis and/or localized peritonitis following umbilical infection.

Treatment

The lamb was treated with procaine penicillin (44,000 iu/kg i/m) for the next two days. There was no improvement in the lamb's clinical appearance and it was euthanased for welfare reasons.

Postmortem examination
Postmortem examination revealed diffuse peritonitis associated with the umbilicus, and early abscesses within the liver.

Action
The importance of careful immersion of the whole of the umbilicus in strong veterinary iodine BP was once again emphasized to the farming staff. It was revealed that the night lambing person was only spraying the umbilicus of lambs with antibiotic spray.

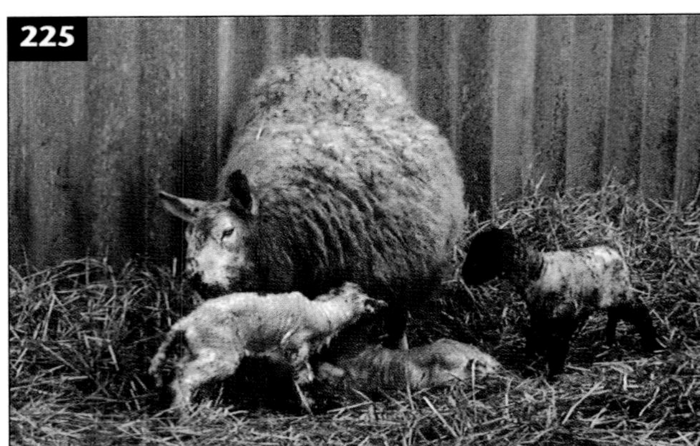

225 A ewe with triplets. What is the immediate fate of these lambs?

CLINICAL PROBLEM 2

A client complains of an unacceptable perinatal lamb mortality rate of 25% in his lowland flock this year, particularly involving triplet lambs (**225**). He asks advice on how to reduce such losses next year.

Describe a possible preventive medicine flock plan, and how the success or failure of the plan could be monitored?

Background
Correct lamb birth weight, together with good ewe body condition and adequate colostrum accumulation at lambing, remain fundamental to ensuring a good start for the lamb during the critical first 36 hours of life. Adequate ewe nutrition during the last six weeks of pregnancy, when 75% of fetal growth occurs, is essential to ensure appropriate lamb birth weights.

Flock plan
Fifteen to 20 ewes due to lamb during the first week should be body condition scored and blood sampled for plasma 3-OH butyrate concentration four weeks before the start of lambing time, thus allowing sufficient time to implement dietary changes. If the flock has been scanned to determine fetal number, an equal number of twin-and triplet-bearing ewes should be sampled. Details of the diet, forage analyses and future alterations should be noted.

Results and interpretation
The target mean 3-OH butyrate concentration is <1.0 mmol/l. 3-OH butyrate concentrations >1.6 mmol/l in individual ewes represent severe energy underfeeding. There is a likelihood of OPT developing as pregnancy advances and fetal energy requirements increase further unless dietary changes are implemented.

Once the mean 3-OH butyrate concentration has been determined, any alteration in the ration can be made with reference to Russel[1] and the farmer advised immediately by telephone, and in writing, regarding any dietary or management changes. The flock should be re-visited and blood samples collected two weeks later to check on progress and further monitor any changes in the body condition scores.

Evaluation of protein status
Blood samples can also be analysed for BUN, which indicates short-term protein intake, and albumin, which reflects longer-term protein status.

Follow-up visit during lambing time
It is important to determine the lamb mortality rate and the causes of these deaths. It should be possible to reduce the lamb mortality rate to single figures.

Measurement (with a spring balance) and recording of lamb birth weights and ewe body condition scores is also essential to determine how successful the flock nutrition advice has been during late gestation. The target birth weight of triplet lambs is 4.5 kg but 4 kg would be acceptable. Lambs <3.5 kg have a very poor survival potential. Postmortem examination of any neonatal deaths will also provide much useful information regarding lamb starvation.

REFERENCE

1 Russel A (1985) Nutrition of the pregnant ewe. *In Practice* 7, 23–28.

5 Digestive System

CLINICAL EXAMINATION OF THE DIGESTIVE SYSTEM

Diagnosis of abdominal disorders in sheep raises numerous difficulties not encountered in cattle:

- Sheep are managed extensively in flocks and individual information such as appetite, defaecation, urination and daily production (milk yield and/or lamb appearance and growth rate) are often unknown.
- Disorders tend to be more chronic and/or severe in sheep than in cattle before detection and presentation to the veterinarian.
- Unlike cattle, rectal examination does not form part of the veterinarian's clinical examination.
- The low economic value of individual sheep frequently limits the veterinarian's scope for detailed laboratory testing.

HISTORY

Examination of the digestive system in sheep should be preceded by obtaining a history of the dietary management, as type and quantity of particular feeds determine the extent of rumen fill, frequency of ruminal contractions and faecal consistency. Sheep fed fibrous diets have a more distended rumen than those fed solely concentrates. They will have one or two full contraction cycles per minute, which is more frequent than sheep fed large quantities of concentrates.

Sheep normally pass pelleted faeces, except when grazing very lush pastures when soft stools are passed; diarrhoea is an abnormal finding under all feeding systems. The presence of dried faeces staining the tail and perineum indicates a prior episode of diarrhoea and is abnormal. Dry, mucus-coated faeces indicate an extended transport time through the gastrointestinal tract.

EXAMINATION OF THE BUCCAL CAVITY

Sheep with lesions within the buccal cavity usually present in poor condition due to impaired feeding. The lower jaw is wet because of drooling of saliva. Lesions affecting the cheek result in obvious firm swellings. Infected lesions of the cheek and/or tongue may cause halitosis and swelling of the submandibular lymph node(s).

Correct dentition is of critical importance to the maintenance of body condition/weight gain in sheep. The importance of examining the mouth fully, with particular reference to the molar teeth, cannot be overemphasized. Overgrown, worn and absent molar teeth cause serious problems with mastication of fibrous feeds.

Sheep have 32 permanent teeth, with a dental formula of 2 (incisors 0/4, premolars 3/3 and molars 3/3). Some textbooks correctly refer to the fourth (lateral or corner) incisor as the canine tooth but in essence it functions as an incisor tooth. The temporary incisor teeth erupt sequentially at approximately weekly intervals from birth. The three temporary premolars erupt within 2–6 weeks. The first permanent molar erupts at three and five months in the lower and upper jaws, respectively. The second permanent molar erupts at 9–12 months and the third permanent molar and permanent premolars erupt between 18 and 24 months.

Examination of incisor teeth alignment is first performed by running an index finger along the dental pad to check incisor teeth contact. This will reveal any teeth projecting forward of (overshot jaw or prognathia) or behind (undershot jaw or brachygnathia) the normal contact on the dental pad. This examination must be undertaken with the mouth closed and the head held in the normal resting position. The incisor teeth can then be viewed by pulling down the lower lip, when the points should still contact with the dental pad in normal sheep.

Molar tooth problems can best be identified by impaction of food in the cheeks and observing short jerky jaw movements with the mouth held slightly open. This results from excessive tooth growth or cheek lesions causing pain during mastication. The sheep will often raise its head to assist movement of the food bolus over the dorsum of the tongue and during swallowing. Where there is frequent quidding, affected sheep often have pieces of fibrous feed protruding from the commissures of the mouth. Careful palpation of the dental arcade through the cheek reveals the sharp irregular ridges of the labial aspect of the upper cheek teeth and any lost upper cheek teeth. There is no enlargement of submandibular lymph nodes associated with molar tooth loss. Examination of the molar teeth with a gag and torch is essential, but lengthy examination is greatly resented by sheep. Radiographs can provide useful information of the jaw and cheek teeth but it can prove difficult not to superimpose the cheek teeth of the contralateral jaw, even using oblique views. Detailed examination of the molar teeth with a view to removal of sharp hooks, and possibly loose teeth, necessitates general anaesthesia, which can be readily and inexpensively achieved using intravenous pentobarbital injection (see Chapter 15: General anaesthesia, p. 315).

Examination of the mandible

The horizontal rami of the mandible can be readily palpated through the skin. Despite the common finding of loose cheek teeth and missing teeth, tooth root abscesses with associated new bone deposition and sinus formation along the ventral margin are uncommon in sheep.

Tumours involving the mandible (e.g. fibrosarcoma) appear over many months as a unilateral, firm, 3–5 cm diameter swelling of the horizontal ramus but they are rare in sheep.

Examination of the pharynx

Pharyngeal trauma is not uncommon following balling gun or drenching gun injury in growing lambs; however, these injuries are often not detected until infection has either extended into the cervical vertebral canal, resulting in tetraparesis, or localized abscess development has caused compression of the larynx with stertorous breathing, by which stage detailed examination of the primary route of infection is of secondary concern. Despite localized infection of the pharynx, it can prove difficult to palpate the enlarged retropharyngeal lymph nodes.

Good visualization of the pharynx can be achieved under general anaesthesia. General anaesthesia is also necessary to permit complete endoscopic examination of the pharynx.

Examination of the oesophagus

Oesophageal lesions are very uncommon in sheep. While choke may occasionally occur within the proximal cervical oesophagus in sheep fed dried sugar beet or similar, this is usually relieved following retching and vigorous head tossing. The cervical oesophagus can be palpated and the presence or absence of an obstruction ascertained by careful passage of a flexible orogastric tube through a suitable mouth gag. Forcing an oesophageal obstruction using an orogastric tube should not be attempted because of the likelihood of causing perforation of the oesophagus.

Examination of the forestomachs

When viewed from behind, the rumen in normal sheep pushes the lower left flank beyond the outline of the costal arch but this is usually masked by the fleece and, therefore, must be palpated. Bloat causing distension of the left sublumbar fossa is uncommon in sheep, except for those ewes with advanced hypocalcaemia.

Auscultation of the rumen is performed in the upper left flank, with the fleece parted to gain good contact between the stethoscope and the skin. The flank is then firmly pressed to contact the dorsal sac of the rumen; any gap between the rumen wall and abdominal wall will greatly reduce transmitted sounds. There are two independent reticuloruminal contraction sequences: a primary biphasic contraction cycle of the reticulum followed by rumen contractions, which occurs approximately once a minute and mixes ingesta and forces small particles into the omasum; and a secondary contraction that does not involve the reticulum but rumen activity pushes the gas cap into the cardia region, with resultant eructation. Typically, one secondary cycle follows two primary cycles so that three cycles occur every two minutes. Due to the fibrous nature of the ration, sheep fed fibrous diets have a more distended rumen, with more frequent contractions, than those fed solely concentrates.

Rumen fluid collection and analysis

With a suitable mouth gag in place, rumen fluid can be easily collected by aspiration through a wide bore orogastric tube. Possible saliva contamination can be reduced by discarding the first few millilitres; a minimum of 20 ml of rumen fluid should be collected. There is no justification for collecting a sample by percutaneous rumenocentesis.

The rumen fluid can be analysed for colour, odour, pH, protozoa, sedimentation rate and methylene blue reduction time. Normal rumen fluid is green, has an aromatic odour, a pH of 6.5–8.0 and many variably-sized motile protozoa per microscope field (×100). The methylene blue reduction time is abnormal if extended beyond 6–8 minutes.

GENERAL EXAMINATION OF THE ABDOMEN

Radiography

Radiography is rarely used to investigate abdominal disorders in sheep because lesions caused by radiodense materials such as ingested sharp metallic objects are rare; fluid accumulations are better demonstrated by ultrasonography and this also avoids the attendant health and safety restrictions.

ABDOMINOCENTESIS

Abdominocentesis is undertaken when excess fluid is identified by ultrasonography. Excess peritoneal fluid associated with peritonitis is very uncommon in sheep because infections are largely confined by the omentum. Large accumulations of peritoneal fluid do occur in sheep with conditions such as subacute fasciolosis and intestinal adenocarcinoma, and in sheep with cor pulmonale. Peritoneal fluid samples can be collected from a midline site immediately caudal to the xiphisternum.

Peritoneal fluid should be collected into tubes containing EDTA. Normal peritoneal fluid has a clear, slightly yellow appearance, a protein concentration of 10–30 g/l and a white cell concentration, comprised mainly of lymphocytes, of $<1 \times 10^6$/l. Infectious peritonitis typically results in a turbid sample with a high protein concentration and a high white cell concentration comprised mainly of neutrophils.

ABDOMINAL ULTRASONOGRAPHY

While ultrasonography has been successfully employed in commercial flocks for the past 20 years to determine fetal number and gestation length, thus permitting more precise ewe nutrition and management during late gestation, transabdominal ultrasonographic examination can also include the peritoneal cavity (ascites, uroperitoneum, peritonitis, abscess involving the body wall), liver, rumen, reticulum, abomasum, bladder, kidney, uterus and fetus(es).

Ultrasonographic equipment

A 5.0 MHz linear transducer connected to a real-time, B-mode ultrasound machine can be used for all abdominal ultrasonographic examinations except examination of the right kidney and liver, where a 5.0 MHz sector transducer is necessary to ensure good contact with the concave flank of the right sublumbar fossa and between the convex intercostal spaces, respectively. The field setting of 10 cm on the linear scanner is appropriate for most abdominal examinations; occasionally, the 20 cm field depth afforded by certain 5.0 MHz sector scanners more accurately determines the extent of fluid accumulation and bladder diameter but this does not significantly alter the diagnosis.

Good contact between the probe head and skin is essential to allow transmission of sound waves. The hair-free area of the abdominal wall in the inguinal region allows examination of the caudal abdomen. Ultrasonographic examination of the cranial abdomen (e.g. reticulum and abomasum in adults) is rarely undertaken in sheep but can be readily achieved after shaving the wool off with a razor or scalpel blade. The skin is then wetted with either alcohol or tap water, and ultrasound gel liberally applied. The probe head is held firmly at right angles against the abdominal wall.

Transrectal examination of the bladder and rectum has been reported in both ewes and rams but this examination has not proved necessary in practice to determine obstructive urolithiasis. Examination of the entire liver may necessitate using a 3.5 MHz convex transducer but this results in loss of definition and image quality.

Ultrasonographic appearance of normal abdominal viscera

The abdominal wall is 1–3 cm thick depending on the site being examined and the BCS of the sheep. There is scant peritoneal fluid in normal sheep and this cannot be visualized during ultrasonographic examination.

Reticular motility can readily be observed in the cranial abdomen immediately caudal to the left costal arch. The liver can readily be visualized from halfway down the right costal arch with the probe head angled towards the left shoulder. Alternatively, the liver can be imaged halfway down the eight to tenth intercostal spaces with the probe head held at a right angle to the chest wall.

The intestines are clearly outlined as broad hyperechoic (white) lines/circles containing material of varying echogenicity. By maintaining the probe head in the same position for 10–20 seconds, digesta can be visualized as multiple small dots of varying echogenicity forcibly propelled within the intestines. Such movement of intestinal contents prevents confusion with other structures, such as an abscess or fluid accumulation within the uterine horns (metritis/pyometra), that may present with a similar sonographic appearance but with the contents remaining static.

The bladder rarely extends beyond the pubis and therefore is not visualized in normal sheep.

Ascites

Ascites can prove difficult to quantify by ballotment, especially in sheep with fluid-distended intestines, but it is readily identified during ultrasonography examination, even in recumbent sheep (**226, 227**). Ascites can be present without significant accumulation of fluid at other sites such as subcutaneous tissue in the submandibular region (bottle-jaw) and brisket. Ascitic fluid appears as an anechoic (black) area with abdominal viscera displaced dorsally.

Ascites must be differentiated from urine accumulation but uroperitoneum is always accompanied by bladder distension, so permitting immediate differentiation from ascitic fluid.

Abdominal wall

The extent of subcutaneous urine accumulation along the prepuce and ventral abdominal wall can be accurately defined in male sheep with urethral rupture. Abscesses involving the body wall, caused by penetration wounds, dog bites and faulty injection/ vaccination technique, occur occasionally. Such abscesses appear as anechoic areas containing multiple bright hyperechoic (white) dots within a well-defined capsule (**228**).

Peritonitis

Significant peritoneal exudation is rarely seen in sheep. Reaction is limited to focal fibrinous/fibrous adhesions and localized accumulation of peritoneal fluid. When present, the hyperechoic lattice-work appearance of the fibrinous reaction within the abdomen contrasts with the anechoic peritoneal fluid.

Localized fibrinous peritonitis has been reported recently in severe cases of subacute fasciolosis (**229**).

Occasionally, the peritoneal reaction is limited to a few fibrinous adhesions, which cannot be visualized. In this situation the intestines proximal to the lesion(s) are distended with fluid (anechoic appearance) rather than containing normal digesta (anechoic appearance containing multiple bright dots), and there are no propulsive intestinal contractions.

Liver

Large liver abscesses caused by *Corynebacterium pseudotuberculosis*, the causal agent of caseous lymphadenitis (CLA), are common in many sheep-producing countries. In the UK, visceral CLA is a rare manifestation of infection. Gall bladder distension is a common finding in cachectic sheep. Hepatomegaly can be identified in sheep with subacute fasciolosis. Fibrinous adhesions between the liver and adjacent intestines have been identified ultrasonographically in sheep with fasciolosis (**229**).

Bladder, kidney and uterus

Further information on ultrasonographic examination of the bladder and kidney can be found in Chapter 9 (p. 236) and of the uterus in Chapter 3: Part 1 (p. 33).

Abomasum in neonates

Ultrasonographic examination of the abomasum of neonatal lambs (**230**) provides an immediate indication as to whether lambs have sucked or not, and may highlight an area for more detailed examination whilst the veterinarian is present on the farm. The difference in lamb abomasal diameter before and after sucking is so large (3 cm versus 8–10 cm) that minor errors in individual lamb recordings should not affect the collection of meaningful data from 20 or more lambs.

TEETH/DENTITION

INCISOR LOSS (*Syn*: broken mouth)

Definition/overview

Premature loss of incisor teeth is a major problem in most sheep-producing countries, including New Zealand and Australia. It leads to early culling because affected sheep are unable to bite short pasture, which results in malnutrition, poor production and weight loss, particularly on marginal grazing and hill pastures. In the UK, culling for reproductive reasons traditionally follows six crops of lambs but incisor tooth loss may affect two-crop ewes on some farms; this represents major production and financial losses.

Incisor wear is the main dental problem of sheep in New Zealand. In some areas early culling of ewes is due to excessive incisor wear.

Aetiology

Incisor loss is preceded by repeated bouts of acute gingivitis, which result in fibrosis and recession of the gingival margin with subsequent damage to the supporting periodontal ligament. While this aetiology implies bacterial involvement, it may not explain the geographic prevalence of broken mouth. The incisor teeth develop an elongated appearance (**231**), become loose and are eventually lost (**232**). This process may take from one to four years.

Clinical presentation

Incisor teeth loss is readily recognized during checks for correct dentition undertaken routinely as part of the selection procedure pre-mating. Broken mouth can lead to chronic weight loss in situations where there is competition for grazing and grass length is short. Loosening of incisor teeth is readily appreciated under gentle digital pressure.

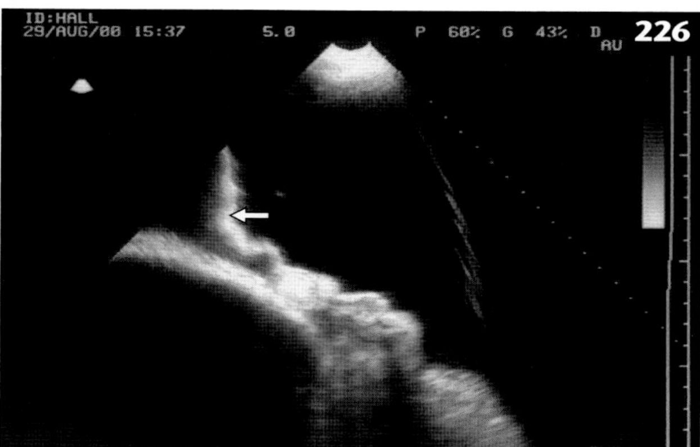

226 Ultrasonogram (5 MHz sector probe). Extensive ascites. The fluid accumulation is seen as an anechoic area; the greater omentum has a broad hyperechoic ribbon-like appearance (arrow). The probe was positioned in the ventral midline and pointed dorsally with the sheep in the standing position. The rumen has been displaced dorsally by the fluid accumulations.

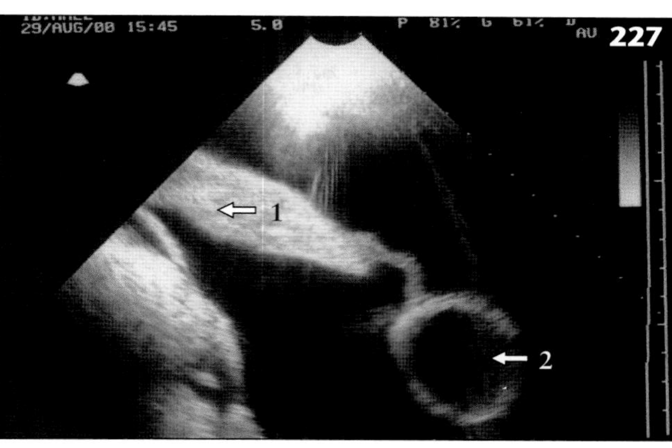

227 Ultrasonogram (5 MHz sector probe). Extensive ascites allowing excellent visualization of the liver (**1**) and gall bladder (wall appearing as a 6 cm diameter circle [**2**]). The liver appears more hyperechoic than normal, consistent with changes resulting from chronic venous congestion.

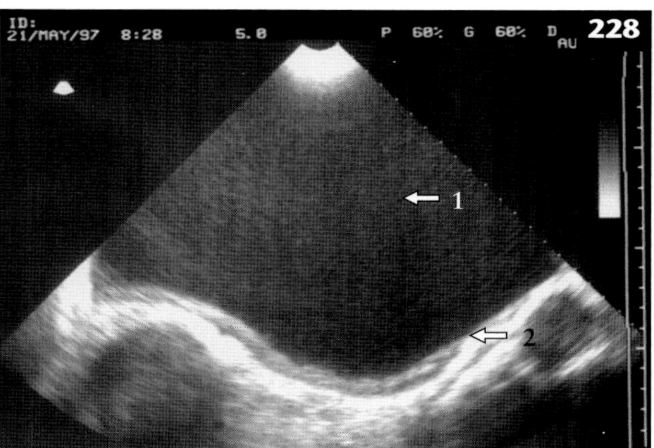

228 Ultrasonogram (5 MHz sector probe). Subcutaneous abscess (**1**) extending for 17 cm from the probe head placed on the ventral abdominal wall. The anechoic area containing multiple white dots represents the abscess, bordered by the broad hyperechoic line of the capsule (**2**).

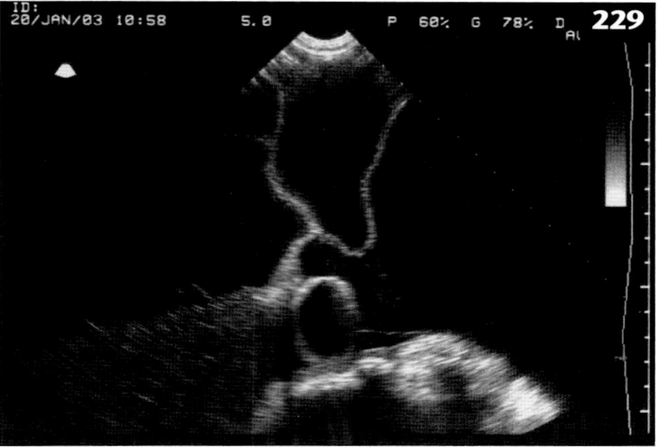

229 Ultrasonogram (5 MHz sector probe). In this case of subacute fasciolosis the hyperechoic lattice-work appearance of fibrinous reaction associated with the liver contrasts with the anechoic peritoneal fluid.

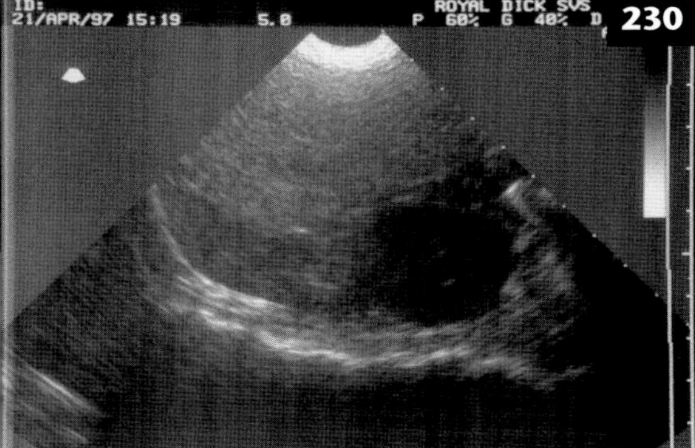

230 Ultrasonogram (5 MHz sector probe). The abomasum in a day-old lamb. The hyperechoic abomasal wall is seen 8 cm from the probe head.

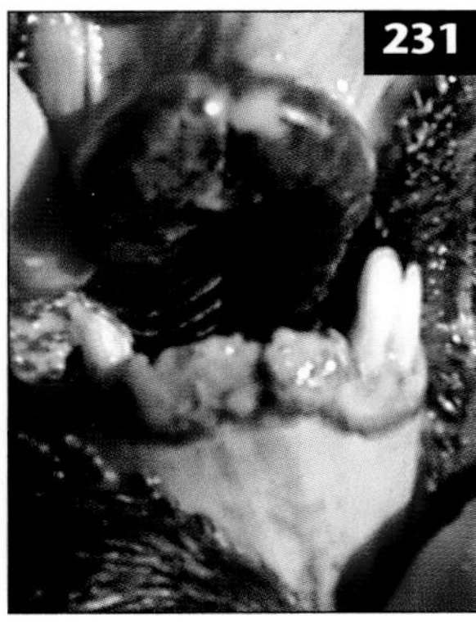

231 Missing central incisors.

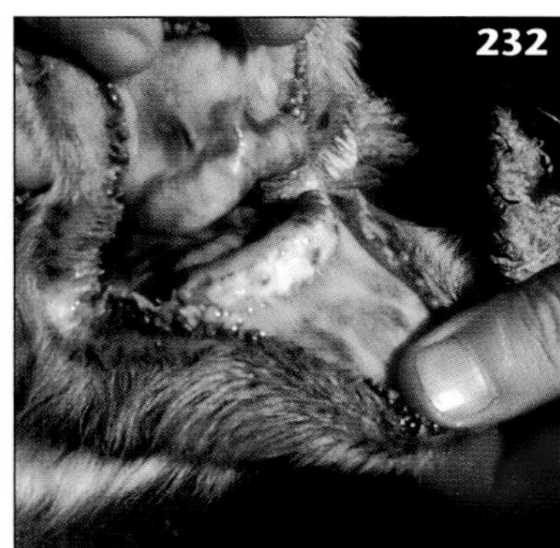

232 All the incisors have been lost.

Diagnosis
Diagnosis is based on the clinical examination.

Treatment
There is no treatment for broken mouth.

Prevention/control measures
There are no recognized control measures for broken mouth. Management factors in the UK include drafting broken-mouthed ewes to lowland pastures where they can be as productive as full-mouthed ewes provided there is an appropriate sward height and/or supplementary concentrate feeding. Traditionally, mountain breeds are drafted off the hill on to lowland pastures after four crops of lambs. They then raise another two crops of lambs.

Shortening overgrown incisor teeth of 3–4-year-old ewes using electric grinders has been promoted in Australia as a means of limiting broken mouth. However, this method is not effective and it raises serious animal welfare issues, with the result that the procedure is banned in many countries.

Economics
Broken mouth can have a serious impact on flock profitability because it necessitates supplementary feeding and premature sale, with a resultant higher replacement rate than normal. Broken-mouthed ewes command much lower prices than similar age ewes with a full mouth. Broken mouth precludes the feeding of root crops.

Welfare implications
There is discomfort and pain associated with gingivitis and periodontal disease in most species but this may be difficult to quantify in sheep. Broken mouth is a cause of emaciation whenever the grass sward has been short for a prolonged period and there has been no supplementary feeding.

Dentigerous (odontogenic) cysts

Definition/overview
Dentigerous cysts occur very sporadically in young adult sheep. Malocclusion leads to weight loss and poor body condition.

Aetiology
The cause of these cysts remains unknown.

Clinical presentation
Affected sheep have a visible swelling of the lower jaw. Sheep aged 2–4 years are typically affected and may present in poor body condition if grazing has been sparse for some months. There is a uniform bony swelling of the mandibular symphysis, measuring 5–6 cm in diameter, which involves the roots of the incisor teeth. Some of the incisor teeth may have been lost while the remaining incisor teeth are often aligned horizontally and at unusual angles to each other. The bony swelling is not painful and there is no discharging sinus or submandibular lymph node enlargement to indicate bacterial infection.

Differential diagnoses
- Osteomyelitis of the mandible.
- Actinomycosis.
- Mandibular fracture.
- Cellulitis.
- Tumour.

Diagnosis
Diagnosis is based on the clinical examination. Radiography reveals loss of normal bone density replaced by a uniform and poorly-mineralized matrix (**233**) but it is rarely undertaken because of cost reasons. The regular appearance of the swelling and the absence of bone lysis suggests that the lesions are not the result of tooth root infection.

Treatment
There is no treatment.

Prevention/control measures
There are no recognized control measures for this sporadic condition. Affected ewes should be managed in a similar manner to broken-mouthed sheep, with preferential grazing and supplementary feeding.

Welfare implications
Sheep with dentigerous cysts require supplementary feeding when grazing is short.

Cheek teeth problems

Definition/overview
Excessive premolar and molar teeth wear leading to malocclusion and poor mastication of fibrous food is a major cause of weight loss and poor condition in older sheep.

Aetiology
Excessive wear is simply a function of the sheep's age and, possibly, diet. Tooth loss, particularly of the first and second premolars due to their shallow roots, is probably preceded by gingivitis and periodontitis, with loss of support structure similar to that recorded for incisor teeth.

Clinical presentation

Cheek teeth problems tend to be of greater significance than incisor teeth loss, due to loss of masticatory function. Cheek teeth problems can best be identified by distant observation of impaction of food in the cheek and swelling caused by overgrown/displaced molar teeth (**234, 235**). There are short jerky jaw movements with the mouth held slightly open. Prehension and initial mastication of food proves difficult. Affected sheep often have pieces of fibrous feed protruding from the commissures of the mouth (**236**) and frequently drop large wads of masticated fibrous food from the mouth (quidding). Sheep with severe teeth lesions may raise their head while masticating in order to assist movement of food over the dorsum of the tongue and into the pharynx.

Careful palpation of the dental arcade through the cheek reveals the sharp irregular ridges of enamel (**237**), and any lost cheek teeth (**238**). Examination of the molar teeth with a gag and torch will confirm such findings but this inspection is resented by sheep. Poorly masticated fibrous feed is typically seen impacted in the cheeks, with sharp enamel ridges on the tooth margins. Significant gum lesions are uncommon. Halitosis is not a common feature. There are rarely any bony lesions associated with cheek tooth loss that could suggest prior tooth root infection.

Cheek teeth problems in multigravid ewes may predispose to pregnancy toxaemia due to reduced forage utilization.

Differential diagnoses

- The common causes of weight loss and poor body condition are described elsewhere in this chapter (see Paratuberculosis, p. 121).
- Food impaction in the cheek(s) is readily differentiated from soft tissue swellings of the face (e.g. an abscess caused by actinobacillosis) and diphtheresis.
- Swelling of the horizontal ramus of the mandible could be caused by osteomyelitis or by a tumour such as a fibrosarcoma or osteosarcoma; both conditions are uncommon in sheep.

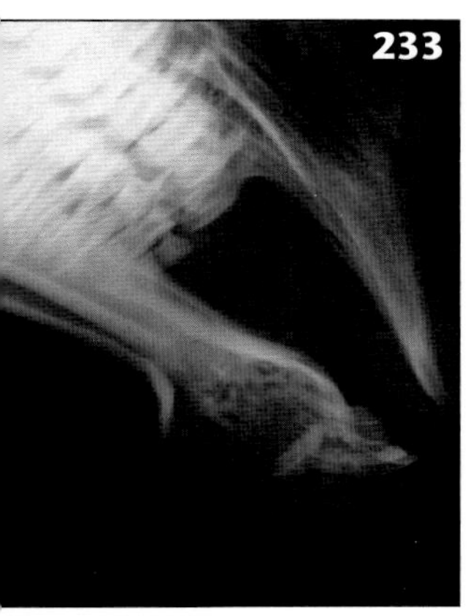

233 Lateral radiograph of the head of a ewe with a dentigerous cyst.

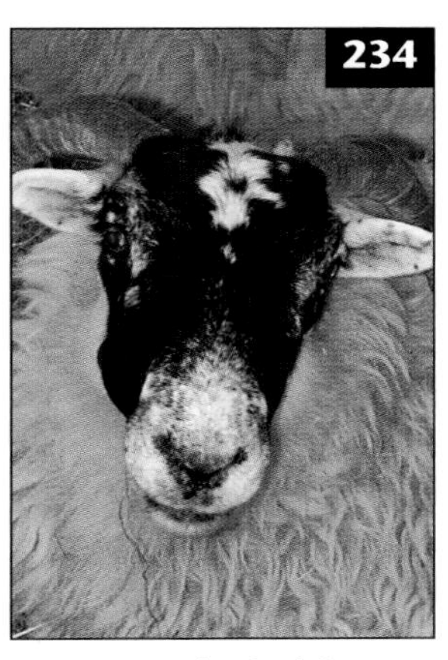

234 Scottish Blackface ewe with molar teeth problems. There is swelling of the right cheek.

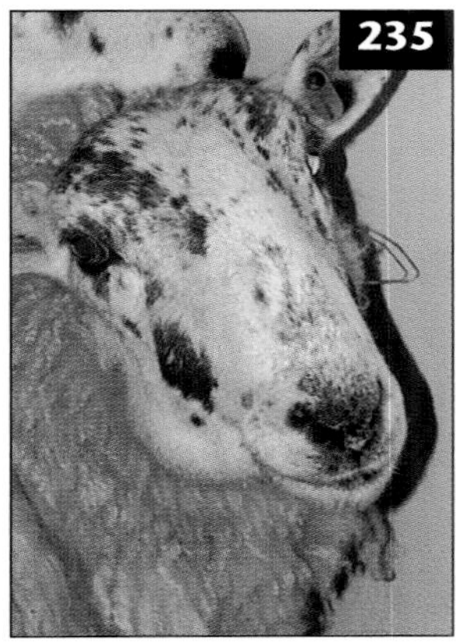

235 Greyface ewe with molar teeth problems. Food material is pouched in the right cheek.

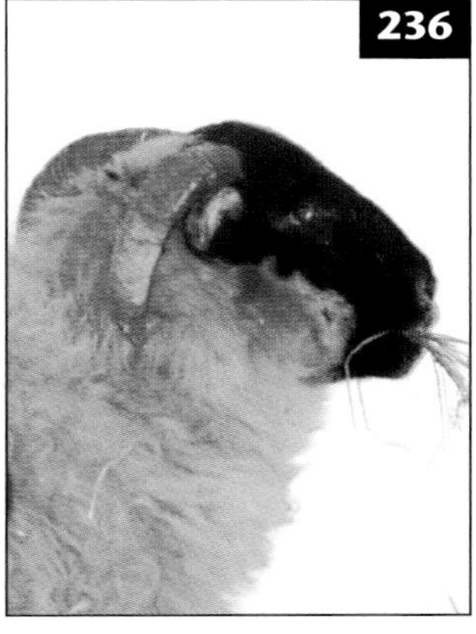

236 Scottish Blackface ewe with molar teeth problems. The ewe has problems masticating fibrous material such as hay.

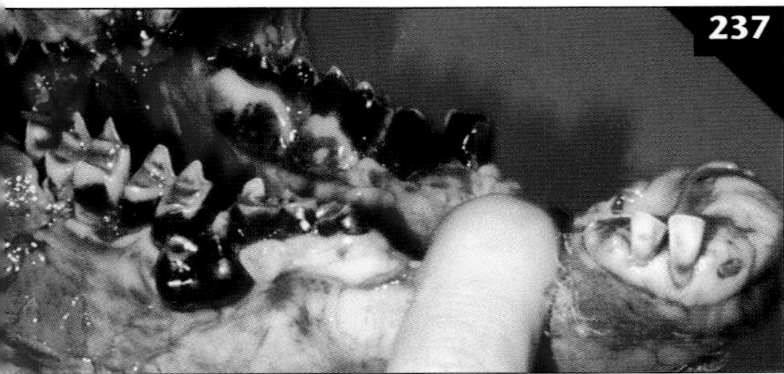

237 Displacement of the lower third premolar on the right side and sharp points on the lingual aspect of all the lower cheek teeth. Several incisor teeth are missing.

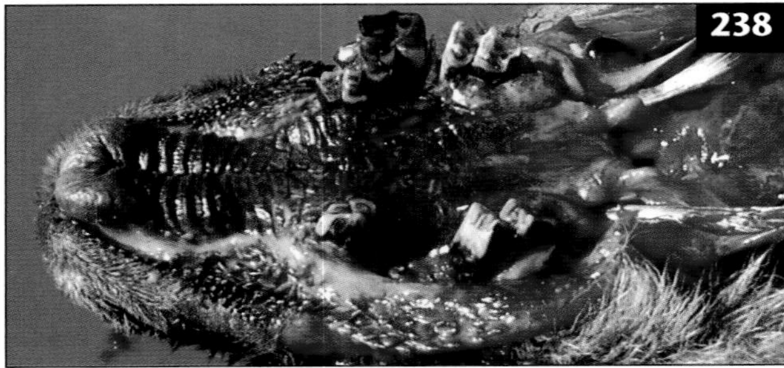

238 Severe upper cheek teeth dentition problems. There are grossly overgrown teeth and missing teeth.

Diagnosis
Diagnosis is based on the clinical findings during examination of the mouth with a gag and torch.

Treatment
There is no treatment and affected sheep should be culled, although their body condition can be improved by generous concentrate feeding (up to 1.5 kg daily) over an 8–12 week period, which should command a better slaughter price.

Prevention/control measures
Excessive wear and molar tooth loss are largely a consequence of the sheep's age. There are no preventive measures. Problems of weight loss caused by poor mastication of fibrous feeds (**239**) can be largely offset by appropriate concentrate feeding, although care must be taken to avoid problems with acidosis when concentrates are first introduced into the ration.

Economics
Cheek teeth problems occur from 5–6 years of age in most flocks, as ewes come to the end of their productive lives. Restoration of body condition can be achieved by supplementary concentrate feeding over 2–3 months to allow sale as mutton.

Welfare implications
Sheep with cheek teeth problems managed on a forage-based ration lose weight and present in poor condition and, possibly, emaciation. Emaciated ewes should be euthanased; ewes in poor condition should be fed concentrates and sold for slaughter when body condition has been restored.

BUCCAL CAVITY

FUSOBACTERIUM NECROPHORUM INFECTION OF THE BUCCAL CAVITY

Definition/overview
Fusobacterium necrophorum causes a necrotic stomatitis in growing lambs. It may be seen as an outbreak in orphan lambs reared on milk replacer and kept in unhygienic conditions with dirty feeding equipment. Lesions may also follow trauma to the buccal cavity caused by dosing gun injuries.

Aetiology
The lesions are due to infection of cuts in the buccal cavity with *F. necrophorum*.

Clinical presentation
Affected lambs present in poor condition due to impaired feeding. The lower jaw is wet because of drooling of saliva (**240**). Lesions affecting the cheek result in obvious firm swellings. These lesions, and those involving the tongue, form large yellow/green diphtheritic lesions with irregular margins and considerable tissue destruction. There is halitosis and swelling of the submandibular lymph node(s). The rectal temperature may be elevated.

Inhalation of infection is not uncommon, resulting in the formation of numerous large abscesses filled with viscous green pus that may extend to the pleural surface and cause an associated pleuritis (**241**). These lambs fail to respond to antibiotic therapy and they remain emaciated and have a poor appetite. Rupture of one of the abscesses may cause death but more commonly results in pyothorax, which eventually may extend to involve all the chest cavity of that side.

239 Rumen contents from two sheep fed the same diet: left side normal dentition; right side from ewe in **238**. The right-hand sample contains long fibres and poorly-masticated hay.

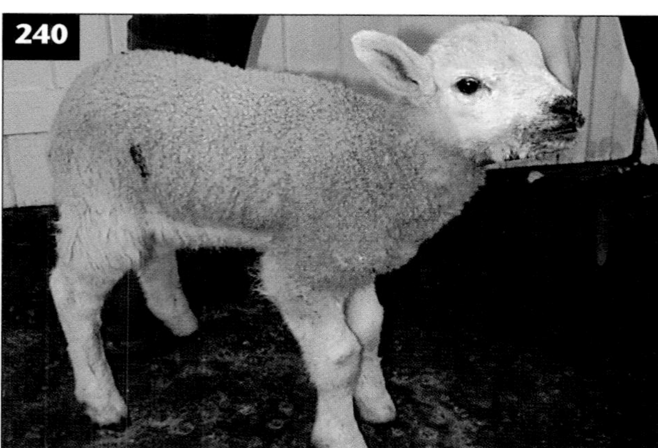

240 Three week-old lamb with *Fusobacterium necrophorum* lesion involving the tongue. Salivation has led to matting of wool on the lower jaw.

Differential diagnoses

- Actinobacillosis may result in cheek lesions.
- Contagious puntular denmatitis virus infection rarely extends from the lips and gingiva of the incisor teeth to involve the tongue.

Diagnosis

Diagnosis is based on the clinical examination.

Treatment

Treatment is with daily procaine penicillin (44,000 iu/kg i/m) for at least seven consecutive days.

Prevention/control measures

The disease is prevented by high standards of hygiene when rearing orphan lambs, and taking care when drenching young growing lambs.

Economics

The disease occurs sporadically and is not a major cause of mortality.

Welfare implications

The oral lesions cause obvious pain and must be treated appropriately. Lambs that fail to thrive after antibiotic therapy should be euthanased.

ACTINOBACILLOSIS

Definition/overview

Actinobacillosis is an uncommon cause of multiple abscesses affecting the subcutaneous areas of the face. The abscesses fistulate to the skin surface and, much less commonly, to the oropharynx, and discharge a viscous yellow/green pus.

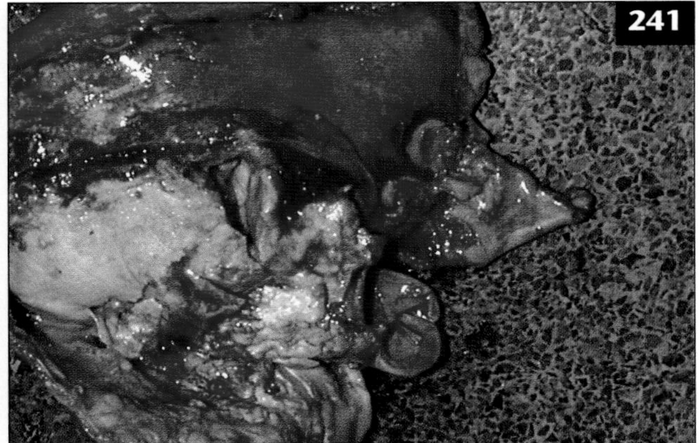

241 Lungs from the lamb in **240**. There are large abscesses on the surface of the lung, one or more of which has ruptured to cause an extensive pleuritis/pleural abscess.

Aetiology

Actinobacillosis is caused by the gram-negative rod *Actinobacillus lignieresi*. A number of cases of abscesses affecting the face may be encountered in sheep grazing pastures containing gorse or similar spiky plants.

Clinical presentation

There are numerous 1–3 cm diameter abscesses on the skin surface of the cheeks, which discharge viscous yellow/green pus. Unlike CLA, the lesions are in the skin rather than the parotid or submandibular lymph node. Enlargement of the drainage retropharyngeal lymph nodes may compress the larynx and cause stertor.

Differential diagnoses

- From an economic standpoint, the important differential diagnosis of actinobacillosis is CLA.
- Stertor could also result from laryngeal chondritis.

Diagnosis

Diagnosis is based on the clinical findings and confirmed following culture.

Treatment

The abscesses cause few problems when confined to the subcutaneous tissue of the face. Antibiotic therapy is unnecessary and, in any case, antibiotics would not penetrate the fibrous capsule of these abscesses. Lancing such abscesses is unnecessary as they will eventually discharge themselves. Lancing is contraindicated in countries with endemic CLA in case the skin lesions are CLA, as this might lead to contamination of the environment.

Sheep with stertor caused by compression of the larynx associated with enlargement/abscessation of the drainage retropharyngeal lymph nodes should be treated with a soluble corticosteroid to reduce associated swelling and procaine penicillin daily for at least ten consecutive days; however, the prognosis is poor.

Prevention/control measures

The condition occurs sporadically, often associated with grazing pastures with spiky plants. There are no specific control measures.

Economics

Actinobacillosis presents no economic concerns.

Welfare implications

There are no welfare concerns unless the swellings prevent prehension and mastication.

Actinomycosis

Definition/overview

Unlike cattle, actinomycosis is a rare disease of sheep.

Aetiology

Actinomycosis is caused by *Actinomyces bovis*.

Clinical presentation

There is marked enlargement of the horizontal ramus of the mandible. One or more sinuses may discharge from the bony swelling. There is enlargement of the ipsilateral submandibular lymph node. The associated pain and physical deformity result in reduced feeding and mastication, with consequent loss of body condition. The swelling is irregular and comprises fibrous tissue with considerable bone remodelling.

Differential diagnoses

- Fracture of the horizontal ramus of the mandible.
- Osteosarcoma.
- Fibrosarcoma.
- Tooth root abscess.

Diagnosis

Diagnosis is based on the clinical findings. Radiography reveals the extent of bone lysis and remodelling.

Treatment

The prognosis even after daily antibiotic injections with penicillin or trimethoprim/sulpha for 4–6 weeks is poor.

Prevention/control measures

The condition occurs rarely and there are no specific control measures.

Economics

Actinomycosis presents no economic concerns.

Welfare implications

Sheep with advanced lesions should be culled.

Pharyngeal abscesses

Definition/overview

Pharyngeal abscesses in growing lambs, and occasionally in adult sheep, result most commonly from trauma caused by incorrect drenching technique (e.g. inappropriate equipment or unskilled administration).

Aetiology

Penetration of the pharyngeal wall by the tip of the drenching gun frequently introduces the contents of the drenching gun (e.g. anthelmintic suspension or trace element capsule/bolus) into fascial planes. Secondary bacterial infection of the penetration site leads to cellulitis, with infection tracking to the cervical spinal canal in some cases.

Clinical presentation

There is rapid loss of body condition in growing lambs. Affected lambs appear dull and depressed and do not suck. There is continuous salivation with staining of the lower jaw. The lambs appear gaunt after 3–4 days' illness, with little abdominal fill. Closer examination of the mouth reveals halitosis and pain on palpation of the pharyngeal region. There may be oedema of the ventral neck, associated with the cellulitis lesion. It is not always possible to distinguish the retropharyngeal lymph nodes even when they are grossly enlarged. Pressure from the abscess/retropharyngeal lymph nodes onto the larynx may cause stertor.

Tetraparesis may result from compression of the cervical spinal cord following extension of the cellulitis into the vertebral canal. There are many reports that describe the typical history of sudden onset of tetraparesis, which rapidly progresses to paralysis and lateral recumbency over 2–4 days, in a number of growing lambs 10–14 days after drenching.

Differential diagnoses

Cellulitis

- Puncture wound such as a dog bite.
- Infection of vaccination site due to poor hygiene standards.
- Oral lesions caused by *Fusobacterium necrophorum*.
- CLA (rarely affects growing lambs).

Weakness

- Vertebral empyema is a common condition of growing lambs.
- Sarcocystosis can present with weakness affecting the hindlimbs.
- White muscle disease.
- Delayed swayback.

Diagnosis

Diagnosis is not simple, especially when the infection has tracked along fascial planes and erupted distant to the entry site in the pharynx. Weakness, with a history of drenching 10–14 days previously and numerous lambs affected, provides strong circumstantial evidence of pharyngeal infection tracking into the cervical spinal canal.

Treatment
The response of cellulitis lesions to 10–14 consecutive days' penicillin treatment is poor and severely affected lambs should be euthanased. Recumbent lambs must be euthanased immediately.

Prevention/control measures
All drenching equipment must be carefully maintained. Shepherds must work patiently amongst small groups of lambs in a confined area, with appropriate restraint to prevent lambs jumping forward when the drenching gun nozzle is introduced into the mouth.

Economics
Pharyngeal abscesses are an avoidable problem and they indicate poor husbandry practice. Lamb losses totalling 2–5% have been reported on occasion from injuries caused by incorrect drenching technique.

Welfare implications
Affected sheep suffer from these painful lesions and should be euthanased.

ABDOMEN

Acidosis (*Syn*: grain overload)

Definition/overview
Acidosis results from the sudden unaccustomed ingestion of large quantities of carbohydrate-rich feeds, typically grain or concentrates and, less commonly, potatoes and by-products such as bread and bakery waste.

Aetiology
Acidosis often results when sheep are turned on to grain stubble that has quantities of spilled grain (**242**); sheep are particularly susceptible to acidosis caused by wheat and barley grain. Too rapid introduction on to a diet of *ad libitum* concentrates may result in acidosis. While the ration may be calculated to supply only 100 g per head per day, if the majority of weaned lambs are slow to start eating the ration, some lambs may eat in excess of 500 g.

The smaller the particle size (e.g. following milling) the more quickly fermentation occurs and the more severe the clinical signs for a given amount ingested by the sheep. Mountain breeds such as the Scottish Blackface (**243**) are more susceptible to acidosis than other breeds.

Pathophysiology
The sudden and unaccustomed ingestion of large quantities of carbohydrate-rich feeds results in a fall in rumen pH, which kills many resident bacteria and protozoa. *Lactobacillus* species multiply rapidly with the production of large amounts of lactic acid, which further reduces rumen pH. There is a marked increase in rumen liquor osmolality, with fluid being drawn in from the extracellular space and causing dehydration. Lactate is absorbed into the circulation, leading to the development of a metabolic acidosis. This metabolic crisis is further compounded by toxin absorption through the compromised rumen mucosa.

Chronic sequelae of rumen acidosis include fungal rumenitis and, occasionally, liver abscessation but the latter condition is less common than in cattle. Laminitis is uncommon in sheep following grain overload.

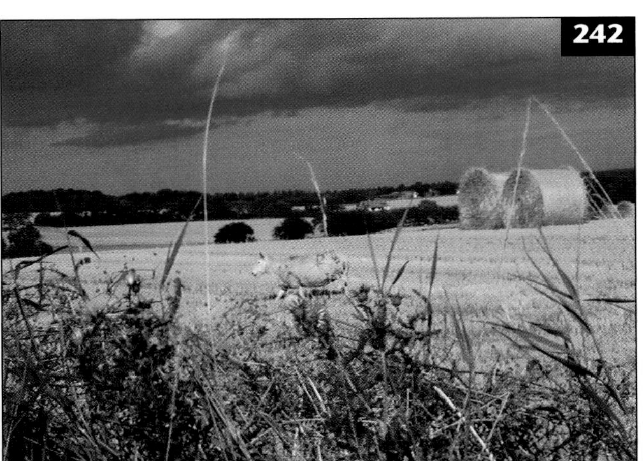

242 Grain spillages on stubble can lead to large grain intakes and acidosis.

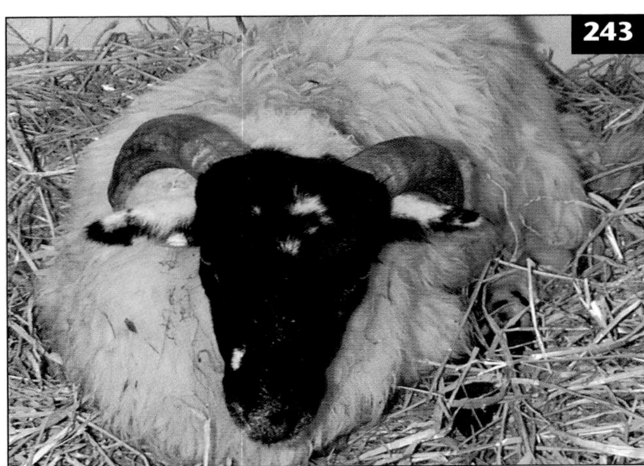

243 Depressed, sternally recumbent Scottish Blackface ram suffering from acidosis.

Clinical presentation

The severity of clinical signs depends on the amount of grain ingested, whether the grain was rolled or whole, the rate of introduction of the dietary change and the breed of sheep. For example, in the UK, weaned Scottish Blackface lambs are particularly susceptible to acidosis and have been found *in extremis* or dead within 24 hours of sudden introduction of barley feeding. It has been reported that colic signs may be observed soon after grain engorgement and that the sheep appear restless. More usually, affected sheep are very dull and depressed and are reluctant to move (**243**). When walking, affected sheep appear ataxic; they may fall and experience difficulty rising due to weakness. They are anorexic and stand with their head held lowered. Bruxism (tooth grinding) is frequently heard. The lambs have a distended abdomen due to an enlarged static rumen. Auscultation reveals no rumen motility; succussion reveals tinkling sounds due to the accumulation of fluid and gas within the rumen. Initially, the rectal temperature may be increased but it falls to subnormal values as the toxaemia progresses. The mucous membranes are congested and there may be enophthalmos and an increased skin tent-up duration of up to five seconds due to moderate/severe dehydration. There may be no diarrhoea for the first 12–24 hours after carbohydrate ingestion; thereafter, there is profuse fetid diarrhoea, which may contain whole grains (**244**). The most severely affected sheep become recumbent and have an increased respiratory rate from the developing metabolic acidosis. The heart rate is increased and the degree of dehydration worsens. Death may follow within 24–48 hours despite treatment. Sheep that recover have a protracted convalescence and occasionally show signs of lameness, associated with laminitis, affecting all four feet.

Differential diagnoses

- Differential diagnoses for profound toxaemia in weaned lambs include systemic pasteurellosis, clostridial disease, especially pulpy kidney disease and black disease, and abdominal catastrophes such as torsion of the small intestine or caecum.
- Redgut should also be considered but it is less commonly associated with grain feeding.
- Polioencephalomalacia and sulphur toxicity may cause initial depression and isolation.
- Subacute fasciolosis can present with recumbency, weakness, anterior abdominal pain and abdominal distension associated with peritonitis and an inflammatory exudate.

Diagnosis

Diagnosis is based on the history and clinical findings, particularly once fetid diarrhoea is evident. Rumen fluid samples can be collected by percutaneous ruminocentesis or, preferably, by orogastric tube. The rumen pH falls below 5.5. There are no live protozoa observed under microscopic examination of rumen liquor, only large numbers of gram-positive rods.

At necropsy the rumen contents are milky-grey and porridge-like and have a rancid odour. The rumen epithelium strips off readily but care is necessary to differentiate this phenomenon from normal autolytic changes present after 4–6 hours.

Treatment

Intravenous fluid therapy is usually cost prohibitive and presents logistical problems when large numbers of sheep are affected. Recumbent sheep could be 7–10% dehydrated and would require from three (30–40 kg fattening lamb) to ten litres (mature ewe or ram) of isotonic saline during the first four hours or so (**245**), followed by mainentance levels.

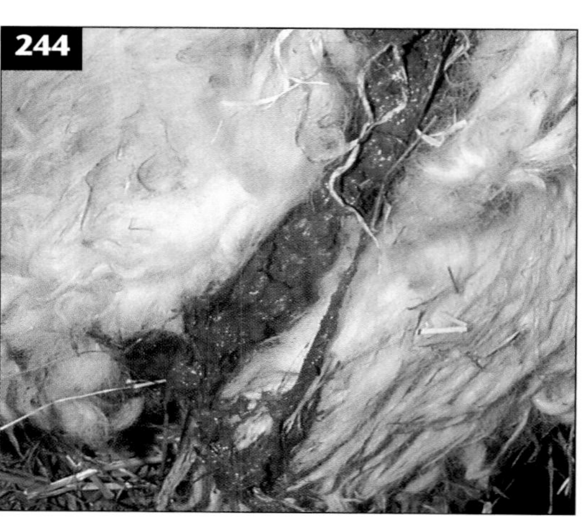

244 Foul smelling diarrhoea in the ram in **243**.

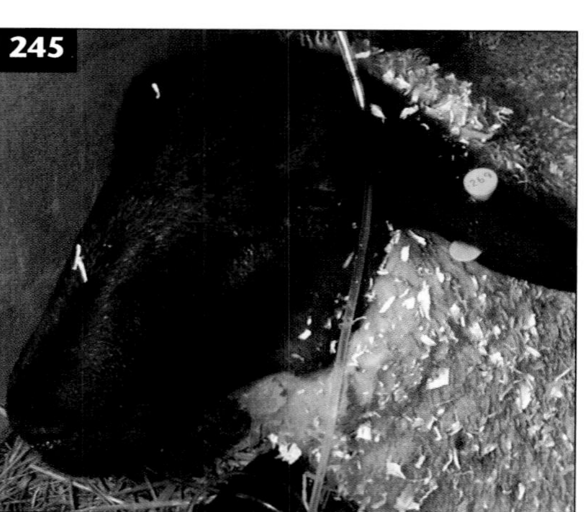

245 Intravenous fluid therapy in a valuable Suffolk lamb suffering from acidosis. The sunken eye is consistent with moderate dehydration.

Intravenous fluids should contain bicarbonate but there are few data for treating acidosis in sheep under field situations. In emergency situations it would be safe to administer 10 mmol/l of bicarbonate over 2–3 hours and monitor progress. In practice, 16 g of sodium bicarbonate = 200 mmol of bicarbonate; therefore, an 80 kg pedigree Suffolk sheep estimated to be 7% dehydrated would require:

> Estimated base deficit × dehydrated body weight × extracellular fluid volume (i.e. $10 \times 74 \times 0.3$) = 222 mmol of bicarbonate.

Therefore, 16 g of sodium bicarbonate would approximate a 10 mmol/l base deficit for a mature Suffolk sheep (8 g for a 40 kg fattening lamb).

Severe metabolic acidosis may cause a base deficit of up to 20 mmol/l, thereby necessitating further intravenous bicarbonate. The response to intravenous fluid therapy should be carefully monitored.

A rumenotomy to remove the rumen contents can be attempted but considerable care is needed to prevent leakage into the abdominal cavity during surgery, because it is usually not possible to exteriorize much of the rumen wall due to the large volume of fluid contents. Attempts to siphon off rumen contents are not as successful as for cattle.

In most practical situations, therapy is restricted to oral fluids, intravenous multivitamin preparations and antibiotic therapy. Diluted oral rehydration solutions can be given by orogastric tube, which is easily achieved in sheep. Sodium bicarbonate can be added to the rehydration solution but this may result in bloat. Some authors have recommended drenching with 15 ml of milk of magnesia every few hours to counter acidosis. Procaine penicillin has been recommended to destroy the ruminal lactobacilli and thereby limit lactic acid production; this should be given by percutaneous injection into the distended dorsal sac of the rumen, or by oral administration.

Some clinicians elect to inject thiamine (vitamin B_1) intravenously rather than a multivitamin injection. Penicillin injections are given daily for up to 10 days to counter potential bacteraemia.

The concentrate feed must be reduced or removed from the remainder of the group, although many farmers reason that as most of the sheep have already adapted to the diet, new cases may occur after reintroduction of the grain ration. Good quality hay should be provided to stimulate rumen function.

Prevention/control measures

Grain/concentrate feeding must be gradually introduced over a minimum of three weeks before *ad libitum* feeding (**246**). If some of the sheep are not coming to the feed troughs, the total allocated amount must be reduced accordingly. The grain can be diluted using sugar beet shreds or similar feed during the acclimatization period. As a rule of thumb, the grain ration can be increased by 50 g per head every 2–3 days provided all the sheep are eating well and all the concentrate feed is eaten within five minutes. Good quality roughage must be available at all times. If roughage is restricted, it must be available to all the sheep at the same time and not restricted to a small bunk/rack. Grain must not be left lying on the floor (**247**) in case sheep escape from their pen.

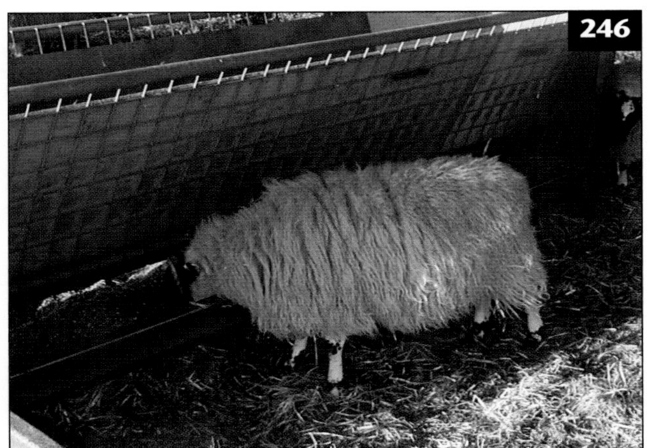

246 *Ad libitum* concentrate feeding in housed fattening lambs.

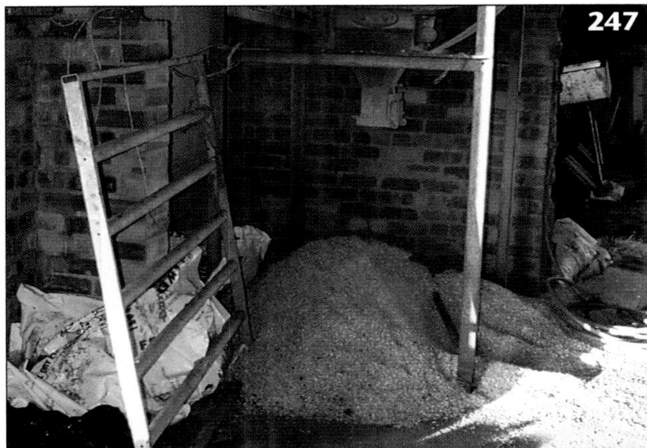

247 Following break-outs, open feed stores are commonly the source of excess grain ingestion.

Economics
Mortality can be high if sheep are suddenly introduced to rations containing high levels of carbohydrates, especially rolled grain. Convalescence is protracted in sheep that develop diarrhoea because of disturbances to the rumen microflora.

Welfare implications
Acidosis is a common problem when concentrates are introduced too quickly. Affected sheep are in obvious pain. Comatose sheep, and those unable to stand within 2–3 days of treatment, should be euthanased.

Bloat

Definition/overview
Bloat is the sudden accumulation of free gas within the rumen, which causes abdominal distension. If untreated, pressure on the diaphragm causes respiratory embarrassment, reduced venous return and, eventually, death. Unlike cattle, bloat in sheep is very uncommon unless secondary to an oesophageal obstruction.

Aetiology
A sudden intake of readily fermented material such as grain can cause bloat. Oesophageal obstruction (choke) occurs sporadically when sheep are fed root crops. Ingestion of legumes may result in the formation of a stable froth in the rumen, preventing presentation of free gas at the cardia for eructation, with consequent bloat.

Clinical presentation
Affected sheep with abdominal distension may simply be found dead following a sudden change in the ration. Other sheep present with predominantly high left-sided abdominal distension; some sheep may become dyspnoeic and show mouth breathing.

Differential diagnoses
- Hypocalcaemia results in recumbency followed by bloat.
- Abdominal catastrophes such as volvulus and redgut present with abdominal distension.
- Chronic causes of abdominal distension may include peritonitis, ascites and uroperitoneum associated with urolithiasis.

Diagnosis
Diagnosis is based on clinical findings and confirmed by release of gas following orogastric tube placement or rumen trocharization.

Treatment
Free gas bloat should be released with an orogastric tube. The administration of dimeticone may assist relief of frothy bloat. Trocharization can be undertaken as an emergency procedure but may not be successful in cases of frothy bloat.

Prevention/control measures
Gradual introduction on to legume or root crops and subsequent restricted grazing should reduce the likelihood of frothy bloat. Choke occurs sporadically.

Economics
Bloat is a significant economic consideration only under specific grazing conditions.

Welfare implications
There are no major welfare concerns provided sheep are treated quickly.

Redgut

Definition/overview
Redgut is a very sporadic condition associated with torsion of the intestine/caecum of weaned lambs and adult sheep. It causes sudden death due to endotoxaemia/ circulatory failure.

Aetiology
Redgut has typically been encountered in sheep grazing legumes or similar crops. This diet results in rapid transit times, reduced rumen volume and secondary fermentation in the lower gut and caecum. The altered proportions of the major abdominal viscera and increased production of gas in the lower gut leads to instability and torsion around the root of the mesentery. This causes sudden death.

Clinical presentation
Affected sheep are usually found dead without premonitory signs. Those that are found alive are very depressed, are recumbent and have abdominal distension with dehydration and toxic mucous membranes.

Differential diagnoses
- Clostridial disease, typically pulpy kidney disease, black disease or struck.
- Bloat.
- Acute/subacute fasciolosis.
- Acute copper toxicity.

Diagnosis
Diagnosis is confirmed at necropsy.

Treatment
There is no treatment. Those sheep found alive should be destroyed for welfare reasons.

Prevention/control measures
Sheep should be introduced gradually on to lush pastures or legume crops. Restricted grazing and provision of good quality fibre should reduce the likelihood of redgut.

Economics
Redgut is a significant economic consideration only under specific grazing conditions.

Welfare implications
Sheep with intestinal torsion die quickly; nevertheless, sheep found alive must be euthanased.

ABOMASAL BLOAT

Definition/overview
Abomasal bloat occurs commonly in orphan lambs fed restricted amounts of milk replacer of variable temperature at irregular intervals during the first four weeks of life.

Aetiology
Abomasal bloat is caused by the sudden fermentation of large amounts of carbohydrate, with gas production that cannot readily escape from the abomasum.

Clinical presentation
Signs of abdominal distension and colic appear within one hour of feeding. Affected lambs alternate between a wide-based stance and lateral recumbency. There is frequent vocalization, tail swishing and kicking at the abdomen. Lambs have a painful expression and a wet lower jaw due to drooling saliva. In some cases, abomasal bloat may lead to volvulus.

Differential diagnoses
Differential diagnoses include:
- Lamb dysentery.
- Abomasal foreign body such as a wool ball blocking the pylorus.
- Abomasal volvulus.
- Urolithiasis in male lambs.

Diagnosis
Diagnosis is based on clinical findings and a history of irregular milk feeding.

Treatment
Attempts to relieve bloat by orogastric tube are rarely successful and offer only temporary remission. Percutaneous needle decompression offers little better success because the needle often becomes blocked with milk clot and/or the abomasal wall moves and the needle comes out of the abomasum. If the lamb survives the initial bloat, leakage of abomasal contents through the needle puncture site(s) in the abomasal wall leads to localized peritonitis. Metaclopramide is unlikely to have any significant affect in advanced cases.

Surgical correction under general anaesthesia could be attempted but it is cost prohibitive.

Prevention/control measures
Excellent results for rearing orphan lambs can be achieved using automated systems that regulate the amount and frequency of milk replacer supply. The early introduction of high quality concentrates will promote rumen function and lessen the risk of abomasal bloat/torsion.

Economics
Rearing orphans lambs presents many disease problems and offers low financial returns, due to the high cost of milk replacer, and high losses unless the management is of the highest standard.

Welfare implications
Lambs with abomasal bloat that cannot be easily relieved should be euthanased.

ABOMASAL EMPTYING DEFECT

Definition/overview
This is an uncommon, yet probably underdiagnosed, disorder reported most frequently in pedigree Suffolk sheep. It also occurs in other breeds and crossbreeds.

Aetiology
The cause remains unknown but its recognition primarily in Suffolk sheep suggests an hereditary component.

Clinical presentation
Signs develop over some months, with gradual weight loss leading to emaciation. There is increasing abdominal distension, especially on the lower right

side when the sheep in viewed from behind (**248**). Affected sheep have a poor appetite and pass firm pelleted faeces, frequently coated with thick mucus. They are afebrile and appear somewhat dull and apathetic. There may be moderate dehydration. Rumen sounds are frequently increased. The abdomen is distended and firm; there is no fluid thrill, hence no ascites.

Differential diagnoses

- Scrapie sheep typically present in poor condition/emaciated and some present with marked abomasal impaction.
- Abomasal impaction resulting in abdominal distension should be distinguished from peritonitis and adenocarcinoma, which may result in accumulations of excess peritoneal fluid.
- Poor cheek teeth with inadequate mastication of fibrous foods may result in rumen distension.
- Vagal indigestion, resulting in ruminal distension with a characteristic 'papple' abdominal silhouette, is uncommon in sheep.

Diagnosis

Determination of rumen chloride concentration gives an indication of reflux of chloride-rich secretions from the abomasum into the rumen. Values in excess of 30 mmol/l are suggestive of this condition (normal values <15 mmol/l). The diagnosis is confirmed at necropsy (**249, 250**).

Treatment

There is no treatment.

Prevention/control measures

There are presently no control measures. While it would be prudent to cull progeny from sheep that develop this condition, this is unlikely to happen because of financial losses in a pedigree flock selling breeding stock.

Economics

The true incidence of this condition has not been determined and its diagnosis is likely to be overlooked in commercial flocks that purchase individual rams.

Welfare implications

Affected sheep should be euthanased when all other treatable alternative conditions have been excluded.

INTESTINAL ADENOCARCINOMA

Definition/overview

Intestinal adenocarcinoma is a sporadic tumour of the small intestine, which causes weight loss and emaciation in adult sheep.

Aetiology

There may be an association between the occurrence of intestinal adenocarcinoma and grazing bracken-infested pasture but such tumours also occur in areas where there is no bracken.

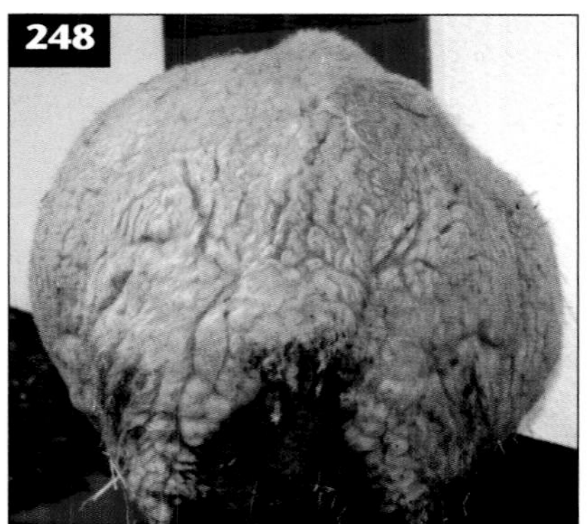

248 Abdominal distension in a Suffolk ram with an abomasal emptying defect.

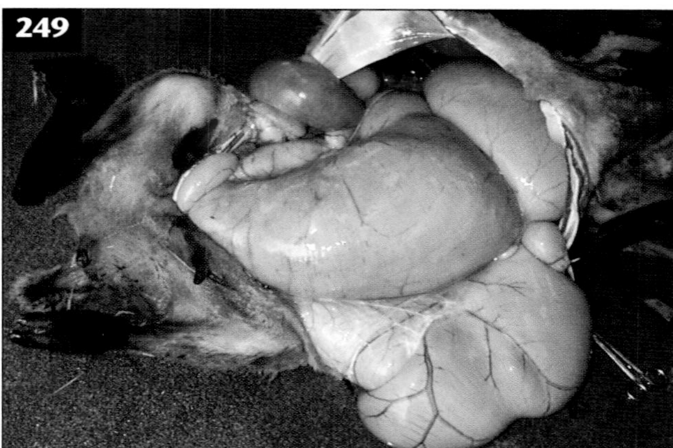

249 Necropsy of the ram in **248**. The abomasum is massively distended.

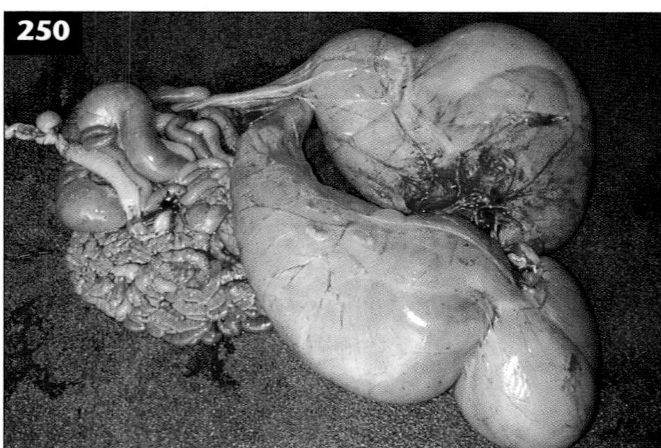

250 Further dissection of the ram in **248** revealing the extent of abomasal distension.

Clinical presentation

An affected adult sheep presents in much poorer condition than other sheep in the group. While ascites is present in most cases, it may prove difficult to assess the extent of the transudate on clinical examination. Ultrasound examination provides a quick and reliable assessment of the amount of peritoneal fluid. In sheep with intestinal adenocarcinoma, ascites appears to result from transcoelomic spread of the tumour, with blockage of lymphatic drainage.

Differential diagnoses

Other conditions that cause weight loss in adult sheep include:

- Subacute and chronic fasciolosis.
- Paratuberculosis.
- Molar dentition problems.
- Chronic suppurative focus such as chronic suppurative pneumonia/mastitis.

Diagnosis

Abdominocentesis, cytospin preparation and staining may yield exfoliated tumour cells but most cases are diagnosed at necropsy (**251**), with confirmatory histopathological examination.

Treatment

There is no recognized treatment and affected sheep should be euthanased when all other treatable alternative conditions have been excluded.

Prevention/control measures

There are no recognized control measures.

Economics

Weight loss and poor condition occurs sporadically in all sheep flocks and losses attributed to various disorders are rarely quantified. Intestinal adenocarcinoma occurs sporadically in flocks and is unlikely to exceed one case every two years.

Welfare implications

Sheep in poor condition despite adequate nutrition should be culled promptly.

Peritonitis

Definition/overview

Infection of the abdominal cavity may result in focal peritonitis, with spread of infection limited by the omentum, or extend to septic peritonitis.

Aetiology

Uterine tears following dystocia are the most common cause of septic peritonitis.

Clinical presentation

Occasionally, adhesions may form between the rumen and the abdominal incision site used for caesarean section. There are few sequelae, although if a subsequent caesarian section is needed, the approach will be more difficult.

The clinical signs depend on the spread of infection within the peritoneal cavity. Initially, focal infections involving leakage of toxins through the uterine wall, with localized adhesion formation, may prove difficult to diagnose because of non-specific signs of poor appetite and weight loss. Affected sheep are rarely febrile. The clinical signs are more pronounced in more generalized cases of peritonitis (**252**).

251 Intestinal adenocarcinoma.

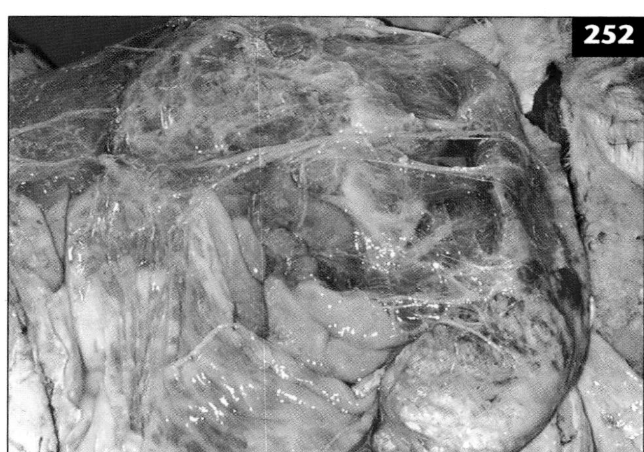

252 Diffuse fibrinous peritonitis associated with septic metritis.

Sheep with septic peritonitis are dull, depressed and anorexic (**253**). Initially, there may be abdominal distension due to gut stasis but inappetence quickly results in a gaunt, drawn-up appearance. Affected sheep may stand with an arched back (**254**) but this is much less of a feature than in cattle with peritonitis. The rectal temperature is rarely elevated but the mucous membranes are congested. There is variable dehydration. The respiratory and heart rates are elevated; there are no rumen contractions. Scant mucus-coated faeces are passed. Affected sheep often stand with their head held over the water trough but drink little (**255**). Death follows within 3–7 days.

Differential diagnoses

- Septic peritonitis frequently follows dystocia/uterine tears; therefore, the most common differential diagnosis is metritis.
- Retained fetus could present with similar signs to peritonitis.
- Hypocalcaemia presents as a dull, recumbent sheep with bloat, which could be confused with peritonitis at initial presentation.
- Subacute fasciolosis may result in focal peritonitis involving the liver and adjacent small intestine.

Diagnosis

Diagnosis of peritonitis is not simple because infection has often been contained by the omentum and therefore cannot be identified by either abdominocentesis or ultrasonography. In chronic cases of peritonitis, fibrous adhesions are the most prominent feature, with scant peritoneal fluid. Careful ultrasonographic examination may reveal fluid-distended static intestines proximal to the lesion; normal intestinal propulsion is prevented by localized adhesions.

Treatment

Antibiotic therapy is hopeless and is only undertaken in case the diagnosis is incorrect and the sheep is suffering from metritis or another infectious disease.

Prevention/control measures

Apart from a correct approach to dystocia management, there are no specific preventive measures. Client education with respect to careful correction of dystocia is indicated in some situations.

Economics

Peritonitis occurs uncommonly in sheep and is not a major economic concern.

Welfare implications

Euthanasia is indicated when the sheep has failed to respond to antibiotic therapy administered because a definitive diagnosis could not be established.

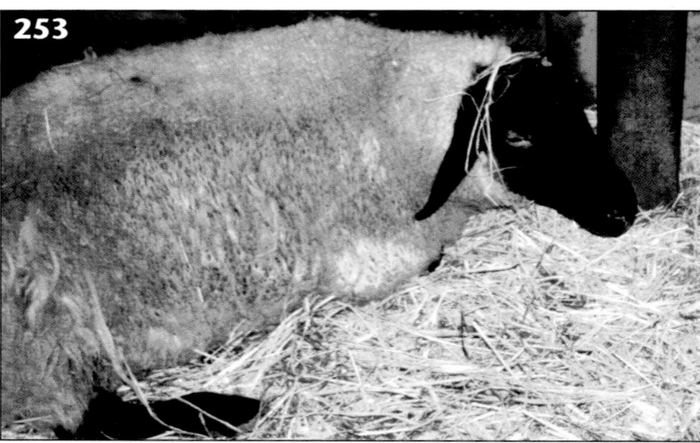

253 Suffolk ewe with acute peritonitis.

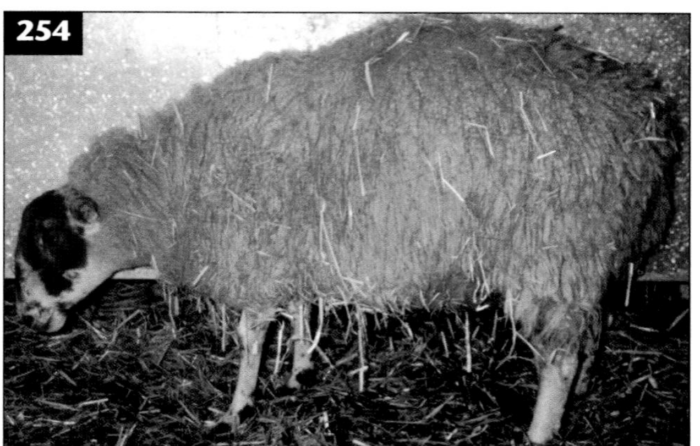

254 Greyface ewe with acute peritonitis. The ewe has a roached back stance.

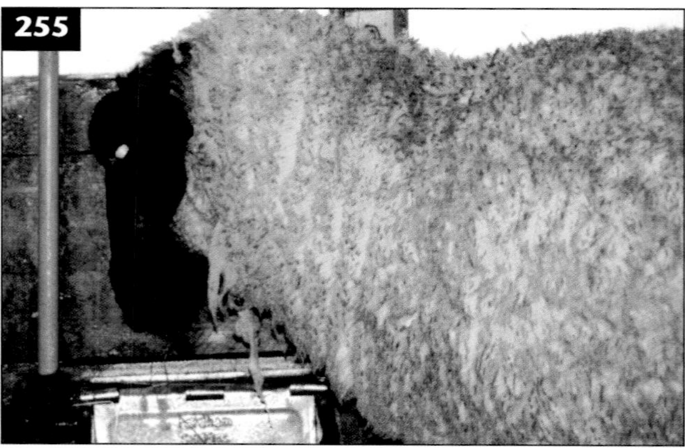

255 The Suffolk ewe in **253** with acute peritonitis often stood with her head over the water trough but drinking little.

INTESTINAL ATRESIA

Definition/overview

Atresia ani is relatively common in lambs, occurring at about one case per 100–500 lambs. Atresia coli is diagnosed much less commonly.

Aetiology

Atresia ani appears sporadically in newborn lambs; there is no recognized hereditary component.

Clinical presentation

Lambs with atresia ani are perfectly healthy for the first 24–36 hours after birth. Thereafter, there is increasing abdominal distension, reluctance to suck, salivation, depression and long periods spent in sternal recumbency (256). Examination usually reveals a bulge beneath the skin where the anus should be. The clinical presentation is largely similar for atresia coli but the diagnosis is much more difficult because there is no swelling under the tail.

Differential diagnoses

Casual inspection of weak neonatal lambs with abdominal distension by the shepherd often results in treatment for watery mouth disease, although the rate of deterioration is slower for lambs with atresia ani.

Diagnosis

Atresia ani is readily recognized on lifting the lamb's tail, which reveals skin covering the site of the anus.

Diagnosis of atresia coli is much more problematic and is based on the clinical findings listed above plus a lack of faeces produced since birth, although such detailed history may not be available.

Treatment

Correction of atresia ani is most easily achieved by a 'X-shaped' stab incision in the skin bulge using a scalpel blade. This is a painful procedure and must only be undertaken after sacrococcygeal lidocaine injection (0.2 ml of 2% solution), which is a simple technique using a 21 gauge 12 mm needle (257). On incision, up to 100 ml of mucus-containing meconium is released (258) under variable pressure. The stab incision in the skin may heal over; therefore, the farmer should be advised to make sure the incision site remains patent by carefully inserting a thermometer coated with liquid paraffin into the rectum twice daily for 3–4 days. The recovery rate is good.

There is no cost-effective surgical correction of atresia coli for non-pedigree lambs and these lambs should be euthanased for welfare reasons.

Prevention/control measures

Even though there is no recognized hereditary component to atresia ani, it would be prudent not to keep these lambs for future breeding replacements.

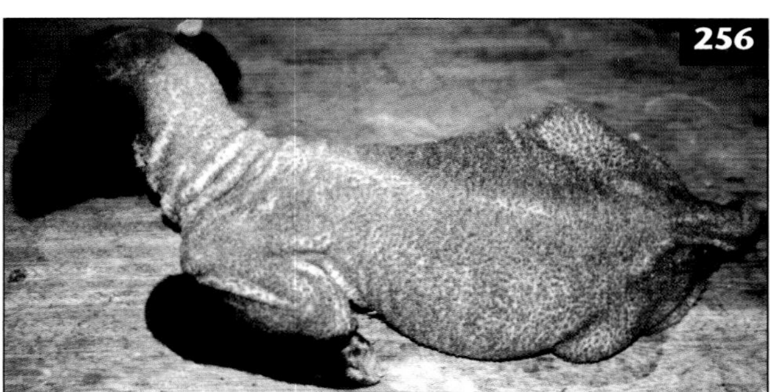

256 Abdominal distension in a three-day-old lamb with atresia ani.

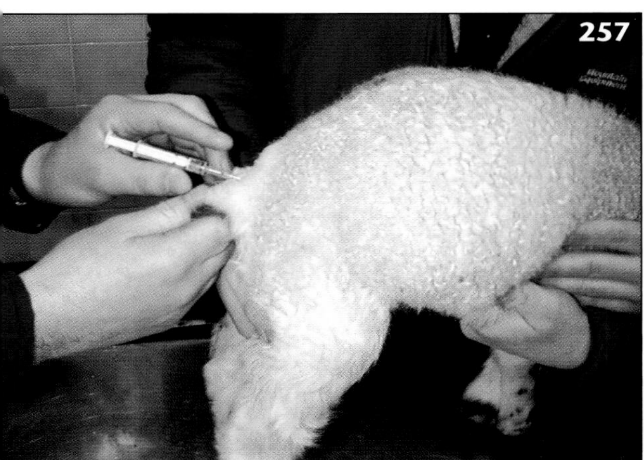

257 Caudal analgesia prior to correction of atresia ani.

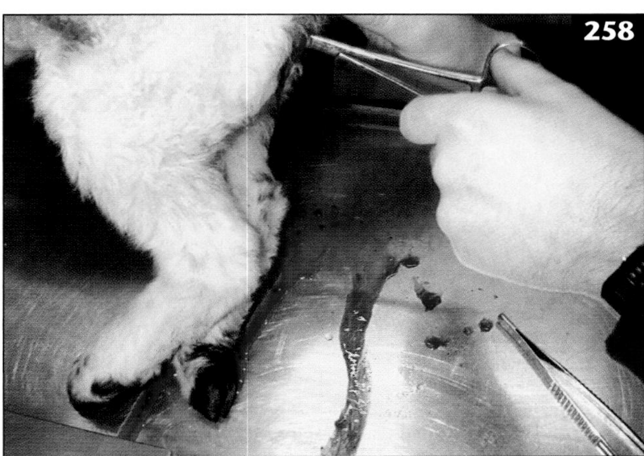

258 Release of meconium following incision of the tissue causing the atresia.

Economics
Atresia ani is not an economic concern to sheep producers.

Welfare implications
With prompt recognition and timely correction there are no specific welfare concerns related to atresia ani.

HERNIATED INTESTINES THROUGH THE UMBILICUS
Definition/overview
Herniation of intestines through the umbilicus occurs very occasionally in newborn lambs due to overzealous licking by the ewe.

Clinical presentation
Soon after the event the lamb is still bright and alert but congestion and trauma to the herniated intestines causes rapid deterioration in the clinical presentation. There is often gross contamination of the intestines/omentum, which proves almost impossible to remove.

Diagnosis
Diagnosis is based on the clinical findings (**259**).

Treatment
The prognosis for such lambs is very poor unless the lamb is brought to the surgery immediately. However, some lambs do survive following replacement and closure of the abdominal defect. The lamb should be injected with 2 mg/kg of ketoprofen intravenously. There are no licensed general anaesthetic drugs for sheep but intravenous alphaxalone/alphadolone combination works remarkably well in neonatal lambs. Gross contamination is removed from the herniated intestines using very dilute povidone iodine solution. Finally, the intestines are flushed with one litre of Hartmann's solution.

An incision is made through the skin/subcutaneous tissues/linea alba using scissors, extending cranially for 3 cm from the hernia site, and the intestines are carefully replaced. The linea alba is closed with interrupted Dexon sutures and horizontal mattress sutures are placed in the skin. The lamb should then be placed in a warming box set at 45°C. The lamb should recover from general anaesthesia within 10–20 minutes, and it should then be carefully stomach tubed with 200 ml of ewe colostrum.

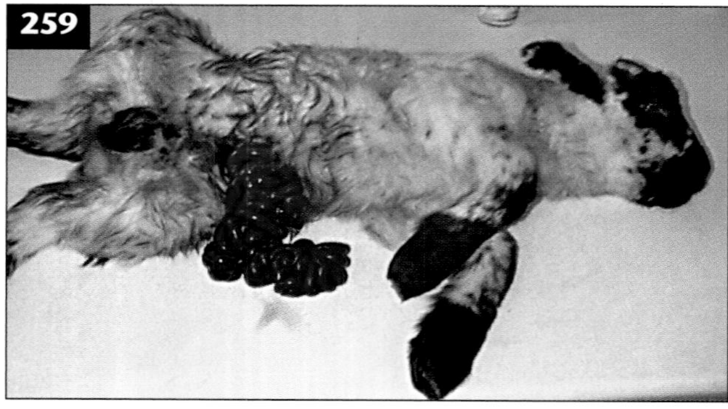
259 Umbilical herniation of intestines in a newborn lamb.

Prevention/control measures
There are no preventive measures as this condition occurs during normal activity by enthusiastic mothers.

CRYPTOSPORIDIOSIS
Definition/overview
Cryptosporidium parvum is a coccidian parasite that has been recognized as a significant cause of diarrhoea in young ruminants only over the past 20 years or so. Cryptosporidiosis is a zoonotic disease and it has been frequently reported in children visiting open farms and 'petting' zoos. Contamination of human water supplies following flooding of pastures grazed by sheep has led to numerous health scares in the UK.

C. parvum is not host specific and severe outbreaks can occur on mixed farming enterprises where there is a build-up of infection towards the end of the lambing period, especially if the same fields or buildings are used for autumn/winter calving then for spring lambing, as the protozoan parasite can remain dormant on pasture for months and is very resistant to environmental stresses. In some instances no clinical disease results from *Cryptosporidium* species infection and the parasites are commonly isolated from clinically healthy animals.

Aetiology
Infection is by the faeco-oral route. Adult sheep may become asymptomatic carriers and shed small numbers of oocysts during stressful periods such as around parturition. Diarrhoea in lambs is caused by the physical loss of villous absorptive area and it exacerbates concurrent gut infections such as rotavirus. Cryptosporidia do not require faecal excretion for sporulation to infective stages and they can invade other villous cells without leaving the intestine. This autoinfection can cause severe disease.

Clinical presentation

Most cases of cryptosporidiosis occur during the second half of the lambing period under intensive management systems. Lambs aged 3–7 days are most commonly affected. There is a profuse yellow/green diarrhoea with some mucus present. Flecks of fresh blood are seen occasionally. Initially, lambs have a distended appearance but they quickly become dull with a tucked-up abdomen, are reluctant to follow their dam and are often found hunched up and sheltering behind walls and hedgerows. There is rapid weight loss and affected lambs develop a gaunt appearance. There is gradual recovery in most lambs over 5–7 days.

Unlike calves, a severe challenge of *C. parvum* can cause high lamb losses if supportive therapy is not administered. There is rapid dehydration in severe cases, leading to recumbency and eventual death. Losses are particularly high during adverse weather conditions such as rain, snow and driving winds. Convalescence of surviving lambs is protracted.

Differential diagnoses

- The clinical signs and epidemiological findings of cryptosporidiosis also fit *E. coli* infections in lambs aged 3–5 days.
- Starvation should also be considered in advanced cases.

Diagnosis

Diagnosis is based on the clinical findings and demonstration of *Cryptosporidium* species oocysts on a faecal smear stained with modified ZN or Giemsa stain; however, other enteropathogens may also be isolated and it may prove difficult to ascertain their relative importance. Identification of *C. parvum* on stained ileal sections of postmortem material is the preferred laboratory method for confirmation.

Treatment

There are no licensed antiprotozoal drugs or antibiotics for the treatment of cryptosporidiosis in neonatal ruminants. Anecdotal reports suggest that long-acting sulphonamides are useful in reducing clinical severity.

Oral fluid therapy is essential for the treatment of dehydrated neonatal lambs and 150–200 ml of a diluted calf oral rehydration solution should be administered 4–6 times daily, although this regimen involves a great deal of labour. Lambs should be left with their dam as they often suck, thus preventing the energy starvation that results from prolonged feeding of oral rehydration solutions, which contain a maximum of 30% of the lamb's daily energy requirements.

Prevention/control measures

Factors to be considered in the control of cryptosporidiosis include:

- Do not use the same fields for calving and lambing.
- Change fields every year or when clinical cases occur in that season.
- Move newborn animals immediately on to clean pasture.

Clinical cases should be isolated wherever possible but this can prove difficult at lambing time. The overall standard of hygiene must be improved for housed sheep, with extra bedding to limit oocyst challenge.

Economics

Losses from cryptosporidiosis can be high during adverse weather and if associated with concurrent bacterial infections of the gut. The lack of adequate farm staff during the lambing period limits effective fluid therapy regimens and this contributes to protracted convalescence and death of lambs. Poor subsequent growth rates lead to delays in marketing and reduced sale prices.

Welfare implications

While losses are generally low, affected lambs have a protracted convalescence and look miserable for a number of weeks before they start to thrive again.

Coccidiosis

Definition/overview

Coccidiosis is a problem worldwide whenever growing lambs are intensively stocked under poor hygiene standards (**260**). In the UK, for example, coccidiosis is becoming a major problem in lambs reared indoors

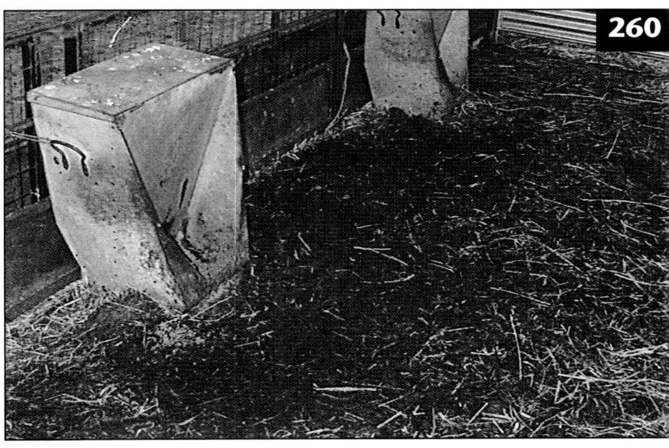

260 Poor hygiene directly contributes to the severity of coccidiosis in lambs.

with high stocking densities for early lamb production. It may also occur in lambs at pasture where there is heavy contamination around feed troughs in creep areas during warm wet weather (**261**). Loss of gut absorptive capacity often results in profuse diarrhoea.

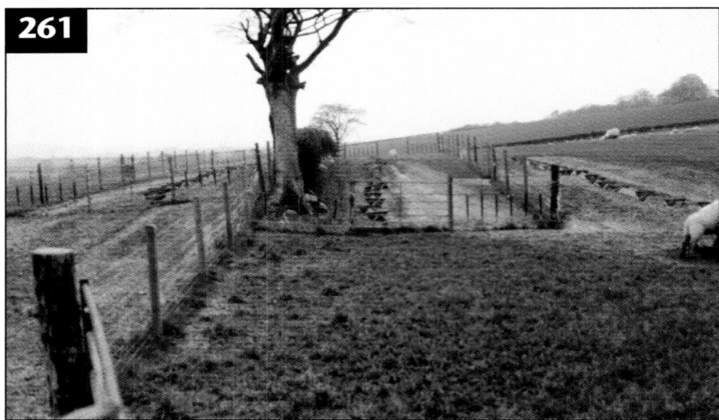

261 Heavy contamination around feed troughs in creep areas during warm wet weather can cause disease.

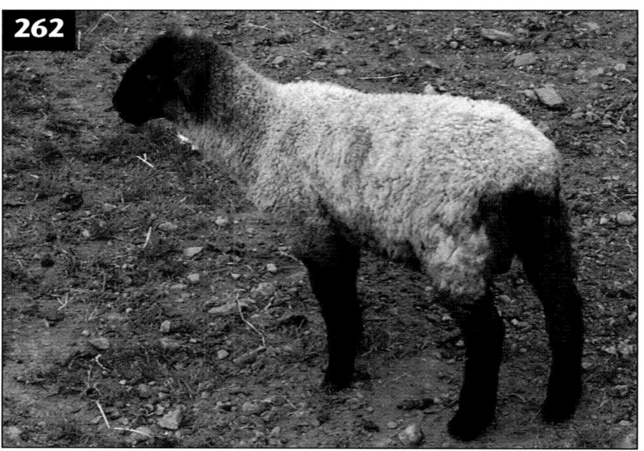

262 Poor condition and fetid diarrhoea in a lamb with coccidiosis.

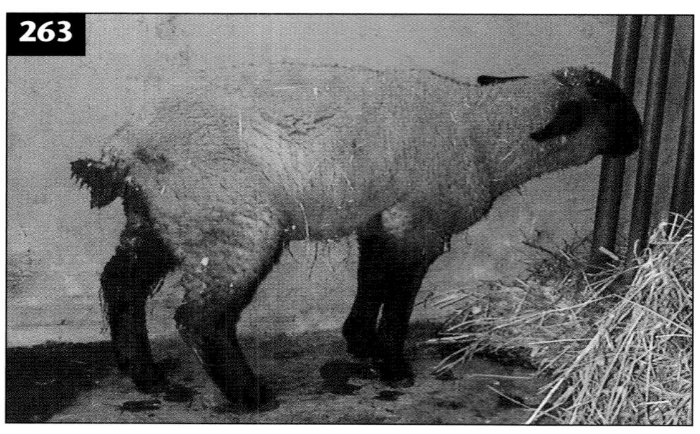

263 Tenesmus and diarrhoea in a six-week-old Suffolk lamb suffering from coccidiosis.

Aetiology

Coccidiosis is caused by infection by the protozoa of the genus *Eimeria*, which parasitize the epithelium lining the alimentary tract. Infection causes a loss of epithelial cells and villous atrophy. There are two pathogenic species in lambs, *E. crandallis* and *E. ovinoidalis*. The ewe is the probable source of the infection, which is then multiplied in young lambs, with a much greater challenge presented to later born lambs. Coccidia must sporulate outside the host to become infective, hence the importance of environmental contamination.

Clinical presentation

Lambs 4–6 weeks old are most commonly affected, with signs of rapid weight loss combined with a tucked-up appearance (**262**). In severe clinical coccidiosis there is a sudden onset of profuse fetid diarrhoea, which contains mucus and flecks of fresh blood. There is considerable faecal staining of the perineum and tail. Tenesmus (**263**) with partial eversion of the rectum is occasionally seen in severe infections. Straining is often accompanied by painful vocalization. Clinical disease is often precipitated by a stressful event such as adverse weather, weaning or dietary change.

More usually, the clinical signs are less severe, with gradual weight loss and poor appetite. Small clots of fresh blood and mucus are passed but the diarrhoea is not so marked. The rectal temperature is often normal. Morbidity is high but mortality is low. Convalescence is protracted in all cases.

There appears to be a synergistic effect between *Nematodirus battus* and *Eimeria* species, with relatively low levels of coccidia associated with clinical disease.

Differential diagnoses

Group problem of scouring lambs

- The major differential for scouring lambs grazing contaminated pasture in many countries is nematodirosis. In the UK, for example, this typically affects 6–8-week-old lambs during May.
- *Strongyloides westeri* infestation can cause diarrhoea in housed lambs kept in unhygienic conditions but this is uncommon.

Problem of poor growth in individual lambs

There are many causes of poor growth in individual young lambs including:

- Poor nutrition of the dam.
- Mastitis or other infectious disease of the dam.
- Liver abscessation.
- Chronic pneumonia.
- Infectious polyarthritis.

Diagnosis

Diagnosis is based on epidemiological and clinical findings plus the demonstration of large numbers of oocysts in faecal samples (often >100,000 oocysts per gram), in which *E. crandallis* or *E. ovinoidalis* predominate. In severe infestations disease may occur before oocysts are shed in the faeces.

At necropsy the caecum is inflamed, empty and contracted, with the wall thickened with hyperaemic mucosa. The ileum and colon may also be affected. Examination of gut sections from clinical cases reveals large numbers of oocysts.

Treatment

Sheep must be moved from infected pastures/premises as soon as disease becomes apparent. Sulphamethoxypyridazine injected subcutaneously once only is a common treatment for coccidiosis in lambs. Sulphadimidine can also be used. Decoquinate and diclazuril can be used but they are considerably more expensive than sulphonamides.

Prevention/control measures

Control involves avoidance of bedding contamination and pasture contamination around feed troughs. Adequate bedding must be provided when sheep are kept indoors. Creep areas at pasture can become heavily contaminated, especially during wet weather; therefore, the troughs should be moved regularly and not only when the area has become heavily contaminated.

Medication of the ewe ration with decoquinate will suppress but not totally eliminate oocyst production; therefore, this regimen is operated in conjunction with medication of the lamb creep feed (**264**). Occasionally, disease may occur because there are problems with ration palatability; the farmer elects to medicate only the lamb ration and the lambs choose to eat the non-medicated ewe concentrate. Indeed, recent developments have suggested that suppressing oocyst production by the ewes may be counter-productive because this only results in a delayed challenge to the lambs, with an increased likelihood of clinical disease in older lambs.

Clinical coccidiosis may also occur in growing lambs once decoquinate-medicated feed has been withdrawn, because active immunity is induced by contact with developing stages in the gut. In this situation, lambs should be moved to clean pasture once the in-feed medication has been discontinued.

Diclazuril can be used for the prophylaxis and treatment of coccidiosis in lambs. For prophylaxis, the whole group is drenched as soon as clinical signs are suspected in a lamb(s). Treated lambs should then be moved to a clean area to prevent re-infection before they have time to develop protective immunity.

In situations where lambs are moved on to suspected heavily contaminated fields, diclazuril should be given 10–14 days later to enable some active immunity to develop during this intervening period.

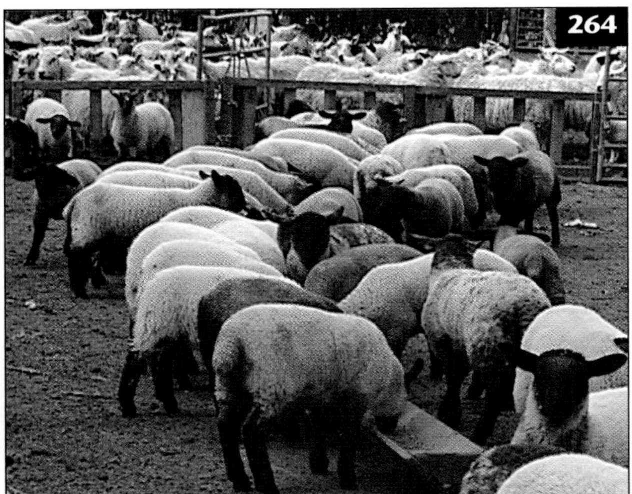

264 Provision of decoquinate-medicated creep feed in intensively reared lambs.

Economics

In-feed medication with decoquinate is expensive, adding approximately 25% to the cost of one tonne of feed. This may add 5–7% to the cost of each lamb reared under intensive conditions. Prophylactic treatment of coccidiosis in one-month-old lambs using diclazuril is an additional but smaller cost.

Welfare implications

Disease prevention is better than treatment/cure but many farmers choose not to use proven prevention strategies for cost reasons, with subsequent adverse effects on lamb well-being when disease occurs.

PARATUBERCULOSIS (*Syn*: Johne's disease)

Definition/overview

Paratuberculosis is a common disease of sheep in many countries worldwide. The disease is characterized by emaciation but not, as in cattle, chronic diarrhoea. Disease is encountered in all sheep husbandry systems including, in the UK, extensively managed Blackface flocks that are rarely housed and are usually confined only to small grass fields during the short lambing period. The annual ewe mortality rate is estimated at between 1–5% in infected flocks but there are few reliable data and underestimation of losses is likely.

Paratuberculosis is notifiable in some countries, including Australia, where annual losses as high as 15–20% have been reported in heavily infected flocks. The incidence of clinical disease is low in New Zealand (estimated to be 0.2%), though there is a higher incidence level in some flocks.

Aetiology

The aetiological agent of paratuberculosis, *Mycobacterium avium* subspecies *paratuberculosis*, is very resistant to desiccation and can survive on pasture for many months. There are a number of strains of this organism, including a pigmented strain. Sheep that develop clinical disease are infected early in life via the faeco-oral route, although infection can also be acquired *in utero* during the advanced stages of disease in the ewe. Infection ingested by adult sheep is unlikely to cause clinical disease. Goats can be an important source of infection when co-grazed with sheep, and this practice has led to very high levels of clinical disease in some sheep flocks. The role of cattle, various wildlife ruminant species and rabbits in the epidemiology of paratuberculosis is currently under investigation in the UK. Whether rabbits are an end-stage host, or act as a reservoir of infection (**265**) without showing clinical signs themselves, remains unclear.

Clinical presentation

Paratuberculosis presents as chronic weight loss/low BCS and poor fleece in individual middle-aged (typically 3–4 year old) sheep with normal dentition and fed an appropriate plane of nutrition. Unusually, disease has been described in yearling sheep. Emaciated sheep are typically detected during routine flock handling procedures such as pre-mating checks, when their BCS of 1.5 or below compares unfavourably with other sheep managed in a similar way (scores of 3.0 or greater) (**266, 267**). Unlike in cattle, chronic diarrhoea is not a feature in the majority of sheep affected by paratuberculosis; sheep often void pelleted faeces until the terminal stages. Affected sheep appear bright and alert (**268**) but may be weak due to their emaciated

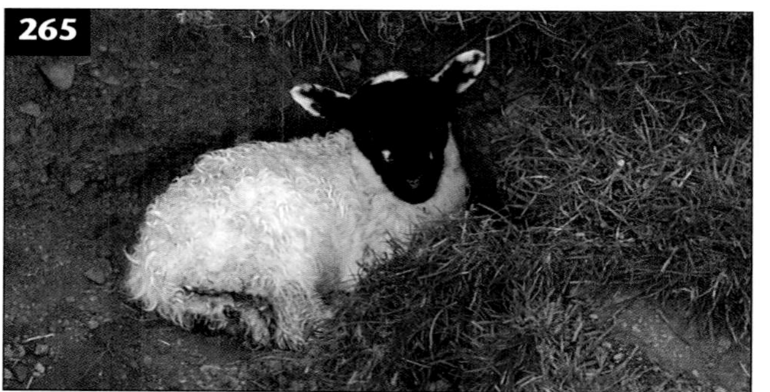

265 The role of rabbits in the aetiology of ovine paratuberculosis is presently under investigation. There is abundant opportunity for neonatal infection as evidenced by this lamb sheltering in a rabbit burrow.

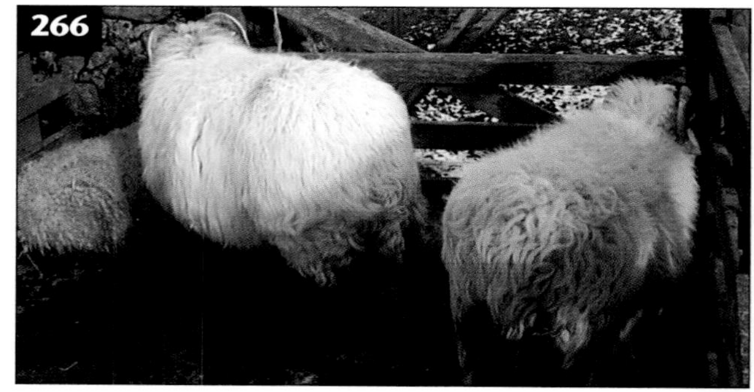

266 Two sheep of the same age from the same group. The ewe with paratuberculosis has a poor, open fleece and low condition.

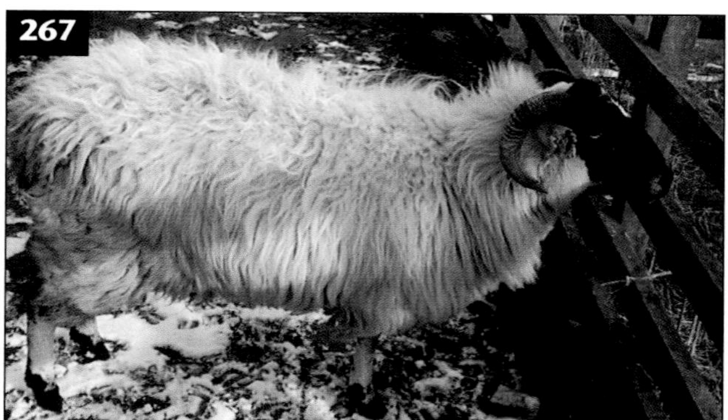

267 The ewe in **266** with paratuberculosis.

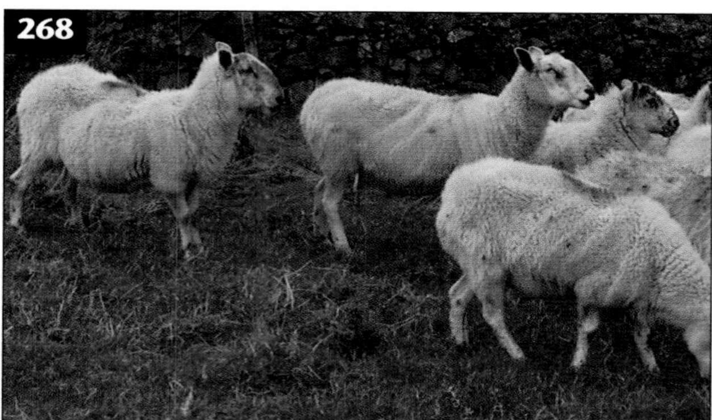

268 Group of young ewes selected for premature culling in a flock with a high prevalence of paratuberculosis. Diagnosis in live sheep can prove problematic.

state. They appear to have a normal appetite but rumen fill is reduced, with sunken sublumbar fossae (**269**). The wool is of poor quality and the fleece appears more open than usual and is easily detached by rough handling. The fleece changes are best appreciated by comparing an emaciated ewe with paratuberculosis with a sheep in good bodily condition (**266**).

During the agonal stages affected sheep may become recumbent and progress to a stuporous state (**270**), which further complicates the clinical diagnosis. Hypoalbuminaemia during the later stages of disease may result in small accumulations of fluid within the peritoneal and pleural cavities and the pericardium, although these are not usually noted during clinical examination. Submandibular oedema presents only in some advanced cases. The severity of clinical disease is compounded by concurrent parasitism, especially fasciolosis.

Lambs born to ewes in the terminal stages of disease have low birth weights (often as low as 2–3 kg) due to chronic intrauterine growth retardation but they are viable. These lambs should be culled immediately; they must not be kept as breeding replacement stock because of the likelihood of transplacental infection. Affected ewes should be culled for welfare reasons, as they will be unable to support even one lamb.

Differential diagnoses

In order of decreasing incidence, the common causes of weight loss and ill-thrift in sheep (in the UK) are:

Group problem

- Poor flock nutrition.
- Virulent footrot.
- Fasciolosis.
- Chronic parasitism due to poor pasture management and erroneous control strategies.
- Chronic parasitism caused by anthelmintic-resistant strains of nematodes.

Individual sheep

- Poor dentition, especially molar teeth.
- Paratuberculosis.
- Chronic suppurative pneumonia, mastitis, septic joint, endocarditis or other septic focus.
- Chronic severe lameness (e.g. septic pedal arthritis).
- Sheep pulmonary adenomatosis.
- Intestinal adenocarcinoma.
- Scrapie.
- Lymphosarcoma.
- Maedi-visna.

In many states in the USA the visceral form of CLA is considered to be the most important cause of chronic weight loss in adult sheep.

Diagnosis

While on-farm postmortem examination of individual ewes will identify gross lesions of many diseases, the intestinal changes caused by paratuberculosis can be easily overlooked, even by experts. More importantly, a single necropsy provides little information regarding the prevalence of certain disease conditions on the farm. In most situations it will prove more useful to investigate weight loss in ten or more ewes than to send a single ewe for detailed postmortem examination. In general practice, with only a limited budget per ewe for laboratory tests, serum albumin and globulin determinations could provide the most useful screening tests for the investigation of chronic weight loss in a number of adult sheep.

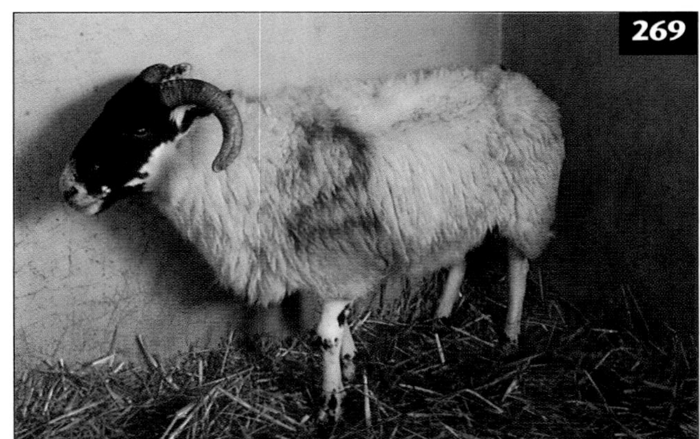

269 Emaciated Scottish Blackface ewe with paratuberculosis. The sublumbar fossae are sunken.

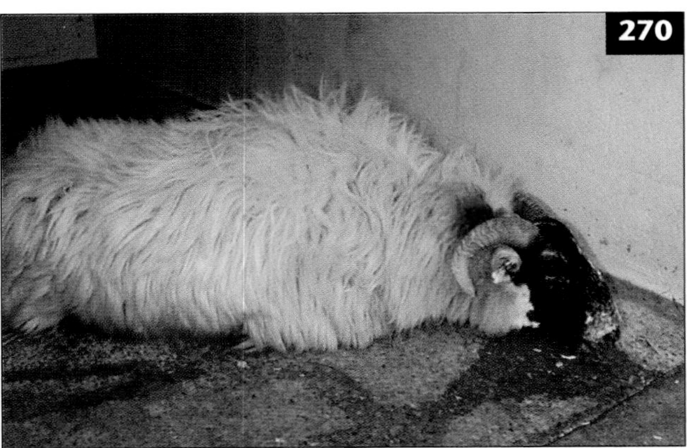

270 Sheep with paratuberculosis can present with vague neurological signs, such as stupor, during the agonal stages.

Serum protein analysis in the investigation of weight loss

Albumin reflects the balance between hepatic synthesis from dietary nitrogenous intake and endogenous demands/losses. Serum globulin is a long-term indicator of the body's response to bacterial infections. Other proteins, such as haptoglobin or fibrinogen, are more useful as indicators of acute disease, with significant increases within 1–3 days and more than 4–7 days, respectively.

Sheep with paratuberculosis have profound hypoalbuminaemia (serum concentration <15 g/l but as low as 6–10 g/l in advanced disease [normal range 30–36 g/l]) and a normal globulin concentration. These changes result from loss of albumin across the damaged intestinal mucosa (protein-losing enteropathy). These serum protein concentrations may also be encountered in cases of severe chronic intestinal parasitism such as haemonchosis, but such infestations are generally group problems. Fasciolosis may result in hypoalbuminaemia but these sheep usually show additional clinical signs such as anaemia and submandibular oedema. In addition, many sheep with subacute and chronic fasciolosis have greatly increased serum globulin concentrations, often exceeding 70 g/l (normal value 35–50 g/l).

It must be remembered that sheep with paratuberculosis often have high faecal egg counts (>1,000 epg) due to immunosuppression. Detailed examination typically fails to reveal significant populations of adult nematodes at necropsy; the high egg output is the result of increased fecundity.

Chronic bacterial infections causing weight loss/ill thrift result in significant increases in serum globulin concentration (often >55 g/l) and low serum albumin concentration (often around 18–25 g/l but rarely <15 g/l). Low albumin/high globulin indicates a probable chronic suppurative disease process/focus (e.g. chronic suppurative pneumonia, endocarditis, liver abscessation, mastitis, infectious polyarthritis, cellulitis). Once the possibility of a chronic suppurative focus has been highlighted, the sheep should be re-examined. Further specific tests can then be selected based on the organ system suspected of being involved: for example, serum gamma glutamyl transferase (GGT) concentrations and faecal fluke egg count for chronic fasciolosis; chest radiographs/ultrasonography if chronic suppurative pneumonia is suspected; abdominocentesis/ultrasonography for peritonitis.

Low serum albumin/normal globulin concentrations (<25 g/l and <45 g/l, respectively) suggest that chronic bacterial infection is unlikely. A dietary effect such as low protein intake is one possible explanation. A lowered serum albumin concentration is also often encountered during late pregnancy in ewes fed poor quality rations at a time when protein metabolism is geared toward immunoglobulin production and transfer into the colostrum in the udder.

Significant serological titres (either AGID or ELISA) are detected in approximately 60% of clinical paratuberculosis cases, resulting in a high false-negative rate (low sensitivity), although the specificity is high (>95%).

Direct faecal examination will not detect the paucibacillary form of ovine paratuberculosis and therefore it provides unreliable results. Cultural isolation takes at least eight weeks, and possibly up to six months, and has very limited practical application.

Postmortem examination

There is an emaciated carcase with gelatinous atrophy of fat depots (**271**). However, gross changes of paratuberculosis can easily be overlooked during a cursory on-farm postmortem examination and great care must be taken not to miss potential lesions. Thickening of the ileum, with prominent ridgeing, is not always obvious in paratuberculosis but the mesenteric lymph nodes are visibly enlarged (**271**). The diagnosis is confirmed by demonstrating clumps of acid-fast bacteria after ZN staining of ileal sections and ileocaecal lymph nodes.

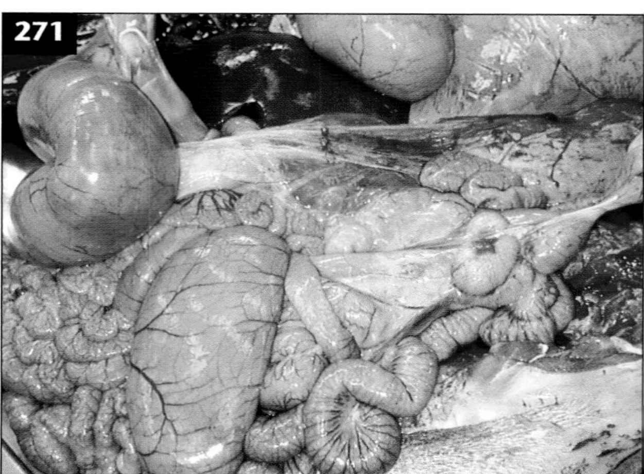

271 Necropsy of the ewe in **270**. The mesenteric lymph nodes are enlarged and there is serous atrophy of the fat.

Depending on the geographic area and the strain distribution, few sheep, if any, present with the yellow/orange pigmented strain of paratuberculosis (272).

Prevention/control measures

The true paratuberculosis incidence in sheep flocks largely remains unknown. In the UK control measures presently operating on some commercial sheep farms are limited to culling suspected clinical cases and, where records permit, their progeny. This measure is unlikely to have a significant impact on paratuberculosis prevalence. The wide host range of *M. a. paratuberculosis*, including wildlife reservoirs, provides many opportunities for disease transmission and may render destocking policies useless.

In several countries, encouraging results, with much reduced disease prevalence, have been reported following adoption of a vaccination programme. Vaccination against paratuberculosis has been practised in flocks in New Zealand since 1987. Vaccinating lambs is useful in controlling and eliminating the disease, but vaccinated lambs have to be permanently identified and the vaccination procedure is dangerous to the administrator. Studies have commenced in Australia using an inactivated *M. a. paratuberculosis* vaccine administered to sheep over one month old.

Presently, vaccination offers the best long-term prospect for control but the high unit cost may restrict this option to replacement pedigree breeding stock. In the UK, for example, the culling rate due to paratuberculosis must exceed 4% to offset the high cost of vaccinating ewe lambs. Vaccinating lambs before they are two weeks of age presents numerous management problems. There is a considerable localized reaction at the injection site in sheep. Care must be exercised not to self-inject with the oil-adjuvant live attenuated vaccine, as this may result in serious local reaction.

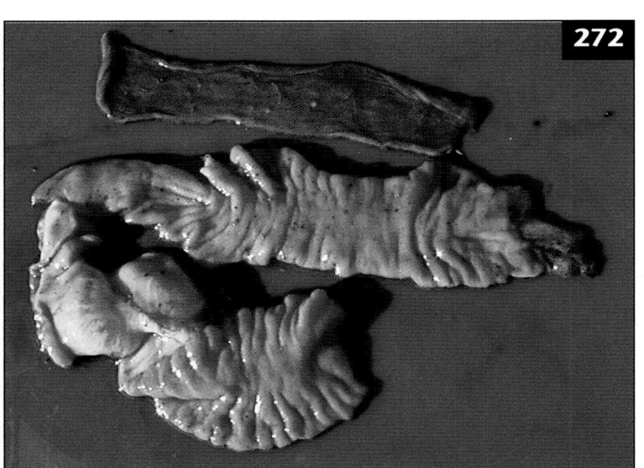

272 Thickened, corrugated and pigmented ileum from a ewe with paratuberculosis (lower specimen) compared with the normal specimen.

Economics

Difficulties with confirmation of the provisional diagnosis of paratuberculosis, coupled with very few ewes culled for poor condition/emaciation submitted to the veterinarian, can lead to a gross underestimation of the prevalence and financial impact of this disease. In the author's experience of some lowland flocks in Scotland (UK), losses and increased culling due to poor body condition in sheep with paratuberculosis approach 5% of adult stock per annum. This figure compares with the UK average ewe mortality rate of 5–7% per annum. Their debilitated state may also render affected ewes more susceptible to infectious disease, parasitic infestations and predation.

Welfare implications

Those suspected/confirmed paratuberculosis-infected sheep during the early stages of disease (poorer body condition compared with that of peers) should be culled immediately to reduce environmental contamination. Emaciated sheep must be destroyed immediately on the farm.

CLOSTRIDIAL DISEASES

Definition/overview

Clostridial diseases remain a serious threat to unvaccinated sheep in all countries worldwide. Typically, death occurs within hours of rapid bacterial multiplication and exotoxin production, although lambs with tetanus can survive for several days. Despite effective control from timely vaccination and the protection afforded lambs by passive antibody transfer, clostridial diseases still occur all too frequently because of management errors. Suprisingly, a recent UK survey revealed that almost 20% of sheep farmers did not vaccinate their sheep on a regular basis. The growth of certain organic food schemes in some countries, including the UK, is a concern when membership prevents clostridial vaccination until these diseases occur on the farm. Such abandonment of proven preventive schemes is grossly irresponsible and merely invites disease, with consequent unnecessary suffering and avoidable deaths.

It is the veterinarian's duty to ensure that all sheep clients operate an effective clostridial vaccination programme for both economic and welfare reasons. With this point in mind the reader is directed to the sections in earlier chapters detailing late gestation ewe nutrition (see Chapter 2: Late gestation ewe nutrition, p. 17) and neonatal lamb management (see Chapter 4: Perinatal lamb mortality, p. 83), because clostridial diseases in young growing lambs are readily prevented by ensuring adequate specific antibody accumulation in colostrum and timely transfer to lambs within the first six hours of life. Such basic husbandry measures must not be overlooked by farmers and veterinarians.

The main clostridial diseases are lamb dysentery caused by *Clostridium perfringens* type B; struck caused by *C. perfringens* type C; lamb dysentery caused by *C. perfringens* type D; black disease (infectious necrotic hepatitis) caused by *C. novyi* type B; braxy caused by *C. septicum*; bacillary haemoglobinuria caused by *C. haemolytica*; and blackleg caused by *C. chauvoei*. Various clostridia, including *C. chauvoei, C. perfringens* type A, *C. septicum*, *C. novyi* type A and *C. sordellii,* are associated with malignant oedema. Tetanus follows the production of a neurotoxin by *C. tetani*. Botulism is caused by the ingestion of preformed toxins of *C. botulinum*.

Aetiology

Clostridia are generally considered to be ubiquitous in the environment, particularly in organic material, with disease triggered by various factors including changes in feeding and parasite damage to tissues. Such microenvironments within the body permit rapid clostridial multiplication and exotoxin production, characteristically leading to death within hours.

Treatment

With the exception of blackleg and bighead, there are no effective treatments for clostridial diseases.

Prevention/control measures

There are well-established vaccination protocols using toxoid vaccines, which prevent all the common clostridial diseases; protection against botulism is not provided by standard polyvalent clostridial vaccines. Clostridial disease invariably results from failure to adhere to vaccination instructions and good management practices.

Initially, two vaccinations are given 4–6 weeks apart, followed by annual vaccination 4–6 weeks before the expected lambing date to ensure adequate accumulation of protective immunoglobulins in the colostrum. Lambs are vaccinated from 3–4 months of age, with the programme completed before weaning, unless they are sold for slaughter before waning of maternal antibody at around 4–5 months of age. Rams are commonly forgotten in vaccination programmes and veterinarians must remind their clients so that this oversight is avoided. It should be assumed that purchased lambs have not been vaccinated unless there is written confirmation from the vendor that this has been correctly undertaken.

In some countries a hyperimmune serum containing lamb dysentery and pulpy kidney disease antibodies can be administered to newborn lambs born to unvaccinated dams in order to afford temporary protection. However, this short-term method of providing protection is expensive, labour-intensive and unnecessary when dam vaccination and passive antibody transfer produces such excellent control. Hyperimmune serum can be used in an attempt to prevent losses in the face of an outbreak of lamb dysentery.

Gradual changes in diet such as a step-wise introduction of concentrate feeding may reduce the incidence of clostridial disease; it will also reduce the risk of conditions such as acidosis and polioencephalomalacia. Prophylactic antibiotic injections following unskilled correction of dystocia may reduce the likelihood of blackleg.

In some countries, vaccination against pasteurellosis is combined with clostridial vaccination.

Economics

Clostridial vaccination is cheap and very effective.

Welfare implications

Illness from clostridial disease has serious welfare implications. Tetanus is a particularly painful condition and affected lambs should be euthanased immediately the condition has been diagnosed.

Lamb dysentery

Aetiology

Lamb dysentry is caused by *C. perfringens* type B.

Clinical presentation

Sporadic cases of lamb dysentry may occur in a flock in those lambs that have received nil or inadequate specific antibody in the colostrum. This may be due to various factors including: individual ewes not vaccinated; insufficient colostrum accumulation in the ewe's udder due to poor feeding/mastitis; large litter; or feeding colostrum supplements/bovine colostrum from unvaccinated donors.

Lamb dysentery is more typically identified as a disease outbreak in lambs born to unvaccinated ewes, with losses approaching 20–30% of susceptible lambs. Lambs less than one week old are affected at the beginning of the outbreak; later, losses occur in older lambs. Initially, lambs are found dead without any observed clinical signs. Thereafter, careful observation reveals lambs that are lethargic, do not suck, have a gaunt appearance (273), show frequent tenesmus with painful bleating and develop dysentery during the agonal stages, which is accompanied by rapid dehydration, recumbency and death within 2–12 hours.

Differential diagnoses

Differential diagnoses of sudden death in young lambs includes:

- Pasteurellosis, colisepticaemia and other acute bacterial conditions.
- Salmonellosis rarely causes disease in young lambs.
- Starvation, exposure, hepatic necrobacillosis, cryptosporidiosis and bacterial enteric infections cause lethargy and a gaunt appearance, often with evidence of diarrhoea, but these signs should be detected before death ensues some days later.

Diagnosis

The provisional diagnosis of lamb dysentery is based on the history of ineffective vaccination and/or failure of passive antibody transfer, clinical findings and postmortem examination. Necropsy findings include a haemorrhagic enteritis with excessive blood-stained fluid within the body cavities and pericardium. The demonstration of specific toxins by ELISA may give a number of false-positive results and such laboratory tests must be interpreted in conjunction with clinical and epidemiological findings.

Treatment

There is no treatment for lamb dysentry.

Pulpy kidney disease

Aetiology

Pulpy kidney disease is caused by *C. perfringens* type D.

Clinical presentation

Pulpy kidney disease occurs in 4–10-week-old lambs born to unvaccinated dams, and in weaned lambs from four months old when passively derived antibody has waned and the lambs themselves have not been vaccinated. Losses in weaned lambs often follow dietary improvements such as the introduction of concentrate feeding or movement to lush pastures.

The major clinical feature is sudden death; losses may exceed 5% before action is taken by the farmer. Affected sheep are initially very dull, almost stuporous, but they progress quickly to seizure activity and opisthotonus, followed rapidly by death (274). Clinical signs are not usually observed by the farmer, as this class of livestock is only inspected daily.

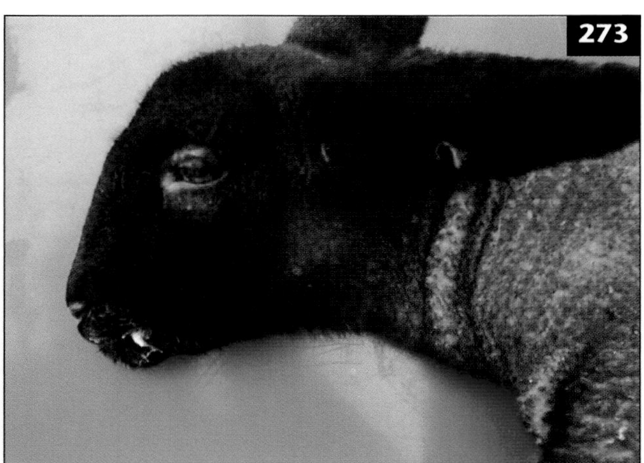

273 Profound depression and painful expression in a young lamb that died six hours later from lamb dysentery.

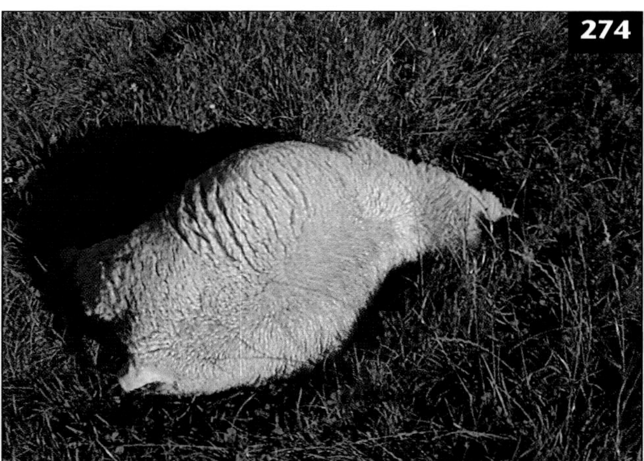

274 Sudden death in a five-month-old lamb, subsequently confirmed at necropsy as pulpy kidney disease.

Differential diagnoses

- Differential diagnoses of sudden death in growing lambs include nematodirosis and pneumonic pasteurellosis.
- The main differential diagnosis in weaned lambs is systemic pasteurellosis. In certain geographic areas acute fasciolosis and black disease must also be considered. Sheep recently introduced on to a concentrate ration or given access to stubble are susceptible to acidosis.

Diagnosis

Diagnosis is based on epidemiology, lack of vaccination history (although this may be uncertain in purchased sheep) and necropsy findings.

There is rapid autolysis of the carcase with excess serosanguinous fluid in the body cavities, more especially the abdomen. The kidneys are very friable. A glycosuria, consequent to hepatic glycolysis, is present and is readily detectable on urinary dipstick (a useful field test). Characteristic lesions of focal symmetrical encephalomalacia can be demonstrated by histopathological examination of brain tissue.

Treatment

There is no treatment for pulpy kidney disease.

BRAXY

Aetiology

Braxy is caused by *C. septicum* and is characteristically seen in unvaccinated weaned lambs during the winter months, associated with ingestion of frosted root crops (275). Although *C. septicum* occurs in New Zealand, braxy as such has never been diagnosed.

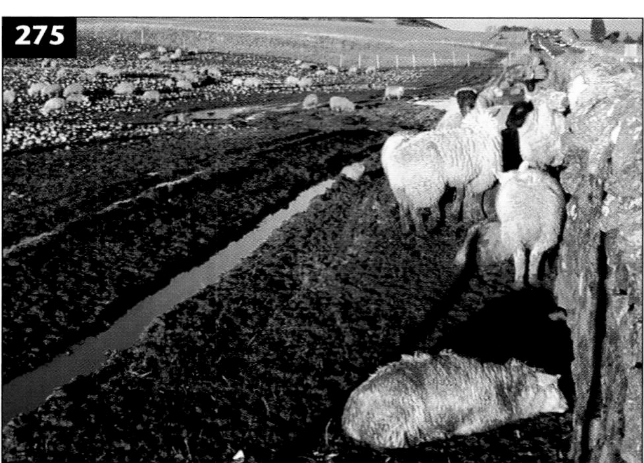

275 Sudden death associated with grazing frosted turnips.

Clinical presentation

Affected sheep are almost invariably found dead. Those that are observed alive are profoundly depressed and may show abdominal pain, but this is difficult to appreciate. There is rapid carcase decomposition despite the prevailing low environmental temperature.

Differential diagnoses

- Other clostridial diseases such as pulpy kidney disease and black disease.
- Other causes of sudden death including systemic pasteurellosis and subacute fasciolosis.
- Sheep recently introduced on to a concentrate ration are susceptible to acidosis.
- Ingestion of root crops may lead to frothy bloat/choke.

Diagnosis

Diagnosis is based on epidemiology, including recent frost, and lack of a vaccination history.

Treatment

There is no treatment.

BLACK DISEASE

(*Syn*: infectious necrotic hepatitis)

Aetiology

Black disease is caused by *C. novyi* type B.

Clinical presentation

In the UK black disease is typically associated with migration of immature liver flukes during late summer/early autumn and it can affect unvaccinated sheep of all ages. In the absence of rapid intervention and appropriate action, losses can be very high in unvaccinated sheep. Sudden death in 2–4-year-old unvaccinated sheep due to black disease is reported in New Zealand and Australia.

Clinical signs are rarely observed and sheep are simply found dead. There is rapid carcase decomposition, accumulation of blood-tinged fluid within body cavities and widespread petechial haemorrhages. The liver is congested and very dark, with areas of necrosis visible on cut section. There is evidence of fluke tracks throughout the liver in those geographical areas where the disease is associated with acute fasciolosis.

Differential diagnoses

- The main differential diagnosis is acute fasciolosis but also includes other clostridial diseases and systemic pasteurellosis.

- Louping ill should be considered in tick-infested areas in certain countries.
- Sheep recently introduced on to a concentrate ration are susceptible to acidosis.

Diagnosis
Diagnosis is based on necropsy findings and lack of a vaccination history. Laboratory tests, such as the fluorescent antibody test (FAT), may yield false-positive results and should not be interpreted in isolation.

Treatment
There is no treatment. An appropriate fluke control plan, combined with an appropriate clostridial vaccination programme, will effectively control black disease, although very occasional deaths may still occur.

Bacillary haemoglobinuria
(*Syn*: redwater)

Aetiology
Bacillary haemoglobinuria occurs sporadically in many countries worldwide. It is caused by *C. haemolytica*.

Clinical presentation
Affected sheep are dull, depressed, inappetent and pyrexic and they have dark red urine. Jaundice is present during the agonal stages and affected sheep die in 2–3 days.

Differential diagnoses
- Copper toxicity and nitrate poisoning.
- Acute fasciolosis can also result in anaemia and death within days from severe infestation.

Diagnosis
Necropsy reveals large infarcts in the liver and haemorrhage into the renal cortex, with red urine in the renal pelvis and bladder. Laboratory tests (e.g. FAT) may yield false-positive results and should not be interpreted in isolation.

Treatment
There is no treatment.

Blackleg (*Syn*: postparturient gangrene)

Aetiology
Blackleg occurs in all countries worldwide. It is caused by *C. chauvoei*, which, in common with the other clostridial organisms causing disease in sheep, can survive in soil for many years. Entry of clostridia occurs through skin wounds, dog bites, shearing cuts, contaminated needles/injection equipment, an untreated umbilicus and trauma to the posterior reproductive tract during attempted dystocia correction. Blackleg has also been reported after tail docking in unhygienic and contaminated handling facilities.

Clinical presentation
Blackleg usually occurs sporadically within a flock. Typically, affected sheep are very dull, depressed, inappetent and febrile (>41.0°C) and they have toxic mucous membranes. Further clinical signs depend on the site of bacterial entry.

Involvement of one limb results in sudden onset severe lameness, with the limb often dragged along. Once recumbent the sheep has great difficulty raising itself. There is marked swelling of the limb (**276**), with oedema, subcutaneous emphysema and purple discoloration of overlying skin, and it often has a crepitant feel. The drainage lymph node is markedly enlarged.

Invasion and infection of traumatized tissues of the posterior reproductive tract result from excessive unskilled interference of dystocia cases without

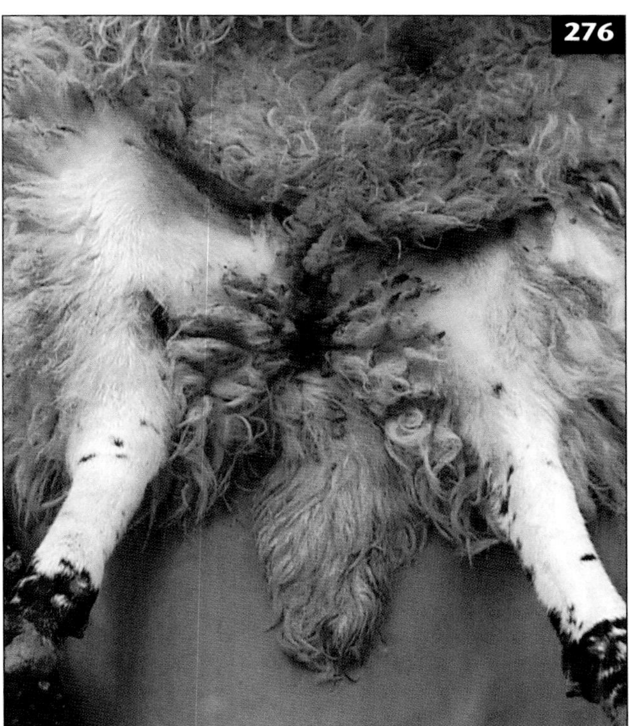

276 Blackleg. The greatly swollen right thigh should be compared with the normal side.

appropriate hygienic precautions. The ewe often spends long periods in sternal recumbency. The ewe has no milk and the lambs are very hungry and gaunt. There may be considerable swelling and oedema of the vulva, with a scant serosanguinous discharge.

Infection of the umbilicus in neonatal lambs leads to rapid death.

Differential diagnoses

- The important differential diagnoses for sudden onset severe lameness include cellulitis from dog bites, long bone fractures and joint trauma. Foot abscesses and septic pedal arthritis can cause severe lameness but are not so acute in presentation.
- The important differential diagnosis for post-parturient gangrene is metritis, which occurs under similar conditions of poor hygiene and unskilled interference. Severe metritis is common after many cases of infectious abortion, particularly *Salmonella typhimurium* and, less commonly, *Chlamydophila abortus*.
- Other differential diagnoses include failure to detect fetal malpresentation (commonly breech presentation), which results in prolonged first stage labour, fetal death and emphysema, with toxin absorption across the compromised endometrium causing illness. Failure to deliver all fetuses and retention of a fetus causes severe toxaemia 36–48 hours after fetal death. Uterine rupture may occur during attempted dystocia correction, with onset of acute septic peritonitis following leakage of bacteria and toxins into the abdominal cavity. Obvious infectious diseases such as gangrenous mastitis will be detected during the clinical examination.
- While much less common after lambing, hypocalcaemia causes recumbency and depression, leading to bloat and stupor, although there is no pyrexia.

Diagnosis

Diagnosis of blackleg is based on typical clinical findings in unvaccinated sheep. Death results in very rapid carcase autolysis and bloat. There is obvious muscle necrosis with associated blood-tinged oedema, although these lesions may be deep-seated within a muscle mass, necessitating methodical sectioning at necropsy.

Treatment

Based on clinical examination alone, it may prove difficult to be certain of a diagnosis of blackleg during the early stages. Penicillin (44,000 iu/kg) is the drug of choice for clostridial disease, with the first dose given intravenously wherever possible. (**NB**: Off-label restrictions may apply in some countries.) NSAIDs such as flunixin or ketoprofen are unlicensed for sheep in many countries but they have potent analgesic and anti-inflammatory actions. Corticosteroids such as dexamethasone assist reduction of oedema and localized swelling.

MALIGNANT OEDEMA (*Syn*: bighead)

Aetiology

Various clostridia, including *C. chauvoei, C. perfringens* type A, *C. septicum*, *C. novyi* type A and *C. sordellii*, are associated with malignant oedema.

Clinical presentation

Malignant oedema is typically seen in rams during late summer/early autumn when head butting is a common behaviour in establishing a hierarchy prior to, and during, the breeding season. Cases often occur within days of introducing purchased rams into an established group. Malignant oedema has been reported after contaminated intramuscular injection and following injection of substances that cause local tissue necrosis.

Affected sheep are dull and depressed and stand isolated from others in the group. The most obvious clinical sign is marked swelling of the head, particularly surrounding the eyes, which forces the eyelids closed (277). There may be skin abrasions to the poll and blood streaked along the wool of the flanks but such indications of fighting are common in groups of rams. There is obvious subcutaneous oedema of the face, and this may extend to the neck. The mucous membranes are congested. It may prove difficult to palpate the submandibular lymph nodes because of the oedema. Affected sheep are febrile (41.0–42.0°C). Occasionally, narrowing of the upper airways may cause inspiratory dyspnoea.

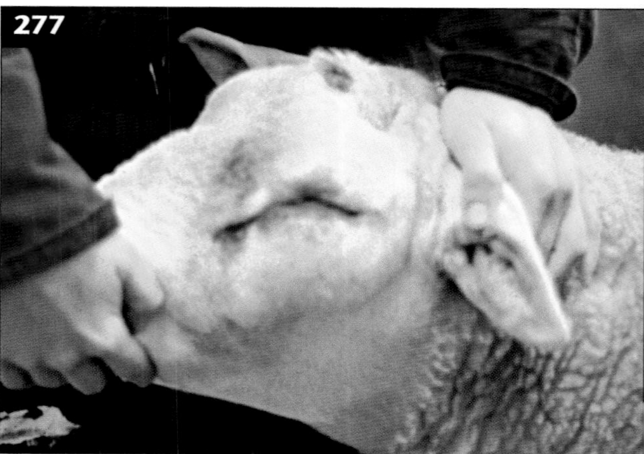

277 Marked facial oedema associated with malignant oedema.

Differential diagnoses

- The main differential diagnosis is cellulitis following infection of head wounds caused by fighting injuries. Myiasis of such head wounds is common.
- Periorbital eczema causes marked swelling and oedema with closure of the palpebral fissure but these sheep are not sick.

Diagnosis

Diagnosis is based on the clinical findings.

Treatment

Malignant oedema is the only clostridial disease that responds well to antibiotic therapy. Penicillin (44,000 iu/kg q12h) is the drug of choice, with the first dose given intravenously. (**NB:** Off-label restrictions may apply in many countries.) Corticosteroids such as dexamethasone assist the reduction of oedema and localized swelling.

Management factors to control malignant oedema are aimed at reducing fighting injuries in rams. Mixing is best achieved by keeping rams confined together in handling pens for a period of time. Such confinement aids spread of odours amongst the rams whilst preventing charging each other and head butting. Many farmers coincide mixing groups of rams with plunge dipping as this is claimed to reduce fighting, presumably due to a 'common odour'. Prompt antibiotic treatment of head wounds will prevent clostridial multiplication but not all wounds are obvious. Collecting areas with large accumulations of organic matter should be avoided but rams actively search out such areas whilst avoiding clean pasture.

TETANUS

Definition/overview

Tetanus is caused by the production of a powerful neurotoxin by *C. tetani*, with clinical signs most frequently encountered in young lambs. The neurotoxin progressively causes spasticity, recumbency, opisthotonus and death. Tetanus has a worldwide distribution but its occurrence depends upon failure of well-established vaccination regimens. All animals, including man, are susceptible to tetanus.

Aetiology

Tetanus is rarely encountered where clostridial vaccination forms an integral part of management practice. However, errors occur and vaccination is forgotten and this can lead to the appearance of clostridial diseases, including tetanus.

Historically, tetanus was observed approximately one week after surgical castration and tail docking, when lambs were 4–6 weeks old. The handling pens rapidly became contaminated with clostridial spores, leading to infection of skin wounds.

Clinical presentation

Lambs show hindlimb stiffness and difficulty following their dam. Difficulty walking leads to long periods spent in sternal recumbency. Affected lambs are hungry and have a gaunt appearance. The condition progresses over 24–48 hours to lateral recumbency, seizure activity progressing to opisthotonus, and death from respiratory failure.

Differential diagnoses

- The initial period of hindlimb stiffness can be differentiated from bacterial polyarthritis on clinical examination.
- Lateral recumbency with extensor tone is observed in lambs with a cervical spinal lesion, typically vertebral empyema affecting C1–C6 in 1–4-month-old lambs.
- Hindlimb ataxia occurs during the early stages of delayed swayback, when lambs are 2–3 months old.
- Louping ill is uncommon in lambs because of protection afforded by maternally-derived antibody.
- Seizure activity and opisthotonus are observed during the agonal stages of bacterial meningoencephalitis, which most commonly affects 2–3-week-old lambs. Bacterial meningoencephalitis occurs only sporadically in lambs and never as an outbreak.
- Polioencephalomalacia is not seen in lambs less than four months old.

Diagnosis

Diagnosis is based on the clinical signs and history of recent castration/tail docking in lambs from unvaccinated ewes.

Treatment

There is no effective treatment and all affected lambs should be euthanased for welfare reasons.

FOCAL SYMMETRICAL ENCEPHALOMALACIA

Definition/overview

Focal symmetrical encephalomalacia (FSE) occurs sporadically in unvaccinated sheep, more commonly in young lambs and in lambs after weaning.

Aetiology

FSE is caused by *C. perfringens* type D.

Clinical presentation
The clinical signs are poorly defined but include depression, lethargy and separation from other sheep in the group, with progression to ataxia, recumbency, opisthotonus and death after a few days.

Differential diagnoses
- Louping ill could occur in sheep introduced on to hill pasture with autumn tick activity.
- Polioencephalomalacia is common in weaned lambs more than four months old, often occurring following pasture change.
- Hepatic encephalopathy has been described in severely cobalt-deficient lambs.
- Nephrosis is uncommon in lambs more than three months old but presents with many of the early clinical signs of FSE.

Diagnosis
Diagnosis is based on clinical signs in sheep from unvaccinated flocks, with confirmation following histological examination of brain tissue.

Treatment
There is no treatment.

Botulism
Definition/overview
The epidemiology of botulism varies from country to country. In the UK botulism is rarely diagnosed in sheep despite the recent upsurge in feeding big bale silage. In some countries (e.g. South America, South Africa and Australia) outbreaks, particularly in cattle, are associated with either pica in phosphorus-deficient animals on extensive grazings or prolonged starvation due to drought.

Aetiology
Botulism is caused by the ingestion of pre-formed toxins of *C. botulinum*.

Clinical presentation
Depending upon the amount of toxin ingested, affected sheep may simply be found dead. Clinical signs are confined to the central nervous system, with ataxia, hyperaesthesia and a characteristic head-bobbing action. This state quickly progresses to flaccid paralysis and death.

Diagnosis
Diagnosis is difficult in individual sheep. In some countries (e.g. Australia) large numbers of dead sheep under extreme grazing conditions should highlight the possibility of botulism.

Treatment
There is no effective treatment. The disease can be controlled by specific vaccination in those areas where botulism occurs but it is not included in standard multivalent clostridial vaccines.

SALMONELLOSIS

Definition/overview
Enteric salmonellosis occurs worldwide, especially in intensively managed production systems, typically feed lots. Salmonellosis is an important zoonosis capable of causing severe disease in vulnerable people.

Enteric disease caused by *Salmonella* species is invariably associated with stress (e.g. transport, post weaning of lambs, close confinement, starvation, dietary change and other stressful conditions). Debilitated sheep are most susceptible to disease. Dysentery and sudden death may occur in neonatal lambs in heavily infected flocks, with infection originating from abortion material, uterine discharges and faeces.

Aetiology
Many *Salmonella* species can cause enteric disease but *S. typhimurium* is the most common isolate, commonly acquired from infected cattle and occasionally human sewage. *S. hindmarsh*, *S. bovis-morbificans* and *S. brandeburg* have been commonly recorded in New Zealand. Birds and carrion may act as vectors. Apparently healthy carrier sheep can also introduce infection into a flock.

Clinical presentation
Typically, disease outbreaks are encountered in recently transported weaned sheep. Starvation, dehydration, fluctuating environmental temperatures and long distances contribute to a high morbidity in susceptible transported sheep. Affected sheep are profoundly depressed and weak and may be unable to stand. Deaths may have already occurred within the group during transportation. The rectal temperature is increased to 41–42°C and there are toxic mucous membranes and episcleral injection. The sheep refuse feed and appear gaunt. There is profuse fetid diarrhoea containing blood clots and mucosal casts. Morbidity rates up to 30% have been reported with mortality rates as high as 25%. Severely affected lambs become recumbent and, in the agonal stages, may show opisthotonus. Death ensues within 2–3 days from dehydration and septicaemia/toxaemia.

Differential diagnoses

- Sudden death in recently weaned lambs may result from pulpy kidney disease and systemic pasteurellosis.
- Diarrhoea may be caused by coccidiosis, yersiniosis, campylobacteriosis and heavy nematode infestations compounded by trace element deficiency.

Diagnosis

The provisional diagnosis of salmonellosis causing dysentery and sudden deaths in recently stressed weaned lambs can be confirmed following culture of faeces and, in septicaemic cases, culture of, for example, mesenteric lymph node, liver, spleen and heart blood.

Treatment

Treatment of individual sheep is limited to injectable antibiotics, NSAIDs and diluted oral electrolyte solutions administered by orogastric tube. The choice of antibiotic can prove problematic, as clinicians should be loathe to use fluoroquinolone antibiotics. Trimethoprim/sulpha is the logical choice in most situations. Water medication may be possible in some feed lot situations but in many countries there are few antibiotics licensed for such use.

Prevention/control measures

Prevention is based on good management practices such as restricted journey times/distances to finishing units, prior weaning and dietary changes, and isolation of groups from different sources at their destination. A vaccine is available in New Zealand and is used annually on sheep at risk. Vaccination is carried out prior to the time of year when salmonellosis can be expected. Clean fresh water must always be available, with feed held in hoppers to prevent faecal contamination. Pens should be free draining to prevent surface water accumulation.

Sporadic cases of salmonellosis arise from contact with cattle, especially calves, and contamination from slurry stores and septic tanks.

Economics

Salmonellosis is not a major problem in sheep except for large, intensive finishing units, where losses can be high.

Welfare implications

Welfare concerns arise from the high morbidity and mortality rates. Recumbent sheep rarely recover and should be euthanased.

INGUINAL/SCROTAL HERNIAS

Definition/overview

Inguinal and scrotal hernias are very uncommon in sheep. The large size of the inguinal ring rarely results in strangulation of the contents, so affected lambs are usually finished for market as normal.

Aetiology

An increased diameter inguinal ring allows passage of omentum and occasionally small intestine into the scrotum in males. Increased abdominal pressure may force abdominal contents through the inguinal ring but this is unlikely unless the ring is already enlarged. Affected sheep should not be kept for breeding because of a possible heritable component of this condition.

Clinical presentation

The hernia presents as a large, soft swelling immediately below the inguinal ring. It can usually be reduced under digital pressure when the sheep is placed in dorsal recumbency. The inguinal ring can be readily appreciated.

Differential diagnoses

- Inguinal hernia can be differentiated from an abscess by careful palpation and by ultrasonography where necessary.
- The major differential diagnosis of scrotal hernia is epididymitis.

Diagnosis

The presence of a hernia is confirmed by demonstration of the hernial ring and, in almost all cases, reduction of the hernia.

Treatment

No treatment is necessary because strangulation is rare. Rams with a scrotal hernia should be culled because of the possible heritable nature of the problem and their compromised fertility.

Prevention/control measures

Affected sheep should be finished for meat and not used as replacement breeding stock.

Economics

Hernias are not a major economic concern to sheep farmers.

Welfare implications

Hernias present no welfare concerns unless they become very large and prove a physical impediment to locomotion.

CLINICAL PROBLEM 1

An emaciated four-year-old Greyface ewe with a poor fleece (**278**) is presented during late winter.

Clinical examination

The ewe is bright and alert. The rectal temperature is normal. The ewe has a full mouth and there are no molar abnormalities. The mucous membranes appear normal but the eyes are slightly sunken due to loss of intraorbital fat. The ewe has a BCS of 1.0; other sheep in the group have scores of 2.5 or greater. There is no evidence of diarrhoea on the tail or the wool of the perineum. Clinical examination fails to reveal any abnormality other than very poor bodily condition.

Which conditions should be considered?
What is a likely provisional diagnosis?
What laboratory tests could be undertaken?

Differential diagnoses

Common causes of weight loss and ill-thrift in individual ewes include:

- Paratuberculosis.
- Chronic fasciolosis (evaded treatment).
- Chronic suppurative pneumonia or other septic focus.
- Lymphosarcoma.
- Intestinal adenocarcinoma.
- Poor dentition, especially molar teeth.
- Peritonitis.
- Sheep pulmonary adenomatosis.
- Maedi-visna.
- Scrapie.

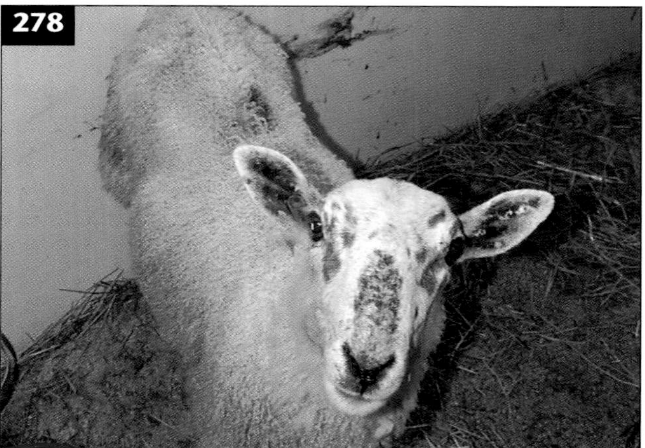

278 Emaciated four-year-old Greyface ewe with a poor fleece.

Common causes of problems involving many sheep in a group include:

- Poor nutrition.
- Virulent footrot.
- Fasciolosis.
- Chronic parasitism including anthelmintic-resistant strains.

Provisional diagnosis

The provisional diagnosis is paratuberculosis, although certain chronic bacterial infections that cause chronic weight loss/ill thrift should not be ruled out.

Laboratory tests

Laboratory analysis revealed a serum albumin concentration of 10.1 g/l and globulin concentration of 36.4 g/l. The faecal egg count was 800 strongyle eggs per gram.

Sheep with paratuberculosis typically have profound hypoalbuminaemia (<15 g/l; normal range 30–36 g/l) and normal globulin concentration, although these protein concentrations may occasionally be encountered in cases of severe chronic internal parasitism. It should also be remembered that sheep with paratuberculosis often have high faecal nematode egg counts (>1,000 epg) due to immunosuppression.

Chronic bacterial infections causing weight loss/ill thrift result in significant increases in serum globulin concentration (often >55 g/l) and low serum albumin concentration (often around 22–25 g/l but rarely <18 g/l). Subacute and chronic fasciolosis cases can present with a similar serum protein profile.

Limitations of laboratory testing

Direct faecal examination will not detect the paucibacillary form of paratuberculosis. Cultural isolation for paratuberculosis takes months and has limited use. Significant titres are detected in only approximately 60% of paratuberculosis cases; therefore, there is a high false-negative rate (low sensitivity).

Postmortem examination

The gross changes of paratuberculosis (e.g. corrugated intestines and enlarged mesenteric lymph nodes) can easily be overlooked by casual examination.

Conclusion

The diagnosis in this case was confirmed after ZN staining of gut sections and lymph nodes demonstrated acid-fast bacteria.

CLINICAL PROBLEM 2

A three-crop Greyface ewe is presented with two three-week-old lambs at foot. The ewe was turned out to pasture three weeks ago amongst a group of 40 recently lambed ewes. The ewes are being fed 1 kg of 18% crude protein nuts per head per day divided into two feeds. The ewe had been brought indoors two days ago to allow closer supervision, although she had not been coming to the feed trough for the past two feeds. The farmer reports that the ewe spends a lot of time kneeling and is generally dull and reluctant to walk (279). The farmer had treated the ewe for two consecutive days with procaine penicillin injected intramuscularly.

Clinical findings

On presentation the ewe appears dull and depressed, adopts the kneeling stance reported by the farmer and has a painful expression (279). The lambs are poorly thriven and appear hungry. The ewe's BCS is 2.0. The rectal temperature is 39.0°C. The skin tent test is extended beyond three seconds and the eyes appear sunken. The mucous membranes appear pale. The heart rate is 90 bpm. The respiratory rate is 22 breaths per minute. No abnormal sounds can be detected during auscultation of the chest. There are no ruminal sounds. There is reduced rumen fill consistent with the inappetence reported. There is scant fetid green/black diarrhoea (280). There is no mastitis. There is no lameness or joint swellings. The prescapular lymph nodes are not enlarged.

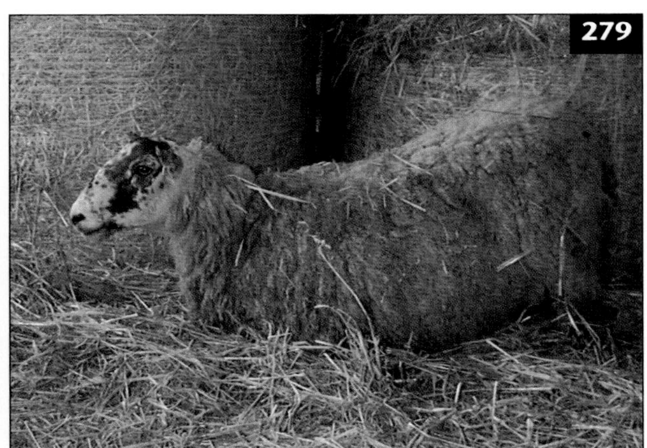

279 The ewe appears dull, with a painful expression, and it adopts a kneeling stance.

What conditions should be considered?
How should this ewe be treated?

Differential diagnoses

- Respiratory disease/pasteurellosis.
- Acidosis.
- Bacteraemia/endocarditis.
- Peritonitis.

Diagnosis

Clinical examination failed to localize the lesion(s). The clinical appearance is not unlike endocarditis but no joint swellings could be appreciated. The lack of pyrexia could be the result of previous antibiotic therapy. The diarrhoea was attributed to endotoxaemia. The farmer reported that the ewe could not have had access to too much concentrates. There are no clinical findings that lead to a specific diagnosis.

Treatment

The ewe was treated symptomatically with 20 mg/kg oxytetracycline injected intravenously.

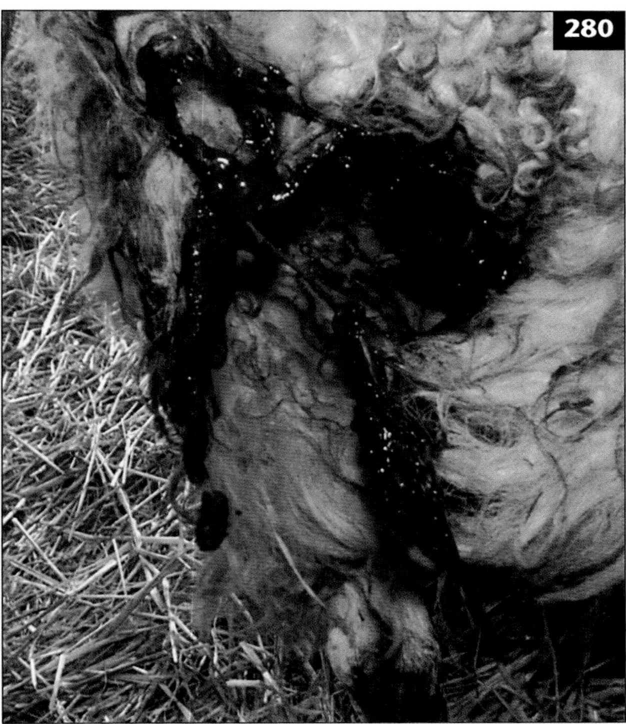

280 There is scant fetid green/black diarrhoea.

Outcome

The ewe was re-examined two days later and as it had not improved it was euthanased.

Postmortem examination

Postmortem examination revealed a localized severe peritonitis with the omentum firmly adherent to the serosal surface of the abomasum (**281**). The abomasum was distended with fetid fluid, which, when emptied, revealed a large area of abomasal ulceration. The cause of such extensive ulceration was not determined.

Discussion

Localized peritonitis can prove difficult to diagnose, especially during the more chronic stages of disease. In hindsight, more attention should have been given to the cause of the diarrhoea, which may have contained digested blood and this would have accounted for the black discoloration and fetid smell. The stance adopted by the sheep presumably reduced tension on abdominal adhesions, thus reducing pain. The provisional diagnosis of endocarditis was suggested because the stance of the sheep and the chronic weight loss were attributed to joint pain (possibly involving the elbows/shoulders, where early lesions can be difficult to detect). Ultrasound examination may have revealed adhesions but these are difficult to identify in the absence of accumulations of peritoneal fluid.

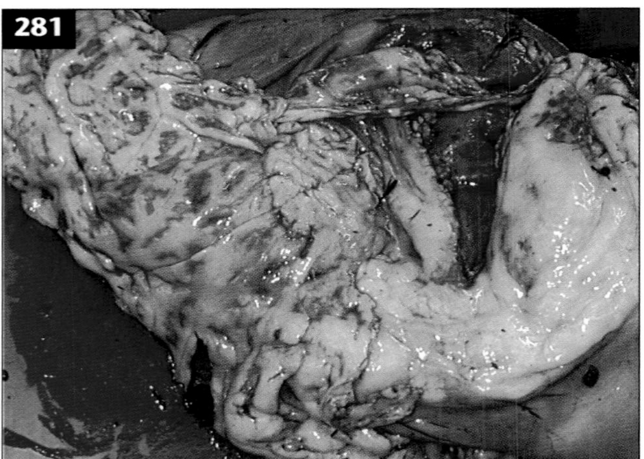

281 Localized severe peritonitis with the omentum firmly adherent to the serosal surface of the abomasum.

6 Cardiorespiratory System

Part 1: Thorax

INTRODUCTION

Respiratory disease is common in sheep but few specific conditions can be diagnosed on clinical examination alone. In most veterinary practice situations the provisional diagnosis of ovine respiratory disease is based on history, clinical examination and response to antibiotic therapy. Fortunately, many infectious respiratory disease conditions respond to antibiotic therapy. Occasionally, the diagnosis of respiratory disease may be supported by on-farm postmortem examination but interpretation of necropsy findings presents many opportunities for error and misdiagnosis. For example, pasteurellosis is a common all-encompassing diagnosis in sheep practice but the necropsy findings require expert interpretation supported by histopathology and bacteriology, especially when some hours have elapsed between death and necropsy. It can prove difficult to differentiate venous congestion of lung tissue from pasteurellosis.

HISTORY

The history comprises the recent management of the sheep including origin, vaccinations and diet. It is important to determine an accurate history for all sheep presented for veterinary examination but because few shepherds can recognize individual sheep, unless tagged, errors occur on a regular basis. Regulatory authorities in many countries require detailed records of all animal treatments but these are not always accurate or contemporaneous. The frequency of flock supervision will also influence the accuracy, and therefore usefulness, of the animal's given history for the current complaint. It is also human nature to report that a sheep's illness has been shorter that its actual duration. In this respect, BCS relative to others in the group may provide some indication of likely duration, although two conditions may co-exist. Alternatively, one disease may precede and/or predispose to another (e.g. sheep pulmonary adenomatosis frequently predisposes to acute illness caused by *Mannheimia haemolytica*).

VISUAL INSPECTION OF THE INDIVIDUAL/GROUP

Sheep must be examined from a distance in order to observe their attitude, response to the observer, respiratory rate and effort, frequency of coughing and the presence and nature of any ocular and nasal discharges. Painful conditions, especially lameness, can have a considerable influence on observed respiratory parameters; therefore, it is essential to note the sheep's stance and gait.

During inspection of sheep under farm conditions, the respiratory rate and lung sounds are variably affected by gathering, handling stresses and BCS. The presence of a full fleece in a hot environment can rapidly induce panting, which may further complicate interpretation of auscultation findings.

CLINICAL EXAMINATION

At least one hour should elapse between gathering and veterinary examination and, whenever possible, the sheep should be left in shade. If doubts exist concerning the effects of recent exercise on a sheep's rectal temperature, it is essential to check some normal sheep from the group that were gathered. Similarly, the rate and depth of respiration should always be compared with those of normal sheep. The effects of forced exercise on rectal temperature (**282**) were all too obvious during the FMD epidemic in the UK in 2001. Groups of gathered sheep, without evidence of clinical disease, often presented with rectal temperatures

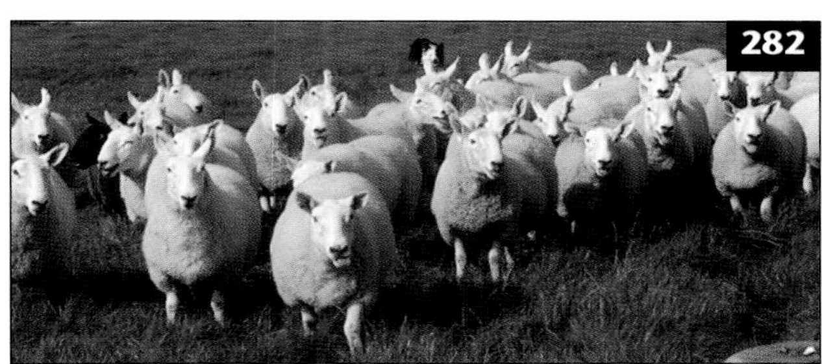

282 The effects of gathering during hot weather on rectal temperature and the respiratory system should not be underestimated.

ranging from 40.0–41.5°C, which returned to the normal range 38.5–39.5°C when re-examined one hour later.

The stethoscope is a grossly overrated tool in the examination of the ovine chest, with poor correlation between auscultation and pathology findings for many conditions. This statement is based on ultrasonographic studies, whereby lung pathology and the auscultation findings can be directly compared in the live sheep (**283**). For example, auscultation of one side of a chest filled by an extensive pleural abscess yields no lung sounds at all. Parietal and visceral pleurae with considerable fibrin deposition do not generate audible 'friction rubs'. It is not possible to detect lung abscesses by auscultation.

Body condition may also influence auscultation findings, with louder breath sounds audible in sheep with low BCSs compared with those in sheep with increased subcutaneous fat deposits. The presence of a full fleece prevents meaningful percussion of the chest in sheep.

Lung sounds

Wheezes are continuous single pitch sounds that usually occur during inspiration and occasionally during both inspiration and expiration. Wheezes result from vibration of airway walls caused by air turbulence in narrowed airways.

Crackles are sudden sounds towards the end of inspiration or, less frequently, during both inspiration and expiration, caused by sudden opening of small airways plugged by mucus, pus and other debris. Crackles are typically heard in sheep with pulmonary adenomatosis in which there are fluid accumulations within the airways.

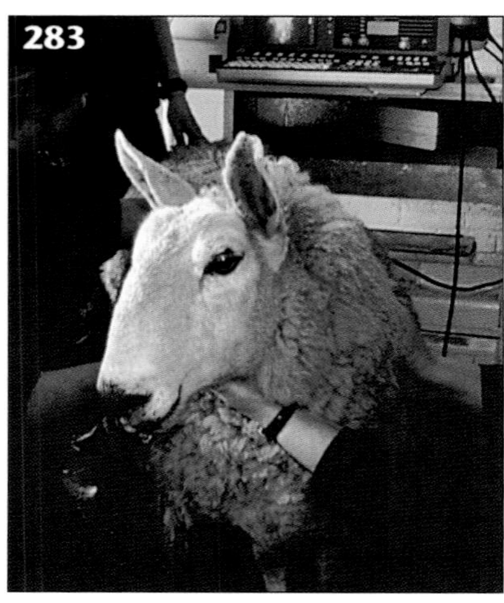

283 Ultrasonographic studies enable auscultation findings to be directly compared with lung pathology.

Laboratory tests

Chronic respiratory disease is common in sheep but few specific conditions can be diagnosed on clinical examination alone. Changes in the leucogram and in the haptoglobin, fibrinogen and serum protein concentrations may indicate an inflammatory response to bacterial infection, but these changes are not specific for respiratory disease. Respiratory disease in adult sheep frequently arises following bacteraemia from another organ such as the udder.

Serological tests are diagnostic for some chronic respiratory tract viral infections (e.g. maedi/ovine progressive pneumonia) but not for sheep pulmonary adenomatosis (SPA). It is possible for flocks to have a high seroprevalence for maedi but also be suffering from another respiratory disease (e.g. SPA), which may prove more important. Once again, interpretation of biochemical results may lead to confusion in the diagnosis of certain respiratory diseases.

Ancillary diagnostic aids such as radiography and ultrasonography are generally limited to valuable pedigree animals where either a definitive diagnosis or extent of the lesion(s) is required, but the practical use of ultrasonography in clinical practice should not be underestimated.

Thoracocentesis

Pleural effusion is rare in sheep with respiratory disease. Fluid accumulation within the chest cavity may result from right-sided heart failure but this is invariably preceded by large accumulations within the abdominal cavity (ascites). Prior recognition of pleural effusion by ultrasonographic examination is essential before attempting thoracocentesis.

Bronchoalveolar lavage

Trans-tracheal bronchoalveolar lavage is rarely indicated in ovine respiratory disease because respiratory pathogens can frequently be isolated from the major airways of healthy sheep with no respiratory disease.

Radiographic examination of the thorax

Radiographic examination of the thorax is expensive and restricted in sheep practice to individual valuable pedigree sheep. Furthermore, the position of the forelimbs and associated musculature in the standing animal largely restricts radiographic examinations to the caudodorsal thorax, when pathological changes associated with aerosol infection more commonly involve the cranioventral lung field.

Ultrasonographic examination of the thorax

Ultrasonographic examination of the ovine chest is inexpensive, non-invasive and, unlike radiography, there are no special health and safety procedures or restrictions and the equipment is readily transportable; therefore, ultrasonographic examinations can be performed on the farm. A 5.0 MHz sector scanner is necessary to achieve sufficiently good contact with the convex chest wall.

A 5–7 cm wide strip of fleece is carefully shaved from both sides of the thorax, extending in a vertical plane from the point of the elbow to the caudal edge of the scapula. The prepared skin overlying the chest wall can be freely moved up to 5 cm, which allows examination of the caudal aspect of the dorsal lung field. The skin is soaked with warm tap water then ultrasound gel liberally applied to the wet skin to ensure good contact.

The transducer head is held firmly against the skin overlying the intercostal muscles of the 6th or 7th intercostal spaces, and the thorax examined in both longitudinal and transverse planes. The dorsal lung field is selected at the start of all ultrasound examinations in an attempt to visualize normal lung tissue, as this area is less commonly affected in the majority of ovine respiratory disease processes. The most cranial aspect of the thorax is scanned by moving the transducer head cranially from the 6th or 7th intercostal space in to the next more cranial intercostal space once or twice as the transducer is moved down the chest wall. The ipsilateral forelimb can be held forward to facilitate access to the ventral aspect of the thoracic wall. The caudodorsal aspect of the thorax is examined by moving the transducer head two or three intercostal spaces more caudally from the 6th or 7th intercostal space to the 9th or 10th intercostal space. The ultrasonographic examinations are made with a depth setting of 6–7 cm, which includes 1–2 cm of chest wall. Good contact between the transducer head and skin overlying an intercostal space is evidenced by the intensity of the ultrasound image.

Interpretation of ultrasonographic findings

The ultrasonograms are presented with the chest wall at the top of the image: dorsal is to the left and ventral to the right of the image. An air interface, created by aerated lung parenchyma, reflects sound waves and appears as a bright white (hyperechoic) linear echo. The sonogram below the white linear echo may contain equidistant reverberation artefacts. The area visualized beyond the linear echo, including the reverberation artefacts, does not represent lung parenchyma. Air contained within a major airway in consolidated lung appears as a hyperechoic spot within the hypoechoic lung parenchyma. Superficial areas of consolidated lung parenchyma, or fluid within an abscess, transmit sound waves and appear more hypoechoic than surrounding lung tissue. Pleural fluid transmits sound waves readily and appears as an anechoic area. Gas-filled pockets within pleural fluid or abscess capsule appear as bright hyperechoic spots within the anechoic area.

Normal sheep

The surface of normal aerated lung (visceral or pulmonary pleura) of normal sheep is characterized by the uppermost white linear echo, with equally spaced reverberation artefacts below this line (**284**). In normal sheep the visceral pleura is observed moving 1–3 mm in a vertical plane during respiration. No pleural fluid is visualized in normal sheep. The chest wall is approximately 1 cm thick in 20–40 kg lambs, extending to 2 cm in adult sheep in good body condition and with a reasonable amount of subcutaneous fat. The intercostal space is too small to obtain good quality ultrasonograms using most large animal ultrasound scanners in lambs <15 kg.

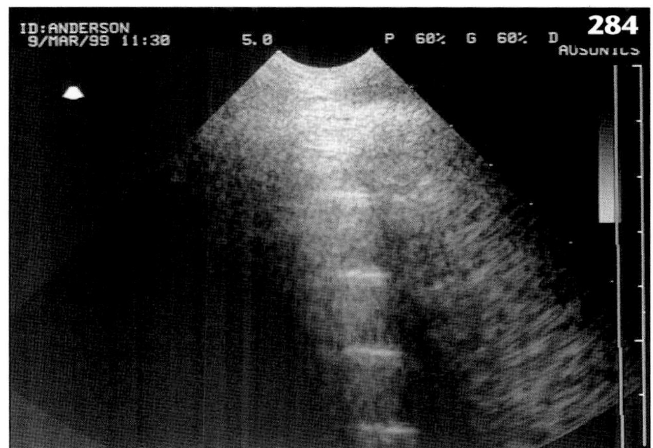

284 Ultrasonographic examination of the thorax. The surface of normal aerated lung (visceral or pulmonary pleura) is characterized by the uppermost white linear echo, with equally spaced reverberation artefacts below this line.

Fibrinous pleuritis

With fibrinous pleuritis, ultrasonographic examination reveals separation of the pleurae and lung lobes by a hypoechoic area (285). There is acoustic enhancement of the visceral pleura, which appears as a broad white line. In more severe cases the fibrin deposits have a hyperechoic lattice-work appearance containing hypoechoic areas. These areas may extend for up to 8–10 cm.

Pleural abscesses

With pleural abscessation there is loss of the white linear echo formed by the visceral or pulmonary pleura. Individual pleural abscesses appear as uniform hypoechoic areas extending up to 4 cm in depth and containing many hyperechoic spots. The pleural abscess may extend up to 16 cm deep (286) and involve one side of the chest. It may contain up to 2 litres of purulent material, with the lung greatly compressed to 1–2 cm thickness against the mediastinum.

Gaining experience with thoracic ultrasonography

Sheep with SPA are excellent patients for gaining confidence with the interpretation of lung pathology (287, 288). Typically, there is a sudden loss of the bright linear echo formed by normal aerated lung tissue (visceral or pulmonary pleura), and this is replaced by hypoechoic areas extending for 6–8 cm in the ventral half of the chest (287) that correspond to lung tissue consolidated by tumour cells (288). The hyperechoic line identifying normal aerated lung dorsally allows the extent of the SPA tumour mass(es) to be defined

285 Ultrasonographic examination of the thorax. Fibrin deposition (**1**) separating the pleurae is represented ultrasonographically by a hypoechoic area, with enhancement of the visceral pleura (**2**) appearing as a broad hyperechoic line.

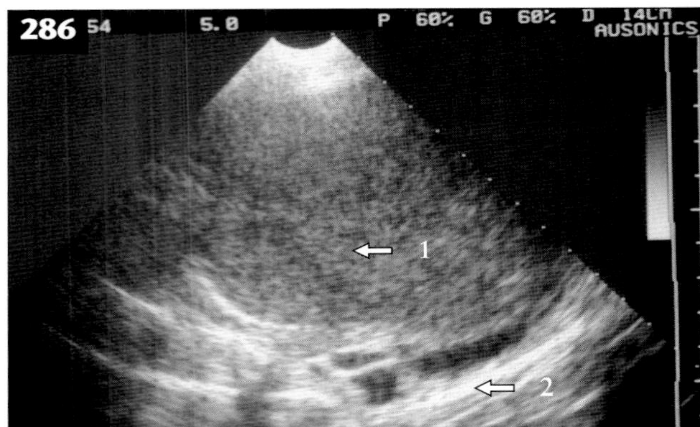

286 Ultrasonographic examination of the thorax. There is loss of the linear echo formed by the visceral pleura (compare with **284**). A large hypoechoic area containing multiple hyperechoic dots extends for 8 cm from the transducer head (**1**); this represents a large pleural abscess. Visceral pleura with compressed lung below (**2**).

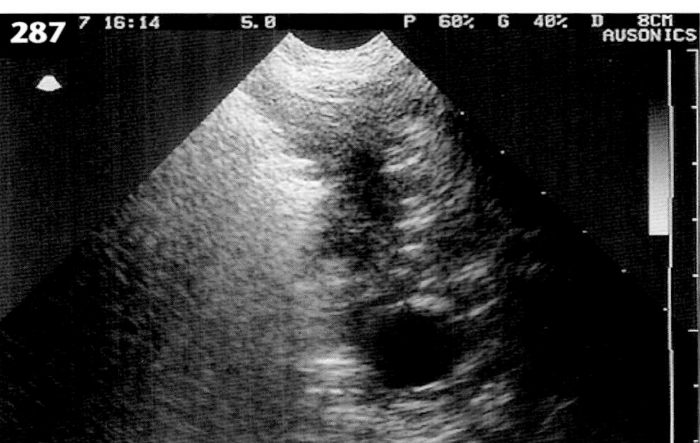

287 Ultrasonographic examination of the thorax. There is loss of the bright line representing the visceral pleura ventrally. This is replaced by a large, sharply-demarcated hypoechoic area ventrally, which is caused by cell proliferation.

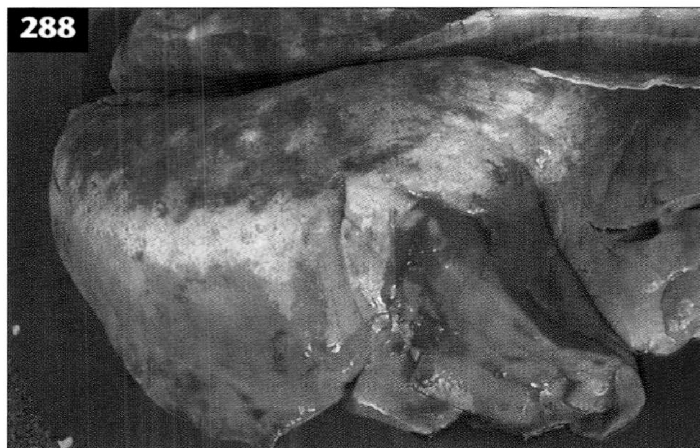

288 The extent of the sharply demarcated SPA tumour mass in **287** is revealed at necropsy.

accurately during the ultrasonographic examination. Focal hyperechoic areas within the tumour mass (hypoechoic area) represent air within large airways. There are no serological tests for SPA; however, it is possible that ultrasonographic examination of the thorax could identify early SPA lung pathology in problem flocks, thereby permitting earlier culling.

ENZOOTIC NASAL TUMOUR

Definition/overview

Enzootic nasal tumour occurs in many countries worldwide (**289**) but has not been recognized in Australia and New Zealand. Only sporadic cases have been reported in the UK.

Aetiology

The condition is caused by an exogenous retrovirus referred to as enzootic nasal tumour virus (ENTV). The condition can be transmitted experimentally by tumour homogenates, which would explain the widespread occurrence of this condition within some flocks.

Clinical presentation

Clinical signs of continuous serous nasal discharge and stridor are noted in sheep aged 2–4 years. The tumour may be unilateral or bilateral. Occlusion of the nasal passage can readily be demonstrated by holding a piece of cotton wool close to the nostril. Weight loss occurs in advanced cases with inspiratory dyspnoea. Rarely, pressure resulting from tumour proliferation from the ethmoid turbinates may cause thinning of overlying bone and deformity and, possibly, exophthalmos. Metastatic spread is uncommon.

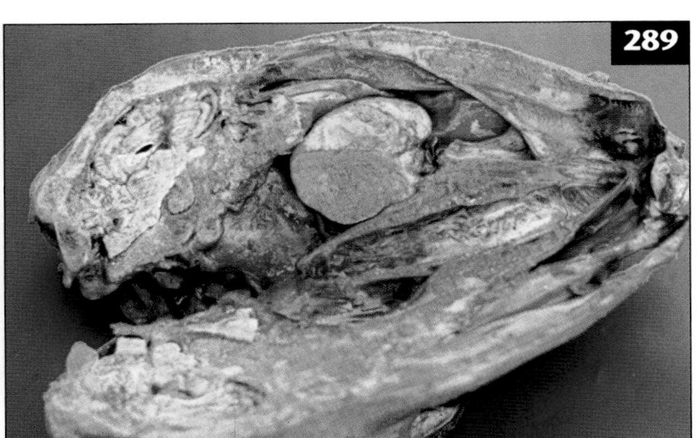

289 Longitudinal section of the head of a Suffolk ewe revealing a well-circumscribed nasal tumour.

Differential diagnoses

The differential diagnoses for nasal discharge and respiratory distress may include:

- Sheep pulmonary adenomatosis.
- *Oestrus ovis* infestation.
- Stridor may also be caused by compression of the larynx by enlarged retropharyngeal lymph nodes associated with abscessation of the head.
- Laryngeal chondritis also results in inspiratory dyspnoea of varying severity.

Diagnosis

Diagnosis is based on clinical findings and, possibly prior occurrence in the flock. Endoscopy reveals occlusion of the caudal part of one or both nasal cavities by a greyish mass, with a granular surface covered by mucus. Radiography may reveal the extent of the lesion but such quantification is not simple. Biopsy of the mass during endoscopic examination and subsequent histopathological examination confirms the provisional dianosis.

Treatment

There is no effective treatment. Affected sheep must be culled immediately because they act as a source of virus for other sheep in the flock, especially when closely confined. Surgical removal of the tumour is not indicated.

Prevention/control measures

Prevention is based on strict biosecurity, with any purchased replacement stock being obtained from flocks with no known history of this condition. There is no vaccine available. In endemically infected flocks, all suspected cases must be isolated immediately and promptly culled once the diagnosis has been confirmed.

Economics

Enzootic nasal tumour is not a disease of major economic importance.

Welfare implications

Affected sheep must be promptly culled once the diagnosis has been confirmed.

OESTRUS OVIS INFESTATION

(*Syn:* nasal bot)

Definition/overview

Oestrus ovis infestation has a worldwide distribution. There are only sporadic infestations in the UK and these are restricted to the warmer south of England and Wales.

Aetiology
Adult flies deposit L1 larvae into the nasal cavity. These migrate to the maxillary, frontal or palatine sinuses, where they develop to the third instar. Third stage larvae are sneezed on to pasture after 30–40 days, where they pupate and emerge as adults 2–10 weeks later.

Clinical presentation
During the summer months adult flies cause irritation, with frequent head shaking and sneezing. Larval infestation of the nasal passages may cause a mucopurulent nasal discharge and, in severe cases, stridor.

Differential diagnoses
Sporadic cases could be confused with enzootic nasal tumour.

Diagnosis
Diagnosis is based on clinical findings affecting a large number of sheep during the summer months.

Treatment
Autumn treatment with ivermectin eliminates larval stages from the nasal cavity, thus preventing build-up of fly numbers.

Prevention/control measures
There are no specific control measures.

Economics
Oestrus ovis infestation is not an economic concern in most situations.

Welfare implications
There are no significant welfare concerns.

PASTEURELLOSIS

Definition/overview
Pasteurella haemolytica (previously termed *P. haemolytica* biotype A but now more correctly called *Mannheimia haemolytica*) is of considerable economic importance to the sheep industry (but not a significant problem in New Zealand), causing septicaemia in young lambs (**290**), pneumonia in older sheep (**291**) and mastitis in ewes (**292**).

Pasteurella trehalosi (previously termed *P. haemolytica* biotype T) causes septicaemia in 4–10-month-old lambs (**293**).

P. multocida only rarely causes disease in the UK but a recent report has described septicaemia in young lambs.

M. haemolytica and *P. trehalosi* are divided into 17 serotypes, with types 3, 4, 10 and 15 identified as *P. trehalosi* and the others as *M. haemolytica*. Serotypes 2 (*M. haemolytica*) and 10 (*P. trehalosi*) are the most commonly diagnosed.

RESPIRATORY DISEASE CAUSED BY *MANNHEIMIA HAEMOLYTICA*

Clinical presentation in adult sheep
The clinical signs of *M. haemolytica* infection include acute sudden-onset depression, lethargy and inappetence (**294**). Affected sheep are typically separated from the remainder of the flock (**295**) and are easily caught and restrained. On approach they may show an increased respiratory rate with an abdominal component. Affected sheep are typically febrile (>40.5°C) but it is important to be aware that periods of exercise before restraint may increase rectal temperature in normal sheep. There may be a scant serous nasal discharge (**294**). The mucous membranes are congested and there may be evidence of dehydration. Auscultation often fails to reveal significant changes other than an increased respiratory rate. Rumen contractions are reduced or absent. Frothy fluid may be noted around the mouth during the terminal stages. In some situations the animal is found dead.

Differential diagnoses
- Clostridial disease must be considered in all cases of sudden death in unvaccinated sheep.
- Farmers frequently mistake hypocalcaemia for respiratory disease because affected sheep are apathetic, anorexic and often have green-stained fluid (rumen contents) at the external nares.
- Subacute fasciolosis may present with some of the clinical signs listed above but anterior abdominal pain is usually present.
- Infections of the respiratory tract including laryngeal chondritis, chronic suppurative pneumonia, pleuropneumonia/pleural abscess and mediastinal abscess caused by CLA.

Diagnosis
Diagnosis of respiratory disease caused by *M. haemolytica* is based on clinical signs but there is no confirmatory test in the living sheep.

Confirmation of diagnosis is made at necropsy, with histopathological examination of lung lesions. There are subcutaneous ecchymotic haemorrhages over

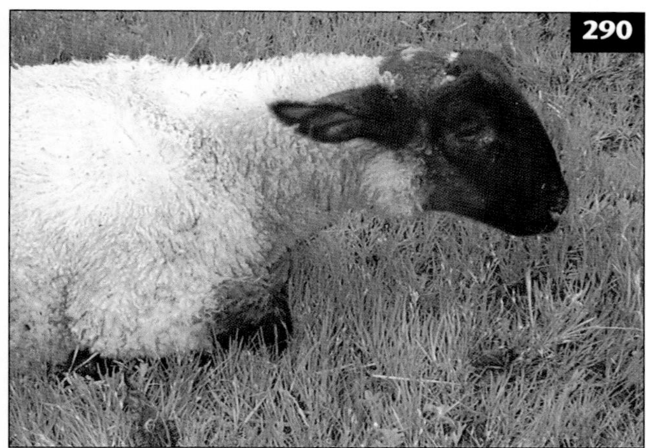

290 Profoundly depressed three-month-old lamb suffering from septicaemic pasteurellosis.

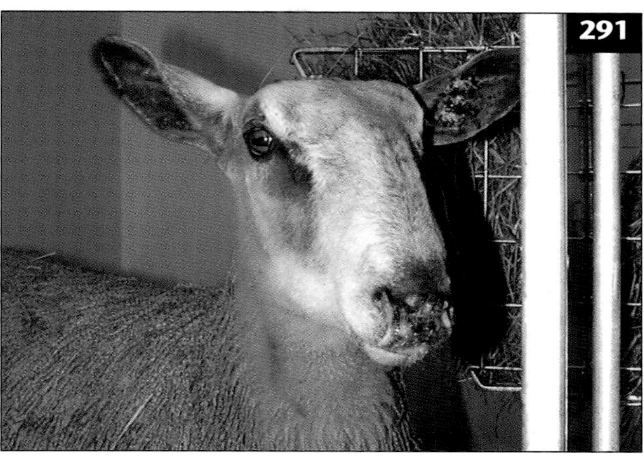

291 Yearling ram with respiratory disease probably caused by *Mannheimia haemolytica*.

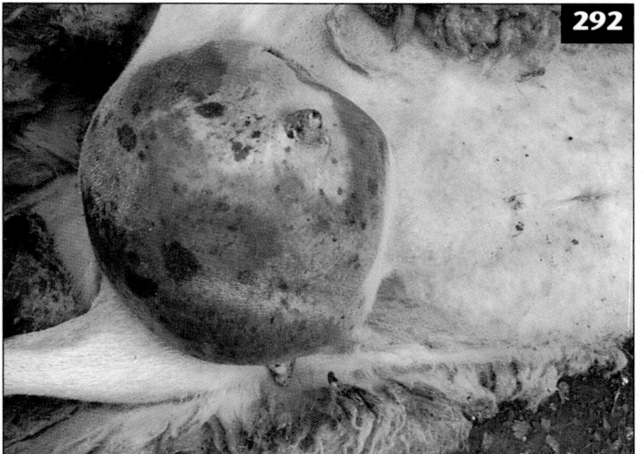

292 Gangrenous mastitis caused by *Mannheimia haemolytica*.

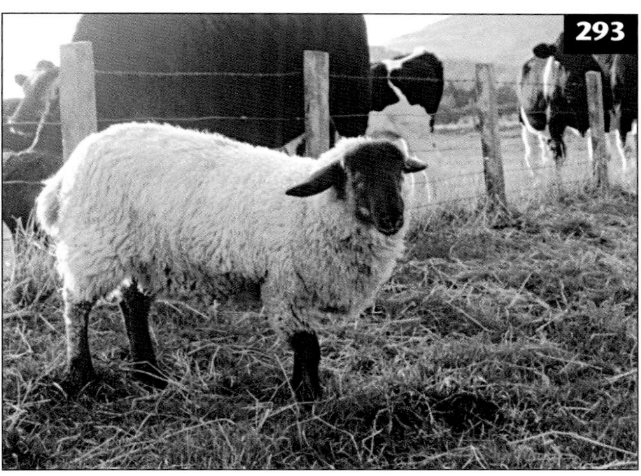

293 Weaned lamb suffering from systemic pasteurellosis. The lamb shows profound depression. It died despite intravenous antibiotic therapy.

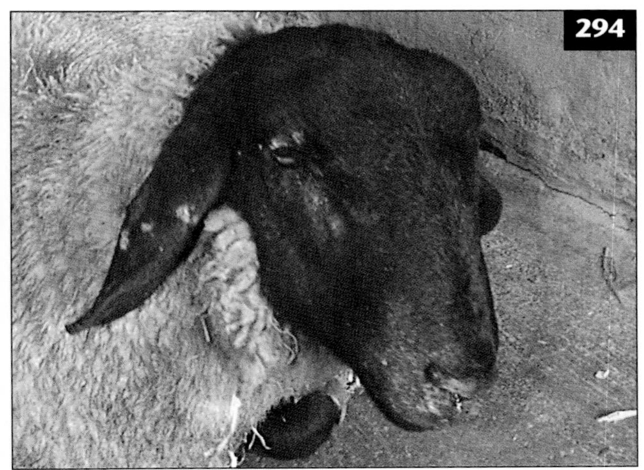

294 Profound toxaemia in a yearling ram with respiratory disease.

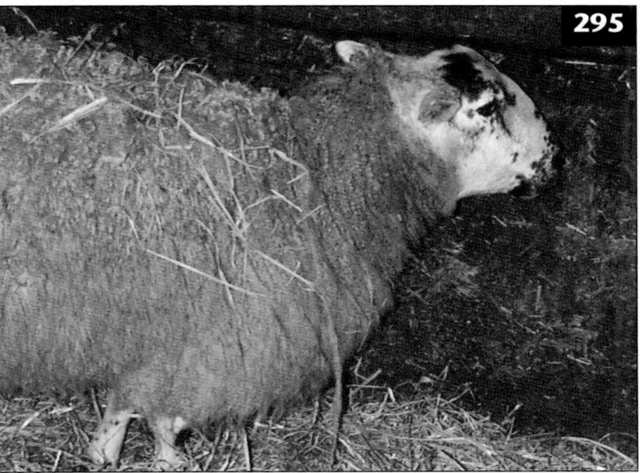

295 Greyface ewe with respiratory disease probably caused by *Mannheimia haemolytica*.

the throat and ribs. The lungs are heavy, swollen and purple-red in peracute cases, and the airways contain blood-stained froth. Cases of longer duration show anteroventral consolidation and fibrinous pleuritis.

Treatment
A good response to antibiotic therapy necessitates rapid detection of sick sheep by the shepherd (**296**). Oxytetracycline, administered intravenously, is the antibiotic of choice for pasteurellosis as there are few antibiotic resistant strains in sheep, unlike in cattle. Tilmicosin can be used but it is considerably more expensive than oxytetracycline.

Prevention/control measures
Prevention is best attempted using vaccines incorporating iron-regulated proteins. Since these iron-regulated proteins are antigenically similar, they confer cross-protection against other serotypes. Breeding ewes require a primary course of two injections 4–6 weeks apart, followed by an annual booster 4–6 weeks before lambing. However, this vaccination regimen only provides passive immunity to the lambs for up to five weeks. Lambs can be protected by two doses of vaccine administered from ten days old, as colostral antibody does not interfere with the development of active immunity.

Economics
The low cost of the vaccine should permit vaccination of all susceptible sheep.

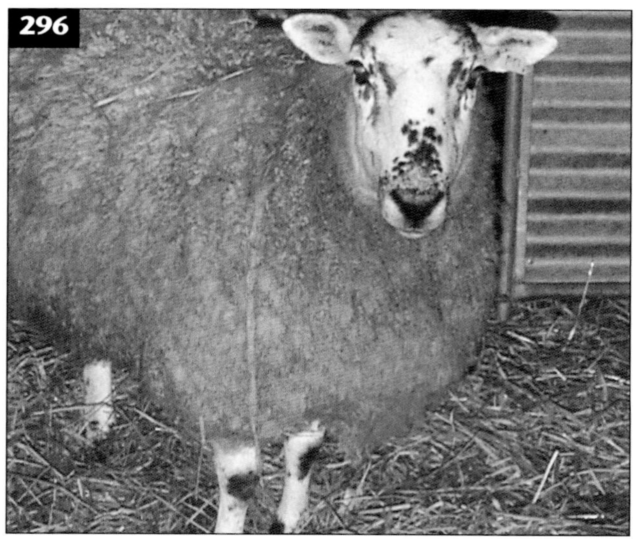

296 The ewe in **295** showing a good response to antibiotic therapy.

Welfare implications
Regulations imposed by various organic lamb production schemes have restricted the use of certain vaccines unless the disease presents a significant problem on the farm. Difficulties in accurately diagnosing pasteurellosis in the field must not deter such a vaccination policy, and any vaccine restrictions must be challenged from an animal welfare standpoint.

SEPTICAEMIC PASTEURELLOSIS

Definition/overview
Septicaemic pasteurellosis, which is also caused by *Mannheimia haemolytica*, is an important cause of sudden death in lambs up to 12 weeks old.

Clinical presentation in growing lambs
Typically, the best lambs in the group are lost over 1–2 weeks, with no obvious predisposing factor(s). Some affected lambs may be found alive; they are profoundly depressed (**297**) and easily caught. They are pyrexic (rectal temperature often >41.0°C) and have injected mucous membranes (**298**) and marked dyspnoea. There is often a large amount of frothy saliva around the mouth and lower jaw.

Differential diagnoses
Causes of sudden death in lambs that have not received sufficient passive antibody, including lamb dysentery and pulpy kidney disease.

Diagnosis
Nasal swabs and serology are of no benefit. Diagnosis is based on clinical signs and postmortem findings, including bacteriology of lung, liver, kidney, spleen, thoracic fluid and heart blood.

In peracute cases there are widespread petechiae over the myocardium, spleen, liver and kidney, and enlarged lymph nodes. Less acute cases are characterized by a considerable fibrinous pleuritis, which may be unilateral and extend up to 1 cm in thickness (**299**).

Treatment
Oxytetracycline is the antibiotic of choice for bacterial respiratory infections in sheep but the prognosis is poor because of the advanced clinical signs when lambs are presented for treatment.

Prevention/control measures
Maternal vaccination using vaccines incorporating iron-regulated proteins provides passive immunity for up to five weeks. Lambs can then be protected

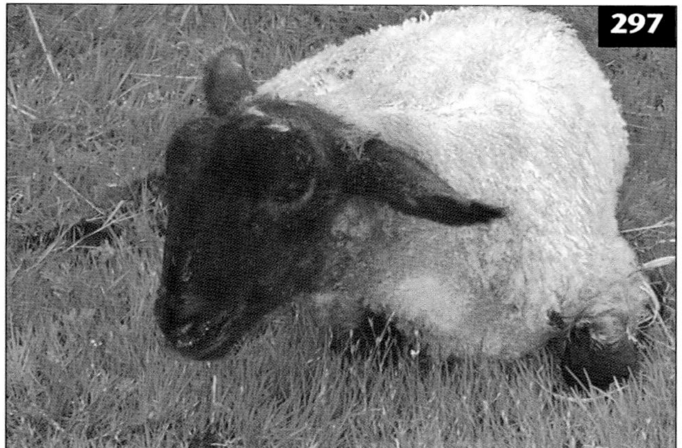
297 Profoundly depressed three-month-old lamb suffering from septicaemic pasteurellosis.

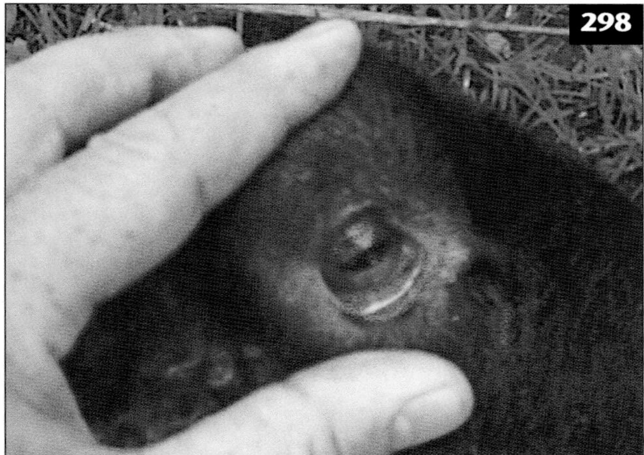
298 Profound toxaemia in a lamb with septicaemic pasteurellosis.

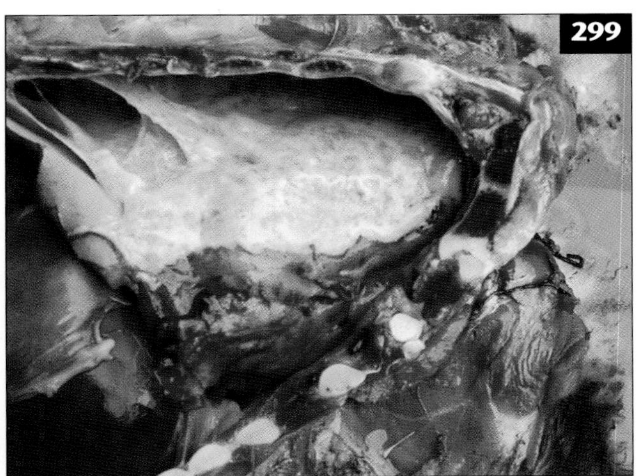
299 Necroposy revealing fibrinous pneumonia in a lamb that died from septicaemic pasteurellosis.

after two doses of vaccine given four weeks apart from ten days old. The role of parainfluenza 3 virus in sheep has been poorly researched but good results for pneumonia control have been reported in some UK flocks after administration of the temperature-specific bovine intranasal PI3 vaccine.

Welfare implications

Lambs in acute respiratory distress should be euthanased for welfare reasons but this is rarely undertaken.

Systemic pasteurellosis

Definition/overview

Systemic pasteurellosis is caused by *P. trehalosi*. It is the most common cause of sudden death in lambs in the UK between August and December. It occurs most commonly in recently weaned lambs. Outbreaks frequently follow weaning, sale and/or movement of lambs on to rape, turnips or improved pastures. Gastrointestinal erosions and ulcers caused by dietary change may be the portal of entry for bacteria, and this leads to septicaemic disease. Mortality averages 2% but may reach up to 10% in severe outbreaks.

Clinical presentation

Any lambs found alive are separated from the remainder of the group and are profoundly depressed (**293**, p. 143). They stand with their neck extended and head held lowered. The respiratory rate is increased, with frothy saliva around the lower jaw during the agonal stages. The mucous membranes are dark red/purple with injected scleral vessels. Auscultation of the chest fails to reveal any dramatic changes in lung sounds.

Differential diagnoses

- The clinical signs should be differentiated from other septicaemic, toxic or stress-induced conditions including clostridial disease (pulpy kidney disease, braxy, black disease), ruminal acidosis, rhododendron poisoning, brassica poisoning and nitrite poisoning.
- Acute and subacute fasciolosis may present as sudden death.

Diagnosis

Confirmation involves isolation of large numbers of *P. trehalosi* from lung, liver or spleen.

Postmortem examination reveals subcutaneous haemorrhages in the neck and thorax and over the pleura, diaphragm and epicardium. The lungs are swollen, with haemorrhages (**300**) and blood-stained froth in the airways. There are necrotic erosions in the pharynx around the tonsils (**301**), the nasal mucosa and the upper alimentary tract. The liver is congested and there are necrotic infarcts in the liver, kidney and spleen.

Treatment
Oxytetracycline is the antibiotic of choice for systemic pasteurellosis but the prognosis is very guarded because of the advanced clinical signs when animals are presented for treatment.

Prevention/control measures
It is important to limit potential predisposing factors that may trigger clinical disease (e.g. handling stresses, long periods held in markets without food, mixing with other stock, repeated journey to markets, sudden dietary changes).

Lambs can be protected by two doses of vaccine given four weeks apart, with the second injection two weeks before weaning and/or sale, but this has rarely been undertaken in most store lambs presented at markets.

Antibiotic metaphylaxis in the face of mounting deaths has produced equivocal results in split-flock trials in the UK, with cost benefits in only one of ten test flocks. Injection with either long-acting oxytetracycline or tilmicosin is often delayed until losses exceed 1%, with total losses unlikely to exceed 2%. The low financial value of many stores lambs and the high cost of antibiotics dictates that mortality must exceed 4% to be cost effective without budgeting for labour costs. It has been reasoned that stresses involved with handling and injection may increase losses.

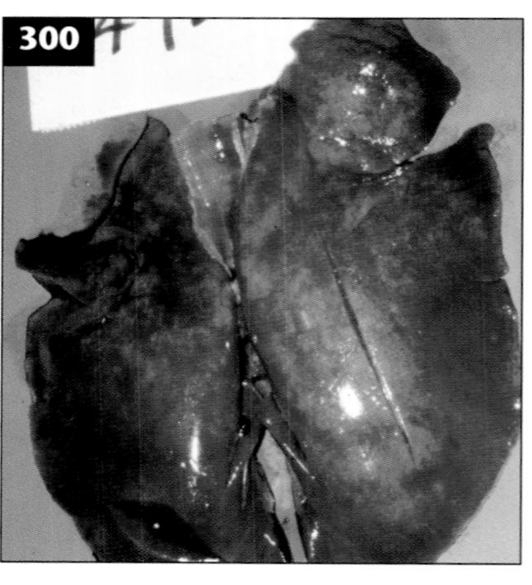

300 Pulmonary congestion and oedema associated with systemic pasteurellosis.

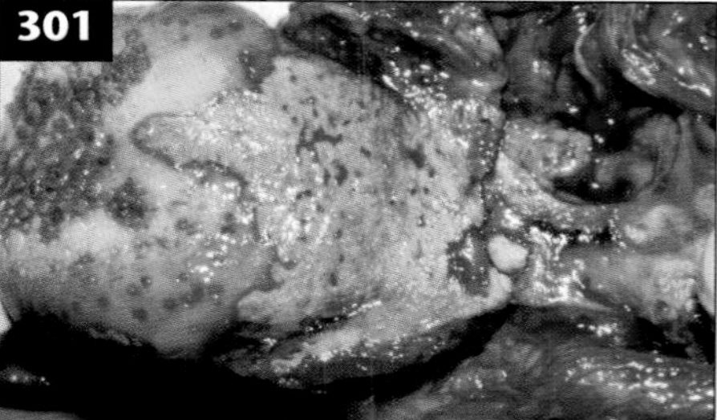

301 Tonsillar necrosis associated with systemic pasteurellosis.

Welfare implications
The treatment response of severely affected lambs is very poor and these sheep should be destroyed. Every effort must be made to convince farmers to vaccinate store lambs against clostridial disease and pasteurellosis before risk periods.

SHEEP PULMONARY ADENOMATOSIS
(*Syns*: jaagsiekte, pulmonary carcinoma)

Definition/overview
Sheep pulmonary adenomatosis (SPA) is a contagious tumour of the lungs of sheep. It is the most common tumour of sheep in the UK. Disease transmission is facilitated by close confinement and this has presented a significant problem in countries where sheep are housed for long periods during the winter months.

Aetiology
SPA is an infectious tumour condition resulting from infection with a lentivirus (jaagsiekte retrovirus [JSRV]). A herpesvirus is also often involved in the lesions.

Clinical presentation
The incubation in naturally infected sheep is long, with clinical disease apparent in 2–4-year-old sheep. Exceptionally, disease is seen in lambs 8–12 months old. These are generally the progeny of infected dams. The early clinical signs include loss of body condition and exercise intolerance, especially during hot weather, which manifests as a markedly increased respiratory rate and brief periods of mouth breathing ('panting'). Appetite remains good. Affected sheep are afebrile unless there is significant secondary bacterial pneumonia. As the disease progresses, affected sheep become increasingly tachypnoeic, with an increased abdominal component to their breathing effort. These sheep have an anxious expression and stand with their neck extended and

the head held lowered (302). Fluid gathers in the respiratory tract. This first appears as a scant serous nasal discharge. A soft cough is often audible. Increased crackles are heard during auscultation over a wide area of the chest, especially involving the ventral portions of the apical and cardiac lobes. During the advanced stages of clinical disease, when the tumour mass may occupy up to 50% of the lung parenchyma, a clear frothy fluid may flow freely from both nostrils when the head is lowered during feeding, and this quantity may exceed 50 ml if the hindquarters are raised when the head is simultaneously lowered (colloquially referred to as the 'wheelbarrow test'). This 'test' causes affected sheep considerable distress and must be discontinued as soon as some clear fluid appears at the nostrils (303). Affected sheep often appear tachypnoeic for some days after this procedure; therefore, euthanasia should be undertaken once the positive result is obtained.

Death may follow a brief illness that manifests as profound depression, inappetence and pyrexia secondary to infection of the compromised lung with *M. haemolytica*. Antibiotic treatment of the secondary bacterial infection often results in improvement of clinical signs but this is only a temporary remission and affected sheep must be culled as soon as the disease in confirmed on clinical examination.

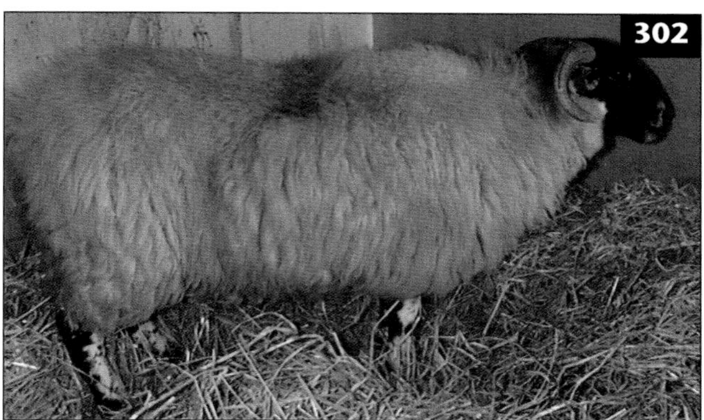

302 Scottish Blackface ewe suffering from SPA. The ewe has an anxious expression and an extended neck with lowered head carriage.

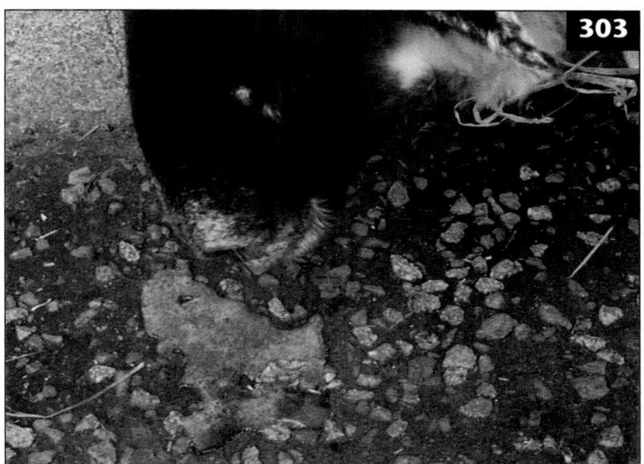

303 Copious discharge of clear frothy fluid from both nostrils when the hindquarters of the Scottish Blackface ewe in **302** were raised (positive 'wheelbarrow' test).

Differential diagnoses

- Chronic suppurative pneumonia.
- Pleuropneumonia/pleural abscess.
- Lungworm infestation.
- Maedi.
- Mediastinal abscess caused by CLA.
- Laryngeal chondritis.
- Enzootic nasal tumour.

These conditions present with tachypnoea, possibly dyspnoea during exercise, nasal discharge and chronic weight loss but none of them would show classical ultrasonographic images of SPA or give a positive 'wheelbarrow test'.

Diagnosis

There is presently no commercial confirmatory serological test for SPA. Radiography reveals the extent of the tumour mass, although such examination is limited to the caudodorsal lung field when the tumour mass is typically distributed anteroventrally (304).

During ultrasonographic examination the normal aerated lung surface (visceral pleura) reflects sound

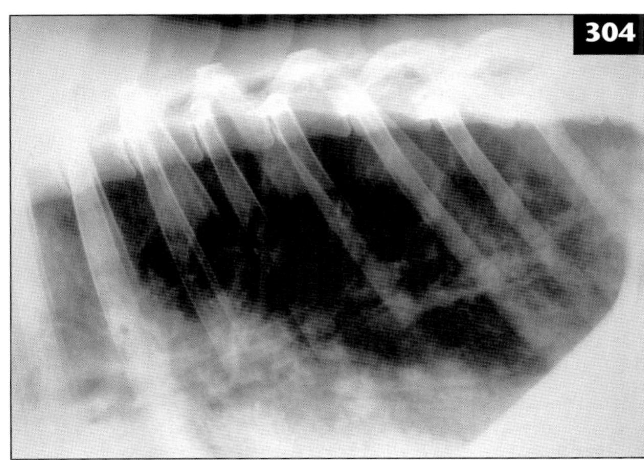

304 Radiograph of a sheep with extensive SPA. The distribution of the tumour is typically anteroventral.

waves and appears as a hyperechoic (bright white) line. Cellular proliferation within the lung parenchyma leading to consolidation, which occurs with SPA infection, facilitates transmission of sound waves and is represented by a hypoechoic (darker) area with bright dots where the sound waves collide with air within bronchioles and smaller airways. Typically, ultrasonographic examination of the chest reveals extensive consolidation due to proliferation of type II pneumocytes, and this can be used to locate accurately the sharply-defined tumour mass (305).

Confirmation of SPA diagnosis is established at necropsy. In advanced cases the lungs are enlarged and heavy (>2 kg), with the tumours occupying the anteroventral lung fields (306, 307). The tumours are solid and grey and are sharply demarcated from normal lung tissue. The lesions may contain abscesses or necrotic centers. The bronchi and trachea contain copious frothy fluid. Histologically, tumour cells replace normal alveolar cells.

Treatment

There is no treatment and affected sheep must be culled as soon as clinical suspicions are confirmed either by copious nasal discharge and/or ultrasonographic examination of the chest.

Prevention/control measures

The disease is introduced into flocks through purchased infected sheep, which shed lentiviruses before illness becomes apparent. The main route of infection is by respiratory aerosol, with housing or trough feeding increasing the rate of spread of infection (308).

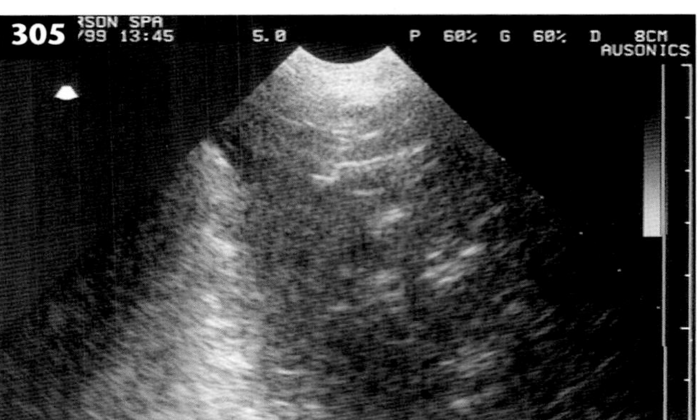

305 Ultrasonogram of a lung affected by SPA. Dorsal is to the left. The normal visceral pleura has been lost and replaced by sharply demarcated consolidated lung represented sonographically by a markedly hypoechoic area extending for 7 cm or more into lung tissue.

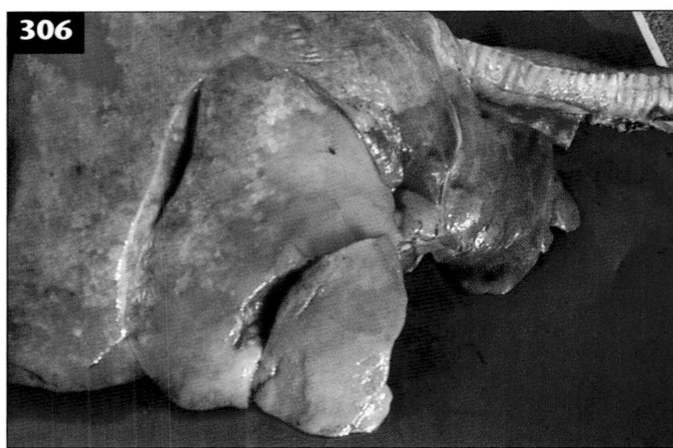

306 Necropsy of a sheep revealing an early SPA lesion. The tumour mass is sharply demarcated.

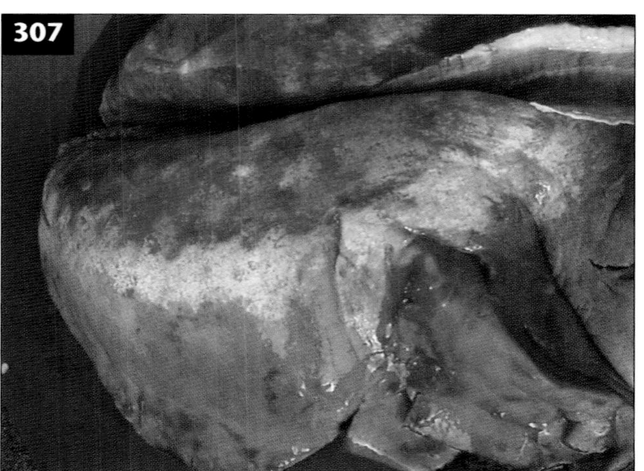

307 Necropsy of the sheep in **305**, revealing extensive SPA lesions, including the sharply-demarcated tumour mass.

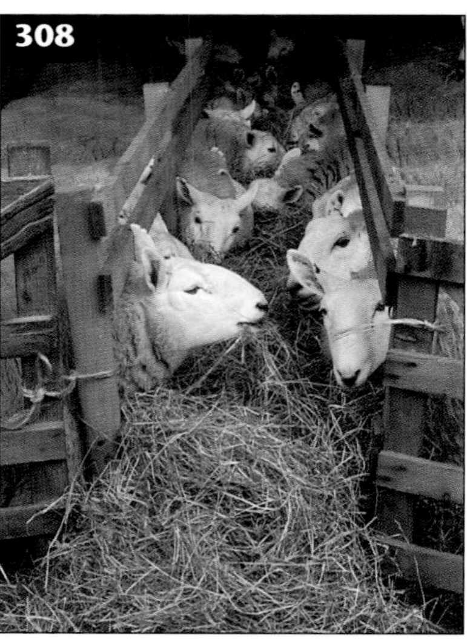

308 Close confinement facilitates droplet spread of the virus.

Regular flock inspection with prompt isolation and culling of lean and/or dyspnoeic sheep may identify early clinical cases and slow the spread of infection. Maintaining sheep in single age groups has been shown to be the most important management factor in reducing clinical disease. The offspring of affected sheep frequently develop SPA and must not be kept as replacement breeding stock.

There appears to be a synergistic effect involving maedi-visna virus (MVV) and SPA, and control measures should involve excluding entry of both virus conditions into the flock. De-stocking is the only practical solution when both infections exist in a flock.

Economics

Serious financial loss can result following the introduction of SPA into a flock, especially if the flock is housed for more than two months of the year. In an endemically infected flock, SPA may contribute up to 50% of ewe deaths (up to 5% of adult sheep per annum), with considerable losses also resulting from an increased culling rate of suspected early cases and their progeny.

Welfare implications

Affected sheep must be culled as soon as clinical disease is suspected.

ATYPICAL PNEUMONIA

Definition/overview

Atypical pneumonia is a non-progressive chronic pneumonia of housed sheep under one year old (**309**) caused by *Mycoplasma ovipneumoniae* and, possibly, other organisms (parainfluenza 3 virus and *Chlamydophila psittaci*). The true prevalence of this disease is unknown because the clinical signs are mild and do not generally warrant veterinary investigation.

Atypical pneumonia (enzootic pneumonia) is a very important disease of weaned lambs and hoggets in New Zealand. Its aetiology is complex and associated with respiratory viruses and mycoplasmas, with *Pasteurella* as a secondary bacterial infection.

Clinical presentation

The significant clinical finding is one of reduced growth rate despite an appropriate ration. A chronic soft cough and nasal discharge spread slowly through the group, most noticeable when the sheep are suddenly disturbed.

Differential diagnoses

- Lungworm infestation.
- Pneumonia caused by other pathogens (e.g. *Pasteurella* species).

Diagnosis

Diagnosis is based on clinical signs and often confirmed at the slaughter plant. Lung changes consist of red-brown or grey collapsed areas in the apical and cardiac lobes (**310**). Histology shows a lymphocytic cuffing pneumonia with pseudoepithelialization of the alveoli and hyperplasia of the bronchial epithelium.

Treatment

Treatment is generally not necessary because the clinical signs are mild. Oxytetracycline should be given to sick lambs.

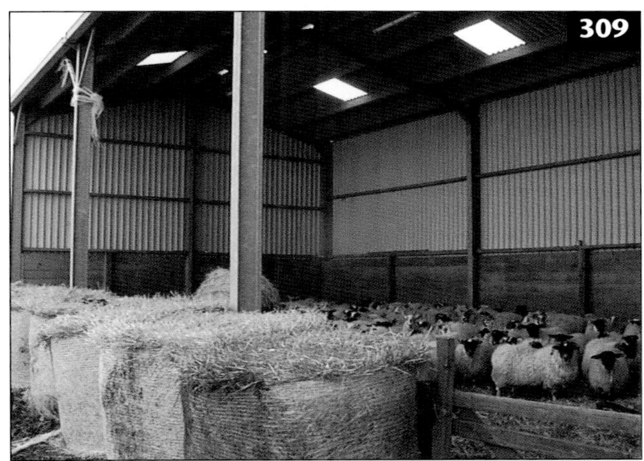

309 Atypical pneumonia with frequent coughing is often encountered in fattening lambs housed in multi-purpose buildings.

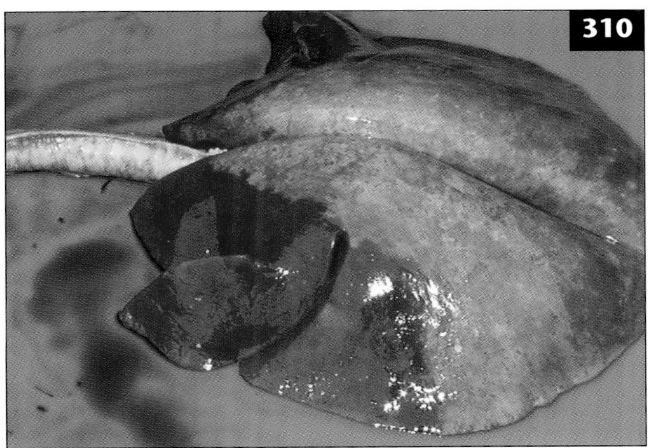

310 Lung changes of atypical pneumonia detected at the abattoir.

Prevention/control measures
Control can be attempted by improving ventilation and reducing the stocking density. The airspace should not be shared with older sheep. Purchased lambs should be housed separately from homebred stock.

Economics
Atypical pneumonia does not usually have a significant adverse effect on growth rate and profitability.

PARASITIC BRONCHITIS

Definition/overview
Unlike cattle, parasitic bronchitis is not a significant problem in sheep, with small infestations found coincidentally at necropsy.

Aetiology
The common nematodes that infest sheep lungs are *Dictyocaulus filaria*, *Protostrongylus rufescens* and *Muellerius capillaris*.

Clinical presentation
D. filaria and, less so, *P. rufescens* may cause coughing and weight loss in heavy infestations but this is uncommon. Young stock are more likely to show clinical signs than adults, especially during late summer/early autumn. *M. capillaris* lesions are common in sheep lungs but are of no clinical significance.

Differential diagnoses
Differential diagnoses would include atypical pneumonia in housed lambs.

Diagnosis
First stage larvae of *D. filaria* can be demonstrated by the Baermann technique in faeces of sheep with patent infestations. Adult *D. filaria* can be demonstrated in the trachea and bronchi at necropsy (**311**).

Treatment
Treatment for lungworm is not necessary.

Prevention/control measures
Control is achieved by the regular anthelmintic treatments used in the management of parasitic gastroenteritis.

Economics
Lungworm infestation is of no economic significance.

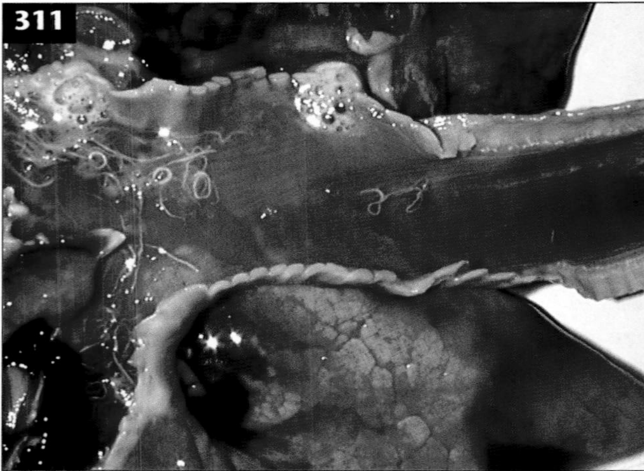

311 *Dictyocaulus* species in the trachea and major airways.

MAEDI

Definition/overview
Maedi-visna virus (MVV) infection is recognized in many countries worldwide. It was first recognized in the UK in 1979. The main economic effect of MVV is not because of the overt clinical disease but because of the poor production that is a result of indurative mastitis and poor body condition, poor reproductive efficiency, high perinatal mortality and poor lamb growth rates. In the USA the respiratory tract form of MVV infection is known as ovine progressive pneumonia.

Aetiology
Maedi (respiratory disease) is caused by a lentivirus, which also causes a nervous disease (visna), mastitis and arthritis. The most important route of transmission of the virus is from mother to offspring via colostrum and milk. The virus establishes infection in the lungs, udder, central nervous system and haematopoeitic organs, despite the immune response. The mechanisms whereby the virus escapes the immune response are complex and not fully understood. A large proportion of the flock (>60%) are likely to be seropositive when the first clinical case is diagnosed.

Clinical presentation
Clinical cases occur in sheep over three years old. In some situations sheep have outlived their productive life span before overt clinical signs of maedi pneumonia develop. The earliest sign of maedi is exercise intolerance noted during gathering. Affected

sheep stand with an extended neck, flared nostrils and an increased respiratory rate with an abdominal component to the breathing effort. As the disease progresses, wasting occurs and dyspnoea becomes obvious even at rest. Any exercise results in tachypnoea and mouth breathing and if affected sheep are severely stressed, cyanosis and collapse may ensue. Auscultation of the chest is largely unrewarding. Sheep remain bright and continue to eat, despite the dyspnoea and weight loss.

Although not a major presenting sign, a large number of affected sheep in the flock also have an indurative mastitis, identified as a flabby udder with diffuse hardening. Milk production is significantly decreased, although the milk produced appears normal. MVV-associated arthritis is important in the USA but to date has not been identified in the UK. A stiff, straight-legged gait with swelling, most commonly of the carpal joints, has been reported.

Differential diagnoses

- Sheep pulmonary adenomatosis.
- Chronic suppurative pneumonia.
- Pleuropneumonia/pleural abscess.
- Mediastinal abscess caused by caseous lymphadenitis.

Diagnosis

Diagnosis relies on detecting antibody to the virus by the agar gel immunodiffusion test (AGIT). This is the basis of the MVV accreditation scheme presently operated in the UK. The ELISA test is a more sensitive screen and is currently being used in several European countries.

On gross postmortem examination the lungs are firm, rubbery and heavy, weighing up to 2 kg (normal = 0.4–0.6 kg). On opening the chest the lungs do not collapse and impressions of the ribs may remain on the pleural surface. The lungs may exhibit mottled or grey areas. Histologically, there is smooth muscle hyperplasia with diffuse interstitial pneumonia, lymphoid infiltration and proliferation of the alveolar septae. The caudal mediastinal lymph nodes are usually greatly enlarged, with marked cortical hyperplasia.

Treatment

There is no effective treatment.

Prevention/control measures

Prevention of infection through adequate biosecurity measures and the purchase of MVV-free stock is the best option at present. A strict culling policy and increased replacement rate can aid control in endemically infected flocks. Control can be attempted in an infected closed flock by regular (3–6 monthly) serological testing and culling of seropositive sheep and removal of their offspring, but this is a costly and protracted business. Alternatively, control can be attempted by the removal of lambs from their dams immediately after birth before they ingest infected colostrum, thus breaking the lactogenic route of transmission.

Economics

The true economic impact of MVV on commercial sheep farms has not been determined. Loss of MVV-accredited status would have potentially disastrous consequences in a pedigree flock selling breeding rams.

Welfare implications

Sheep showing respiratory distress should be culled.

CHRONIC SUPPURATIVE PNEUMONIA/LUNG ABSCESSES

Definition/overview

Lung abscesses are common in sheep but are difficult to diagnose on clinical examination alone.

Aetiology

Chronic suppurative pneumonia/lung abscesses can result from bacterial infection of viral-compromised lung tissue (**312**); inhalation of infection from the

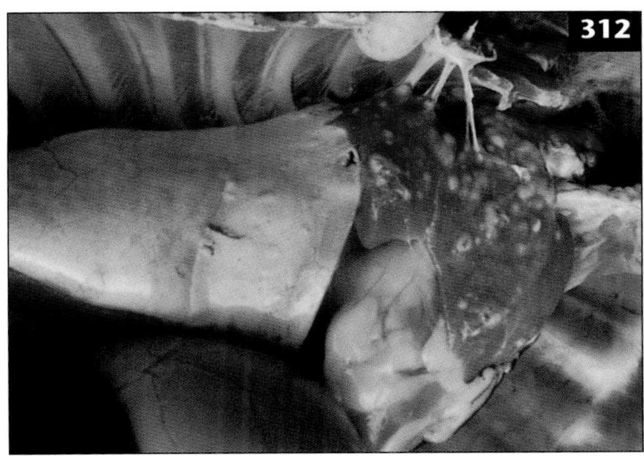

312 Viral-induced consolidation of the right apical and cardiac lung lobes with secondary abscessation and pleuritis in a two-month-old orphan lamb.

oropharynx, typically associated with *Fusobacterium necrophorum* infection in young lambs (**313, 314**); or haematogenous spread from a septic focus elsewhere in the body (e.g. the udder, the uterus or a cellulitis lesion). Tick pyaemia is a common cause of lung abscessation in lambs. *Arcanobacterium pyogenes* is a common isolate from lung abscesses.

Clinical presentation

There is a wide spectrum of clinical presentation depending on the number and size of the lesions. Sheep with significant chronic suppurative pneumonia lesions present with a history of weight loss (**315**). Affected sheep are often dull and depressed, although appetite may appear normal. The rectal temperature is often within the normal range or slightly elevated (up to 40.0°C). At rest, affected sheep are tachypnoeic compared with normal sheep in the group, and they cough occasionally. There may be an occasional scant mucopurulent nasal discharge. Depending on the site and extent of the lesion(s), auscultation may reveal absence of normal lung sounds and muffled heart sounds.

Differential diagnoses

In many cases it can prove difficult to identify the lung as the major site of bacterial infection; therefore, the differential diagnosis list should include the common causes of weight loss in individual sheep:

- Paratuberculosis.
- Suppurative mastitis.
- Sheep pulmonary adenomatosis.
- Endocarditis.
- Mediastinal abscess caused by caseous lymphadenitis.
- Chronic parasitism including fasciolosis.

Diagnosis

Routine haematological analyses are rarely helpful in the diagnosis of chronic bacterial infections in sheep. Increases in acute phase proteins, including haptoglobin and fibrinogen, and serum protein concentrations may indicate inflammation caused by bacterial infection but these changes are not specific for respiratory disease. Serological tests are diagnostic for some chronic respiratory tract viral infections (e.g. maedi-visna) but not for SPA.

Radiography

Pathological changes associated with aerosol infection, typically respiratory viruses and secondary bacterial infection in young lambs, more commonly involve the anteroventral lung field; however, the position of the forelimbs and associated musculature in the standing

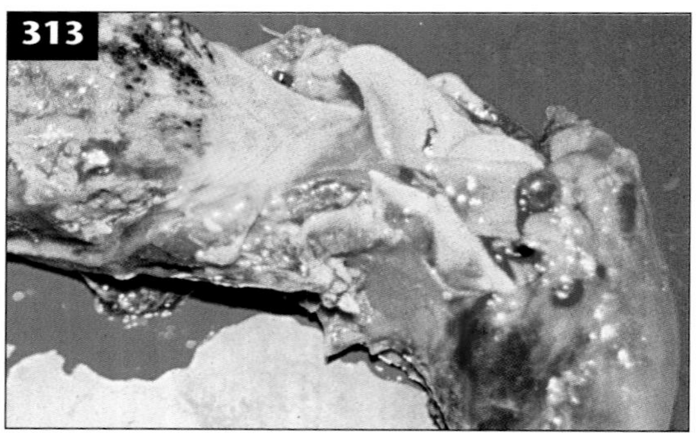

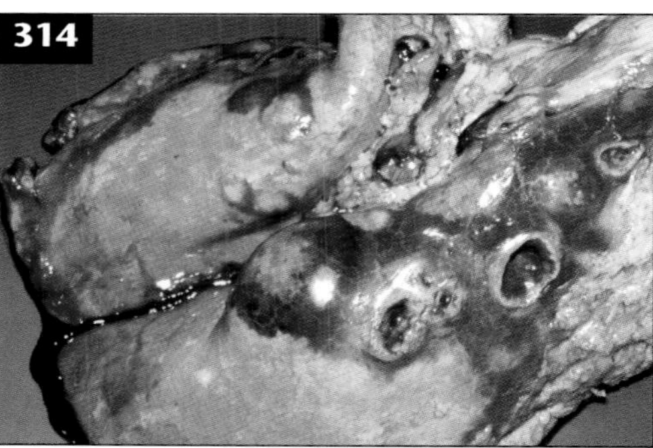

313 Severe tongue lesions caused by *Fusobacterium necrophorum*.

314 Pleural and superficial lung abscess in a six-month-old lamb.

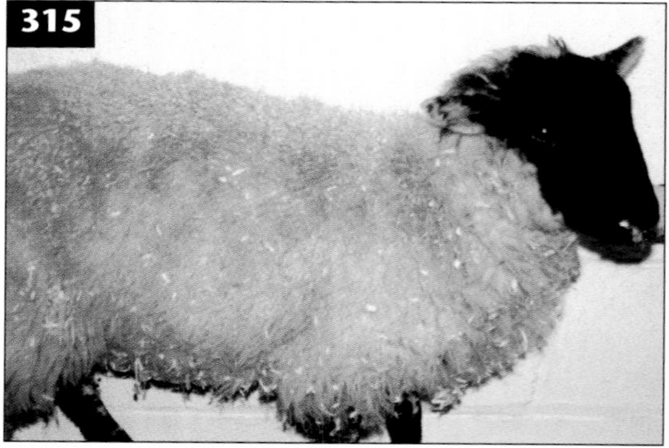

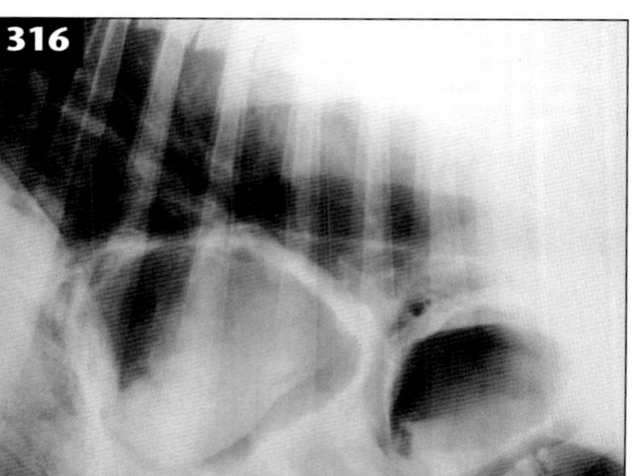

315 Six-month-old lamb with *Fusobacterium necrophorum* infection presenting with weight loss.

316 Radiograph revealing two large well-encapsulated lung abscesses.

sheep largely restricts radiographic examination. Following bacteraemic spread to the lung, the lesions tend to be distributed to the caudodorsal lung field and large abscesses can therefore readily be identified (**316**). Radiographic examination of the ovine thorax is limited by cost considerations, availability of equipment and problems associated with the sheep's fleece.

Ultrasonography

Ultrasound examination is a cheap and portable alternative to radiographic examination of the chest and it is useful for pleural lesions such as abscesses (**317, 318**). The abscess capsule can be readily identified in well-encapsulated lesions (**317**) or it may extend to occupy all of that side of the chest (**318, 319**).

Treatment

Penicillin is the antibiotic of choice for chronic respiratory disease because of the frequent isolation of *Arcanobacterium pyogenes*. Treating valuable breeding stock with multiple pleural and superficial lung abscesses, identified by ultrasonographic examination, for 20–30 consecutive days has produced encouraging results.

Prevention/control measures

Prevention is aimed at prompt treatment of bacterial infections such as mastitis, metritis and cellulitis lesions before significant bacteraemic spread to the lungs occurs. *F. necrophorum* infection of the lungs is not uncommon in orphan lambs reared in unhygienic conditions.

Economics

The total cost of daily administration of 44,000 iu/kg procaine penicillin for three or more weeks may well exceed the value of non-pedigree sheep.

Welfare implications

Sheep with significant lung pathology should be euthanased.

LARYNGEAL CHONDRITIS

Definition/overview

Laryngeal chondritis is an acute onset restriction of the upper airway that causes severe dyspnoea and, in many cases, death of the sheep.

Aetiology

Laryngeal chondritis is most commonly encountered in 18–24-month-old meat breed rams such as the Suffolk, Beltex and Texel (**320**) during the late summer and autumn months. It is often associated with high

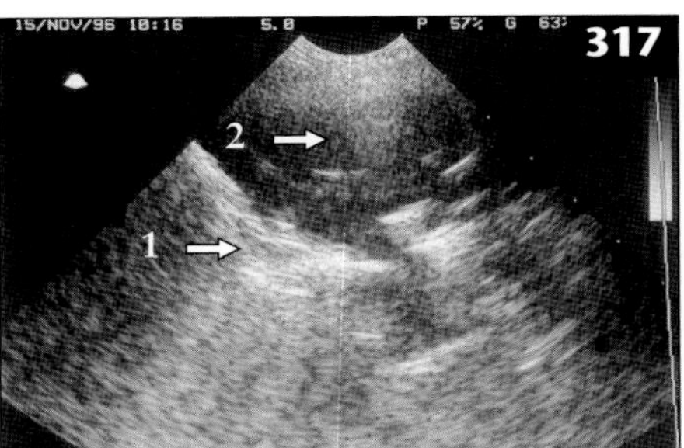

317 Ultrasonogram of the pleural abscess shown in **314**. The bright white (hyperechoic) line formed by normal visceral pleura (**1**) has been replaced by an anechoic area containing multiple hyperechoic dots typical of an abscess. (**2**).

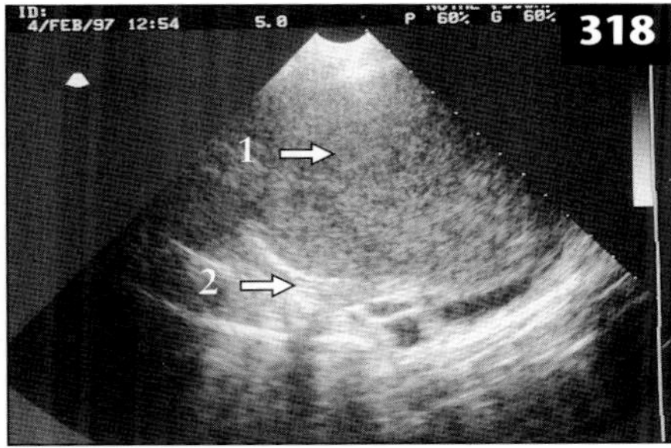

318 Ultrasonogram of a pleural abscess (**1**) that extends for 10 cm. (**2**, visceral pleura.)

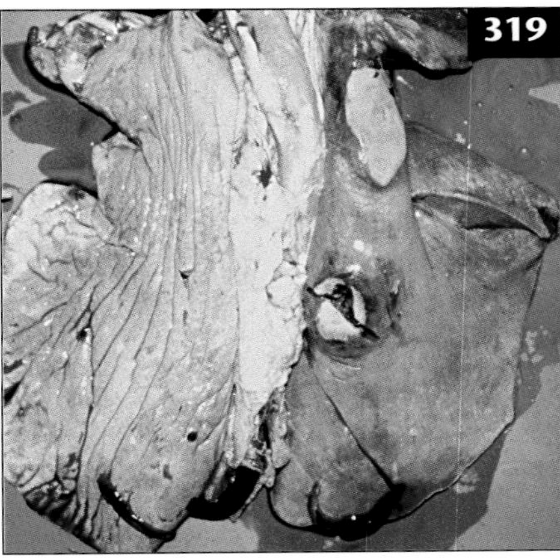

319 Necropsy of the lamb in **318**. The extensive pleural abscess occupies one side of the chest.

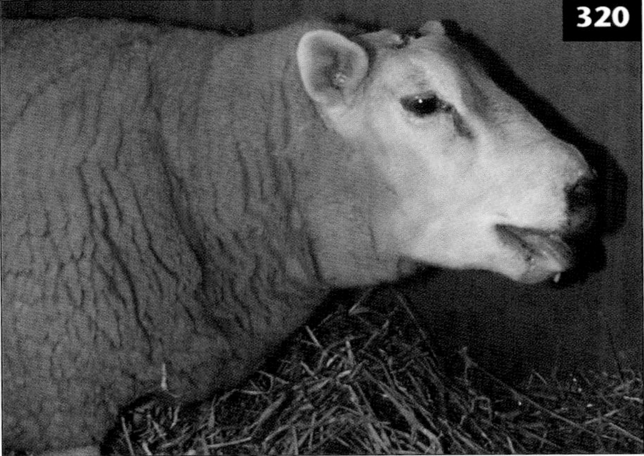

320 Inspiratory dyspnoea in a Texel ram suffering from laryngeal chondritis.

levels of concentrate feeding in preparation for sale. The condition appears somewhat later in the year in ram lambs, perhaps related to later maturity. Laryngeal chondritis is rare in ewes.

During the rut, under the influence of testosterone and other male hormones, the ram's head becomes enlarged, with obvious oedema of the skin folds. It has been suggested that similar changes in the voice box also occur at this time. Such changes may explain the seasonal occurrence of laryngeal chondritis in rams. Similar changes in the larynx have been noted in species such as the elk and moose, which bugle during the rut to attract females. Turbulent air passage through the reduced diameter larynx aggravates this problem, leading to further localized oedema and erosion of the lining epithelium, with secondary bacterial infection causing swelling of the arytenoid cartilages and further restriction of air flow.

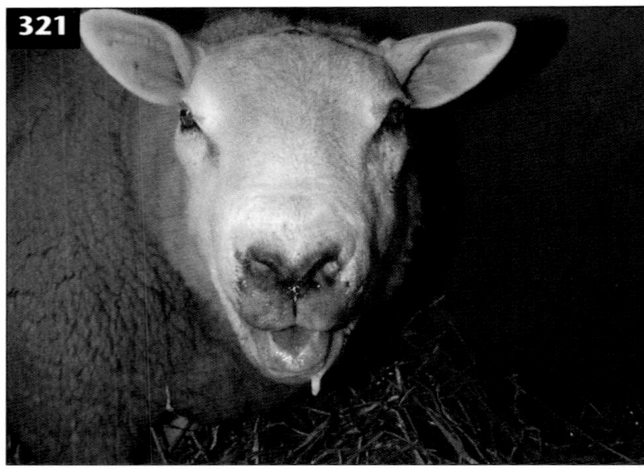

321 Mouth breathing in the Texel ram in **320**.

Clinical presentation

There is acute onset severe respiratory distress (**321**, **322**). Affected sheep are reluctant to move and they stand with the head held slightly lowered and the neck extended (**320**, p. 153). The respiratory rate is greatly increased to over 90 breaths per minute (often panting), with a marked inspiratory effort and associated noise (stertor), which is audible from a considerable distance. The nostrils are flared and the mouth is held open with the tongue partially protruded (**321**). There is frothy saliva around the mouth and lower jaw (**322**). There is no nasal discharge or halitosis. The rectal temperature is normal or only marginally elevated. The mucous membranes appear cyanotic. There is no palpable enlargement of the submandibular lymph nodes. Auscultation over the larynx reveals very loud crackles, which are transferred over the whole lung field. The heart rate is increased to over 120 bpm. Affected sheep are in such distress that they are unable to eat or drink. Handling exacerbates the respiratory distress, which may precipitate death.

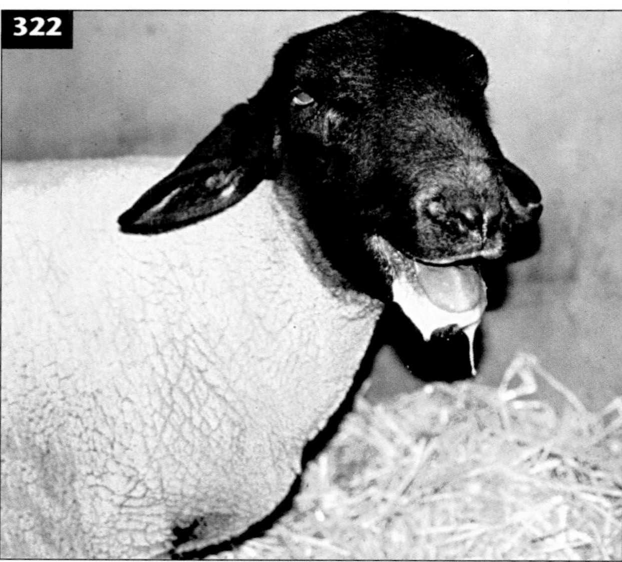

322 Severe inspiratory dyspnoea in a Suffolk ram suffering from laryngeal chondritis.

Swelling of the arytenoids (with or without erosion/infection of the overlying epithelium), which causes severe narrowing of the larynx, can be visualized during endoscopic examination (**323**). Endoscopic examination is not routinely performed but it could be considered in particularly valuable rams that have failed to respond to initial treatment or where the condition has recurred.

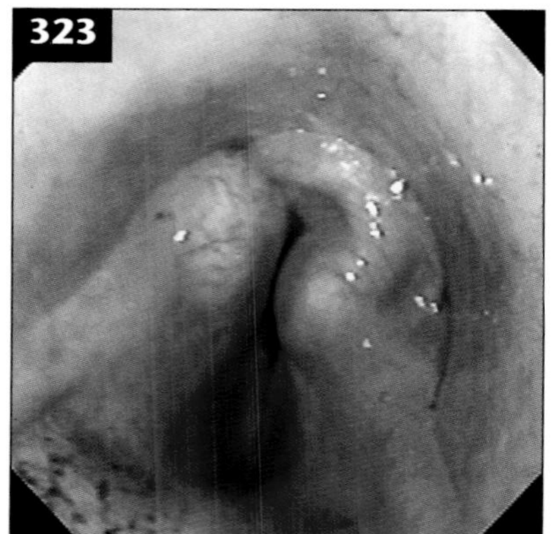

323 Marked oedema of the artyenoid cartilages observed during endoscopy. The airflow is severely restricted by the oedema.

Laryngeal chondritis will recur within 2–4 weeks in approximately 30–50% of rams affected by this condition. Less than 50% of these sheep fully recover after a second treatment course.

Differential diagnoses

- Swollen retropharyngeal lymph node(s) causing laryngeal compression.
- Foreign body in the pharynx/pharyngeal abscess.
- Choke.
- Pasteurellosis.
- Advanced cases of maedi.
- Sheep pulmonary adenomatosis.
- Enzootic nasal tumour.
- Severe lungworm infestation.

Diagnosis

Diagnosis is based on the clinical findings and can be confirmed during endoscopic examination. Approximately 20% of cases are refractory to antibiotic and corticosteroid therapy; in these cases postmortem examination reveals swelling of the arytenoid cartilage(s), which almost occlude the airway. The fibrous nature of these swellings and/or abscessation of the cartilages (**324**) indicate that medical treatment would not resolve this problem successfully.

Treatment

Treatment involves dexamethasone (20 mg i/v or i/m once only at presentation) to reduce the oedema and a broad-spectrum antibiotic, preferably lincomycin (i/m for 7–10 days).

In severely dyspnoeic sheep a tracheostomy can be considered as an emergency procedure, but this is not a simple operation because the handling stresses further exacerbate the dyspnoea. Intranasal oxygen insufflation should be given where available.

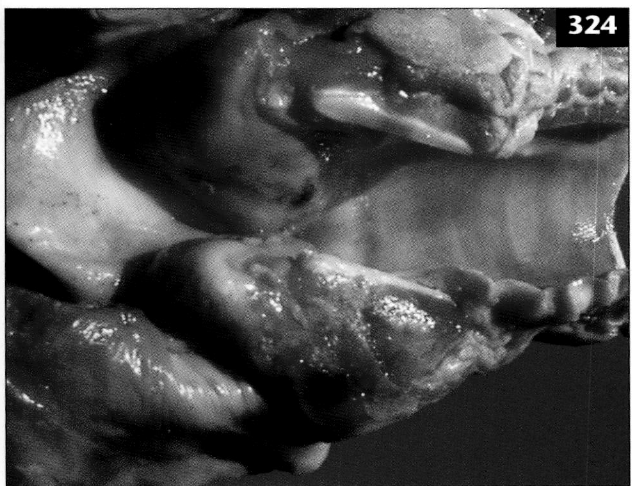

324 Abscessation and fibrosis involving the right arytenoid cartilage of the Texel ram in **320**.

Alternatively, trans-tracheal oxygen administration via a wide bore needle (14 gauge of larger) distal to the tracheostomy could be considered. In many situations it is best to administer 20 mg dexamethasone intravenously and wait for 4–6 hours, by which time some reduction in laryngeal oedema and improvement in clinical signs would be expected.

Prevention/control measures

The sporadic occurrence of laryngeal chondritis means that little constructive advice can be given to breeders regarding prevention. Early identification and treatment are essential. Reducing the level of supplementary feeding may reduce the prevalence of this problem but farmers are most reluctant to have their rams not in top condition for the sales.

The prevalence of laryngeal chondritis would appear to be increasing in the Suffolk breed within the UK. A predisposition for this condition may be selected for coincidentally alongside other characteristics such as 'a bold head' and other spurious, yet fashionable, phenotypic considerations.

Economics

Laryngeal chondritis occurs sporadically in rams. Losses result from deaths and the inability to present recovered rams for sale. The loss of even a small number of yearling rams can have a serious economic impact on a ram stud.

Welfare implications

Severely dyspnoeic rams must be monitored and careful consideration should be given for euthanasia of those sheep that do not respond within 24 hours to treatment. Cases of laryngeal chondritis that recur within two weeks have a guarded prognosis.

CLINICAL PROBLEM 1

A six-crop Greyface ewe is presented with a history of chronic weight loss (BCS 1.0, whilst the others in the group of recently weaned ewes are within a range from 2.0 to 2.5). The ewe had lambed eight weeks ago and the lambs have just been weaned on to an intensive finishing ration in order to reach slaughter weight (34–42 kg at 10–14 weeks old). The ewes had been fed approximately 2.0 kg concentrates per day plus *ad libitum* hay. The lambs had been offered creep feed *ad libitum* from two weeks of age.

Clinical examination

The ewe is slightly dull and depressed (**325**), although her appetite is quite good and she comes forward to the feed trough with the other sheep. The ewe has been observed cudding normally. She has no incisor teeth (broken mouth) and the molar teeth are worn but with sharp points on the labial aspect of the upper molars. The rectal temperature is 40.0°C. At rest the ewe is tachypnoeic (40 breaths per minute), with an occasional cough. Auscultation of the chest reveals an absence of lung sounds on the left-hand side and muffled heart sounds. Normal heart and lung sounds can be auscultated on the right-hand side of the chest. There is a chronic mastitis with numerous large 2–4 cm diameter abscesses within the udder. There are numerous orf lesions on the teats. No clear frothy nasal discharge is produced when the hindlimbs are raised (negative 'wheelbarrow test').

What conditions should be considered (differential diagnoses)?
How can the diagnosis be confirmed?
What is the prognosis for this ewe?

Differential diagnoses

Primarily a unilateral lung lesion:

- Chronic suppurative pneumonia
- Pleuropneumonia/pleural abscess
- Mediastinal abscess caused by CLA

The negative 'wheelbarrow test' suggests that SPA (jaagsiekte) is unlikely.

Further tests to determine a specific diagnosis

Ultrasonographic examination of the left chest revealed that the normal hyperechoic line formed by the visceral pleura (**326**) had been replaced by an extensive hypoechoic area with a slightly hyperechoic latticework matrix throughout (**326, 327**). In the anteroventral area of the chest this hypoechoic area extended from the chest wall for a depth of almost 12 cm (see scale in **328**), indicating that there would be little normal left lung tissue remaining. This large fibrin deposit in the left chest could explain the displacement of the heart towards the right chest wall and why the heart sounds were poorly audible on the left-hand side of the chest. Ultrasonographic examination of the right chest revealed the normal hyperechoic line formed by the visceral pleura at a depth of approximately 1.5 cm from the probe head. The heart was more easily visualized than normal, with the right heart chambers pushed adjacent to the right chest wall.

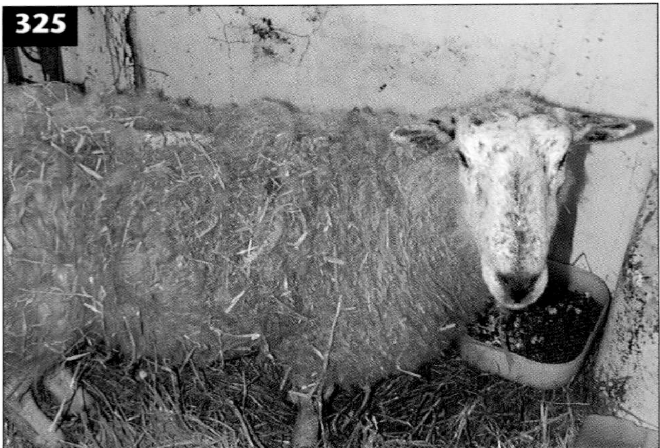

325 Greyface ewe presenting in poor condition and with no lung sounds on the left side of the chest.

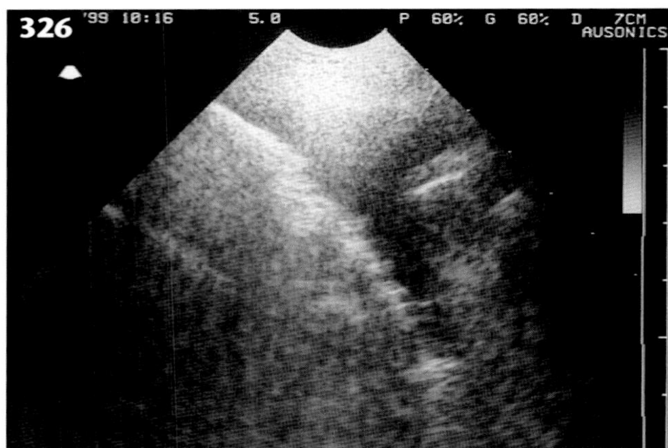

326 Ultrasonogram of the dorsal lung area, revealing separation of the pleurae and lung lobes by an anechoic area extending up to 2 cm thick. There is acoustic enhancement of the visceral pleura (broad white line).

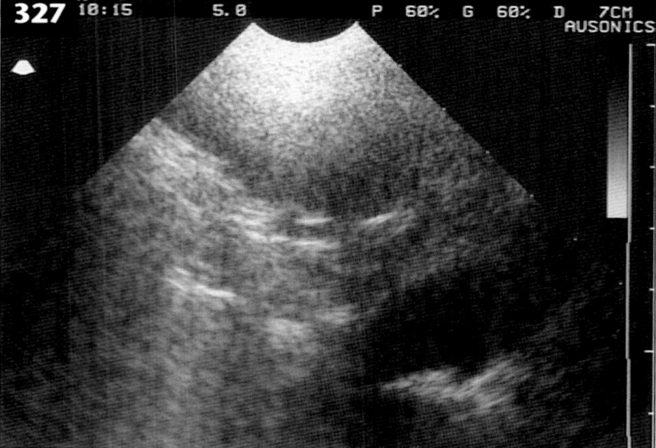

327 Ultrasonogram taken as the probe head travels ventrally, revealing increased separation of the pleurae and an irregular lung surface.

Diagnosis

On the basis of the ultrasonographic findings a diagnosis of extensive pleuritis of the left chest was made. The right side of the chest was considered to be normal.

Prognosis

A hopeless prognosis was given and the ewe was euthanased.

Postmortem examination

Postmortem examination confirmed the diagnosis of extensive pleuritis of the left chest (**329**, **330**). The right side of the chest was normal. Numerous large abscesses were present in the udder parenchyma. Interestingly, *Streptococcus dysgalactiae* was isolated from the pleuritis lesions and the mastitis lesions.

Discussion

At necropsy, it is not unusual to find single or multiple lung abscesses in cull ewes that also have chronic mastitis. It is possible that the development of bacteraemia from a chronic mastitis lesion(s) is underestimated in sheep and greater care should be taken with the treatment of such lesions. Chronic mastitis lesions should not be dismissed as a simple abscess but should be regarded as a potential source of bacteraemia seeding the lungs and, possibly, the endocardium. In this case it was not possible to determine why the bacteraemia, presumably originating in the udder, gave rise to such a severe unilateral pleuritis.

CLINICAL PROBLEM 2

A three-crop Wensleydale ewe is presented with a history of chronic weight loss (**331**) (BCS 1.5, whilst the remainder of the small group of ewes belonging to a hobby farmer are within a range from 3.0–3.5). The ewe had reared twin lambs that season and they had been weaned four months ago. The ewes are at pasture with plenty of late autumn grass still available.

Clinical examination

The ewe is slightly dull and depressed and unable to stand, although her appetite is good. The mucous membranes appear normal. The rectal temperature is 40.1°C. At rest the ewe is tachypnoeic (42 breaths per minute) with an obvious abdominal component. There is a scant mucoid nasal discharge. Auscultation

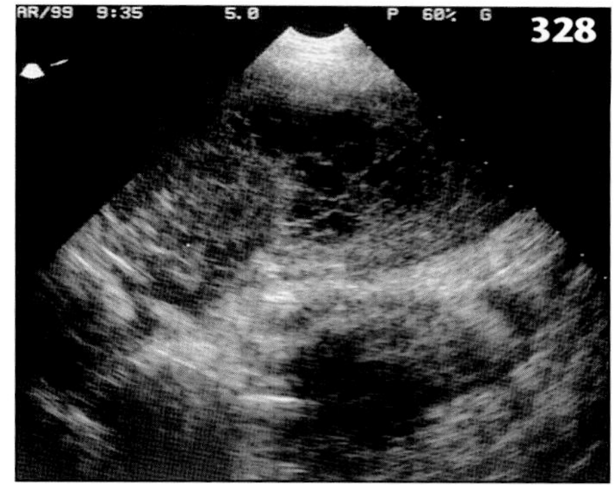

328 Halfway down the left chest wall, ultrasonographic examination reveals an extensive hyperechoic latticework within an anechoic mass extending for up to 10 cm from the parietal pleura.

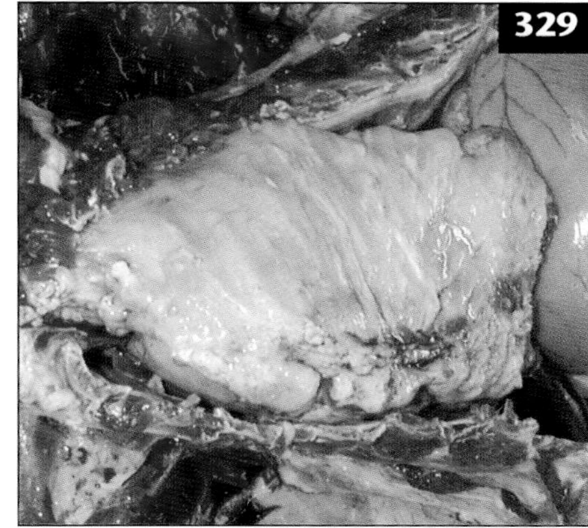

329 Necroposy reveals the extensive fibrinous pleuritis seen in the ultrasonograms **326** and **327**.

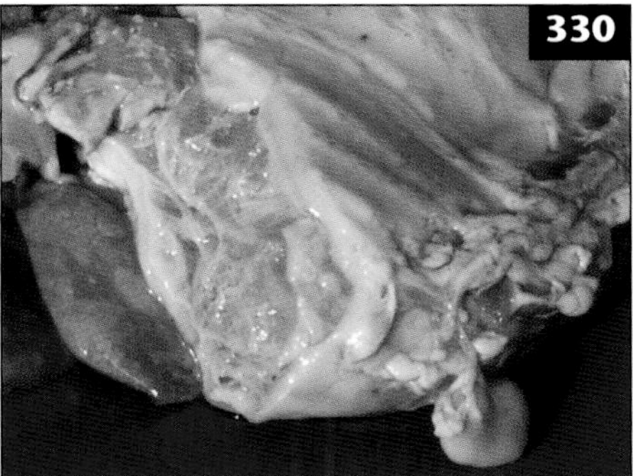

330 Section revealing the extent of the fibrinous pleuritis. Compare the pathology specimen with the ultrasonogram in **328**.

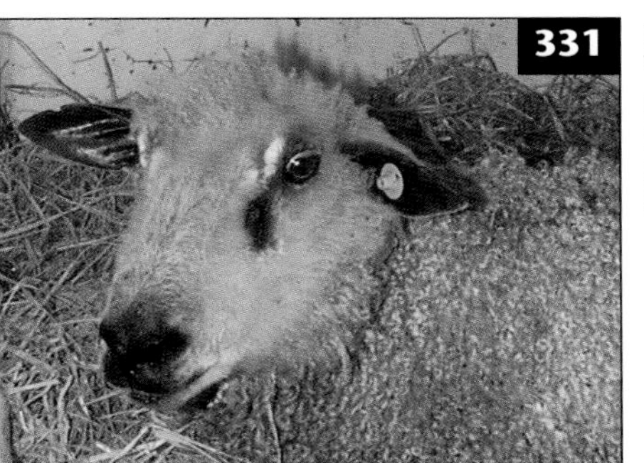

331 Wensleydale ewe with a history of chronic weight loss.

of the chest reveals much reduced lung sounds on the right-hand side and muffled heart sounds. Increased lung sounds (wheezes) can be auscultated on the left-hand side of the chest. No clear frothy nasal discharge is produced when the hindlimbs are raised (negative 'wheelbarrow test' for SPA). The abdomen appears distended and it is possible to appreciate a fluid thrill. The rumen sounds are increased in frequency, occurring every 20 seconds. The ewe has passed normal pelleted faeces.

What conditions should be considered (differential diagnoses)?
How can the diagnosis be confirmed?
What is the prognosis for this ewe?

Differential diagnoses

Primarily a unilateral pleural/lung lesion causing consolidation:

- Chronic suppurative pneumonia.
- Pleuropneumonia/pleural abscess.
- Mediastinal abscess caused by CLA.

The negative 'wheelbarrow test' suggests that SPA (jaagsiekte) is unlikely. The abdominal distension could be caused by ascites as a consequence of:

- Right-sided heart failure associated with the thoracic/pulmonary lesion.
- Tumour of the gastrointestinal tract (e.g. adenocarcinoma).
- Hypoproteinaemia.
- Inflammatory exudate associated with sub-acute fasciolosis.

Further tests to determine specific diagnosis

Haematological examination

Routine haematological examination revealed changes consistent with dehydration (total RBC count 16.6×10^{12}/l [normal = 5–9 $\times 10^{12}$/l]; Hb 142 g/l [normal = 80–140 g/l]; PCV 0.44 l/l [normal = 0.26–0.36 l/l]). There was a leucocytosis (12.9×10^9/l [normal = 4–10 $\times 10^9$/l]) resulting from a marginal neutrophilia (10.4×10^9/l [81%]) with 16% lymphocytes and 3% monocytes. There was a marginal reduction in the serum albumin (24.3 g/l [normal = 30–36 g/l]) and normal globulin concentration (45.3 g/l [normal = 35–50 g/l]). The serum haptoglobin concentration was 0 g/l (normal = <0.1 g/l).

Ultrasonographic examination

Ultrasonographic examination of the left chest revealed the normal hyperechoic line formed by the visceral pleura at a depth of approximately 1.5 cm from the probe head. The heart could be clearly imaged and was displaced caudodorsally and towards the left chest wall. Examination of the right chest, commencing dorsally, revealed an anechoic area with multiple bright spots (typical of an abscess) extending up to 14 cm from the chest wall (**332**). The mediastinum, which contained major blood vessels, could be imaged distal to the probe head at a depth of approximately 12–16 cm. There was no evidence of any normal lung tissue. Examination of the abdomen revealed ascites extending to a depth of 18 cm from the probe head (**333**), with the omentum clearly visible floating within the fluid. The bladder could not be imaged.

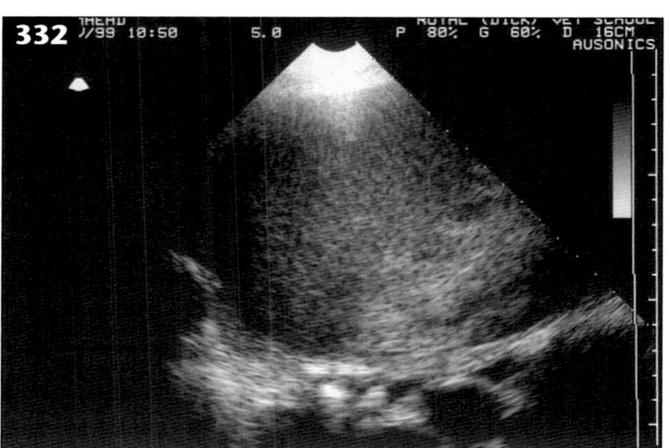

332 Ultrasonographic examination of the right chest, commencing dorsally, reveals an anechoic area with multiple bright spots (typical of an abscess) extending for up to 14 cm from the chest wall.

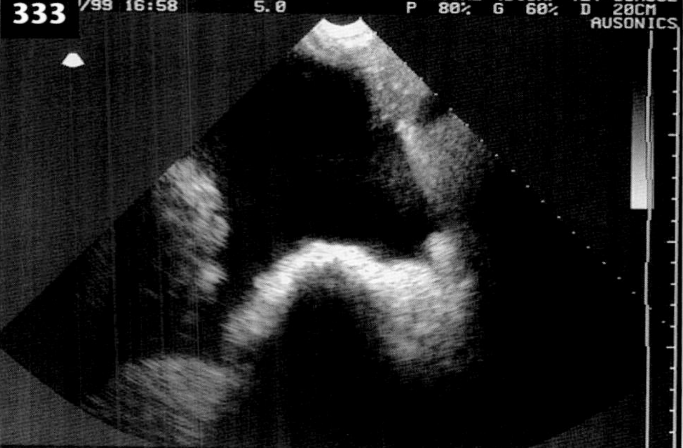

333 Ultrasonographic examination of the abdomen reveals ascites (anechoic area) extending to a depth of 18 cm from the probe head. The omentum appears as a hyperechoic broad ribbon-like structure.

Abdominocentesis
Abdominocentesis yielded a large quantity of colourless, odourless fluid with a stable foam suggestive of a high protein concentration. Laboratory analysis revealed a protein concentration of 44.3 g/l, suggestive of an exudate. The white cell concentration was normal (0.5×10^9/l), with 64% neutrophils, 16% lymphocytes and 20% histiocytes.

Diagnosis
Based on the ultrasonographic findings, a diagnosis of a massive pleural abscess occupying the entire right chest was made. It was estimated that the abscess could contain up to two litres of purulent material. The left side of the chest was considered to be normal except that the heart was displaced towards the left chest wall. The ascites was considered to be secondary to right-sided heart failure, although the protein concentration was higher than expected for a transudate (normal = <25 g/l). The haematological findings were not indicative of such chronic severe bacterial infection.

Prognosis
A hopeless prognosis was given and the ewe was euthanased.

Postmortem examination
The ascites was clearly discernible when the skin had been removed; this also revealed anterior oedema. The extent of the ascites was revealed on incising the abdominal wall (**334**). Bulging of the diaphragm, caused by increased pressure in the right chest, was clearly visible (**335**). The liver was enlarged, with rounded borders (**335**).

There were extensive fibrinous adhesions between the pleurae of the right chest (**336**) and the extent of the pleural abscess was clearly demonstrated (**336**). The heart was displaced towards the left chest wall. The pericardium contained excess pericardial fluid.

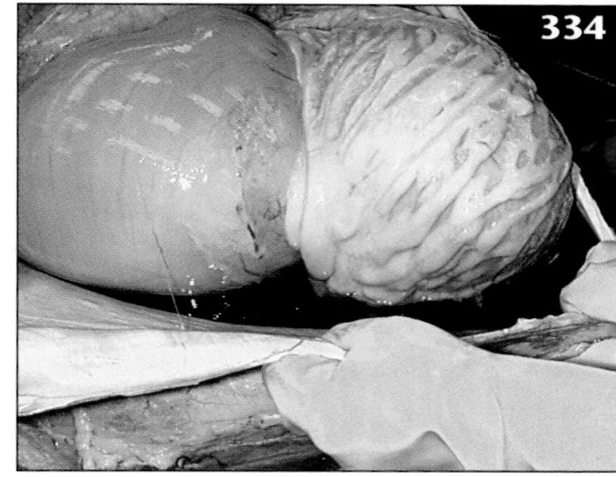

334 The extent of the ascites is revealed on incising the abdominal wall (see **333**).

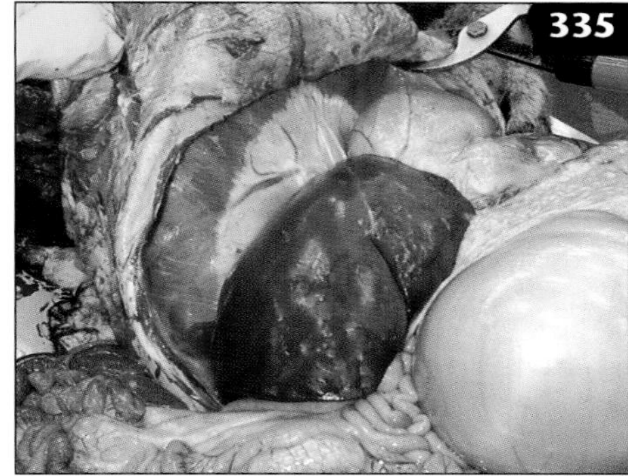

335 Bulging of the diaphragm, caused by increased pressure in the right chest, is clearly visible.

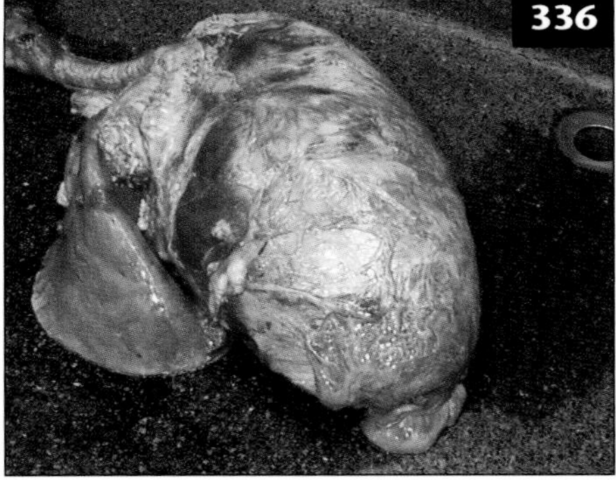

336 Fibrinous deposits are visible on the visceral pleura. The extent of the pleural abscess is clearly demonstrated (see **332**).

CLINICAL PROBLEM 3

A sick lamb (**337**) is noticed in a pen with 20 other orphan lambs. There are three dead lambs in an adjacent pen awaiting collection. The sick lamb is approximately six weeks old. The lambs have been weaned off milk and are being fed a ewe concentrate *ad libitum*.

The lamb is very dull and emaciated. The rectal temperature is 41.1°C. The respiratory rate is 44 bpm and the heart rate is 120 breaths per minute. There is a slight mucoid nasal discharge. Occasional coughing

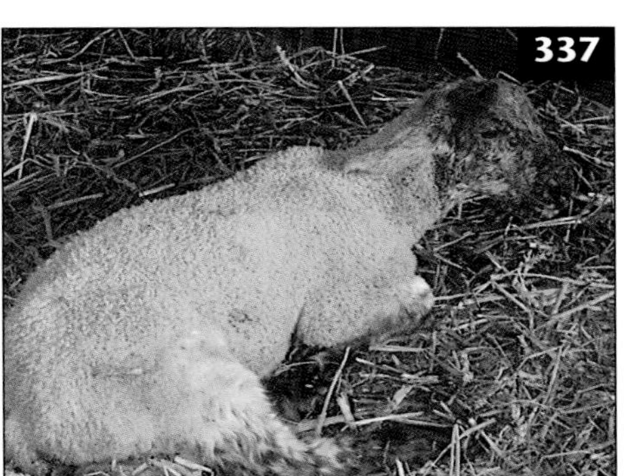

337 Sick lamb in a pen with 20 other orphan lambs.

has been heard in this group of lambs. The mucous membranes are congested. Auscultation of the chest reveals widespread crackles and wheezes. There is little abdominal fill. There is evidence of faecal staining of the tail and perineum. Many of the lambs in the group have crusting lesions over the muzzle and surrounding the eyes.

What conditions should be considered (differential diagnoses)?
What is a likely diagnosis?
What is the prognosis for this lamb?

Differential diagnoses

- Septicaemic pasteurellosis.
- Flare-up of chronic suppurative pneumonia.
- Pleuropneumonia/pleural abscess.

Alimentary tract signs:

- Coccidiosis.
- Acidosis.
- *Strongyloides westeri.*

Diagnosis

A diagnosis of chronic suppurative pneumonia was based on the pyrexia and depression and the widespread crackles heard on auscultation of the chest. Coccidiosis may explain the diarrhoea, especially when the creep feed does not include any coccidiostat, the pen is very poorly drained and there is a lack of dry bedding material (**338**). The ewe concentrate is in a large hard pellet form, which is wholly unsuitable for recently weaned lambs. Malnutrition is a major factor contributing to the losses in this group of orphan lambs (three dead from 25 lambs).

Treatment

The lamb was treated with oxytetracycline (20 mg/kg i/v). The sheherd was instructed to inject the lamb with oxytetracycline for five more days (10 mg/kg i/m).

Prognosis

The prognosis is hopeless and there is a strong case that this lamb should be euthanased for welfare reasons.

Further advice

The shepherd was advised to feed the lambs an appropriate lamb pencil ration containing decoquinate to prevent coccidiosis. This suggestion was declined. The shepherd was informed that coccidiosis would be likely and that treatment would be necessary if mucoid diarrhoea containing fresh blood clots, inappetence, weight loss and tenesmus were observed in the lambs.

Vaccination of the dam with a *Pasteurella* vaccine will provide some passively derived immunity for the first four weeks or so of life but orphan lambs often fail to ingest sufficient colostrum; therefore, there may be no circulating specific immunoglobulin in these orphan lambs to afford protection. Alternatively, lambs can be vaccinated with a live attenuated bovine PI3 intranasal vaccine once only. Such vaccination against the most common viral cause of respiratory disease in young lambs is claimed to reduce the prevalence of pasteurellosis in the flock, especially housed sheep.

Outcome

The lamb died within 12 hours.

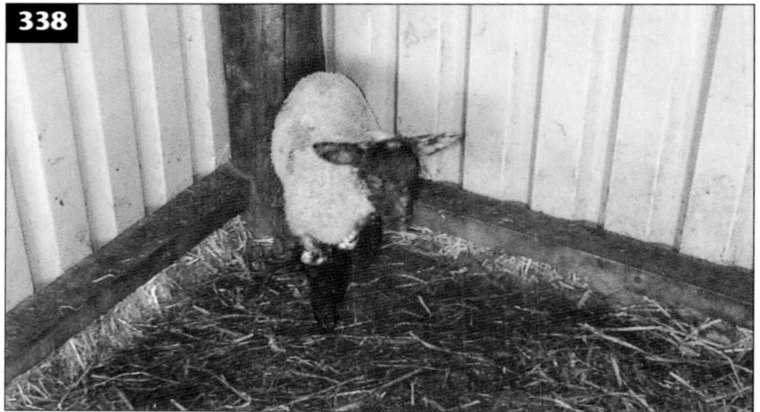

338 There is very poor pen drainage and a lack of dry bedding material.

Part 2: Cardiovascular System

INTRODUCTION

There are few conditions affecting the cardiovascular system in sheep; many reference textbooks do not include this body system. Congenital cardiac disorders are very uncommon in lambs. Unlike calves, where ventricular septal defect is relatively common and can be diagnosed with reasonable accuracy on clinical examination, this condition is rarely reported in lambs. Septic pericarditis secondary to traumatic reticulitis, while common in cattle, is not seen in sheep. Vegetative endocarditis is encountered occasionally in weaned lambs and adult sheep.

Clinical examination

The rate, rhythm and intensity of heart sounds are determined by auscultation over the chest in the region immediately beneath the elbow joints. It is essential to listen to both sides of the chest because unilateral space-occupying lesions in the cranial thorax frequently displace the heart, leading to marked disparity in intensity and origin of heart sounds. The heart rate of neonatal lambs may approach 180 bpm; older lambs and adult sheep have a heart rate of 65–80 bpm. Handling and other stresses may increase the heart rate by more than 50% but it returns to near normal within 5–10 minutes. The heart rate should be re-assessed at the end of the clinical examination. While the heart rate is usually regular, it is not uncommon to find every fourth or fifth beat dropped in otherwise healthy adult sheep.

Peripheral pulses are not easy to find in sheep and they are not usually assessed during the clinical examination; the femoral artery affords the best opportunity. Blood gas analysis, electrocardiography and echocardiography are rarely undertaken in sheep; echocardiography would be most useful in the diagnosis of vegetative endocarditis, the most common condition affecting the ovine heart.

VEGETATIVE ENDOCARDITIS

Definition/overview

Compared with cattle, there are few detailed clinical reports of ovine vegetative endocarditis because the condition in sheep commonly presents with no audible murmur. Furthermore, unlike in cattle, polyarthritis is relatively common in growing sheep; therefore, this common pointer to endocarditis in cattle is often attributed to erysipelas or other infectious causes. The provisional diagnosis of vegetative endocarditis is based on clinical findings of chronic weight loss, pain, pyrexia and, commonly, an associated polyarthritis. A detailed necropsy is rarely undertaken in farm animal practice, leading to underreporting of endocarditis. Lesions involving the tricuspid valve may result in ascites and peripheral oedema.

In the author's experience, vegetative endocarditis is typically encountered in ewes 2–4 months after lambing. The occurrence of cases at this time may suggest that the uterus is one potential source of infection; however, this cannot apply to endocarditis in rams, where another septic focus must be the origin of the bacteraemia. It is uncommon to find clinical evidence of concurrent focal infection such as mastitis in ewes with endocarditis.

Aetiology

Vegetative endocarditis is caused by bacteraemia with localization in the heart valve, more commonly the tricuspid valve.

Pathophysiology

Vegetative growths on the tricuspid valve may be associated with dilation of the right ventricle and a thinner wall than usual. There may be evidence of bacteraemic spread to other viscera (e.g. the lungs). Right-sided heart failure has been described in association with vegetative lesions on the tricuspid valve.

Clinical presentation

Affected sheep typically present with depression and weight loss that manifests as poorer body condition compared with that of other sheep in the group. The rectal temperature is elevated, typically within the range 40.0–40.5°C. The sheep spends long periods in sternal recumbency and, when standing, adopts a roached-back appearance (**339**) and continually shifts weight from one limb to another because of the joint pain. The respiratory rate is usually normal. The heart rate may be irregular and s lightly elevated (up to 100 bpm) but no murmur is audible. There may be a marked jugular pulse. Typically, there is effusion of the hock, carpal and all four fetlock joints (**340**) but no thickening of the joint capsule. There may be palpable enlargement of the drainage lymph nodes of these joints.

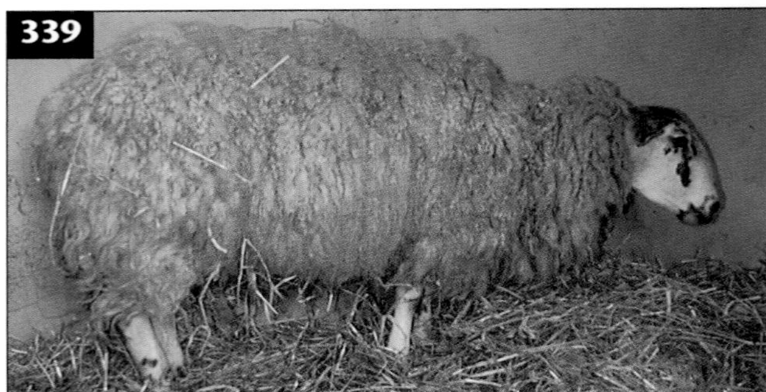

339 Depressed Greyface ewe suffering from endocarditis. The ewe has a roached back stance.

Differential diagnoses

- Bacterial polyarthritis is the most important differential diagnosis but such infections are uncommon in adult sheep.
- Bacterial infection of a single joint does occur, usually via a puncture wound, and this will cause severe lameness.
- Peritonitis may present with a roached back and some clinical features similar to endocarditis.

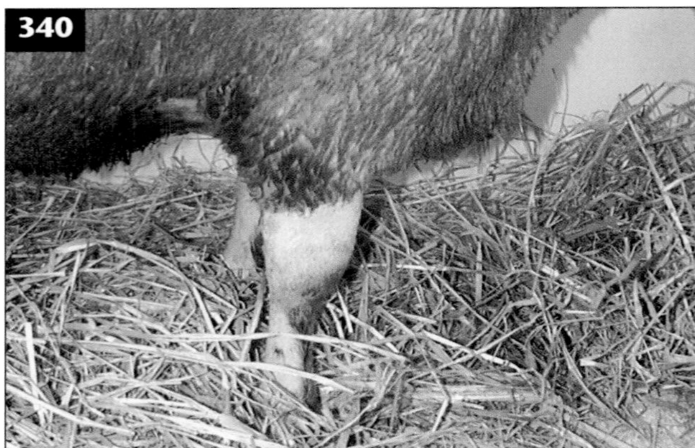

340 Swollen right carpus in a lame Scottish Halfbred ewe suffering from endocarditis.

Diagnosis

Diagnosis is based on clinical findings of chronic weight loss, pyrexia and associated joint effusions, and confirmed at necropsy (**341**).

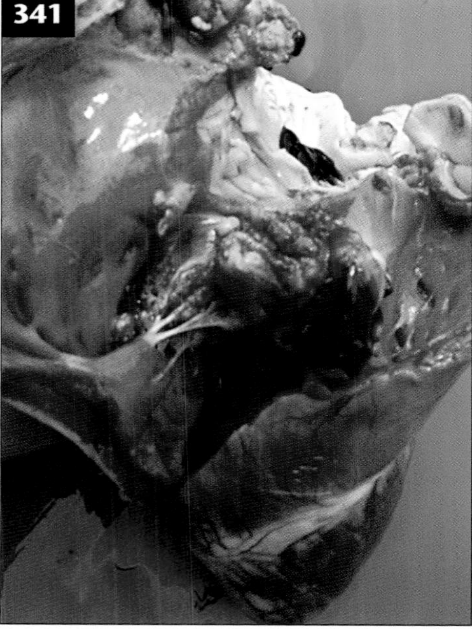

341 Large vegetative lesions on both the tricuspid and pulmonary valves.

Treatment

Treatment of ovine vegetative endocarditis with procaine penicillin (44,000 iu/kg daily for 10 days or more) has been singularly unsuccessful. As in cattle, a marked reduction in joint effusions and clinical improvement follows dexamethasone injection but the condition deteriorates after 2–3 days.

Prevention/control measures

Prevention of endocarditis is based on timely and effective treatment of focal bacterial infections but these may, in themselves, not present with outward clinical signs (e.g. metritis, mastitis, foot abscess, grain overload/bacteraemia from gut).

Economics

Vegetative endocarditis occurs sporadically in adult sheep and is not a disease of major economic concern.

Welfare implications

The joint effusions associated with vegetative endocarditis cause marked lameness and affected sheep should be euthanased for welfare reasons if the condition suspected as being vegetative endocarditis remains refractory to an extended course of penicillin therapy (at least ten consecutive days).

CLINICAL PROBLEM

A very valuable Blueface Leicester stud ram presents with depression and weight loss (BCS 2.5 compared with other rams in the group [BCS 3.5–4]). The ram spends long periods in sternal recumbency and, when standing, it adopts a roached-back appearance (**342**) and continually shifts weight from one limb to another.

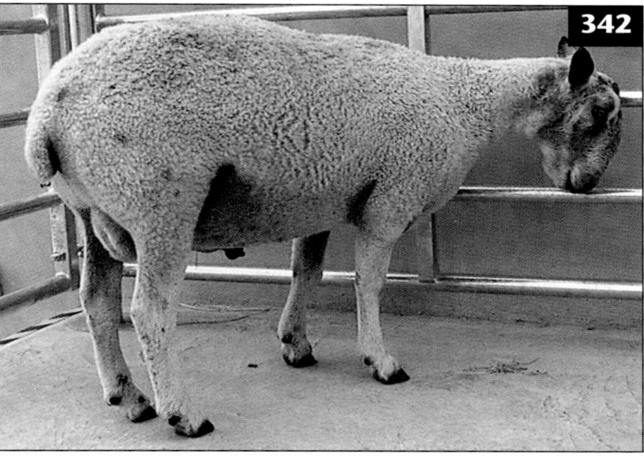

342 Depressed Blueface Leicester ram with multiple joint effusions. The distended abdomen is caused by ascites.

Clinical examination

The rectal temperature is 40.2°C. There is marked distension of the abdomen with an obvious fluid thrill on ballotment. There is slight submandibular oedema and obvious brisket oedema to a depth of 4 cm. The respiratory rate is 25 breaths per minute. The heart rate is irregular and elevated to 84 bpm but no murmur is audible. There is a marked jugular pulse. No ruminal contractions are audible. There is effusion of both hock joints and all four fetlock joints. There is no palpable enlargement of the regional lymph nodes.

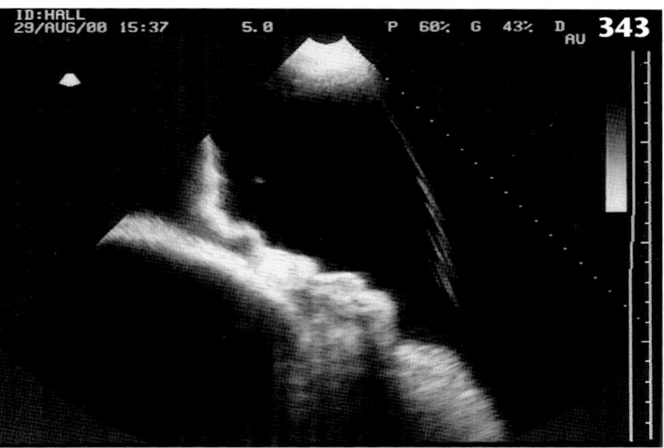

343 Ultrasonographic examination of the caudal abdomen revealing extensive transudate resulting from right-sided heart failure. The omentum and rumen wall appear as broad white lines.

What conditions should be considered and how would this case be investigated further?

Further investigations

Ultrasonographic examination of both sides of the chest with a 5.0 MHz sector transducer connected to a real-time, B-mode ultrasound machine reveals the normal hyperechoic line formed by the visceral pleura at a depth of approximately 1.5 cm from the probe head. There is slight pericardial effusion but the 5 MHz sector scanner does not permit detailed examination of the heart valves.

Ultrasonographic examination of the abdomen immediately caudal to the xiphisternum, with the probe head pointed dorsally, reveals ascites extending to a depth of 20 cm, with dorsal displacement of viscera (**343**) including the liver (**344**). The liver appears more hyperechoic than normal (**344**), consistent with cirrhosis. The gall bladder is distended and its wall appears oedematous. Numerous fibrin

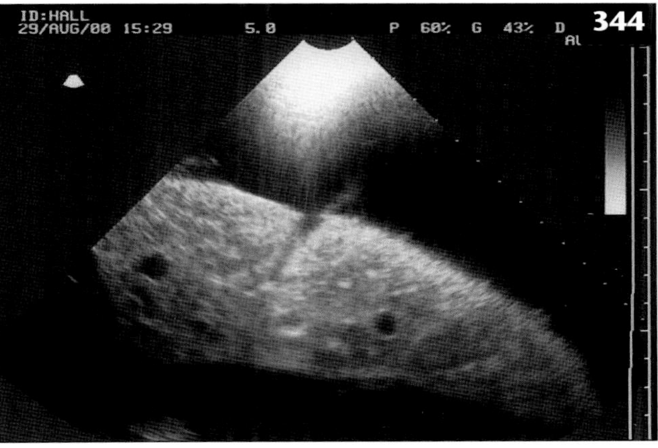

344 Ultrasonographic examination of the cranial abdomen. The liver appears more hyperechoic than normal and is clearly visible within the ascitic fluid.

tags are visible adherent to the liver capsule. The liver is also scanned via the ninth to eleventh intercostal spaces half way up the right chest. The liver appears more hyperechoic and heterogeneous than normal, with poorly defined vessels typical of chronic hepatic congestion. The bladder cannot be imaged when the abdominal cavity is searched immediately cranial to the pubis.

Routine haematological examination reveals changes consistent with moderate dehydration (total RBC count 16.8×10^{12}/l [normal = 5–9 $\times 10^{12}$/l]; haemoglobin 148 g/l [normal = 80–140 g/l]; PCV 0.45 l/l [normal = 0.26–0.36 l/l]). There is a marked leucocytosis (32.3×10^9/l [normal = 4–10 $\times 10^9$/l]), resulting from a mature neutrophilia (27.1×10^9/l, 84%), with 12% lymphocytes and 4% monocytes. There is a reduction in the serum albumin (18.7 g/l [normal 30–36 g/l]) but normal globulin concentration (37.0 g/l [normal = 35–50 g/l]). Increased liver enzymes (AST 184 U/l [normal = 45–134 U/l]) and GGT 78 U/l [normal = 0–44 U/l]) indicate ongoing mild hepatic insult. Abdominocentesis yields a colourless, odourless fluid with a protein concentration of 24.3 g/l, which suggests a transudate.

Diagnosis

On the basis of the polyarthritis, fever and ultrasonographic findings of extensive ascites, a diagnosis of right-sided congestive heart failure caused by vegetative endocarditis is reached. The absence of a distended urinary bladder ruled out a diagnosis of urolithiasis.

Outcome

The ram was euthanased for welfare reasons.

Postmortem examination

Postmortem examination confirmed the presence of 30 litres of ascitic fluid (**345**). The liver was enlarged and mottled (nutmeg liver), consistent with congestive heart failure. The right ventricle was dilated, with a thinner wall than usual, and there were vegetative growths on the tricuspid valve (**346**).

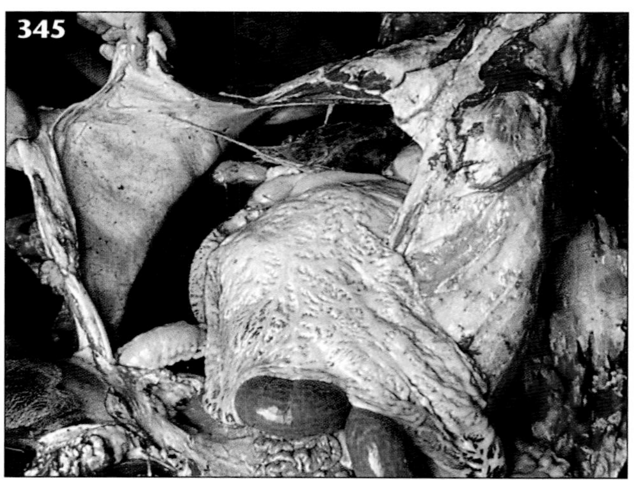

345 Necropsy revealing the extent of the ascitic fluid in **343** and **344**.

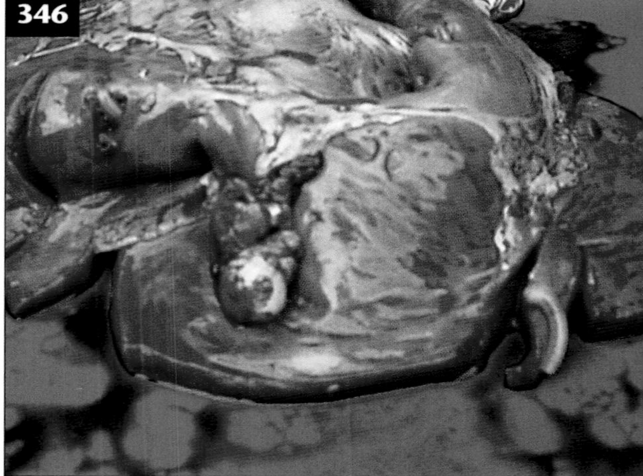

346 Large vegetative lesion on the tricuspid valve.

7 Neurological Diseases

INTRODUCTION

The central nervous system (CNS) consists of the brain (encephalo) and spinal cord (myelo). Nerve cell bodies from the grey matter (polio) and collections of nerve cell processes make up the white matter (leuco).

At certain times of the year (e.g. during late gestation) neurological disease is one of the more common ovine disease syndromes presented to the busy general practitioner, and includes conditions such as listeriosis (**347**), acute coenurosis, polioencephalomalacia (PEM), sarcocystosis, scrapie and ovine pregnancy toxaemia (**348**). Many neurological diseases, including listeriosis, PEM, OPT and border disease virus-induced cerebellar hypoplasia (see also Chapter 3: Part 1: p. 67), can occur as outbreaks.

Rapid diagnosis permits appropriate therapy early in the clinical course of disease before irreversible changes have occurred. A number of factors, which are unique to the CNS, considerably hinder treatment. These factors include lack of effective drainage, low white blood cell counts in cerebrospinal fluid (CSF) and poor penetration of the blood/brain barrier by antibiotics. Few antibiotics are capable of achieving minimum bactericidal concentrations (MBCs) within the CSF at normal recommended dose rates.

CLINICAL EXAMINATION OF THE CENTRAL NERVOUS SYSTEM

It is important to perform a complete clinical examination in order that important clinical signs are not overlooked. Rectal temperature is not a useful guide to infectious conditions of the CNS as most diseases are afebrile. Cases of neonatal bacterial meningitis, which are comatose at veterinary examination, may present with a subnormal rectal temperature. Conversely, muscle activity and opisthotonus, as observed in PEM, may raise the rectal temperature. Respiratory function may be influenced considerably by acid/base disturbances. Digestive tract dysfunction may be influenced by fluid and acid/base disturbances associated with cranial nerve V and VII deficits, which cause loss of saliva, as observed in listeriosis.

Many neurological diseases have a breed, sex, age and management system predisposition. It is essential to inspect the whole group of sheep, as subtle changes in other animals in the group may not have been noticed by the farmer.

It is essential to ascertain recent management changes, particularly changes in the animals' environment and nutrition, and the duration of clinical signs and rate of progression or deterioration in the sheep's clinical condition.

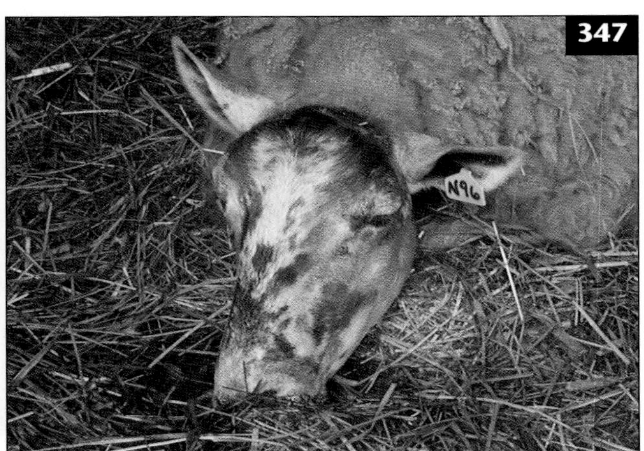

347 Disorientation, recumbency and depression in a Greyface gimmer with listeriosis.

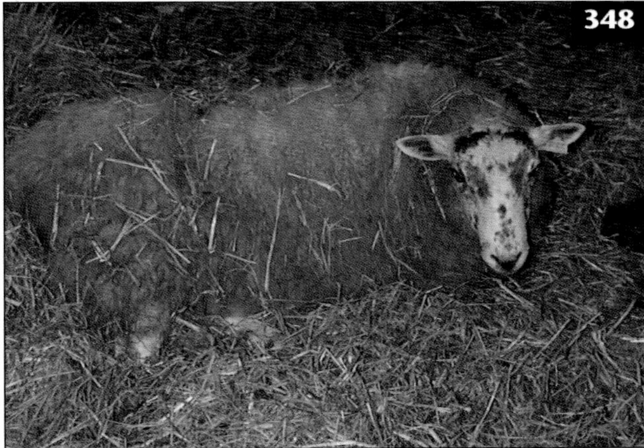

348 Disorientation and recumbency in a Greyface ewe suffering from ovine pregnancy toxaemia. This ewe is from the same group as the gimmer in **347**.

NEUROLOGICAL SYNDROMES

The brain is conveniently divided into six areas, each with a recognized neurological 'syndrome'. However, some overlap of the clinical signs of some 'syndromes' may result because of the complex pathways in the brain. Of the six neurological syndromes only four, the cerebral, cerebellar, pontomedullary (brainstem) and vestibular syndromes, concern the ovine practitioner. The midbrain and hypothalamic syndromes are uncommon in sheep.

CEREBRAL SYNDROME

Cerebral dysfunction is the most common neurological syndrome encountered in sheep. The cerebrum is concerned with mental state, behaviour and, in conjunction with the eye and optic nerve (II), vision. Clinical signs that suggest cerebral dysfunction include:

- Blindness, but with normal pupillary light reflex.
- Compulsive walking, circling, constant chewing movements.
- Severe depression, dementia, yawning, head pressing.
- Hyperaesthesia to auditory and tactile stimuli, opisthotonus.
- Contralateral proprioceptive defects.

The common ovine neurological conditions that present with diffuse cerebral signs include PEM, bacterial meningitis and OPT. Clinical signs attributable to a cerebral lesion localized to a cerebral hemisphere are seen in space-occupying lesions, such as a brain abscess or coenurosis, and include compulsive circling, deviation of the head (not a head tilt) and contralateral blindness and proprioceptive deficits.

Approximately 90% of efferent nerve fibres cross at the optic chiasma; therefore, animals with a left-sided space-occupying lesion are blind in the right eye. The pupillary light reflex is normal. The menace response is not always reliable in cases of unilateral space-occupying lesions and this test can be supplemented with unilateral blindfolding.

CEREBELLAR SYNDROME

The cerebellum is primarily concerned with fine coordination of voluntary movement. In cerebellar disease all limb movements are spastic (rigid), clumsy and jerky. Initiation of movement is delayed and may be accompanied by tremors.

Cerebellar disease is characterized by a widebased stance and ataxia (incoordination), particularly of the hindlimbs, but with preservation of normal muscle strength. In addition to ataxia, dysmetria (problems associated with stride) may be observed. Hypermetria, a Hackney-type gait, is the more common form of dysmetria observed in cerebellar disease. With hypometria the animal will frequently drag the dorsal aspect of the hoof along the ground.

Cerebellar disease may result in jerky movements of the head, especially when the animal is aroused or at feeding times when affected animals will often overshoot the feed bowl. This condition is often referred to as 'intention tremors'.

VESTIBULAR SYNDROME

The major clinical sign associated with a vestibular lesion is that of a 5–10° ipsilateral (same side) head tilt, which is best determined when the animal is viewed from a distance of 5–10 metres. The poll is tilted down to the affected side and this may be exaggerated by blindfolding the animal. Circling may also be observed. Normal positional nystagmus can be induced by rapid movements of the head in vertical or horizontal planes. The fast phase of the nystagmus is in the direction of the head movement. Positional nystagmus may be depressed or absent in animals with a vestibular lesion when the head is moved towards the side of the lesion (head tilt). Resting nystagmus is present and permits differentiation between the two forms of vestibular disease:

- Peripheral vestibular disease – fast phase away from side of lesion.
- Central vestibular disease – fast phase in any direction, including dorsal or ventral.

In addition, Horner's syndrome and facial nerve paralysis are common in peripheral vestibular disease, since both facial and sympathetic nerves fibres pass close to the middle ear.

PONTOMEDULLARY SYNDROME

As most of the cranial nerve nuclei are present in the brainstem, dysfunction, referred to as the pontomedullary syndrome, is characterized by multiple cranial nerve deficits. In brainstem disease, depression is attributed to a specific lesion in the ascending reticular activating system. Ipsilateral hemiparesis is common (**349**), with sheep leaning against objects to support themselves (**350**). Circling results from involvement of the vestibulocochlear nucleus. Involvement of the facial nucleus results in ipsilateral facial nerve paralysis. Facial palsy is evident as a drooped ear (**349**), drooped upper eyelid (ptosis) and a flaccid lip. Involvement of the trigeminal nerve or the trigeminal motor nucleus results in paralysis of the cheek muscles and decreased facial sensation. Abnormal respiratory patterns may result from damage to the respiratory centres in the medulla.

Cranial nerves

Cranial nerves leave the forebrain and brainstem and have a variety of specialized functions. Assessment of normal function tests the cranial nerves and their associated centres (**Table 4**).

Table 4 Relationship between assessment of normal function and the relevant cranial nerves and their associated centres.

Test	**Cranial nerve(s) and associated centres**
Vision	Eye, II, cerebrum (contralateral)
Pupillary light response (pen torch)	II, III
Pupil size and symmetry (pen torch)	II, III, brainstem, sympathetic nervous system
Menace response (rapidly approaching object)	II, VII, cerebrum, brainstem, cerebellum
Eyeball position	II – lateral strabismus IV – dorsal and medial strasbismus VI – medial strabismus
Normal head/cheek muscle tone	V
Touch cornea, eyeball retracts	V, VI
Touch medial canthus, eye closes	V, VII
Ears held in normal position	V, VII
Nostrils – normal sensation	V
Eyelids in normal position	III, VII, sympathetic nervous system
Hearing	VIII
Normal head position	VIII, cerebrum
Deglutition, tongue movement	IX, X, XII

Olfactory nerve (I)

Assessment of the olfactory nerve has little clinical application in ruminant species.

Optic nerve (II)

The visual pathway is usually tested by observing individual sheep encountering obstacles and by evaluating the menace response – the eyelids close quickly in response to a rapidly approaching object. The menace response can be difficult to evaluate in depressed animals and should be interpreted with caution.

Up to 90% of optic nerve fibres decussate at the optic chiasma; therefore, vision in the right eye is perceived in the contralateral cerebral hemisphere. Incoming (afferent) fibres recognize the menace response in the left eye, travel along the left optic nerve to the optic chiasma and then cross to the right optic tract and right occipital cortex. The motor (efferent) pathway is from the right visual

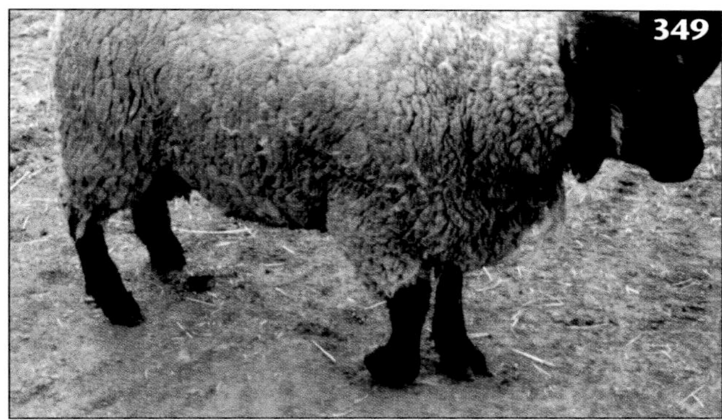

349 Ipsilateral hemiparesis in a Suffolk ram with listeriosis. There is right-sided hemiparesis and ear drop.

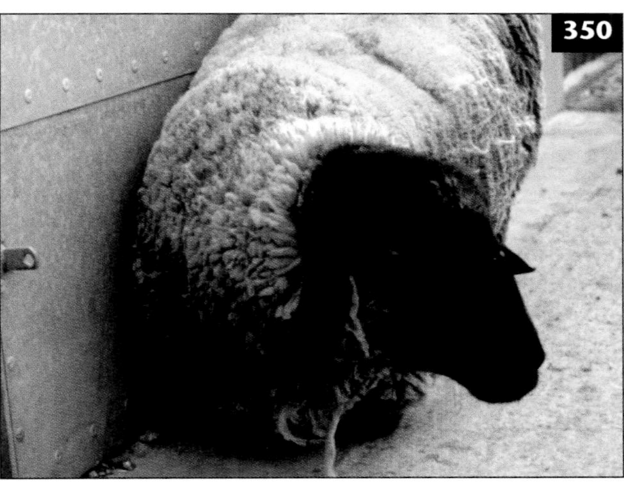

350 Right-sided hemiparesis in the Suffolk ram in **349**.

cortex to the left facial nucleus, resulting in closure of the left eye.

Lesions of the eye and optic nerve result in ipsilateral blindness. Lesions of the optic tract or nucleus cause contralateral blindness. Therefore, an abscess in the right cerebral hemisphere affecting the nucleus will result in blindness of the left eye.

Oculomotor nerve (III)

Pupillary diameter is controlled by constrictor muscles innervated by the parasympathetic fibres in the oculomotor nerve, and by dilator muscles innervated by the sympathetic fibres from the cranial cervical ganglion.

The normal response to light directed into one eye is constriction of both pupillary apertures, with a direct response in the stimulated eye and a consensual response in the contralateral eye.

A dilated pupil in an eye with normal vision (menace response) would suggest a lesion in the oculomotor nerve. The contralateral eye with normal oculomotor nerve function will respond to both direct and consensual stimulation. If a lesion involves primarily one cerebral hemisphere, increased pressure to one oculomotor nerve presents as different pupillary aperture diameters (anisocoria), with the affected side displaying pupillary dilation.

Horner's syndrome

Horner's syndrome refers to the clinical appearance of slight ptosis (drooping) of the upper eyelid, constriction of the pupil (miosis) and slight protrusion of the nictitating membrane caused by damage to the sympathetic nerve supply to the eyeball. The menace response (vision) and pupillary light response are normal.

Oculomotor nerve (III), trochlear nerve (IV) and abducens (VI) nerve

These cranial nerves are responsible for normal position and movement of the eyeball within the bony socket. Abnormal position of the eyeball is rarely seen as an acquired syndrome in sheep. An abnormal eyeball position is referred to as strabismus:

- Paralysis of the oculomotor nerve – lateral strabismus.
- Paralysis of the trochlear nerve – dorsomedial strabismus.
- Paralysis of the abducens nerve – medial strabismus.

Many cerebral lesions can result in strabismus. If there is a unilateral cerebral lesion, the strabismus is directed to the ipsilateral side. Dorsomedial strabismus is classically seen in PEM, lead poisoning, salt poisoning and acute bacterial meningitis of neonates. In such diseases, dorsomedial strabismus is not a specific lesion of trochlear nerve damage but a reflection of cerebral oedema involving upper motor neuron pathways.

Trigeminal nerve (V)

The trigeminal nerve has three branches: mandibular, maxillary and ophthalmic. They supply motor fibres to the muscles of mastication and sensory fibres to the face.

Loss of motor function of the mandibular branch of the trigeminal nerve results in rapid atrophy of the temporal and masseter muscles, which are responsible for mastication. Unilateral lesions result in deviation of the lower jaw and muzzle away from the affected side. Responses to stimulation of the skin around the face are mediated through sensory fibres in the trigeminal nerve and motor fibres in the facial nerve. These reflexes require intact cranial nerves V and VII, trigeminal and facial nuclei, and brainstem.

Abducens nerve (VI)

Lesions of the abducens nerve result in constant medial strabismus and loss of the ability to retract the eyeball into the bony socket (corneal reflex).

Facial nerve (VII)

The facial nerve is concerned primarily with motor supply to the facial muscles. The facial nerve contains the lower motor neurons for movement of the ears, eyelids, nares and muzzle and the motor pathways of the menace response and the palpebral reflex.

When the periocular skin is touched, the normal reflex is that the animal will close the palpebral fissure. Lack of the palpebral reflex may indicate a lesion in:

- The facial nerve or facial nucleus (motor pathway).
- The trigeminal nerve or trigeminal nucleus (sensory pathway).
- Or both nerves or nuclei involved.

If the facial nerve only is involved, skin sensation of the face is normal due to normal trigeminal nerve function.

Facial nerve paralysis is characteristically seen as drooping of the upper eyelid and ear. With a unilateral lesion there is deviation of the muzzle towards the unaffected side due to loss of facial muscle tone in the affected side.

Differentiation between central or peripheral facial nerve involvement can be attempted by identifying involvement of other central structures such as the trigeminal and vestibulocochlear nuclei.

Vestibulocochlear nerve (VIII)
Deafness in ruminants may be difficult to determine. The vestibular system controls orientation of the head, body and eyes. Nystagmus refers to movement of the eyeball within the bony socket. Normal vestibular nystagmus refers to horizontal movement of the eyeball as the head is turned laterally, with the fast movement phase towards the side to which the head is turned. Pathological changes that result in nystagmus originate in the vestibular system.

Spontaneous nystagmus refers to nystagmus when the head is held in the normal position. Positional nystagmus results when the head is held in various abnormal positions.

Glossopharyngeal nerve (IX) and vagal nerve (X)
Damage to these nerve nuclei results in dysphagia and associated salivation. Affected animals cannot swallow or drink.

Accessory nerve (XI)
In ruminants the accessory nerve appears to have little specific function.

Hypoglossal nerve (XII)
The hypoglossal nerve provides motor supply to the muscles of the tongue. With a unilateral lesion there is atrophy of musculature but the sheep is still able to retract the tongue within the buccal cavity. In the case of a bilateral lesion the sheep is unable to prehend and masticate food and the tongue remains protruded.

Midbrain syndrome

The midbrain syndrome is relatively uncommon in ruminants and is characterized by depression/coma, possible limb rigidity and opisthotonus. Most affected animals have normal vision, ventrolateral strabismus and a mydriatic pupil that is unresponsive to light. The most common causes of midbrain syndrome in sheep are cranial trauma or a hepatic encephalopathy.

Hypothalamic syndrome

Hypothalamic syndrome is a relatively uncommon syndrome. Animals may manifest altered behaviour or mental state such as hyperaesthesia, aggression and disorientation. Vision is impaired and the pupils are dilated and poorly responsive to light stimulation. There may be alterations in appetite and thermoregulation. The most common causes of hypothalamic syndrome include abscesses and tumours of the pituitary gland.

MENINGITIS

The CNS is covered by three layers of membrane. Inflammation of the meninges is divided into pachymeningitis (inflammation of the dura mater) and leptomeningitis (inflammation of the leptomeninges – the pia mater and arachnoid). Most cases of meningitis involve the leptomeninges, when extension into the underlying cerebral cortex is common. Such infections are more correctly referred to as meningoencephalitis.

COLLECTION AND ANALYSIS OF CEREBROSPINAL FLUID

CSF collection and analysis provides rapid and, in some situations, instant information to the veterinarian investigating a disease problem in the living animal. CSF analysis is particularly useful for confirming the presence of an inflammatory lesion involving the leptomeninges (e.g. bacterial meningoencephalitis [**351**]).

To collect CSF it is necessary to puncture the subarachnoid space in the cerebellomedullary cistern (cisternal sample) or at the lumbosacral region (lumbosacral sample). In the absence of a focal spinal cord compressive lesion there is usually no substantial difference between the composition of cisternal and lumbosacral CSF samples.

Collection of lumbosacral CSF is facilitated when the animal is positioned in sternal recumbency with the hips flexed and the hindimbs extended alongside the

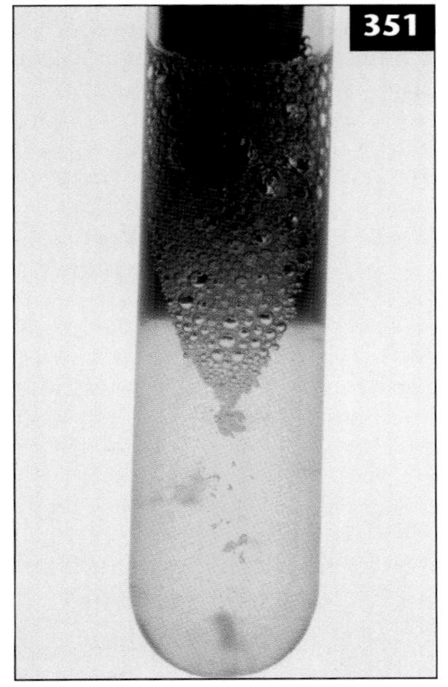

351 Turbid lumbar CSF sample from a lamb with bacterial meningitis.

abdomen. Aversion of the sheep's head against one flank may assist in maintaining sternal recumbency during CSF collection.

The site for lumbosacral CSF collection is the midpoint of the lumbosacral space, which can be identified as the midline depression between the last palpable dorsal lumbar spine (L6) and the first palpable sacral dorsal spine (S2). The site must be clipped, surgically prepared and 1–2 ml of local anaesthetic injected subcutaneously. The needle is slowly advanced either at a right angle to the plane of the vertebral column or with the hub directed 5° caudally. It is essential to appreciate the changes in tissue resistance as the needle point passes sequentially through the subcutaneous tissue and interarcuate ligament, and then the sudden 'pop' due to the loss of resistance as the needle point finally exits the ligamentum flavum into the extradural space. Once the point of the needle has penetrated the dorsal subarachnoid space, CSF will well up in the needle hub within 2–3 seconds. Failure to appreciate the change in resistance to the needle travel may result in puncture of the conus medullaris.

One to two millilitres of CSF are sufficient for laboratory analysis and, while the sample can be collected by free flow, it is more convenient to employ gentle syringe aspiration over 10–30 seconds. Care must be taken not to dislodge the point of the needle from the dorsal subarachnoid space when the syringe is attached to the needle hub. Stabilizing the position of the needle can be assisted by resting the wrist firmly on the sheep's back. The seal on the syringe should be broken before it is connected to the needle hub, which must be anchored firmly between the thumb and index finger. Selection of the correct needle length (**Table 5**) ensures that the needle hub is close to the skin, thereby assisting stabilization.

Analysis of CSF

Specific gravity

Specific gravity results are not sufficiently precise to be useful in the investigation of ovine neurological disease.

Protein concentration

Many CSF samples have first to be concentrated due to low protein content. The normal range for CSF protein concentration is <0.4 g/l.

White cell concentration

White cell concentration in CSF can be determined using a haemocytometer. Cytological examination of CSF should be performed within two hours of collection and is greatly facilitated if the sample is first concentrated by cytospin. The sample is then air dried and stained with Leishman stain. The differential white cell count should be based on a minimum of 20 cells. Alternatively, a sedimentation chamber can be used to examine CSF cellular morphology. Normal CSF contains less than 0.012×10^9/l cells, which are predominantly lymphocytes with occasional neutrophils.

Table 5 Guide to needle length and gauge for lumbar CSF sampling.

Lambs <30 kg	2.5 cm, 21 gauge
Ewes 40–80 kg	4.0 cm, 19 gauge
Rams >80 kg	5.0 cm, 19 gauge

Presence of bacteria in cerebrospinal fluid

Samples of CSF can be examined microscopically for the presence of bacteria following preparation with Gram's stain. This technique is most useful for the confirmation of neonatal meningoencephalitis.

Other cerebrospinal fluid constituents

Concentrations of glucose, creatine kinase, lactate dehydrogenase and other CSF constituents are not routinely determined, as they provide little additional information in the diagnosis of the common sheep CNS diseases.

RBCs may be present in the CSF following pathological haemorrhage into the subarachnoid space, but this is very uncommon and is most confidently diagnosed by the presence of phagocytosed RBCs within CSF macrophages. Much more commonly, RBCs in the CSF sample result from haemorrhage caused by the sampling technique; they appear as streaking of blood in clear fluid. If the CSF sample is left to stand for approximately two hours, the RBCs gravitate and form a small plug at the bottom of the collection tube (**352**). Release of pigment following lysis of RBCs, referred to as xanthochromia (**353**), appears within a few hours after subarachnoid haemorrhage and may persist for 2–4 weeks.

SWAYBACK

Definition/overview

Swayback is a congenital condition affecting newborn lambs; the delayed form of swayback (enzootic ataxia) most commonly affects lambs aged 2–4 months.

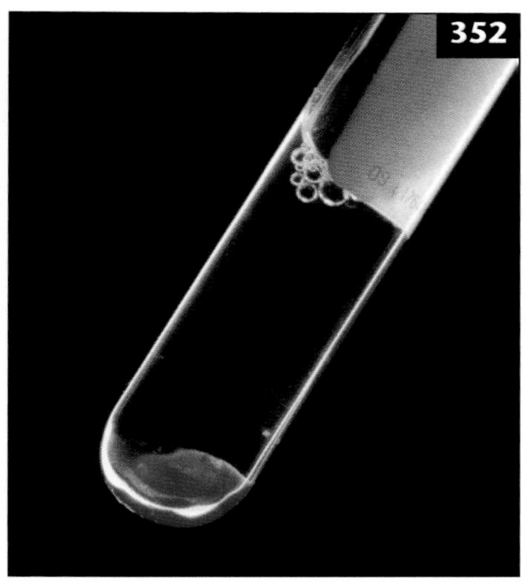

352 Turbidity caused by recent haemorrhage into the CSF will clear after the sample has been centrifuged to leave a clear supernatant.

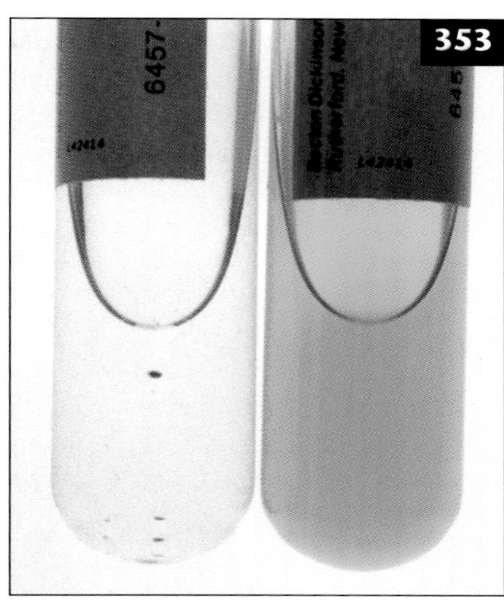

353 Orange discoloration of the CSF (xanthochromia) appears within a few hours after subarachnoid haemorrhage.

Aetiology

Swayback is associated with low copper status of the dam and/or growing lamb. The condition occurs within well-defined geographic areas, usually upland and hill pastures, where it is often related to pasture improvement, including liming, fertilizer application and reseeding.

Clinical presentation

Congenital form

Severely affected lambs are small and weak and may be unable to raise themselves or maintain sternal recumbency. Some affected lambs show a fine head tremor, which is increased during periods of activity such as feeding. Less severely affected lambs have poor coordination and experience difficulty finding the teat, leading to starvation.

Delayed form

In the delayed form of swayback (enzootic ataxia) the lambs are normal at birth but show progressive weakness of the hindimbs from 2–4 months of age. Weakness is first noted during gathering or movement when affected lambs lag behind the remainder of the flock. The hindlimbs are weak, with reduced muscle tone and reflexes, and show muscle atrophy.

Differential diagnoses

Congenital form

Differential diagnoses of the congenital form of swayback include:

- Septicaemia.
- Hypoglycaemia/hypothermia.
- Border disease.

Delayed form

- Vertebral body empyema involving the thoracolumbar spinal cord (T2–L3) is common in 2–4-month-old lambs, causing hindlimb paresis with progression over 4–7 days to paralysis.
- Hindlimb paresis has also been reported in sheep with thoracolumbar spinal cord lesions associated with *Sarcocystis* species infestation and coenurosis.

Diagnosis

Clinical diagnosis of swayback is based on clinical findings, confirmed by histopathological examination of the brain and spinal cord, and supported by liver copper determination, where concentrations <80 mg/kg indicate low copper status. Care must be taken to ensure that cases of enzootic ataxia have not received copper supplementation prior to liver copper determinations.

Treatment

Treatment of lambs with congenital swayback is hopeless and affected lambs must be humanely destroyed for welfare reasons. There is limited evidence that copper supplementation of lambs with enzootic ataxia slows the progress of the condition.

Prevention/control measures

Prevention of swayback by copper supplementation must be carefully considered because of the risk of toxicity. Factors that should be considered before supplementation include the prevalence of confirmed or suspected swayback cases in the flock, the breed of sheep, supplementary feeding during gestation, and the geographical area, including soil analysis. Determination of serum copper and copper-dependent enzyme concentrations (e.g. superoxide dismutase in pregnant ewes) provides some indication of copper status but liver copper concentration is the most useful measurement. Subcutaneous or intramuscular injection of chelated copper presents the most convenient method for supplementation of extensively managed ewes during mid-gestation but is not without risk of toxicity.

Economics

The cost of administration of copper either by injection or by oral administration of copper oxide needles to ewes during mid-gestation is 0.5% of the value of the ewe.

Welfare implications

Newborn lambs with swayback fail to thrive. They should be euthanased for welfare reasons and a healthy lamb fostered onto the ewe. Lambs with delayed swayback should be confined to lowland pastures and not returned to hill pastures. Supplementary feeding will aid finishing, and these lambs should be slaughtered at the nearest slaughter plant to limit transport distances.

BACTERIAL MENINGOENCEPHALITIS

Definition/overview

Bacterial meningoencephalitis occurs sporadically in young lambs, rarely exceeding 0.5% of lambs at risk.

Aetiology

Bacterial meningoencephalitis most commonly affects young lambs aged 2–4 weeks, after localization of bacteraemia arising from the upper respiratory tract or intestine. Failure of passive antibody transfer predisposes neonates to bacteraemia, with subsequent localization of pathogenic bacteria. *Escherichia coli*, *Pasteurella* species, *Staphylococcus pyogenes* and *Arcanobacterium pyogenes* have all been isolated from clinical cases of meningoencephalitis.

Clinical presentation

Initial clinical signs include depression (**354**), lethargy, a gaunt appearance and separation from the dam. Affected lambs are rarely pyrexic. The head is often held lowered in rigid extension, and gentle forced movement of the neck causes pain and evokes abnormal (pitiful) vocalization. Affected lambs are hyperaesthetic to tactile and auditory stimuli and seizure activity may be precipitated during intravenous antibiotic injection. Episcleral injection, congested mucous membranes and dorsomedial strabismus are consistent findings. The menace response may be reduced or absent but can be difficult to interpret in depressed or stuporous lambs. Advanced stages of the disease process are characterized by lateral recumbency with seizure activity (**355**), opisthotonus and odontoprisis.

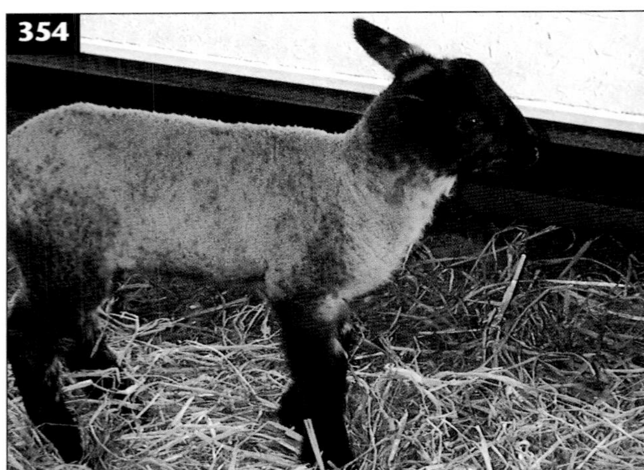

354 Disorientated, depressed three-week-old lamb with impaired vision during the early stages of bacterial meningoencephalitis.

Differential diagnoses

Differential diagnoses of bacterial meningoencephalitis in young lambs include:

- Cerebellar hypoplasia (caused by border disease virus).
- Infection of the atlanto-occipital joint causing recumbency.
- Hepatic necrobacillosis.
- Starvation.
- Septicaemia.
- Nephrosis.

Diagnosis

Diagnosis is based on a thorough clinical examination. Gross inspection of lumbar CSF reveals a turbid sample caused by the huge influx of white cells, and a frothy appearance visible after gentle sample agitation due to the increased protein concentration (**351**, p. 169). If necessary, laboratory analysis reveals an average 100-fold increase in white cell concentration, comprised mainly of neutrophils (neutrophilic pleocytosis), and a five-fold or greater increase in protein concentration. Culture of lumbar CSF is largely unrewarding.

Treatment

Few lambs respond to treatment (**356**) and lambs showing seizure activity should be humanely destroyed once the diagnosis has been confirmed by CSF examination. Antibiotics that could be used include trimethoprim/sulphonamide combination, ceftiofur and florfenicol (**NB**: off-label use). It is recommended that antibiotic therapy be continued for 4–6 weeks; however, the treatment response is very poor, so such theoretical consideration rarely arises. The role of high doses of soluble corticosteroid (e.g. 1.1 mg/kg dexamethasone) remains controversial in the treatment of bacterial meningoencephalitis.

Prevention/control measures
Control should be directed at general preventive measures for all bacterial infections in the perinatal period, and should include high standards of hygiene in the lambing environment and timely passive antibody transfer.

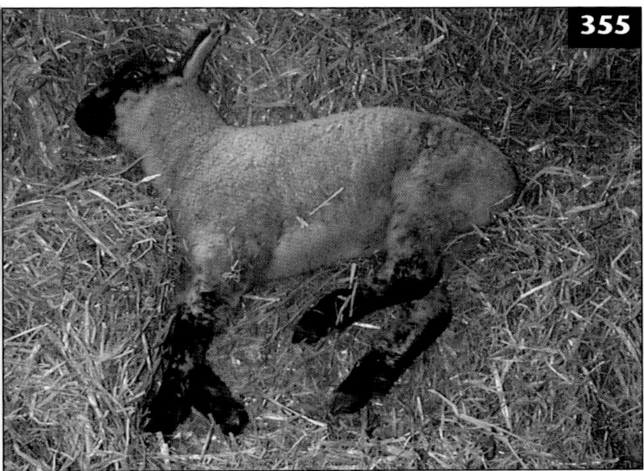

355 Six-week-old lamb with bacterial meningoencephalitis showing seizure activity.

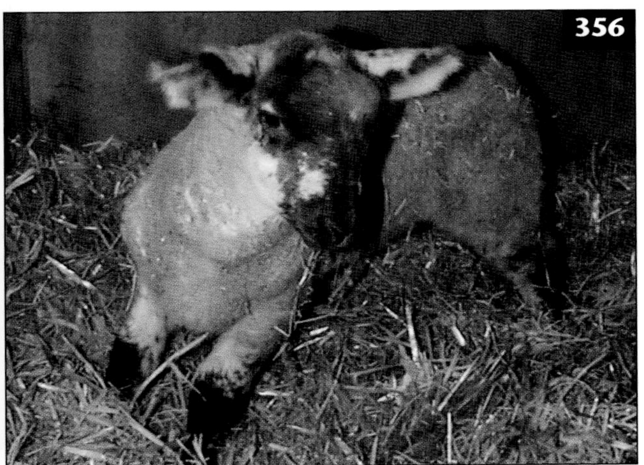

356 Lamb in **355** two days after intravenous antibiotic therapy.

Economics
Bacterial meningoencephalitis occurs sporadically in young lambs and rarely exceeds 0.5% of lambs at risk, compared with perinatal lamb losses totalling 15–25% in many flocks.

Welfare implications
Affected lambs should be humanely destroyed once the diagnosis has been established.

BRAIN ABSCESSATION

Definition/overview
Brain abscesses are very occasionally diagnosed in lambs aged 2–4 months.

Aetiology
Brain abscesses arise following bacteraemic spread but it is unusual to find evidence of another septic focus.

Clinical presentation
The clinical signs of brain abscessation are slowly progressive and result from the space-occupying nature of the lesion rather than any associated inflammatory response. Depression is commonly observed, with the head turned towards the lamb's chest (357). There may be compulsive circling but affected sheep often stand motionless or appear trapped with the head pushed into a corner. The lesion commonly affects one cerebral hemisphere; as a consequence, the animal often presents with

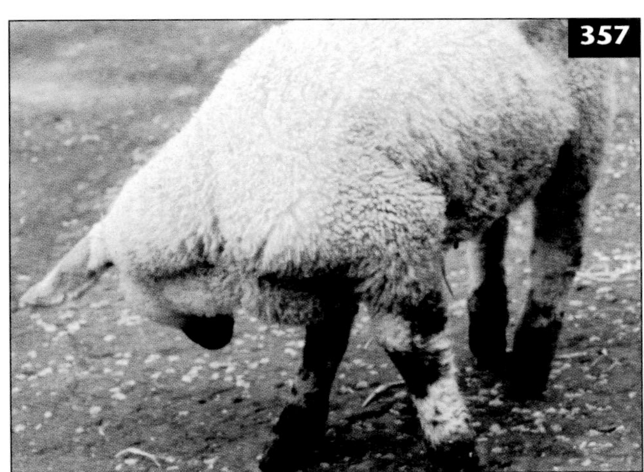

357 Depressed three-month-old lamb suffering from a cerebral abscess.

contralateral blindness and proprioceptive deficits but normal pupillary light reflexes. Proprioceptive deficits, with hyperflexion of the fetlock joint (knuckling) of the contralateral limb, are commonly observed.

Basillar empyema (pituitary abscessation) occurs rarely in adult sheep. The clinical findings include depression (358), anorexia and ataxia followed by head pressing, dysphagia (bilateral trigeminal nerve paralysis), eye drop (359) and blindness.

Differential diagnoses

The common differential diagnoses causing depression/stupor of some days' duration in growing lambs include:

- Nephrosis.
- Possibly sulphur toxicity.
- Coenurosis, although coenurosis is uncommon in lambs less than six months old.
- Polioencephalomalacia has a more acute clinical course than brain abscessation.
- Circling behaviour is encountered in listeriosis but there is also evidence of multiple cranial nerve deficits (especially V and VII), which may be bilateral in young lambs.

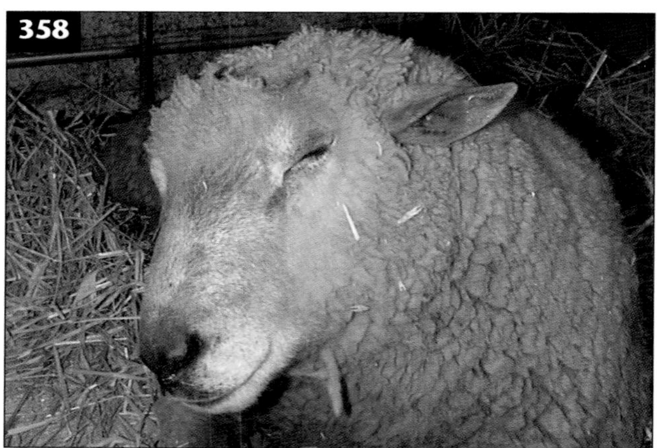

358 Depression in a Charollais ram with basillar empyema.

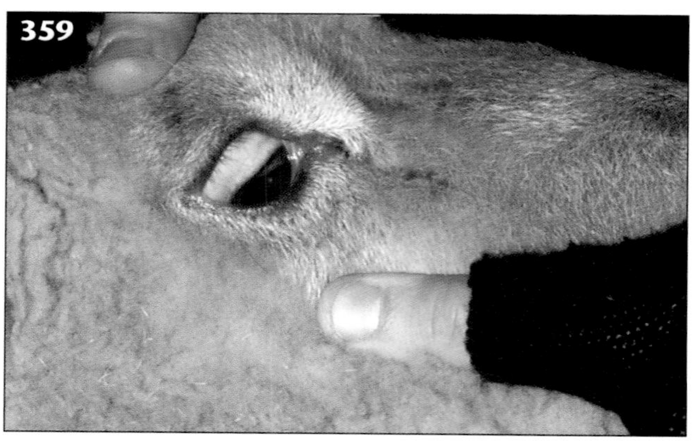

359 Eye drop in a Charollais ram with basillar empyema.

Diagnosis

Diagnosis is based on a careful neurological examination. Lumbar CSF analysis may reveal a small increase in protein concentration and increased white cell concentration.

Treatment

Treatment of brain abscessation is hopeless and affected lambs should be euthanased for welfare reasons.

Prevention/control measures

Good husbandry practices in the neonatal period will ensure adequate passive antibody transfer and reduce environmental bacterial challenge.

Economics

Brain abscesses are uncommon and therefore not a major financial concern to sheep producers.

Welfare implications

Affected lambs should be euthanased for welfare reasons.

POLIOENCEPHALOMALACIA

(*Syn*: cerebrocortical necrosis)

Definition/overview

PEM is a common neurological disease of weaned lambs aged 4–8 months but it is also seen sporadically in adult sheep. The disease is characterized by blindness, initial depression and dorsiflexion of the neck, progressing rapidly to hyperexcitability, seizure activity and opisthotonus.

Aetiology

Changes in the diet alter the rumen microflora, with proliferation of thiaminase-producing bacteria and reduction in numbers of thiamine-producing bacteria. Thiamine is an essential co-factor involved in glucose metabolism, including transketolase and pyruvate decarboxylase enzymes.

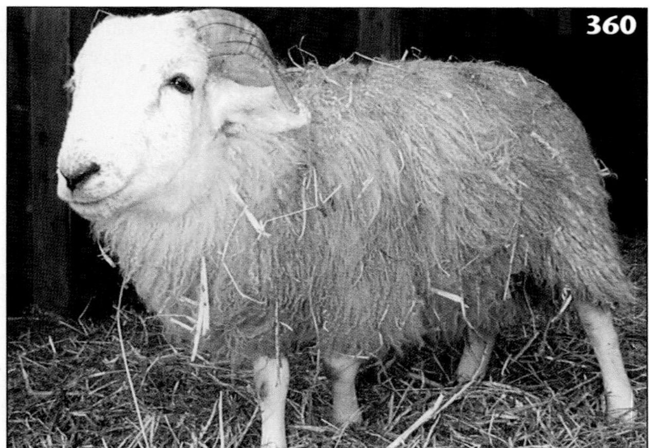

360 Blind, disorientated weaned lamb with dorsomedial strabismus.

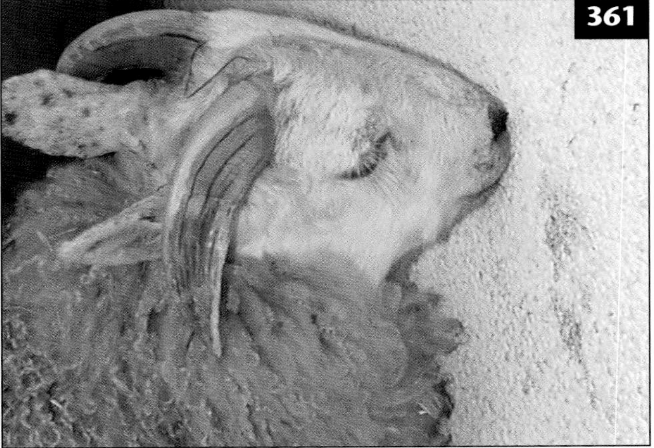

361 Head pressing behaviour in the lamb in **360**.

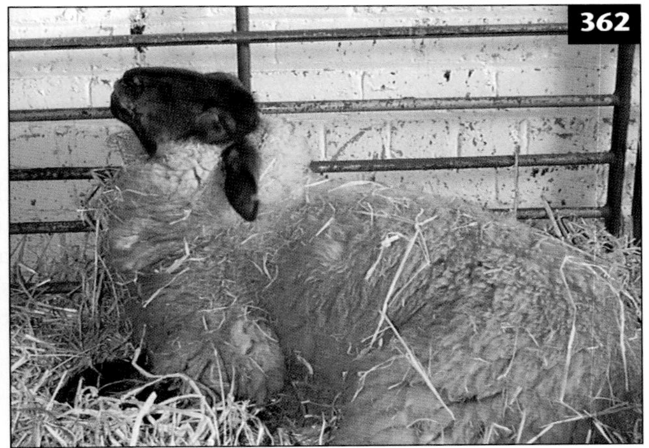

362 'Star-gazing' behaviour in a housed Suffolk lamb.

Clinical presentation

Individual lambs are usually affected approximately two weeks after movement to another pasture or other dietary change; either event may be associated with routine anthelmintic treatment. During the early stages of PEM, affected sheep are blind (**360**) and become isolated from the group, may wander aimlessly and show head-pressing behaviour (**361**). There is marked dorsiflexion of the neck ('star-gazing') when stationary (**362**). The condition deteriorates within 12–24 hours to lateral recumbency with opisthotonus. Affected sheep are hyperaesthetic to auditory and tactile stimuli, which may precipitate seizure activity during handling. Dorsomedial strabismus and spontaneous horizontal nystagmus are frequently observed. Trauma to the peripheral facial nerve on the dependent side may result in ptosis and drooped ear. Death follows within 3–5 days in untreated sheep.

Differential diagnoses

- A common differential diagnosis is focal symmetrical encephalomalacia in unvaccinated weaned lambs.
- Very occasionally, the occurrence of numerous lambs in lateral recumbency, as a result of drenching gun injury, which progresses to involve the cervical spinal cord, may briefly be confused with PEM.
- Ovine pregnancy toxaemia, acute coenurosis and listeriosis represent the more common differential diagnoses in adult sheep.

Diagnosis

Diagnosis is based on clinical findings and response to parenteral administration of thiamine. Diagnostic biochemical parameters for PEM, including thiaminase activities in blood, rumen fluid or faeces, are rarely used in farm animal practice.

Affected areas of the cortex may exhibit a bright white autofluoresence when cut sections of the cerebrum are viewed under ultraviolet light (Wood's lamp; 365 nm). This property has been attributed to the accumulation of lipofuchsin in macrophages, but not all PEM cases fluoresce. Definitive diagnosis relies on the histological findings in the cortical lesions of vacuolation and cavitation of the ground substance, with astrocytic swelling, neuronal shrinkage and necrosis.

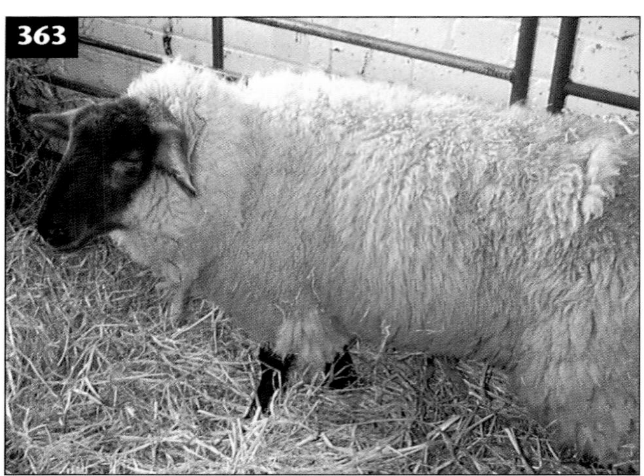

363 Lamb in **362** three days after the start of intravenous thiamine therapy.

Treatment

The treatment response during the early clinical stages of PEM to high doses of thiamine (10 mg/kg q12h, i/v for the first occasion) is generally good. Successfully treated sheep are able to stand and commence eating within 24 hours (**363**), although normal vision may not return for 5–7 days. Treatment should be continued for three consecutive days. Intravenous injection of high doses of a soluble corticosteroid such as dexamethasone (1 mg/kg) at the first treatment to reduce cerebral oedema remains controversial. Affected sheep should be housed in a quiet, dark, well-bedded pen and propped in sternal recumbency between straw bales or similar. If unable to maintain sternal recumbency, the sheep must be turned regularly to prevent scalding.

Prevention/control measures

There are no specific preventive measures.

Economics

PEM occurs sporadically, with a good treatment response during the early stages (**363**). Thiamine is inexpensive (5% of the value of the ewe for a course of treatment).

Welfare implications

Sheep that are unable to stand unaided after two days' treatment are unlikely to fully recover and should be euthanased for welfare reasons.

SULPHUR TOXICITY

Definition/overview

A small number of outbreaks of a disease with a clinical presentation not dissimilar to PEM and affecting groups of weaned lambs fed high levels of concentrates have been recorded in the literature.

Aetiology

An outbreak of sulphur toxicity has been reported affecting 21 of 71 weaned lambs aged 4–6 months 15–32 days after they were introduced to an *ad libitum* concentrate ration containing 0.43% sulphur. No further cases were identified after all the remaining lambs were given a single intramuscular injection of vitamin B_1. Similarly, an outbreak of sulphur toxicity was reported in a group of fattening lambs fed a ration containing ammonium sulphate as a urinary acidifier.

Clinical presentation

The clinical signs are acute in onset and include depression (**364**), bilateral lack of menace response (**365**) and head pressing behaviour (**366**). However, hyperaesthesia, nystagmus, dorsiflexion of the neck and opisthotonus, typical of spontaneous cases of PEM, are not observed.

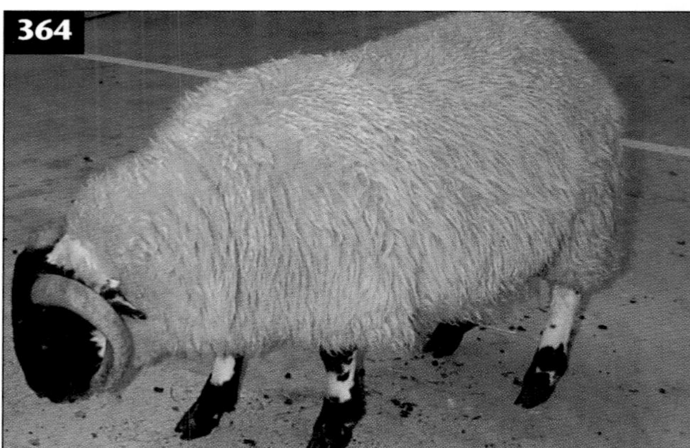

364 Stupor in a ram lamb with sulphur toxicity.

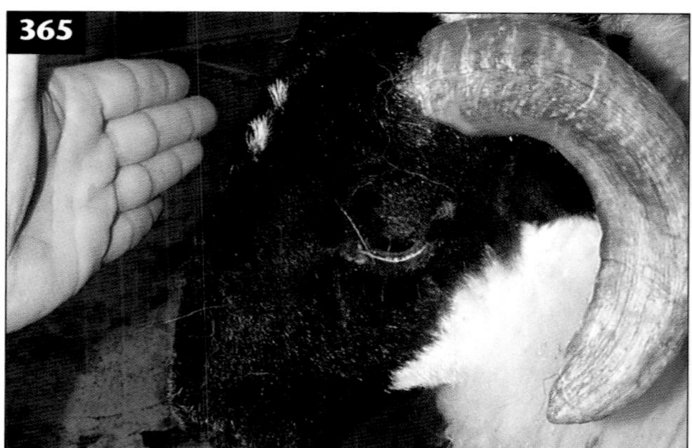

365 Lack of menace response in a ram lamb with sulphur toxicity.

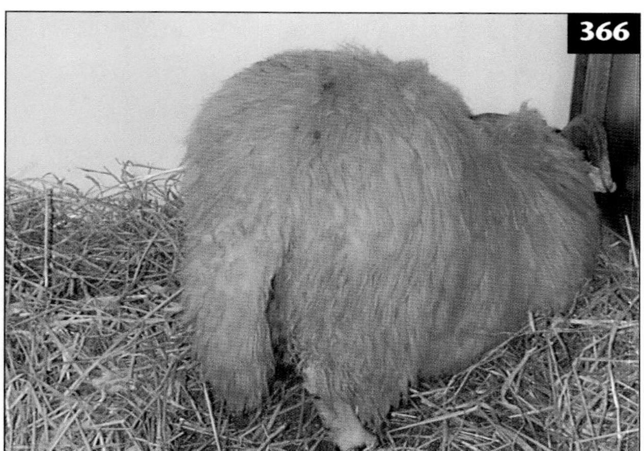

366 Head pressing behaviour in a ram lamb with sulphur toxicity.

Differential diagnoses

- Polioencephalomalacia.
- Hepatic encephalopathy associated with cobalt deficiency.
- Acidosis/grain overload.
- Urolithiasis.

Diagnosis

The response to the standard treatment regimen for PEM is poor. The diagnosis is confirmed on histopathological examination of brain tissue.

The pathology of sulphur toxicity cases includes widespread areas of malacia in the brain, with a clearly defined periphery. Areas of the thalamus and mid-brain are also involved but no lesions are observed in the cerebellum or hippocampus.

Treatment

There is a poor response to intravenous treatment with vitamin B_1 and dexamethasone. Affected lambs may regain a normal appetite but remain dull with impaired vision.

Prevention/control measures

Care should be taken with respect to sulphur content when formulating intensive rations for fattening lambs. While no further cases have been identified in some outbreaks after all the remaining lambs were given a single intramuscular injection of vitamin B_1, some anecdotal reports have questioned such a metaphylactic approach.

Economics

Whilst not commonly reported, production losses due to sulphur toxicity can be considerable.

Welfare implications

Sheep that do not respond to treatment should be slaughtered for welfare reasons.

VESTIBULAR DISEASE

Definition/overview

Peripheral vestibular disease occurs sporadically in sheep of all ages but particularly in growing and weaned lambs.

Aetiology

Unilateral peripheral vestibular lesions are commonly associated with otitis media, and ascending infection of the eustachian tube is not uncommon in growing lambs. Haematogenous spread may also result from a localized infection elsewhere in the body. There may be a history of head trauma, including fighting injuries in rams. *Pasteurella* species, *Streptococcus* species and *Arcanobacterium pyogenes* have been isolated from infected lesions.

Clinical presentation

The vestibular system helps the animal maintain orientation in its environment and maintain the position of the eyes, trunk and limbs with respect to movements and positioning of the head. Clinical signs depend on whether there is unilateral or bilateral involvement and if the disease process involves the peripheral or central components of the vestibular system.

Sheep with unilateral vestibular disease present with a head tilt towards the affected side (**367**) and horizontal nystagmus with the fast phase directed

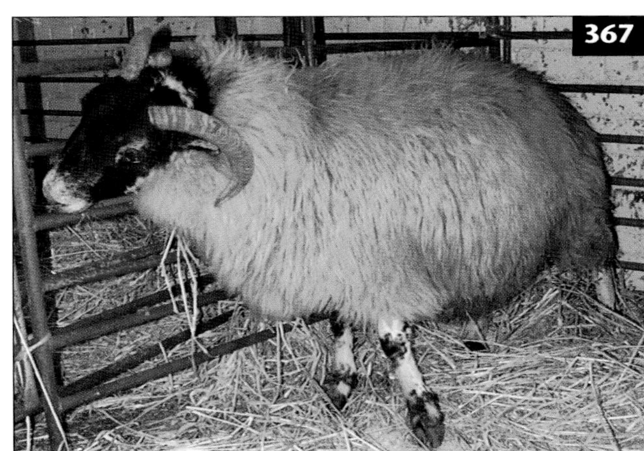

367 Lack of balance and left head tilt in a Scottish Blackface ewe with a left-sided vestibular lesion.

away from the side of the lesion, although this may regress with time. Circling behaviour towards the affected side may be present. Eye drop on the affected side is usually present. Ipsilateral peripheral facial nerve paralysis frequently results from otitis media and causes ptosis and drooping of the ear. There may be evidence of otitis externa with a purulent aural discharge in some cases, but rupture of the tympanic membrane is not a common portal of infection.

Differential diagnoses

- Unilateral peripheral vestibular lesions with associated superficial facial nerve trauma should be differentiated from listeriosis because of the different treatment regimens and control measures.
- Circling may also be caused by coenurosis and a cerebral abscess.

Diagnosis

Diagnosis is based on the clinical examination.

Treatment

A good treatment response is achieved with five consecutive days' treatment with procaine penicillin (44,000 iu/kg q24h) when the disease is recognized during the early stages (**368**). Alternatively, trimethoprim-sulphonamide combination can be used to similar effect.

Prevention/control measures

Vestibular disease occurs sporadically and there are no specific control measures.

Economics

Vestibular disease is of no economic significance in sheep flocks.

Welfare implications

Prompt detection and treatment achieve a good recovery.

LISTERIOSIS

Definition/overview

Listeriosis typically occurs as an outbreak in silage-fed sheep. A 2% prevalence is not uncommon and, in exceptional circumstances, the prevalence may reach 10% of the flock.

Aetiology

Listeriosis is caused by *Listeria monocytogenes*. Organisms are ingested or inhaled and may cause septicaemia, abortion and latent infection. Infection of trigeminal nerve roots via minute wounds in the buccal mucosa ascends the nerve and causes encephalitis.

Clinical presentation

Listeriosis is found classically in sheep fed poorly conserved silage and it affects all ages, sometimes as an epidemic in feedlot sheep. In the UK, sheep aged 18–24 months are most commonly affected. This is associated with cheek teeth eruption facilitating infection of buccal lesions and silage feeding during the winter housing period. Listeriosis can occasionally be encountered in young lambs that have had no access to silage.

Listeric encephalitis is essentially a localized infection of the brainstem that occurs when *L. monocytogenes* ascends the trigeminal nerve. Clinical signs are generally unilateral in sheep more than four months old and vary according to the degree of dysfunction of the damaged nerve nuclei. Signs also include depression, due to involvement of the ascending reticular activating system, and circling (vestibulocochlear nucleus).

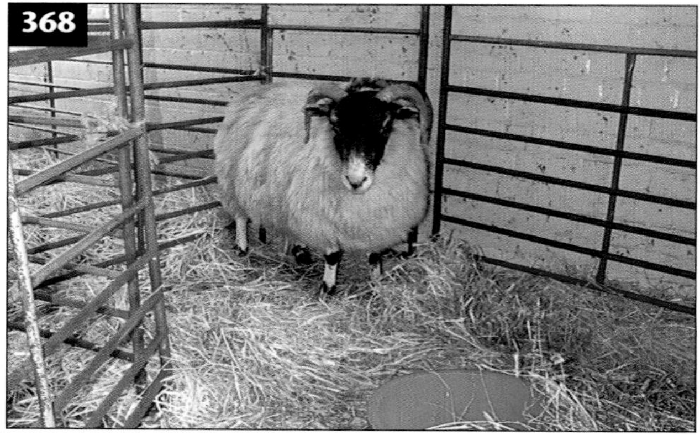

368 Ewe in **367** four days after start of antibiotic therapy.

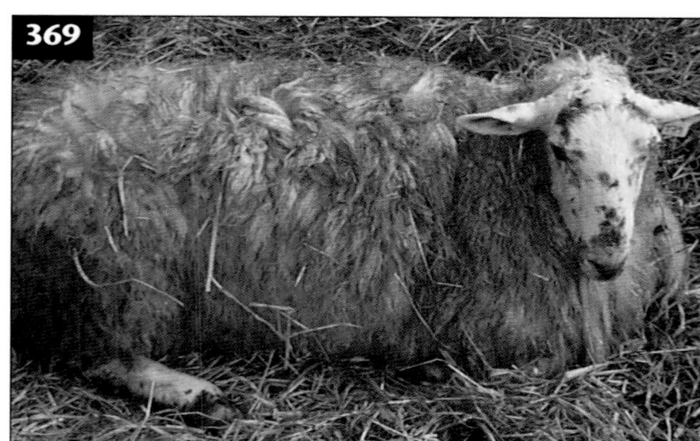

369 Sudden onset stupor in a Greyface gimmer with listeriosis. There is right-sided facial paralysis with drooped ear and ptosis.

Initially, affected animals are anorexic, depressed (**369**) and disorientated and they may propel themselves into corners or under gates (**370**). This propulsive tendency must be differentiated from the head pressing behaviour observed in sheep with cerebral dysfunction (e.g. as in OPT). They may lean against objects due to hemiparesis (weakness affecting same side of body), with knuckling at the fore fetlock joint occasionally present. Affected animals may move in a circle towards the affected side but this is by no means pathognomic of listeriosis. There is profuse, almost continuous, salivation (**371**), with food material impacted in the cheek of the affected side due to trigeminal nerve paralysis, which also results in loss of skin sensation of the face. Facial paralysis results in a drooped ear, deviated muzzle (**371**), flaccid lip and lowered eyelid on the affected side. There is a unilateral lack of blink response and exposure keratitis may arise after 2–3 days. During the terminal stages affected animals are unable to rise or maintain sternal recumbency, and they lie on the same side. Involuntary running movements are common, leading rapidly to the development of superficial trauma. Typical cases of listeriosis in adult sheep, summarizing the clinical signs described above, are featured in **372–376**, and in lambs in **377–379**.

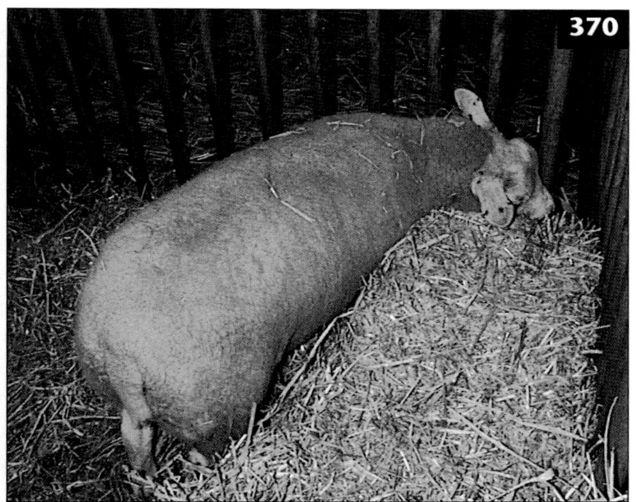

370 Texel gimmer with propulsive tendency and its head forced into the corner of the pen. There is right-sided facial paralysis with drooped ear.

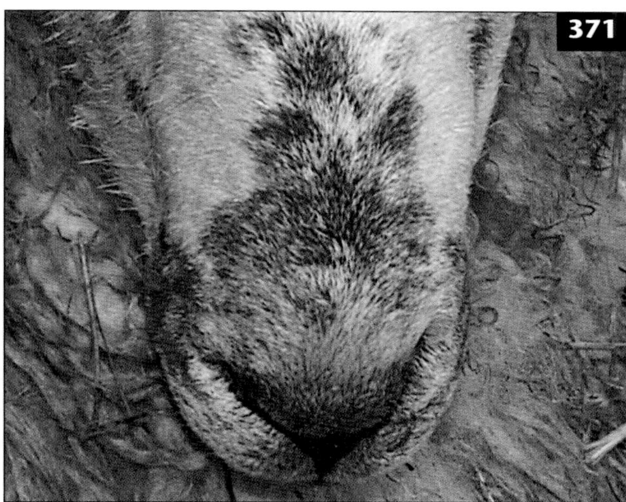

371 Close-up of the gimmer in **369**. The muzzle is deviated towards the normal left side and there is profuse salivation.

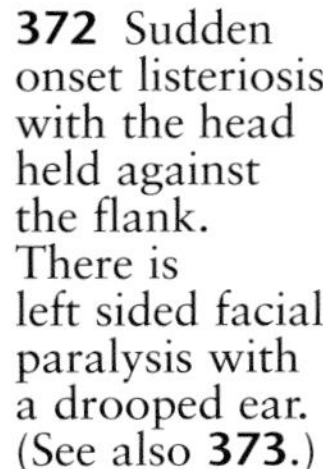

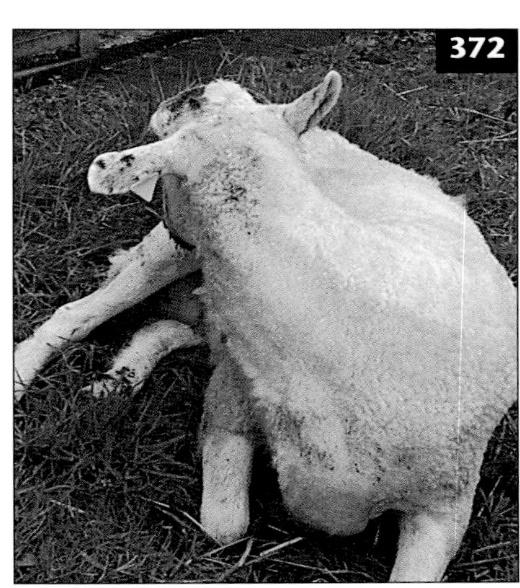

372 Sudden onset listeriosis with the head held against the flank. There is left sided facial paralysis with a drooped ear. (See also **373**.)

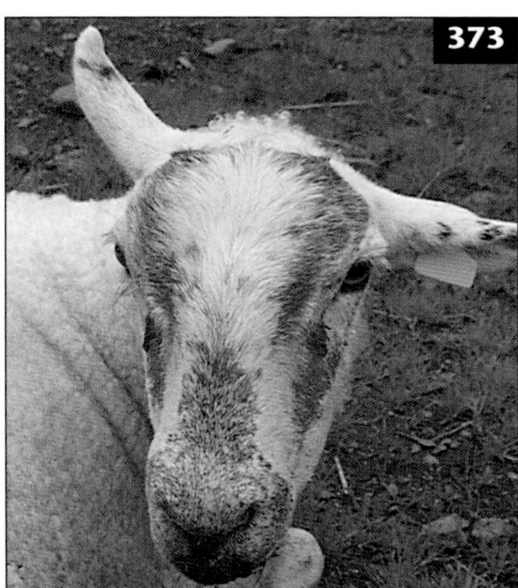

373 Listeriosis. There is salivation and the muzzle is deviated towards the normal right side, with a drooped left ear and upper eyelid. (Compare the angle of the upper eyelashes.)

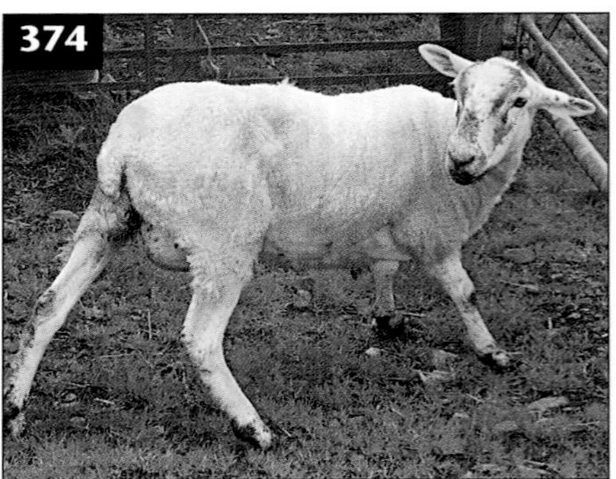

374 Sheep with listeriosis showing slight head tilt to the left. There is an unsteady gait and abnormal stance.

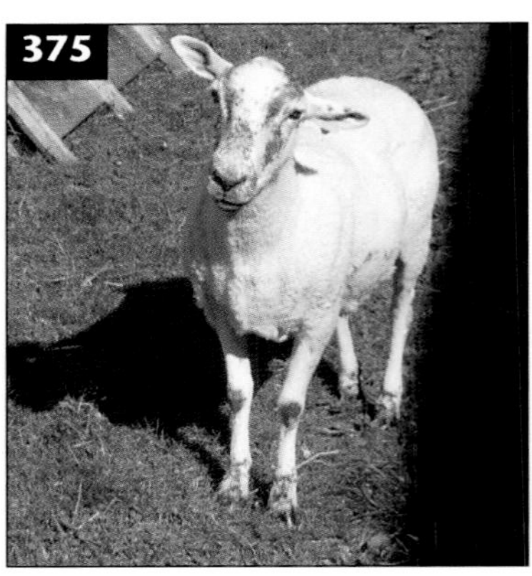

375 Ewe in 374 five days later.

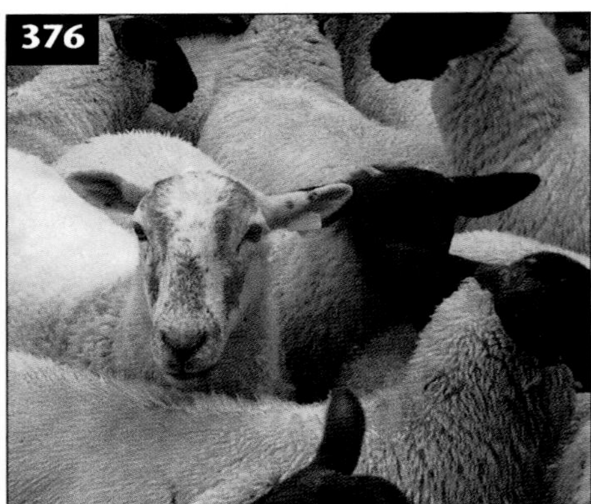

376 Ewe in 375 one month later.

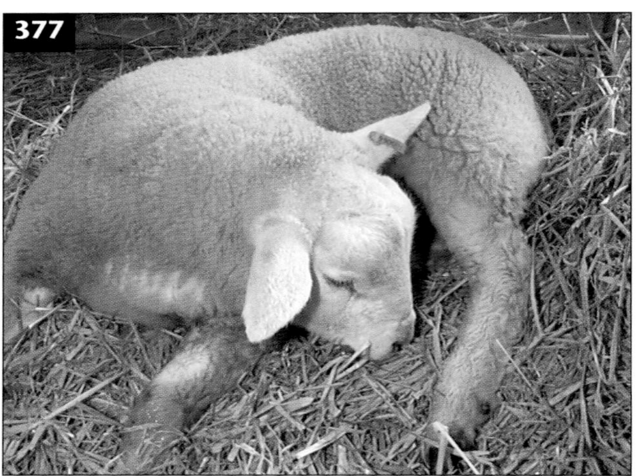

377 Listeriosis affecting a six-week-old Texel lamb. There is stupor, and profuse salivation is visible over the left forelimb.

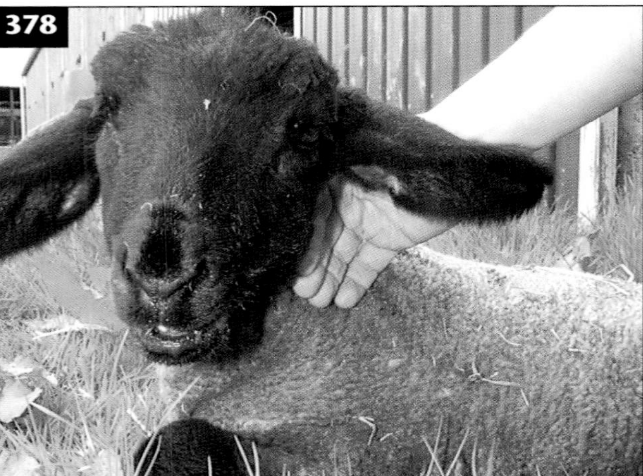

378 Stupor with bilateral trigeminal and facial paralysis in a six-week-old lamb suffering from listeriosis.

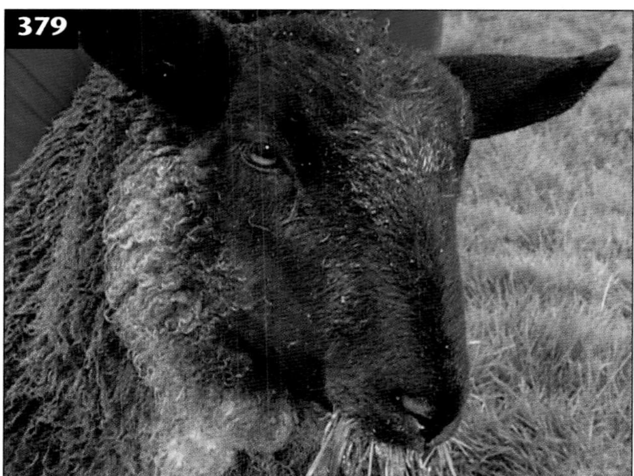

379 Weaned lamb with listeriosis. The lamb is depressed and has poor ability to prehend food.

Differential diagnoses

- Ovine pregnancy toxaemia.
- Peripheral vestibular lesions.
- Brain abscessation.
- Coenurosis.
- Early stages of hypocalcaemia.
- Trauma to the superficial facial nerve frequently results after short periods spent in lateral recumbency caused by a number of conditions, and it is important that the drooped ear and ptosis that can result are not mistaken for the involvement of the facial nerve nucleus present in listeriosis.
- Radial nerve paralysis should not be mistaken for hemiparesis, which is observed in some sheep with listeriosis.

Diagnosis

Sheep with listeriosis present with an elevated CSF protein concentration (**380**) in the range 0.8–4.0 g/l (n = <0.4 g/l) and a mild increase in white cell concentration (pleocytosis) comprised of large mononuclear cells.

Listeriosis can be confirmed only by isolation and identification of *L. monocytogenes*. Specimens of choice are brain tissue from animals with CNS involvement and aborted placentae and fetuses. If primary isolation attempts fail, ground brain tissue should be held at 4°C for several weeks and re-cultured weekly. Serology is not used routinely for diagnosis because many healthy sheep have high anti-*Listeria* antibody titres.

Treatment

Recovery of sheep from listerial encephalitis depends on early detection of illness by the shepherd, accurate diagnosis and prompt aggressive antibiotic treatment by the veterinary practitioner (**376**). *L. monocytogenes* is susceptible to various antibiotics including penicillin, ceftiofur and trimethoprim/sulphonamide.

The author's treatment for a 75 kg ewe affected by listeriosis comprises two vials of crystalline penicillin (each vial contains 5 mega-units [3 g] of benzylpenicillin) given intravenously, plus 20 ml procaine penicillin (300,000 iu/ml) injected intramuscularly divided between two sites at the first examination, followed by 5 ml procaine penicillin q24h for the next five days. A single intravenous injection of a soluble corticosteroid such as dexamethasone (1.1 mg/kg) may reduce the associated severe inflammatory reaction and improve the prognosis; however, this treatment is based on clinical observations and there are no supportive clinical studies reported in the literature. High-dose corticosteroid treatment is expensive but could be considered for valuable individual sheep. (**NB:** injection of more than 16 mg of dexamethasone after day 136 of pregnancy will cause abortion/premature birth). Propylene glycol, or a concentrated oral rehydration solution containing dextrose, should be administered as per the manufacturer's data sheet to prevent development of a severe energy deficit and the possibility of OPT in multigravid ewes. Fresh palatable foods and clean water must always be available. A topical antibiotic eye ointment should be applied four times a day.

The response to successful antibiotic treatment is slow and initially appears only to arrest deterioration of clinical signs (**374, 375**). After a few days the ewe attempts to eat but may experience difficulty masticating food and swallowing. Soft food such as soaked sugar beet pulp plus some rolled barley in a shallow bowl placed at shoulder height is helpful. Rumen impaction is common after prolonged periods of inappetence and large volumes of warm water and 'rumen stimulants' by orogastric tube assist restoration of rumen function. If available, the transfer of rumen contents from a healthy animal aids recovery. Facial paralysis slowly improves over some weeks (**376**).

The overall recovery rate in sheep can be up to 30% when sheep are presented early in the clinical course but if signs of encephalitis are severe (lateral recumbency, seizure activity), death usually occurs despite treatment.

Prevention/control measures

Outbreaks may occur more than ten days after feeding poor quality silage (**381**). Affected animals should be segregated and if silage is being fed, use of that

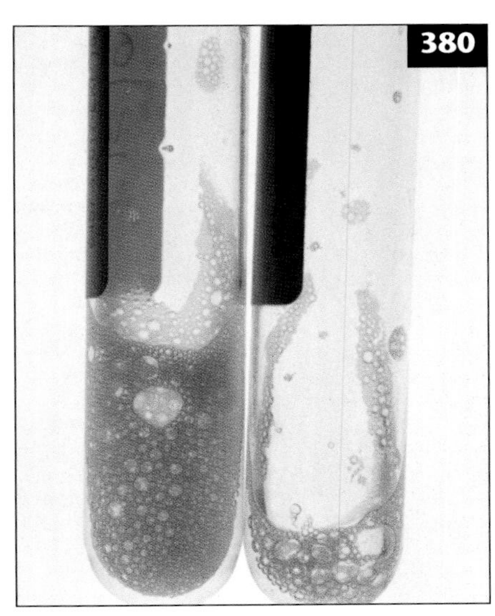

380 Two lumbar CSF samples after agitation. There is much greater 'foaming' in the left sample (sheep with listeriosis), resulting from a higher protein concentration, than the right sample (normal sheep).

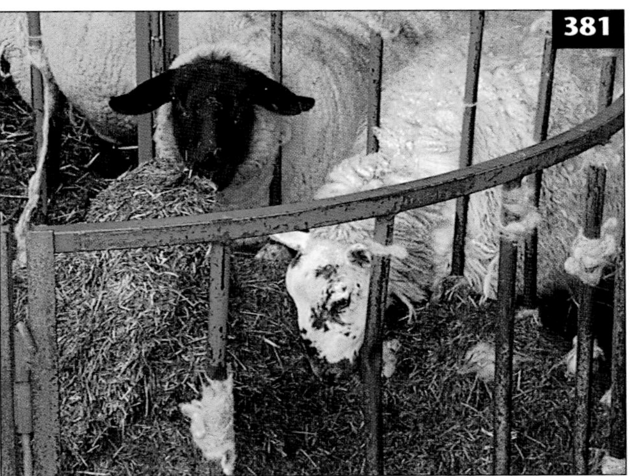

381 Listerial organisms can multiply rapidly in silage exposed to air.

particular silage should be discontinued whenever possible. Spoiled silage should be discarded routinely, or fed to growing cattle at the farmer's risk (382–384).

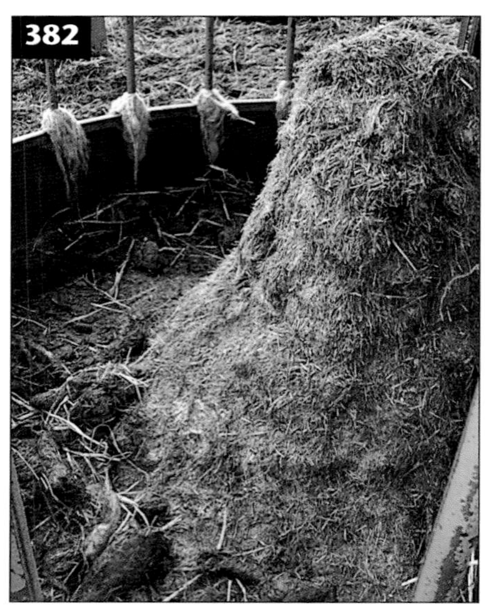

382 An outbreak of listeriosis in gimmers was attributed to multiplication of bacteria in the centre of this feeder. The silage was added every 2–3 days and the core was pushed over by the farmer after one week or so to prevent wastage.

The use of additives for grass silage is likely to produce a more acid pH, which discourages multiplication of *L. monocytogenes*. Silage clamps must be rolled continuously during filling (385) and then sheeted (386) to prevent entry of air. A block cutter operating along a short silage face (387) limits air entry and secondary fermentation once the clamp has been opened. Every effort must be taken not to puncture wrapped silage bales during handling and storage (388), and all punctures must be sealed immediately. Stores of wrapped silage bales must be fenced against farm stock and vermin.

The usefulness of a single intramuscular injection of procaine penicillin, or other antibiotic, to all at-risk sheep during an outbreak of listeriosis (antibiotic metaphylaxis) has not been reported.

Results with vaccines in sheep are limited, and the sporadic nature of the disease questions the cost benefit of vaccination. Some authors argue that vaccines are contraindicated for listeriosis.

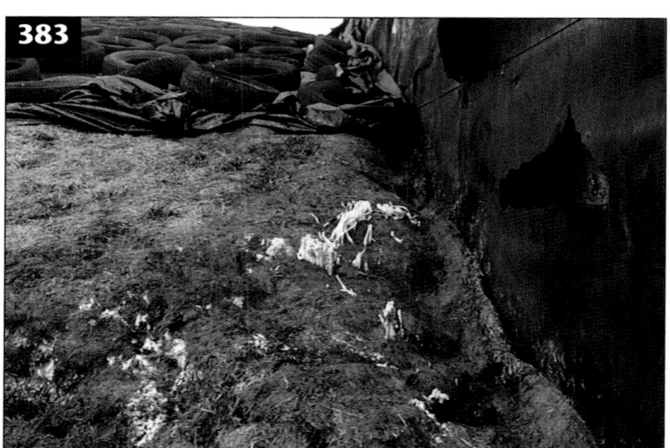

383 Spoilage of grass silage due to a poor seal along the clamp.

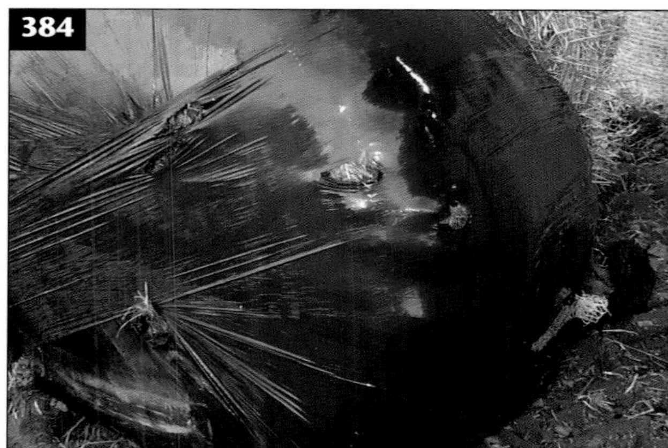

384 Punctures to silage bags/wraps must be sealed immediately.

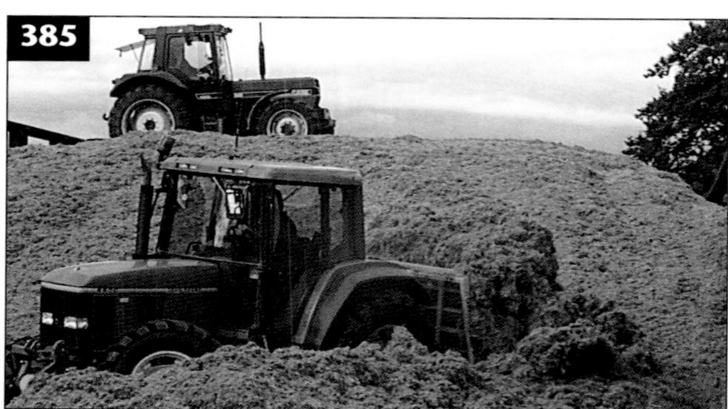

385 Compaction of harvested grass to exclude air, which promotes anaerobic fermentation.

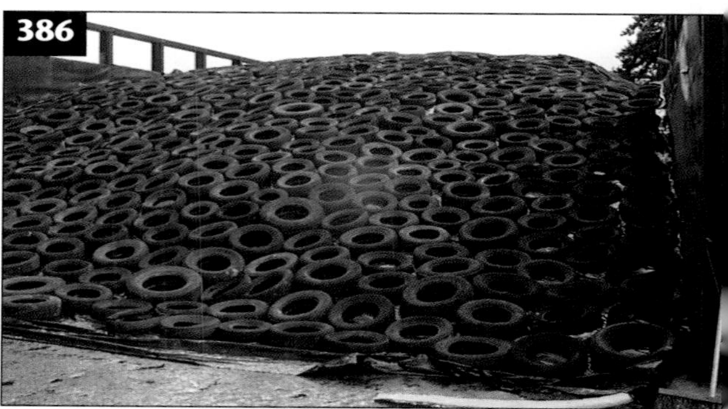

386 Correct sheeting of silage clamp.

Economics

Farmers acknowledge the risk posed by listeriosis when feeding silage but these can be limited by attention to detail when ensiling grass, and by prompt recognition and appropriate treatment of clinical cases.

Welfare implications

Sheep presenting with seizure activity and unable to maintain sternal recumbency, and those that deteriorate despite 2–3 days' antibiotic therapy, should be humanely destroyed.

VISNA

Definition/overview

Visna is an uncommon manifestation of MVV infection, often appearing some years after the diagnosis of maedi in the flock, although there are few reliable surveillance data. Recent (1996) UK data showed a MVV seroprevalence of 0.5% with 2% of flocks showing serological evidence of infection. Interestingly, clinical disease was rarely reported until the flock seroprevalence exceeded 60%. Visna is exotic to New Zealand and Australia.

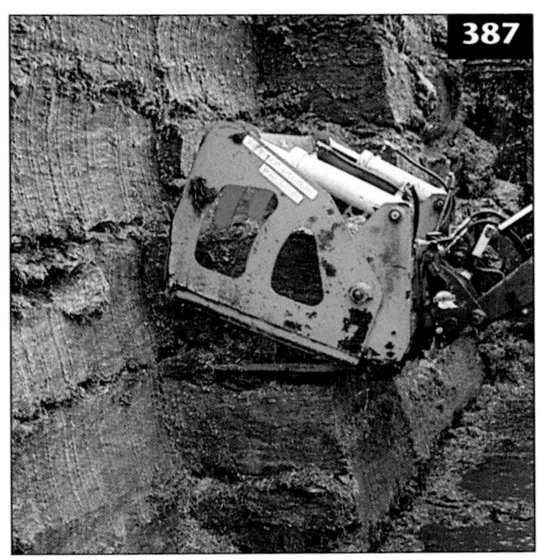

387 Use of a block cutter to limit exposure at the silage face.

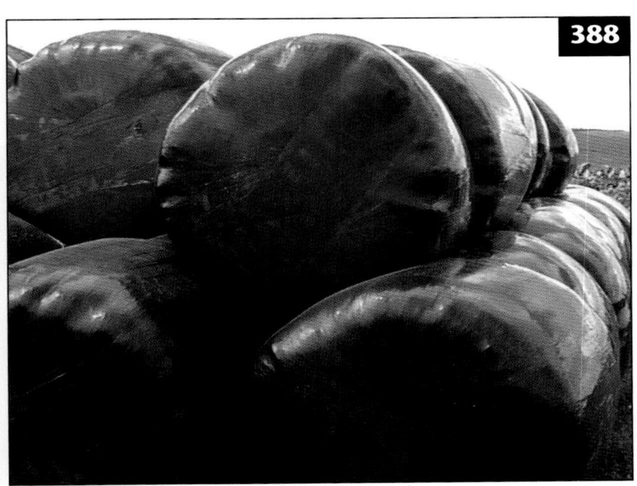

388 Correct big bale storage. A vermin proof fence in essential to prevent damage to the plastic wrapping.

Aetiology

MVV is a lentivirus related to caprine arthritis encephalitis virus, with cross-infection possible between species.

Clinical presentation

The incubation period is protracted and clinical disease is more common in 4–5-year-old sheep. There are essentially two forms of visna: a brain form and a spinal cord form. In each form the neurological signs are insidious in onset, with gradual deterioration over a period of months.

Brain form

The neurological signs are insidious in onset and present as a head tilt of approximately 5–10° from the vertical plane and circling towards the affected side. The clinical signs result from lesions within the lateral ventricles. Some affected sheep may display hypermetria and hindimb ataxia. There is a slow deterioration of the neurological signs and affected sheep are usually destroyed for humane reasons within two months of initial recognition of the condition.

Spinal cord form

The initial neurological signs are hypometria, reduced flexion of the hindimb joints, reduced weight bearing affecting one hindimb and conscious proprioceptive deficit (389). As the condition progresses the dorsal

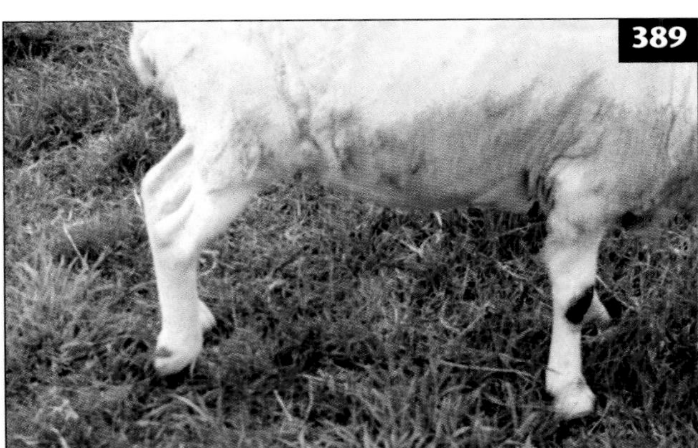

389 Texel ewe displaying unilateral hindlimb conscious proprioceptive deficit typical of visna.

surface of the hoof remains in contact with the ground when the limb is weight bearing, there is characteristic knuckling of the fetlock joint and finally hindimb paralysis (**390**).

Differential diagnoses

Brain form

- Peripheral vestibular lesion.
- Scrapie.
- Space-occupying brain lesions such as abscess formation or coenurosis.

Spinal cord form

- Vertebral empyema.
- Hindlimb joint lesion.
- Peroneal nerve paralysis.
- Sarcocystosis.

Diagnosis

Diagnosis is based on the clinical examination findings supported by positive MVV serology.

Treatment

There is no treatment and all clinical cases, seropositive stock and their progeny should be culled, although this recommendation must be tempered where MVV infection is considered endemic.

Prevention/control measures

The impact of MVV on sheep production is disputed between countries. This, in addition to national seroprevalence rates, largely determines the adoption of prevention and control measures. In countries such as the UK, MVV flock control measures are limited to a relatively small number of pedigree flocks. No specific control measures have been adopted by commercial UK farmers other than the rudimentary biosecurity measures adopted since the 2001 FMD epidemic.

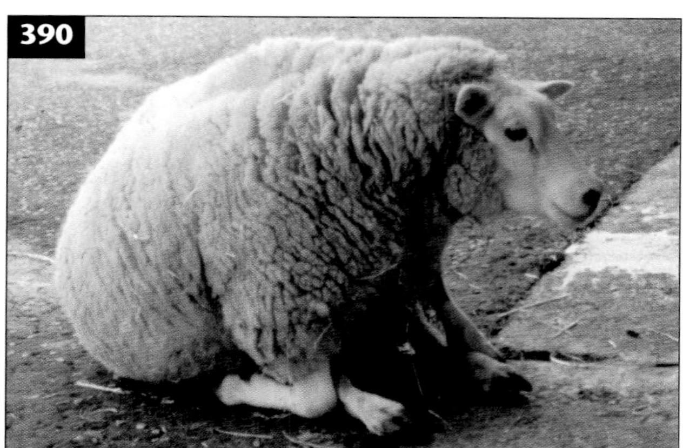

390 Texel ewe, which had displayed unilateral hindlimb conscious proprioceptive deficit progressing to hindlimb paralysis.

Economics

Loss of MVV accreditation status prevents the sale of pedigree rams to other pedigree breeders and this incurs a severe financial penalty. There are no recent reliable data on potential losses from MVV infection in commercial flocks. Such losses in MVV infected flocks could accrue from culling of clinical cases, poor lamb growth rate resulting from the dam's chronic indurative mastitis and, possibly, lameness.

Welfare implications

There are no specific welfare problems related to MVV infection other than timely culling during the early stages of clinical disease.

SCRAPIE

Definition/overview

Scrapie is an infectious disease whose incubation period is determined genetically. Scrapie belongs to a small group of diseases called transmissible spongiform encephalopathies (TSEs). These are characterized by certain physical properties including a protracted incubation period, a relatively short clinical course, lack of host immune response but no immune system suppression, and experimental transmission of infection to a range of species. Other important members of this group are bovine spongiform encephalopathy (BSE), variant Creutzfeldt-Jacob disease (vCJD), kuru, chronic wasting disease of deer and elk, and transmissible mink encephalopathy.

Since 1st January 1993, scrapie has been a notifiable disease in the UK (and since 1994 within the European Union [EU]), with the clinical diagnosis confirmed by histopathological examination of brain tissue at necropsy and the demonstration of characteristic neuronal vacuolation and astrocytic hypertrophy. Scrapie is exotic to New Zealand and Australia, although it has occurred in the past in both countries but was recognized and successfully contained and eliminated. In some EU countries, retrospective culling has been introduced in an attempt to eradicate scrapie.

Aetiology

There remains considerable debate regarding the causal agent of scrapie, with the infectious protein or prion theory most widely accepted. There is considerable genetic variation in susceptibility to infection.

Clinical presentation

Natural cases of scrapie are rarely encountered in sheep less than two years old. The median age is three years, although this depends on the genetically determined incubation period, age at infection and infectious dose. Affected sheep present with poorer bodily condition compared with that of the remainder of the flock, despite an adequate plane of nutrition and lack of significant metabolic demand of advanced pregnancy or lactation. Cheviots, Swaledales and Suffolks appear to be overrepresented.

The fleece is in poor condition. In the majority of sheep with scrapie there are areas of loss over the flanks and tailhead caused by rubbing (**391**). In a small number of cases, regrowth of the fleece, with hyperpigmentation (black wool), has occurred in areas where the fleece had been rubbed out. Cutaneous stimulation of the skin over the dorsal sacral area (provocative scrapie test) elicits a nibble response that manifests as manic lip smacking and swaying of the hindquarters in the majority of scrapie sheep. However, this response is not pathognomic of scrapie, as ectoparasite infestations can provoke a similar response.

A common behavioural abnormality observed during the early stage of scrapie is that affected sheep, when stressed during gathering, appear to 'collapse' and assume sternal recumbency, with the neck extended and the head held on the ground for up to ten minutes. In this narcoleptic state (**392**) the sheep cannot be prompted to regain its feet but will do so unaided soon afterwards and appear normal.

The neurological findings can be attributed to cerebral and cerebellar dysfunction. Cerebral dysfunction is indicated by an altered mental state, with depression and a vacant, detached appearance but hyperaesthesia to visual, auditory and tactile stimuli. The neck is often extended with the head held lowered (**393**). The mental state is best judged in suspected cases once the group has settled down, and by comparison with normal sheep. Vision and pupillary light reflexes are normal. Cerebellar dysfunction is indicated by postural and gait abnormalities, namely hindlimb ataxia but with preservation of muscle strength, dysmetria, most commonly hypermetria of the forelimbs, and a

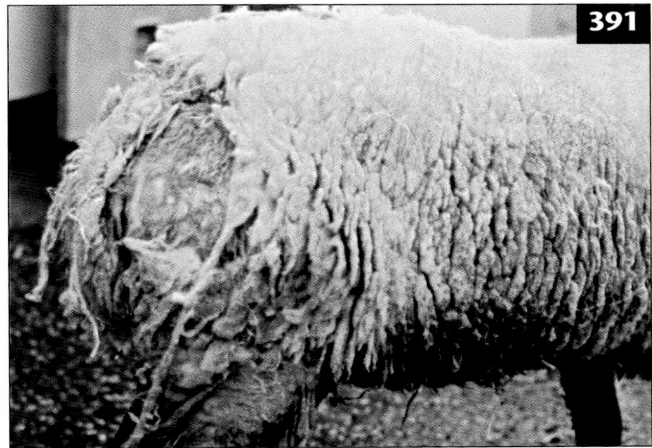

391 Wool loss due to pruritus in a Suffolk ewe suffering from scrapie.

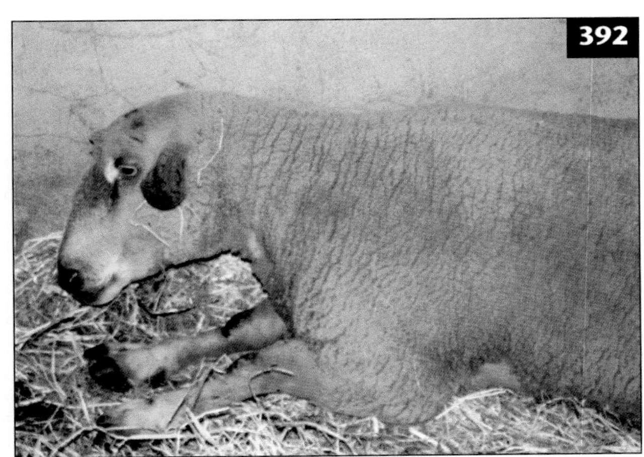

392 Onset of narcolepsy in a Charollais ram suffering from scrapie.

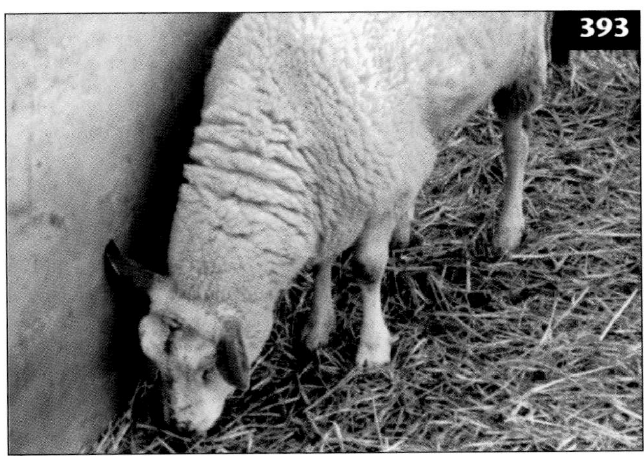

393 Detached attitude in a Texel ewe suffering from scrapie.

wide-based stance. The gait abnormalities are most obvious when the animal is made to trot downhill or turn acute angles, when hopping with both hindlimbs is frequently observed.

As the clinical course progresses over several weeks to months, affected sheep spend increasing periods in sternal recumbency. They have a drawn-up abdomen with sunken sublumbar fossae. Appetite is poor and sheep prefer concentrate feedstuffs and eat little hay. Faeces are generally dry, pelleted and coated with mucus. Frequent teeth grinding (bruxism) is a non-specific finding that can be attributed to ruminal impaction with dry fibrous material. While scrapie cases may die suddenly during the terminal stages of disease, most sheep are killed for welfare reasons before they reach an emaciated state.

Differential diagnoses

- Ovine pregnancy toxaemia.
- Meningoencephalitis caused by *L. monocytogenes*.
- Brain abscessation.
- Coenurosis.
- Sheep affected with sheep scab (psoroptic mange) may become emaciated and present with fleece loss and a positive nibble response, but they show none of the gait and behavioural signs observed in scrapie.

Diagnosis

A provisional diagnosis of scrapie is based on an accurate history of the animal and a thorough clinical examination, with particular attention being paid to the neurological examination and findings of cerebral and cerebellar dysfunction.

The clinical diagnosis is confirmed following histopathological examination of brain tissue at necropsy, with the demonstration of characteristic neuronal vacuolation and astrocytic hypertrophy.

Treatment

There is no treatment and affected sheep should be euthanased as soon as the condition is suspected on clinical examination.

Selection for genotypes with delayed onset of clinical signs of scrapie (as is the case with the UK National Scrapie Plan) is no guarantee that such sheep do not incubate the disease, and the infectious agent may still be present in the reticuloendothelial system before replicating in brain tissue. In addition, reducing the gene pool will only hinder attempts to develop natural resistance to the important challenges facing the sheep industry.

Economics

Scrapie is of economic importance to pedigree sheep breeders who are unable to sell breeding stock with genotypes encoding for susceptibility/shortened incubation periods. For example, the New Zealand experience in 1972 has seriously affected the trade in UK live sheep exports to New Zealand and Australia.

Welfare implications

Affected sheep should be euthanased for welfare reasons.

COENUROSIS (*Syn:* gid)

Definition/overview

Coenurosis is an uncommon disease of the CNS in sheep, although in the UK during the 1980s, slaughter-house surveys in certain geographical areas reported prevalence rates of *Coenurus cerebralis* from 0.5–5.8%.

Aetiology

Coenurus cerebralis is the larval stage of *Taenia multiceps*, a tapeworm that infests the small intestine of carnivores. Contamination of pastures grazed by sheep with dog faeces can result in larval invasion of the CNS and clinical disease. The life cycle is completed when the carnivorous definitive host ingests infested sheep's brain.

Clinical presentation

Both acute and chronic forms of coenurosis have been described, although chronic disease is more readily identified and more frequently reported.

Acute coenurosis has been reported in a flock of sheep introduced on to a pasture heavily contaminated by dog faeces. Clinical signs appeared within ten days and ranged from mild to severe, with death occurring within 3–5 days of onset of neurological dysfunction. Acute coenurosis has also been reported in 6–8-week-old lambs where clinical signs ranged from pyrexia, listlessness and head aversion to convulsions and death within 4–5 days.

Chronic coenurosis is more commonly reported in growing sheep aged 6–18 months, where it presents as a slowly progressive focal lesion of the brain, typically involving one cerebral hemisphere. Chronic coenurosis has rarely been reported in sheep over three years of age. The time taken from larval hatching, migration to the brain and evidence of neurological dysfunction ranges from 2–6 months. The cyst is located in one cerebral hemisphere in 80% of cases, the cerebellum in approximately 10% and affecting multiple locations in 8%. Individual cases of coenurus cyst within the spinal cord have been reported but such cases could be more prevalent as the clinical presentation is similar to vertebral body empyema.

Localization of the coenurus cyst

Compulsive circling behaviour is commonly observed in sheep with coenurosis. Narrow diameter circles (1–2 metres) suggest involvement of the basal nuclei at a deep location within the forebrain, whereas wide circles are suggestive of a more superficial location for the cerebral cyst. There is a tendency for sheep to circle towards the side of superficial cysts and away from the side of more deeply sited cysts. Depression and head-pressing behaviour occur with cysts involving the frontal lobe of the cerebrum.

The presence of a cyst in one cerebral hemisphere causes loss of the menace response in the contralateral eye; therefore, blindness in the right eye indicates that the lesion is in the left hemisphere, and vice versa. Blindness can also be investigated by unilateral blindfolding. Unilateral proprioceptive deficits suggest a contralateral cerebral cyst, whereas bilateral deficits more likely indicate a cerebellar cyst.

A head tilt towards the affected side may result if the cyst involves either the vestibular or cerebellovestibular pathways. Cerebellar lesions are characterized by dysmetria, ataxia, but with preservation of strength, and a wide-based stance. Bilateral postural deficits and lack of menace response are usually also present with a cerebellar cyst. Deterioration of the clinical condition occurs more rapidly with a cerebellar cyst.

Differential diagnoses

- Listeriosis, louping ill and PEM should be considered when formulating a diagnosis of acute coenurosis.
- Brain abscessation should be included in the differential diagnosis list but the clinical signs tend to remain relatively static and do not deteriorate, as occurs in chronic coenurosis.

Diagnosis

The presumptive diagnosis is confirmed at surgery after the lesion has been localized to either the right or left cerebral hemisphere following a thorough neurological examination. Softening of the frontal bone, as a consequence of a generalized increase in intracranial pressure, may be palpable but is not a reliable guide to the precise location of the cyst. The bone softening may be either ipsilateral or contralateral to the cyst position, and in some cases there is softening on both sides in the presence of only a unilateral cyst. Real-time B-mode ultrasonography has been described as an aid to *C. cerebralis* cyst localization.

Treatment

Many farmers may elect to slaughter sheep that are fit for marketing for economic reasons. An 85% surgical success rate for removal of the coenurus cyst can be achieved after accurate localization of the lesion.

It has been recommended that the dose rate of pentobarbital sodium for sheep with coenurus cysts should be approximately two-thirds of the normal calculated dose. Whenever possible, feed and water should be withheld for 24 hours before surgery. The sheep is placed in sternal recumbency with the head held lowered to allow drainage of saliva from the mouth throughout the operation. Pre-operative intravenous dexamethasone injection is recommended in an attempt to reduce brain oedema, which may result from the surgical procedure and complicate the animal's recovery. Procaine penicillin (44,000 iu/kg) should be administered two hours before surgery; alternatively, crystalline penicillin can be given intravenously 20–30 minutes before surgery. Pre-operative analgesia should include an NSAID and should be continued for three consecutive days thereafter.

The surgical approach is based on the neurological findings. For a cerebral cyst the trephine site is 1–2 cm lateral to the midline and immediately rostral to the coronal (parietofrontal) suture line. The trephine site for a cerebellar cyst is midline between the nuchal line and the suture line between the occipital and parietal bones. The dura mater is incised once the 1 cm diameter bone core has been removed. At this point the increased intracranial pressure caused by the cyst forces brain tissue into the trephine hole. An 18 gauge intravenous catheter connected to a 20 ml syringe is used to drain the cyst and withdraw a portion of the cyst wall to the trephine hole, where it can be grasped with forceps and the entire cyst wall and protoscolices carefully removed. Recovery after successful surgical cyst removal is rapid and there is a return to full neurological function within one week.

Prevention/control measures

Control of coenurosis can be effected by regular dosing of farm dogs at 6–8-week intervals with an effective taenicide and correct disposal of all sheep carcases to prevent scavenging by dogs belonging to the general public, as these dogs may not receive regular anthelmintic treatment.

Economics

While the recovery rate following removal of a cerebral cyst is good, the poor clinical condition of the sheep at the time of presentation to the veterinary surgeon, and the low financial value relative to the cost of general anaesthesia, cause most farmers to slaughter those sheep fit for marketing for economic reasons, and euthanase those in poor condition.

Welfare implications

Timely treatment, slaughter and/or humane destruction resolve any welfare concerns.

SARCOCYSTOSIS

Definition/overview

The prevalence of neurological disease caused by *Sarcocystis* species is probably underdiagnosed, because the clinical signs are easily mistaken for vertebral empyema. All ages of sheep may be affected but neurological signs of spinal cord disease are more commonly observed in 6–12-month-old lambs, where up to 10% can be affected.

Aetiology

Sarcocystis species are obligate, two-host protozoon parasites. The two potentially pathogenic microcyst species in sheep (*S. arieticanis* and *S. tenella*) have either a sheep/ dog or sheep/fox cycle.

Clinical presentation

Affected sheep remain bright and alert with a normal appetite. Hindlimb ataxia and paresis have been described (**394**), with affected sheep frequently adopting a dog-sitting posture. Some sheep may die without premonitory signs, whilst less severely affected sheep may recover with supportive care.

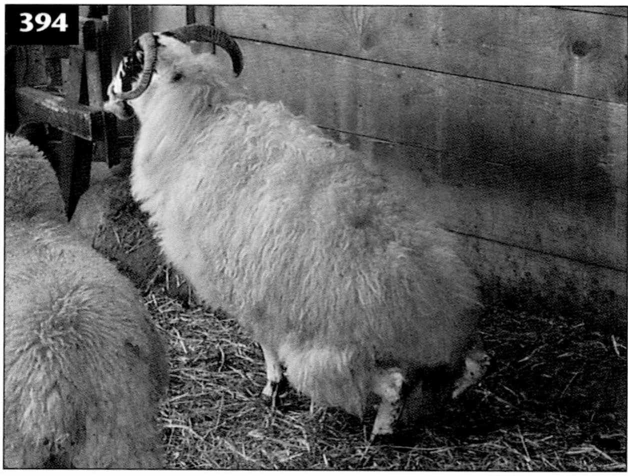

394 Hindlimb paresis in a ewe suffering from sarcocystosis.

Diagnosis

Diagnosis in farm animal practice is difficult because compressive spinal cord lesions present with similar neurological findings. Serology is unhelpful as the majority of sheep have titres to *Sarcocystis*, and the provisional diagnosis can only be confirmed by demonstration of characteristic histological lesions in the CNS. The use of CSF *Sarcocystis* antibody titres has not been determined. A high eosinophil count is suggestive of a parasitic invasion.

There is a non-suppurative encephalomyelitis characterized by multifocal perivascular cuffing and gliosis in the brain. Histopathological examination of the spinal cord has revealed axonal swelling and oedema but no significant demyelination. Despite intensive searches, few cells containing protozoa may be found and further investigations using immunocytochemistry may be necessary.

Treatment

Treatment of naturally occurring cases is unlikely to be effective; however, there are anecdotal claims of cure following drenching with diclazuril daily for six weeks at the dose rate quoted for coccidiosis treatment, although such a regimen is expensive (approximately 50–60% of the value of a mature sheep).

Prevention/control measures

Control is based on preventing completion of the sheep/dog life cycle, including prevention of faecal contamination of pasture and bedding material by dogs, especially litters of puppies, correct disposal of sheep carcases and not feeding uncooked sheep meat or offal to dogs.

Economics

The disease occurs sporadically but may have a significant financial impact if neurological disease occurs in pedigree breeding stock.

Welfare implications

Sheep with hindlimb paralysis should be confined to deeply bedded straw pens and given supportive care including being turned regularly. If there is no improvement within ten days, affected sheep should be euthanased.

GENETIC DISORDERS

DANDY-WALKER MALFORMATION

Definition/overview

Dandy-Walker malformation (**395**) has been reported in Suffolk sheep. The prevalence of Dandy-Walker malformation can be high, with reports of 16 affected lambs from 22 ewes and 17 lambs from 60 ewes.

Aetiology

The occurrence of Dandy-Walker malformation (agenesis of the caudal cerebellar vermis [**396**]) in Suffolk flocks following the introduction of a particular ram into the breeding programme indicates a strong genetic component.

Clinical presentation

The associated hypertensive hydrocephalus and doming of the skull frequently causes dystocia even when the lamb is presented normally. Many affected lambs are either stillborn or die during the neonatal period because of failure to ingest colostrum, with death resulting from starvation/hypothermia and/or septicaemia.

Diagnosis

The occurrence of numerous progeny of one ram with doming of the skull is strongly suggestive of Dandy-Walker malformation.

On postmortem examination there is marked distension of the ventricular system, including the lateral ventricles and the third and fourth ventricles (**396**). The cerebellum is abnormal with no visible vermis.

Treatment

Dystocia results from the skull being too large to enter the maternal birth canal. The veterinary surgeon is presented with two options: either deliver the lamb by caesarean section or crush the thinned cranium and deliver the lamb *per vaginam*. While the author has always selected the former course of action, it is reported that crushing the thinned bones comprising the cranium requires little force because of the pressure exerted by the hypertensive hydrocephalus during fetal development.

Affected lambs that are delivered alive by either method must be humanely destroyed.

Prevention/control measures

Careful examination of breeding records in pedigree flocks may identify the affected lambs as the progeny of a ram introduced into the flock for that breeding season. It is important that this ram and his progeny are not used for further breeding.

Economics

The occurrence of Dandy-Walker malformation has serious financial implications for a pedigree flock offering studs rams for sale; however, this condition is rarely, if ever, declared by vendors.

Welfare implications

Affected lambs with gross hydrocephalus should be delivered by caesarean section because *per vaginam* delivery is likely to result in trauma to the ewe's posterior reproductive tract.

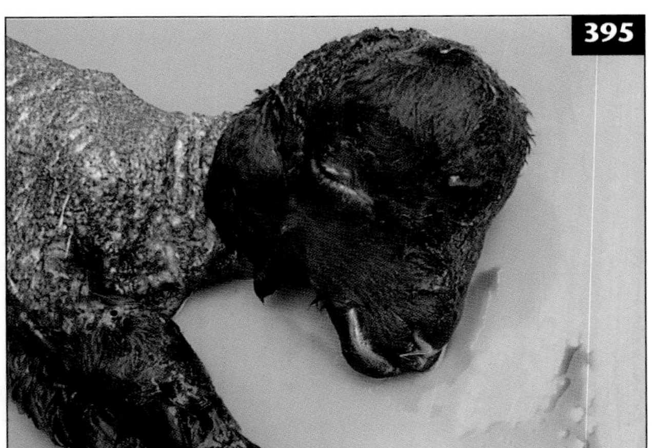

395 Hypertensive hydrocephalus and doming of the skull in a newborn Suffolk lamb with Dandy-Walker syndrome.

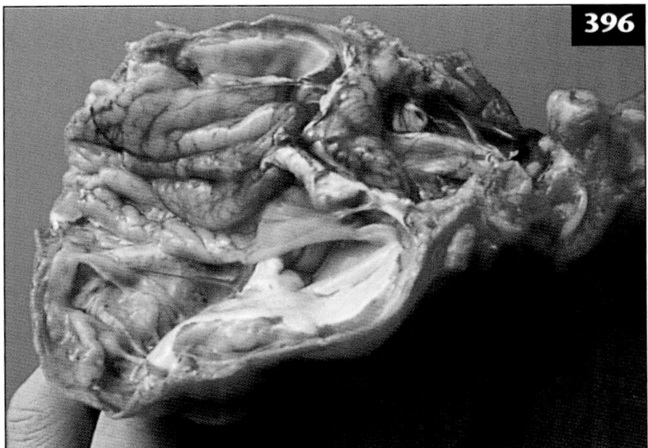

396 Agenesis of the caudal cerebellar vermis and hypertensive hydrocephalus in the brain of a newborn Suffolk lamb with Dandy-Walker syndrome.

Cerebellar abiotrophy

Definition/overview

Cerebellar abiotrophy is a familial syndrome. It has been described occasionally in Charollais sheep in the UK. Problems with establishing a clinical diagnosis probably lead to underreporting of this condition.

Aetiology

The mode of inheritance has not been established but is likely to be an autosomal recessive condition.

Clinical presentation

Clinical signs of progressive cerebellar abiotrophy may be present from birth or occur in adults. More recent reports in the UK have described lambs with a normal gait for the first 4–8 weeks of life; thereafter, there is progressive deterioration of clinical signs. The clinical signs are typical of cerebellar dysfunction and include lowered head carriage, intention tremors, a wide-based stance, ataxia, but with preservation of strength, and dysmetria. The hindlimb ataxia may result in the animal falling over, especially when turning quickly. Fine muscle fasciculations, which are present in the head and neck, may become more pronounced following arousal and resemble coarse muscle tremors, causing frequent vigorous jerky movements of the head.

Differential diagnoses

- Border disease.
- Bacterial meningoencephalitis.
- Delayed swayback.

Diagnosis

Clinical diagnosis is based on the history of progressive deterioration in neurological function, with signs indicative of a cerebellar lesion. There is no antemortem test.

Pathology

At necropsy the major histological findings include widespread degeneration of Purkinje cells, with associated hypocellularity of the granular layer and degeneration of myelin in cerebellar foliae and peduncles.

Treatment

There is no treatment.

Prevention/control measures

The probable inherited nature of this metabolic defect underlines the importance of an accurate diagnosis, especially in a stud ram, which may contribute significantly to the genetic profile of the flock. The parents and siblings of the affected lamb should be sold for slaughter and not kept as breeding replacements.

Economics

It is important that any ram with affected progeny is not used for further breeding and that his progeny are not presented for sale. This could result in considerable loss for a pedigree breeder.

Welfare implications

Affected lambs should be humanely destroyed as soon as the diagnosis has been established.

SPINAL CORD LESIONS

Definition/overview

Traumatic and infective lesions of the vertebral column causing spinal cord compression and dysfunction are common in sheep. Infective lesions are more common in growing lambs between one and four months old (**397**) but they can occur in all age groups. Traumatic lesions involving the cervical vertebrae are not uncommon in rams following head butting during the breeding season.

Aetiology

Vertebral empyema occurs as a sequela to an infectious focus elsewhere; however, macroscopic evidence of localized infection of another organ system is uncommon. A high incidence of vertebral body empyema may be associated with tick bite pyaemia in areas with tick-borne fever. *Arcanobacterium pyogenes* and *Staphylococcus* species have been

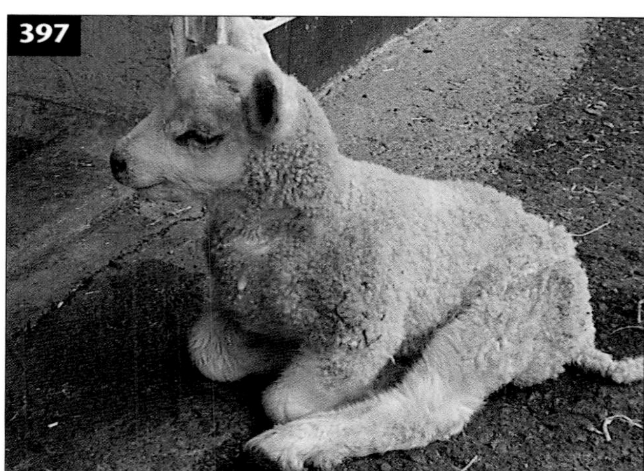

397 Dog sitting posture in a five-week-old lamb suffering from a compressive thoracolumbar lesion.

isolated from typical lesions. Lesions caused by dosing gun injuries, and those associated with intramuscular injection of a potentially irritating substance into the neck muscles, may give rise to infective lesions tracking to involve the cervical spinal cord.

Traumatic lesions involving the cervical region, caused by fighting injuries prior to the seasonal breeding period, occur in rams. Tumour conditions affecting the spinal cord (e.g. meningioma) have occasionally been reported.

Clinical presentation

Localization of a spinal cord lesion involves evaluation of the withdrawal and tendon jerk reflexes of the fore- and hindlimbs, and assessment of the panniculus reflex. The simple spinal reflex arc is the basis of the spinal cord examination. Under field situations it may prove difficult to undertake a satisfactory examination in large rams and heavily pregnant ewes that are recumbent.

The presence of a lesion at the level of the reflex arc results in lack of muscle contraction in response to stimulation. Denervation of the effector muscle results in flaccid paralysis with atony. This type of lesion is referred to as lower motor neuron disease.

The presence of a lesion cranial to the reflex arc removes the normal inhibitory controlling inputs from the descending upper motor neuron pathways and results in spastic paralysis (stiffness). There is similar loss of voluntary motor function but stimulation of the reflex arc results in an exaggerated response referred to as upper motor neuron disease. Determination of fore- and hindlimb responses aids in the localization of a spinal lesion. Flexion of the stimulated limb with extension of the contralateral limb is referred to as a 'crossed extensor reflex' and indicates the presence of a CNS lesion above the reflex arc.

The clinical signs depend on the degree and location of spinal cord compression. Localization of a spinal cord lesion is achieved by evaluating the reflex pathways.

Cervical spinal lesions (C1–C6)

Cervical spinal lesions may result from vertebral body fractures associated with fighting injuries in rams, pharyngeal perforation in growing lambs, with infection tracking into the cervical vertebral canal, and vertebral body empyema (**398–401**) following pyaemia.

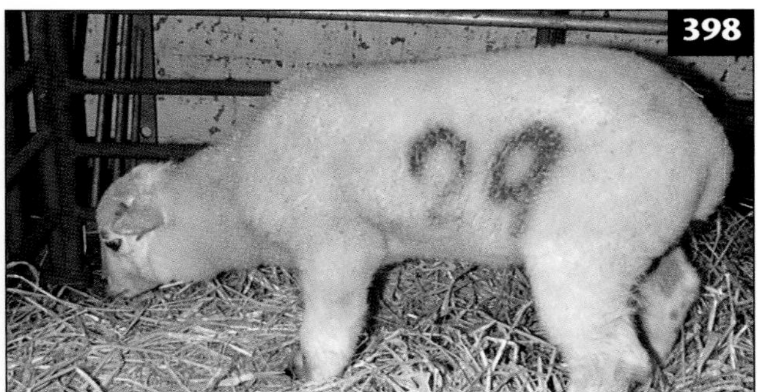

398 Tetraparesis and low head carriage in a four-week-old lamb with a compressive cervical spinal lesion.

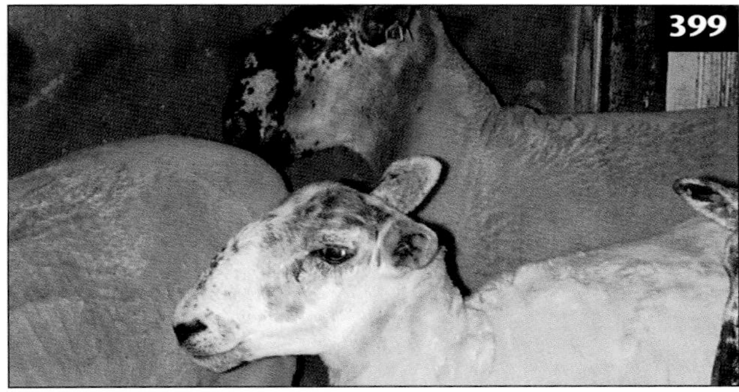

399 Compressive cervical spinal lesion in a gimmer. Compare the abnormal head carriage with the normal ewe in the background.

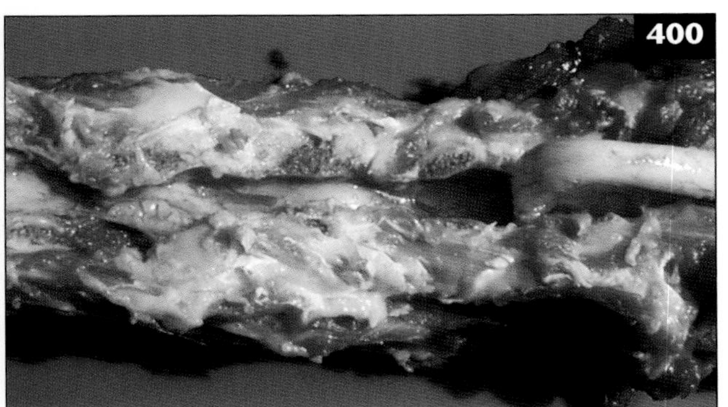

400 Necropsy revealed the lesion in the gimmer in 399.

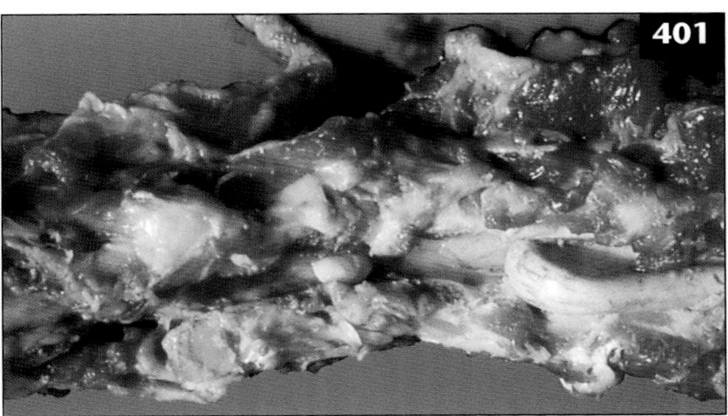

401 Further dissection of the lesion protruding into the spinal canal revealed an abscess.

In mildly compressive cervical lesions there is ataxia and weakness involving all four limbs (**402–404**), although the hindlimbs are usually more severely affected. There are hopping, placing and conscious proprioceptive deficits. The fore- and hindlimb reflexes are increased (upper motor neuron signs). Severely affected sheep may not be able to maintain sternal recumbency and will need to be supported.

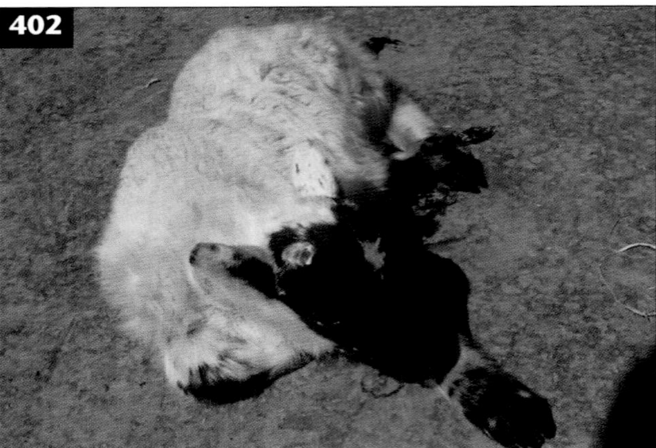

402 Tetraparesis in a two-week-old lamb suffering from cellulitis in the neck muscle resulting from a fox bite.

Brachial intumescence (C6–T2)
Spinal cord lesions involving the brachial intumescence may result in more severe deficits in the forelimbs than in the hindlimbs (**405**). Forelimb weakness is judged by the resistance to lateral movement of the animal by pushing the animal's shoulder away.

T2–L3
Animals with a spinal lesion caudal to T2 have normal forelimb function. These animals frequently adopt a dog-sitting posture with the hips flexed and the hindlimbs extended alongside the abdomen (**406, 407**)

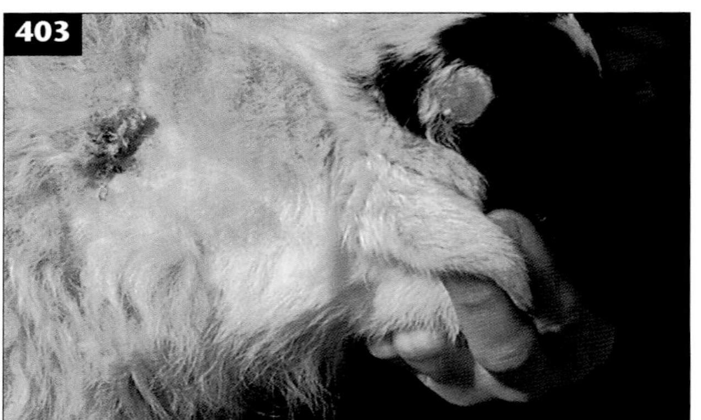

403 Abscess/cellulitis lesion in the lamb in **402**.

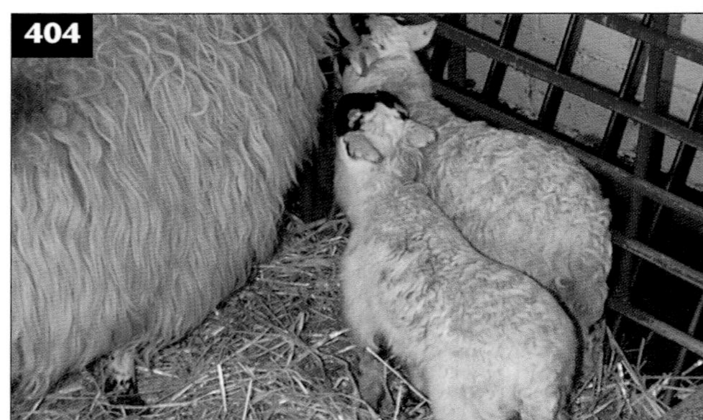

404 The lamb in **402** three days after antibiotic therapy and lancing the abscess.

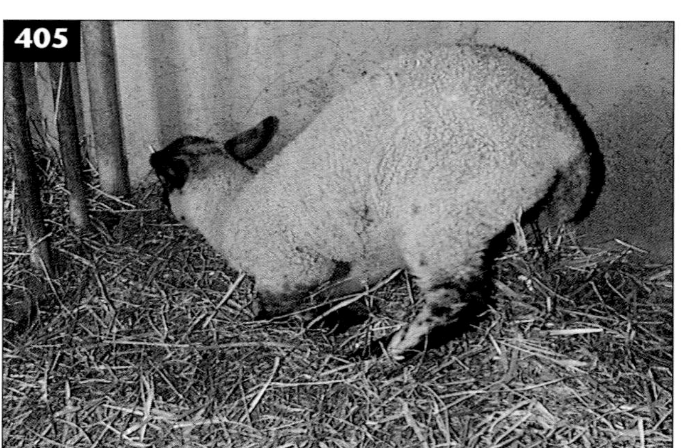

405 Compressive spinal lesion affecting C6–T2. The forelimbs are more severely affected than the hindimbs.

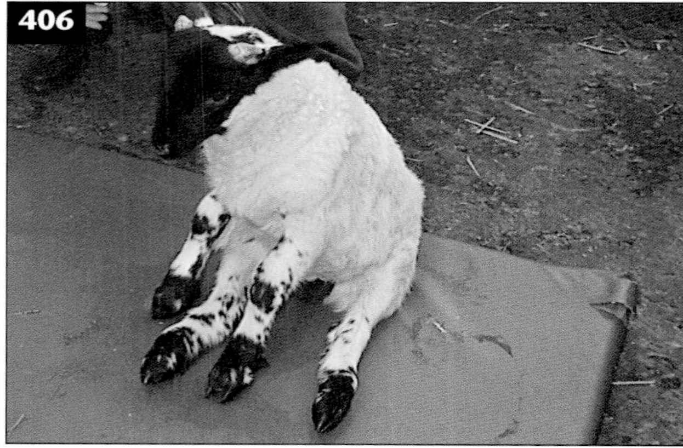

406 Dog-sitting posture in a four-week-old Scottish Blackface lamb with a compressive thoracolumbar lesion caused by tick bite pyaemia.

rather than in their normal flexed position underneath the body. The clinician's attention is immediately drawn to this abnormal posture because normal sheep always raise themselves with the hindlimbs first.

The presence of a spinal cord lesion in the thoracolumbar region (**408–410**) results in upper motor neuron signs of increased tendon jerk and withdrawal reflexes in the hindlimbs. There are conscious proprioceptive deficits and weakness of the hindlimbs.

The panniculus reflex is a useful means of localizing a thoracolumbar spinal lesion. The sensory stimulus travels to the spinal cord at the level of stimulation. The absence of reflex muscle contraction indicates the caudal aspect of the spinal lesion.

L4–S2

Lesions in the L4–S2 region result in flaccid paralysis of the hindlimbs with reduced or absent reflexes.

S1–S3

Lesions affecting S1–S3 cause hypotonia of the bladder and rectum, resulting in distension with urine and faeces, respectively.

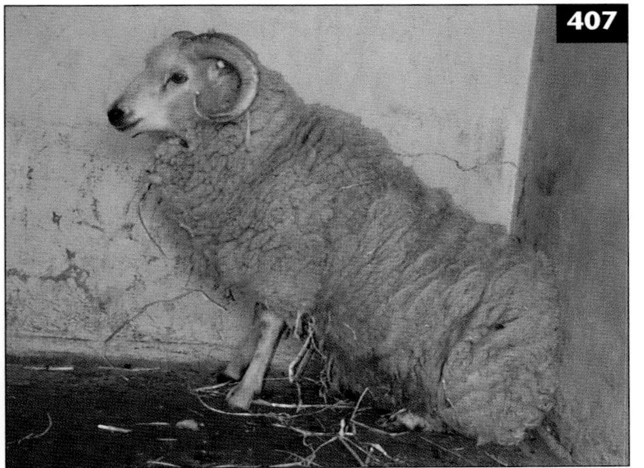

407 Dog-sitting posture in a yearling suffering from a compressive thoracolumbar lesion.

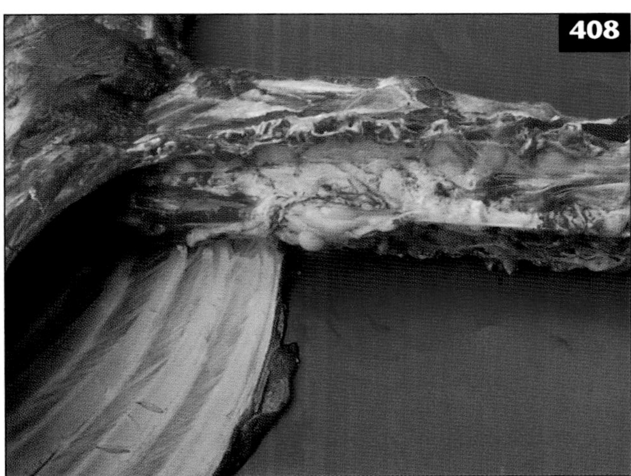

408 Vertebral empyema in the yearling in 407.

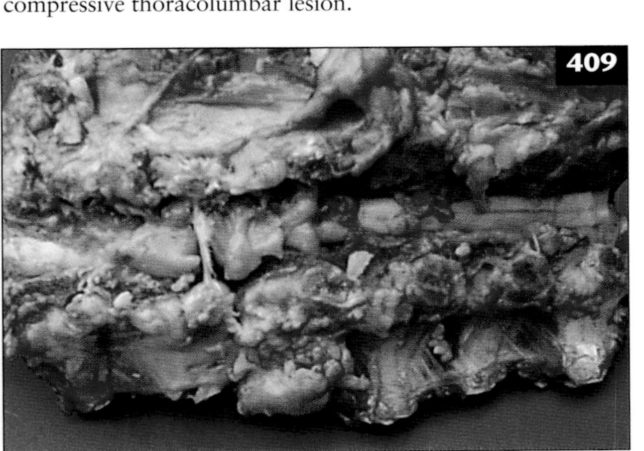

409 Further dissection of the lesion from the yearling in 407.

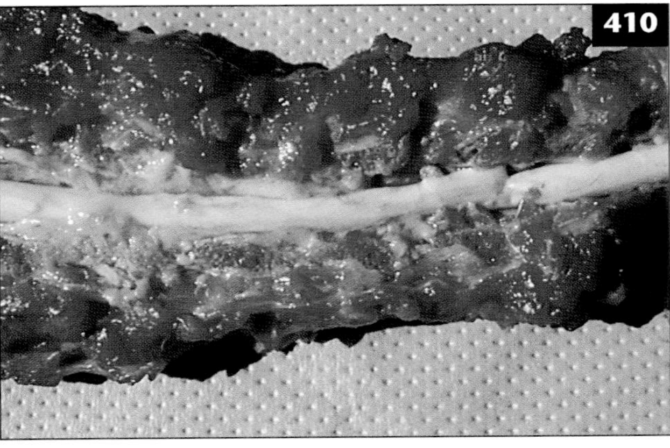

410 Vertebral empyema in the lumbar region causing cord compression.

Differential diagnoses

- Recumbency can be caused by a variety of conditions including limb fractures and painful joint lesions (e.g. bacterial polyarthritis, osteoarthritis and associated with endocarditis).
- Metabolic conditions causing recumbency and altered mentation, including OPT and hypocalcaemia, should be carefully considered in recumbent ewes during late gestation.

Diagnosis

A careful neurological examination should identify the section of the spinal cord involved in the disease process. Rapidity of onset, duration and change in clinical presentation, in addition to age and recent management practices of the animal, such as mixing mature rams, may provide some useful information.

Inflammatory lesions extending into the vertebral canal and causing spinal cord compression result in elevations in lumbar CSF protein concentration, typically >1.5 g/l (normal = 0.4 g/l).

Once the suspected lesion has been localized to a region of the spinal cord, radiography may allow identification of vertebral osteomyelitis. Myelography can be undertaken under general anaesthesia, but these more specific diagnostic procedures are too expensive except for particularly valuable breeding stock. Radiography may be helpful in identifying suspected fracture(s) of a cervical vertebra in a valuable ram.

Treatment

The extent of the vertebral empyema that precedes spinal cord compression, and the appearance of neurological dysfunction, is so severe that antibiotic treatment will never effect a cure; therefore, affected sheep must be humanely destroyed for welfare reasons.

Prevention/control measures

Prevention of tick bite pyaemia is described in Chapter 14 (Tick-borne diseases, p. 308). Vertebral empyema occurs sporadically in many other flocks where there are no specific prevention or control measures in place.

Economics

Significant losses may occur when infective lesions arise from tick bite pyaemia. Valuable breeding rams may occasionally be lost to cervical vertebral body fracture.

Welfare implications

Lambs with vertebral body empyema should be humanely destroyed once the condition has been determined. Predation may occur in extensive management systems.

KANGAROO GAIT

Definition/overview

Kangaroo gait is a rare locomotor disturbance, primarily of ewes during lactation, with spontaneous recovery after weaning. The condition has been reported occasionally in New Zealand and the UK but it has no economic or flock health implications. It is probable that the condition is greatly overdiagnosed due to incomplete clinical examination.

Aetiology

The cause of this condition is unknown.

Clinical presentation

There is bilateral forelimb weakness with the hindlimbs held well forward under the body. This propels the sheep forward with a characteristic bounding or 'kangaroo gait'.

Differential diagnoses

- Vertebral empyema compressing the brachial intumesence (C6–T2).
- Elbow arthritis.
- Virulent footrot or other painful condition affecting both forefeet.

Diagnosis

Careful clinical examination should exclude other possible causes of bilateral forelimb locomotor dysfunction. There is no confirmatory diagnosis and a diagnosis of kangaroo gait should be made with caution.

Treatment

There is no treatment and affected ewes recover spontaneously after weaning of their lambs.

Prevention/control measures

The rare occurrence of this disease and uncertain aetiology do not justify any action.

Economics

Kangaroo gait is of no economic significance.

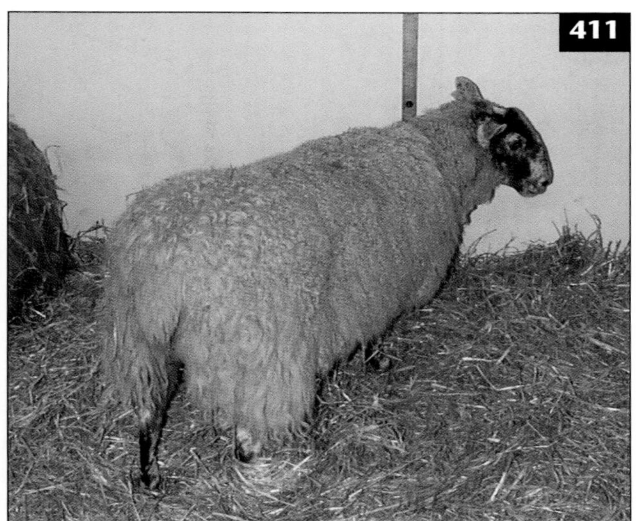

411 Greyface gimmer circling towards the right side with drooped right ear.

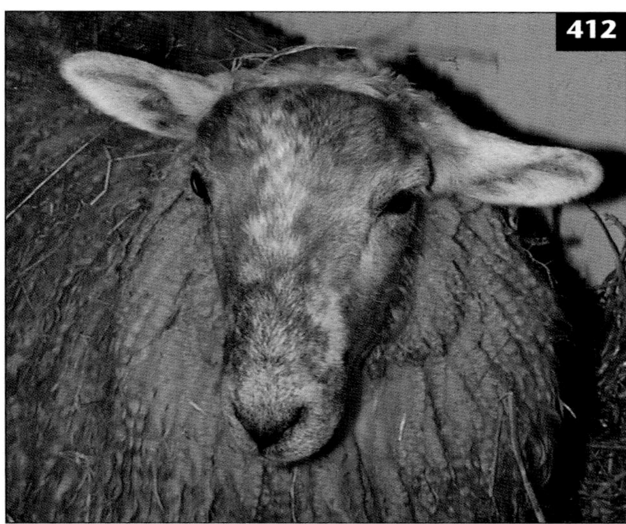

412 Drooping of the left ear, deviated muzzle towards the right, flaccid left lip and lowered left upper eyelid.

Welfare implications

If kangaroo gait is suspected, the ewe should be housed and fed appropriately and the lambs weaned as soon as practicable.

CLINICAL PROBLEM 1

Two gimmers (two year olds) (**411, 412**) are presented because they are displaying abnormal behaviour. The farmer reports that yesterday they were anorexic and appeared disorientated. Both gimmers are in good body condition (BCS 3.0).

Clinical examination

One gimmer is circling towards the right side, which has resulted in balling of straw around the right hindlimb (**411**). Closer examination reveals drooping of the right ear, muzzle deviated towards the left, flaccid right lip and lowered right upper eyelid. There is lack of menace response involving the right eye and drooling of saliva. The gimmer frequently pushes herself into a corner of the pen.

The other gimmer is less severely affected and shows drooping of the left ear, muzzle deviated towards the right, flaccid left lip and lowered left upper eyelid (**412**). There is lack of menace response involving the left eye, and drooling of salivation.

The farmer reports that four other sheep from his flock of 600 ewes have shown similar clinical signs during the past week. The signs progressed such that the sheep became unable to rise or maintain sternal recumbency and lay on one side. Involuntary running movements were common, leading rapidly to the development of pressure sores. All four sheep had died despite treatment with long-acting penicillin.

What conditions should be considered as differential diagnoses?
What is a possible provisional diagnosis?
What laboratory tests could be undertaken to confirm the provisional diagnosis?
What treatments should be administered?
What control measures should be recommended?

Differential diagnoses

Ovine pregnancy toxaemia

OPT commonly affects multigravid ewes (three or more fetuses) in poor body condition during the last four weeks of pregnancy rather than in primiparous sheep. Clinical examination reveals diffuse cerebral signs including central blindness, head pressing and depression, but there is frequently hyperaesthesia to tactile and auditory stimuli. Facial and trigeminal nerve paralysis are absent. 3-OH butyrate concentrations exceed 3.0 mmol/l, often >5.0 mmol/l.

Peripheral vestibular lesion
Peripheral vestibular lesions can present with head tilt, loss of balance, spontaneous horizontal nystagmus and, commonly, damage to the facial nerve causing ptosis and drooped ear. The appetite remains good and there is no depression or signs indicative of trigeminal nerve involvement. The response to conventional-dose antibiotic therapy is very good.

Brain abscessation/coenurosis
Brain abscessation and coenurosis generally involve only one cerebral hemisphere, and are uncommon in adult sheep. Affected sheep commonly present with circling, contralateral blindness and proprioceptive deficits, but no cranial nerve deficits.

Polioencephalomalacia
Sheep with PEM show signs of diffuse cerebral involvement such as blindness and altered mental state.

Listeriosis
Unilateral cranial nerve deficits involving trigeminal and facial nerves (often nerve nuclei much less frequently). Often show depression and propulsive tendency and may circle to the affected side.

Provisional diagnosis
A provisional diagnosis of listeriosis is based on the clinical examination, which can be supported by CSF collection and analysis and, in fatal cases, by histopathological examination of the brainstem and bacteriology.

Laboratory tests
Gross examination of CSF collected from these gimmers revealed protein concentrations of 1.6 and 1.8 g/l (normal = <0.4 g/l), with a mild increase in white cell concentration comprised of large mononuclear cells.

In unsuccessful cases, listeriosis can be confirmed only by isolation and identification of *L. monocytogenes*. If primary isolation attempts fail, ground brain tissue should be held at 4°C for several weeks and re-cultured weekly.

Treatment
The gimmers were treated with penicillin G (200,000 iu/kg i/m followed by 44,000 iu/kg i/m q12h for 4 consecutive days). Dexamethasone (1.1 mg/kg i/v) was also given at the time of the first antibiotic injection.

Outcome
Both gimmers made an uneventful recovery.

Control measures
While outbreaks of listeriosis often stop abruptly even when there have been no management changes, feeding of second cut silage of dubious quality was discontinued and the sheep were fed first cut silage. The poorer silage was fed to adult cattle without any problem of listeriosis. Despite the change in silage, two further cases of listeriosis occurred in the sheep flock in the next ten days from infection gained when the poorer quality silage was fed.

CLINICAL PROBLEM 2

A five-week-old Blackface-cross lamb is presented. It is unable to bear weight on its hindlimbs and frequently dog sits (**413**). The flock is inspected daily and this abnormal posture was first noted by the farmer three days ago.

What is the probable cause?
How could the provisional diagnosis be confirmed and what action should be taken?
How could this condition be prevented?

Clinical examination
The lamb is bright and alert and adopts a dog-sitting posture (**413**). There are no cranial nerve deficits. The patellar reflex is increased in both hindlimbs.

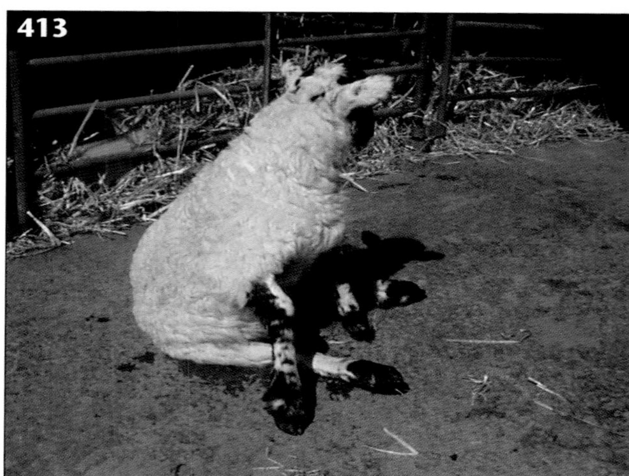

413 Dog-sitting posture in a Blackface lamb.

Pinching the coronary band with artery forceps elicits an exaggerated response characterized by rapid, forceful withdrawal. The stimulated limb remains flexed for a short period and there is extension of the contralateral hindlimb. This reaction, coupled with the increased patellar response, indicates loss of the upper motor neuron pathways to the limb (upper motor neuron signs). No other abnormalities are found during the clinical examination. Forelimb function is normal.

Diagnosis

Upper motor neuron signs to the hindlimbs with normal forelimb function could be explained by a spinal cord lesion between T2 and L3. Vertebral empyema would be the most likely cause, resulting in compression of the spinal cord affecting both hindlimbs.

Other conditions to consider include delayed swayback and white muscle disease but these can be excluded during the clinical examination. Sarcocystosis is uncommon in such young lambs.

Further diagnostic tests

Lumbar CSF protein concentration was 2.6 g/l (normal = <0.4 g/l), consistent with a compressive lesion resulting from vertebral empyema.

Action

The lamb was destroyed for welfare reasons. Postmortem examination revealed a vertebral body empyema at T13/L1 (**414**).

Prevention

Appling good hygiene measures in the lambing shed and ensuring passive antibody transfer should help to prevent such infections. There is no conclusive evidence to suggest that such infections arise as a consequence of bacteraemia originating from tail docking wounds using elastrator rings.

In areas where tick bite pyaemia is a problem and causes vertebral empyema, prevention should include the application of a synthetic pyrethroid preparation to control ticks and, possibly, an injection of long-acting oxytetracycline to help control tick-borne fever when the lambs are turned on to potentially infested pastures.

CLINICAL PROBLEM 3

A five-month-old weaned Suffolk-cross wether lamb is presented. It is isolated from other sheep in the group and appears blind (**415**). The lambs in the group had been weaned two weeks previously, drenched with an anthelmintic at that time, and vaccinated for a second time against clostridial diseases.

Clinical examination

The lamb is bright and alert but blind and wanders aimlessly bleating to attract other sheep in the group. There is bilateral loss of menace response but no cranial nerve deficits. Presently, there is no dorsiflexion of the neck or strabismus. The rectal temperature is normal.

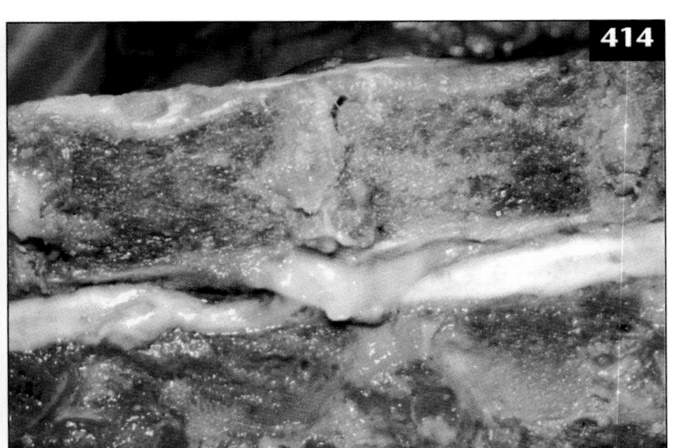

414 Vertebral body empyema at T13/L1.

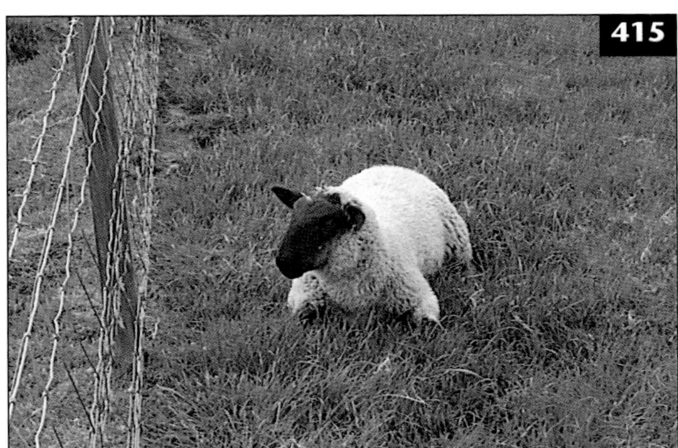

415 Five-month-old weaned Suffolk-cross wether lamb, which is isolated from other sheep in the group and appears blind.

No abnormalities are heard during auscultation of the chest. There is very little rumen content and no evidence of diarrhoea. There is occasional teeth grinding. No other abnormalities are detected during clinical examination.

What conditions should be considered?
What treatment should be administered?

Differential diagnoses

- Polioencephalomalacia.
- Nephrosis.
- Focal symmetrical encephalomalacia.
- Sarcocystosis.
- Listeriosis.
- Brain abscessation.
- Coenurosis.

Diagnosis

Early stages of polioencephalomalacia.

Treatment

The lamb was injected with thiamine (10 mg/kg i/v q12h). There is anecdotal evidence from field studies that giving dexamethasone (1.0 mg/kg i/v), or a similar short-acting corticosteroid, on initial examination aids recovery. Twice daily intramuscular injections of thiamine were given for the next three days.

Outcome

There was a rapid response to intravenous thiamine and the lamb was much improved 24 hours later. One further case of PEM occurred in this group of 340 lambs one week later.

8 Musculoskeletal System

INTRODUCTION

The musculoskeletal system comprises the skeleton, joints, ligaments, tendons and muscles. Together with the nervous system, it is responsible for the animal's stance and gait. Infections of the musculoskeletal system are common in sheep; polyarthritis is common in neonates and footrot is especially common in growing lambs and adults. Arthritic changes, commonly predisposed by trauma, are largely confined to the elbow and stifle joints. Clinical involvement of the musculoskeletal system is manifest as lameness and, much less commonly, as weakness.

ASSESSMENT OF THE PROBLEM(S)

While the history is important it is not always correct, as farmers invariably understate both the severity and duration of any problem. In addition, individual sheep may not be recognized, and their lameness not recorded, in an extensive management system.

The extent of the lameness problem within the group must be defined by the veterinarian before the sheep are penned, otherwise the lameness of many sheep will be masked by their close confinement. It is best to walk quietly through the sheep while they are still at pasture in order to quantify accurately the extent and severity of the problem(s).

It may be possible to select lame sheep from the group by slowly walking the sheep through a gate into another field; lame sheep will trail behind their sound peers and may even lie down if the lameness is severe, so the majority of the lame sheep can be separated from the group. This method is not always successful as the flocking instinct and fear of separation may temporarily override the pain of the lameness. Diseases of other organ systems, such as respiratory disease, may also cause exercise intolerance.

ASSESSMENT OF THE HANDLING FACILITIES

While on the farm it may be advisable to check the sheep handling facilities and those used for foot bathing, their suitability for the number of sheep, and their care and maintenance. Treatment records, if kept, should be consulted.

OBSERVATION

Sheep with moderate to severe lameness and weakness spend increased time in sternal, or even lateral, recumbency. Prolonged periods in sternal recumbency result in carpal and brisket sores, which are slow to heal. Brisket sores in rams can also be caused by poorly fitted harnesses.

Distant observation of sheep for the presence of muscle atrophy is often masked by the presence of a full fleece. Painful lesions affecting the forelimb often result in increased extension (or reduced flexion) of the joints when the sheep is in sternal recumbency; the forelimb is held forward of the chest rather than in its normal position flexed alongside the chest. Painful lesions affecting the foot and distal joints, as well as elbow arthritis, cause sheep to graze on their knees, leading to abrasions and thickening of the skin overlying the knees. Repeated skin trauma over the cranial aspect of the carpal joints may result in discoloration of the hairs at the periphery of these callused areas; typically, black hairs re-grow grey or white. Painful forelimb lesions result in the hind feet being drawn forward under the body to achieve greater weight bearing.

Painful lesions affecting a hindlimb generally result in the affected hindlimb being uppermost when a sheep is in sternal recumbency. This position allows the sheep to use its lower hindlimb to propel itself forward and up during rising.

Lameness is best defined when the animal is made to trot slowly in a straight line on a firm level surface both towards and away from the observer. While this is possible in horses, such assessment is not possible in sheep. Individual sheep often fear the presence of humans and either do not move or attempt to escape by jumping at fences etc. The best compromise is to walk the lame sheep with another sheep from the same group on a firm level surface in a confined area and observe them from a distance of 15–20 metres. It is not usual for a sheep to be lame on more than one limb. Lambs with polyarthritis and sheep with endocarditis may be lame on all four limbs.

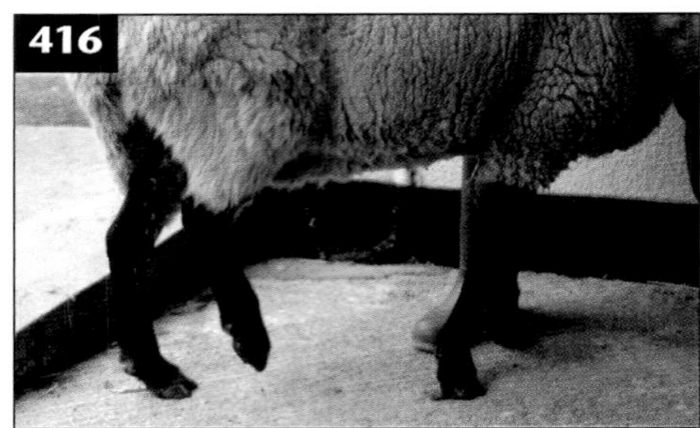

416 Severe lameness (10/10 lame) in a Suffolk lamb.

The extent of the lameness is scored subjectively on a 10 point scale; 1 being very slight lameness up to 10, which is non-weight bearing even at rest (**416**) with the sheep unwilling to take even one or two steps forward. Typically, long bone fractures and septic joints result in severe (10/10) lameness but so too can white line abscesses, especially those that track up to the coronary band. Therefore, the degree of lameness does not necessarily determine prognosis.

CLINICAL EXAMINATION

The clinician must always remember that lameness originates from a painful lesion and that manipulations should be kept to a minimum and undertaken with care and empathy. In particular, joint lesions are especially painful; manipulations to elicit crepitus are unnecessary and cruel. The clinical examination must not exacerbate the degree of lameness; this merely reflects poor examination technique. Gentle digital palpation will reveal much more information regarding joint effusion and thickness of the joint capsule than trying to elicit crepitus by forceful movement of the joint. The more sensitive the palpation process, the more information is gleaned.

The extent of muscle wastage depends on both the severity and the duration of lameness. Muscle wastage can be reliably detected after 5–7 days of moderate to severe lameness by careful palpation over bony prominences such as the spine of the scapula and the head of the femur for forelimbs and hindlimbs, respectively. Visual detection of muscle wastage is usually prevented by the presence of a full fleece. Comparison of changes with the contralateral limb, if sound, is recommended. In cases of elbow arthritis where there is considerable enthesophyte formation, the breadth of the affected joint should be measured with callipers and compared with measurements from sound sheep of similar breed, sex and age.

Enlargement of the prescapular lymph node (2–5 times normal size) can be readily appreciated within 3–7 days of bacterial infection of forelimb joints and cellulitis lesions. White line and sole abscesses and footrot lesions do not usually cause such obvious drainage lymph node enlargement. Infected lesions distal to the stifle joint cause enlargement of the popliteal lymph node but this node is not readily palpable unless there is considerable muscle atrophy. Infection proximal to the stifle joint results in enlargement of the deep inguinal lymph nodes within the pelvic canal.

Casting the sheep to permit detailed examination of the foot/feet is performed as the last component of the examination. This must not be undertaken if there is a painful joint lesion or suspected fracture. The interdigital space is examined and any impacted foreign material removed. All overgrown horn from the abaxial walls and toes is removed with shears or a sharp hoof knife. Then, all underrun horn, commencing at the axial margin of the sole, should be removed. This underrun horn is often soft and rubbery and difficult to cut with a hoof knife or shears. A scalpel blade (or Stanley knife) can be used to excise the underrun sole horn once it has been lifted clear of the corium using forceps.

Underrunning of the sole horn associated with virulent footrot is very painful and it may be best to treat these lesions topically with oxytetracycline and, perhaps, parenteral antibiotics, returning to the foot trimming 2–3 days later when the lesions are less aggressive and less painful. It is important not to damage the sensitive corium as this will lead to delayed regeneration of epithelium and extended healing time. Exposure of the sensitive corium to irritant chemicals, such as formalin, may result in excess granulation tissue and the development of a toe fibroma.

Turning crates are commonly used to facilitate turning and restraint of sheep in dorsal recumbency during foot paring, and they are well tolerated.

ARTHROCENTESIS

Arthrocentesis is not commonly undertaken in sheep because joint infection with the common bacterial pathogens *Streptococcus dysgalactiae* and *Erysipelothrix rhusiopathiae* does not cause marked joint effusion. Attempts can be made to collect synovial fluid from distended joints under local anaesthesia but anaesthetic can only be given subcutaneously; the joint capsule/synovial membrane cannot readily be desensitized. The arthrocentesis site is shaved and prepared aseptically. In general the joint capsule is punctured where it is most distended, as this 'pouching' occurs away from structures such as ligaments and tendons.

Normal synovial fluid is pale yellow, viscous, clear and does not clot. The protein concentration is <18 g/l, with a low white cell concentration comprised mainly of lymphocytes. Septic arthritis is characterized by a turbid sample caused by an increased white cell concentration, which is comprised almost exclusively of neutrophils. The protein concentration is increased to >40 g/l.

Samples collected from chronically infected joints frequently fail to grow bacteria. Direct smears of the aspirate can be made on to a glass slide and stained with Gram's stain to gain some information of the potential pathogen(s) involved. When investigating a flock outbreak, the best means of establishing the cause is to sacrifice a typical early case, which has received no antibiotic therapy, and submit a sample of synovial membrane from several affected joints to the laboratory.

RADIOGRAPHY

Radiography is most useful in the investigation of long bone fractures distal to the elbow and stifle joints. Deep sedation or, preferably, general anaesthesia may be required to allow correct positioning of the sheep for radiography of the humerus and femur. Enthesophyte formation is common in the elbow joint of adult sheep, and the best radiographic results are obtained from an oblique view. Radiography may prove useful in the investigation of chronic cases of septic pedal arthritis, where new bone formation may have led to arthrodesis of the distal interphalangeal joint.

Radiography adds little new information to the investigation of most cases of septic arthritis other than to reveal widening of the joint space and osteophyte formation. Indeed, radiography of a septic joint, which reveals only widening of the joint space, may be mistakenly interpreted as little pathology being present. In such cases ultrasonography, and arthrocentesis if the joint is distended, are more informative.

ULTRASONOGRAPHY

Ultrasonography using a 7.5 MHz linear array scanner can provide useful information regarding the thickness of the joint capsule and the extent and nature of any joint effusion. The skin overlying the joint is shaved to ensure good contact. A stand-off may be required for examination of smaller joints. Affected joint(s) should be compared with the contralateral joint where normal. Ultrasonography has numerous advantages over radiography for joint examination in that the procedure is cheap, reveals more detail of soft tissue, involves no health and safety concerns and is readily portable for on-farm examinations.

Ultrasound examination of the joint should be undertaken prior to arthrocentesis to determine the presence of an effusion.

NERVE BLOCKS

Unlike horses, nerve blocks and intra-articular anaesthesia are rarely, if ever, used in sheep.

OVINE INTERDIGITAL DERMATITIS

Definition/overview

Ovine interdigital dermatitis is an acute necrotizing infection of the interdigital skin caused by *Fusobacterium necrophorum*. It is most commonly seen affecting intensively managed, densely stocked lambs aged 4–10 weeks, causing considerable lameness and a morbidity rate that can rapidly exceed 50% in less than one week. Infection is much more common during periods of warm wet weather.

Aetiology

Infection with *F. necrophorum* is predisposed by wet conditions and trauma to the interdigital skin.

Clinical presentation

Ovine interdigital dermatitis causes severe lameness, particularly of the forelimbs (**417**), resulting in lambs grazing on their knees or spending long periods in sternal

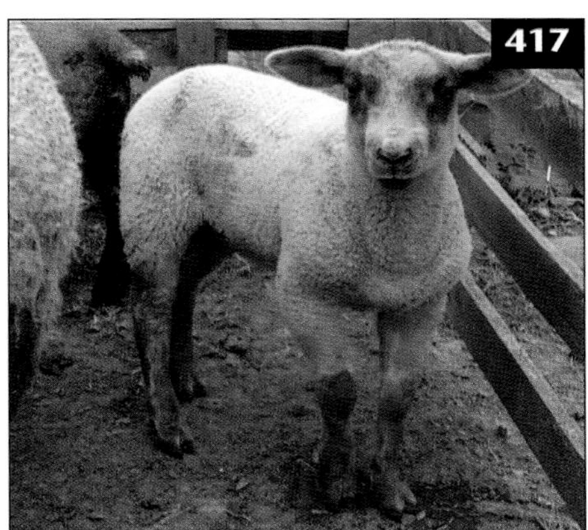

417 Ovine interdigital dermatitis in a six-week-old lamb causing marked forelimb lameness.

recumbency. There is sudden-onset severe lameness, such that lambs may not put the affected foot to the ground.

Close examination reveals marked hyperaemia of interdigital skin, with superficial accumulations of moist, whitish necrotic material (**418**). Much less commonly, the infection may extend into the subcutaneous tissues. Unlike footrot, there is no underrunning of the horn of the axial hoof wall.

Differential diagnoses

Sudden-onset severe lameness affecting one or more growing lambs could also be caused by erysipelas, which can be readily differentiated on clinical examination.

Diagnosis

Diagnosis is based on clinical examination and rapid response to topical oxytetracycline spray or other bactericidal agent.

Treatment

If possible, the flock should be moved to dry pasture, where spontaneous recovery may occur, but this is not an option in most situations. In the UK, for example, the method of choice is to turn every lamb and treat all affected feet with topical oxytetracycline aerosol but this is very labour intensive. Affected lambs are identified and topical treatment repeated two days later if necessary. Surprisingly, despite the severe lameness at treatment, there is return to full soundness within days of first treatment.

The use of 5% formalin footbaths produces acceptable results but young lambs do not go through a footbath easily. Lambs are often considerably lamer for a short period after formalin foot bathing. Zinc sulphate, as a 10% solution with sodium lauryl sulphate added as a wetting agent, has largely replaced formalin in footbaths.

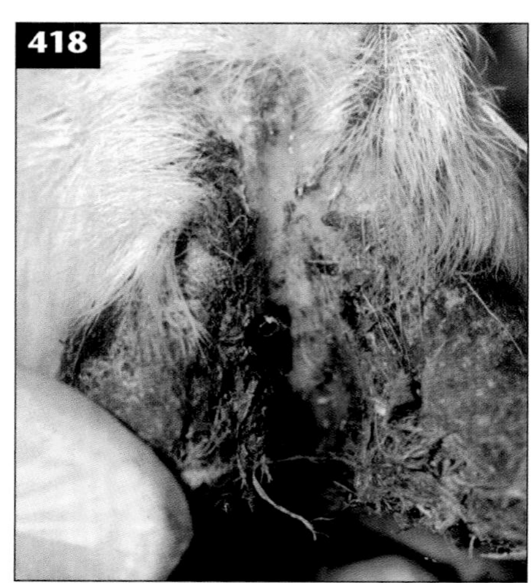

418 Marked hyperaemia of interdigital skin with superficial accumulations of moist whitish necrotic material.

Prevention/control measures

Footbaths can be used at weekly intervals to control foot infections, although less frequent foot bathing (e.g. every two weeks) will usually contain the problem.

Economics

Ovine interdigital dermatitis can cause severe lameness and an abrupt check in growth rate in growing lambs, with a consequent extended interval to marketing if left untreated for a week or more. Footbaths are an inexpensive means of treatment, although extra labour may be necessary to handle young lambs when they are passing through the footbath for the first time.

Welfare implications

Ovine interdigital dermatitis can cause severe lameness, which necessitates prompt treatment. Zinc sulphate is preferred to formalin in the footbaths.

FOOTROT

Definition/overview

Footrot is the term used to describe the highly contagious foot disease caused by the synergistic action of *Dichelobacter nodosus* and *Fusobacterium necrophorum*. Footrot is a major concern in all countries where sheep are managed intensively. It causes serious welfare concerns and leads to significant lost production due to lameness. Losses result from reduced wool production, poorer wool quality, lowered live weight gain/poorer body condition and reduced reproductive performance. Ram lameness during the breeding season can cause a significant reduction in reproductive performance, with rams reluctant or unable to serve ewes. Footrot eradication schemes are in operation in a number of countries, most notably Australia, and some drier area of New Zealand, where the climatic and environmental conditions are more conducive to such programmes than in the UK.

There is a wide range of clinical signs attributed to these two organisms. Two forms of the disease are generally described:

- **Benign footrot or scald:** inflammation and superficial infection of the interdigital skin, which extends only to involve the hoof horn of the axial wall. Such infection is caused by strains of *D. nodosus* with low protease activity.
- **Virulent footrot:** extensive separation and underrunning of the hoof horn. Lesions start at the junction of the skin and axial wall horn and spread abaxially to underrun the sole and, possibly, the

abaxial wall. There is a characteristic smell of necrotic horn/exudate. The whole hoof capsule may be shed in severe cases. Chronic infection leads to grossly misshapen hooves.

The role of spirochaetes in the aetiology of severe dermatitis of the digits in sheep is currently under investigation. This condition has been referred to as ovine digital dermatitis because of similarities in the clinical appearance and, perhaps, aetiology to the condition of digital dermatitis reported in cattle.

Aetiology

Outbreaks of virulent footrot are typically seen in warm wet conditions during late spring/early summer and they are also often encountered in housed sheep during the winter months (**419**).

F. necrophorum invades the interdigital skin following wet underfoot conditions and superficial trauma. *F. necrophorum* produces both endotoxins and exotoxins, which result in epidermal necrosis. The resultant inflammatory reaction is commonly referred to as ovine interdigital dermatitis. The inflamed and compromised skin is then susceptible to *D. nodosus* infection. *D. nodosus* is an obligate anaerobic organism found only in the feet of ruminants affected by footrot but it can survive in the environment for no longer than 7–14 days. Therefore, disease is introduced into a flock by the purchase of infected carrier sheep. This carrier state may persist for 2–3 years.

The synergistic effect of *D. nodosus* and *F. necrophorum* causes lysis of the epidermal matrices, leading to the separation of hoof horn typically seen in virulent footrot. *D. nodosus* invasion leads to slow but persistent infection. Strains of *D. nodosus* vary in the extent to which they produce keratinolytic proteases and this property directly determines their invasive capacity. Strains of *D. nodosus* with low protease activity cause mild lesions affecting only the hoof of the axial wall (benign footrot); strains of *D. nodosus* with high protease activity may extend to cause complete separation of the hoof capsule from the corium in severe cases (virulent footrot).

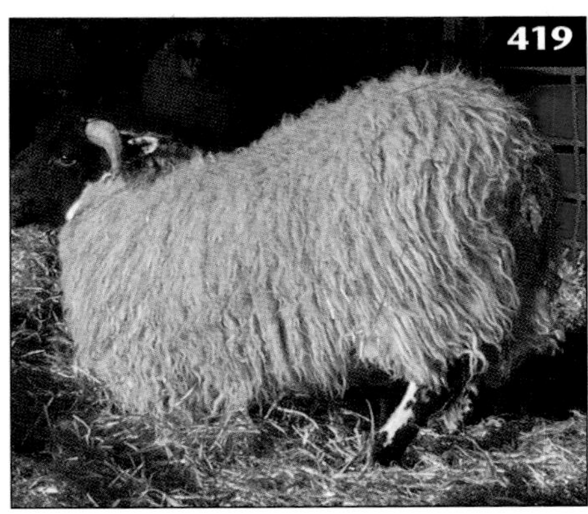

419 Severe bilateral forelimb lameness in a housed Scottish Blackface lamb.

Clinical presentation

Benign footrot

The clinical appearance of benign footrot is not dissimilar to ovine interdigital dermatitis, although limited involvement of the hoof horn of the axial wall does result. The lameness is mild to moderate and very much less severe than that encountered in cases of virulent footrot.

Virulent footrot

The initial stage comprises an interdigital infection with hyperaemia, swelling and moistening of the interdigital skin. The axial hoof horn margin becomes separated from the skin, appearing as a thin irregular white strip 2–3 mm wide. Separation and erosion of horn at the heel region of the axial wall progresses until it underruns abaxially and towards the toe (**420, 421**). The axial margin of the solar horn has a multilayered, ragged appearance and is soft and pliable. The solar

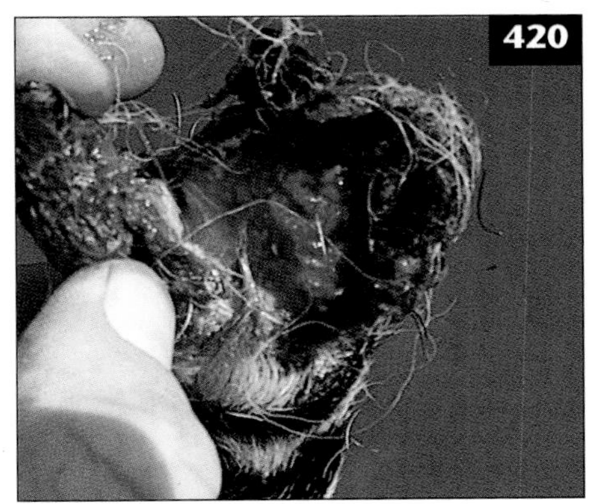

420 Virulent footrot with underrunning of the horn of the sole extending to the abaxial wall.

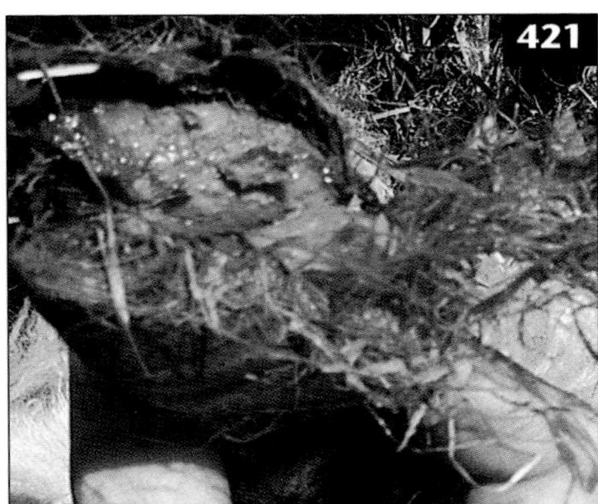

421 Virulent footrot with underrunning of the horn extending up the abaxial wall.

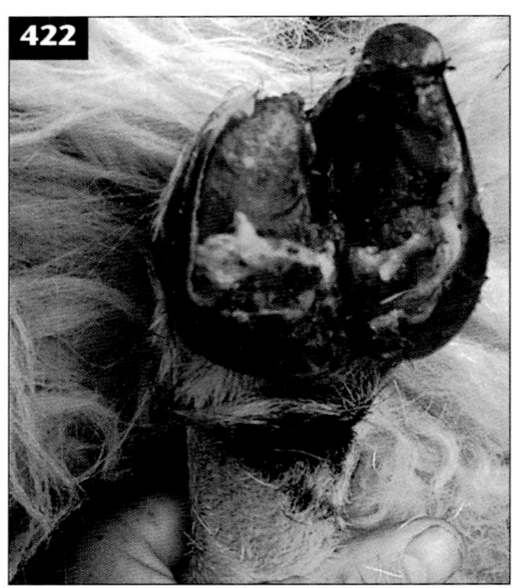

422 Virulent footrot with underrunning of the horn of both soles.

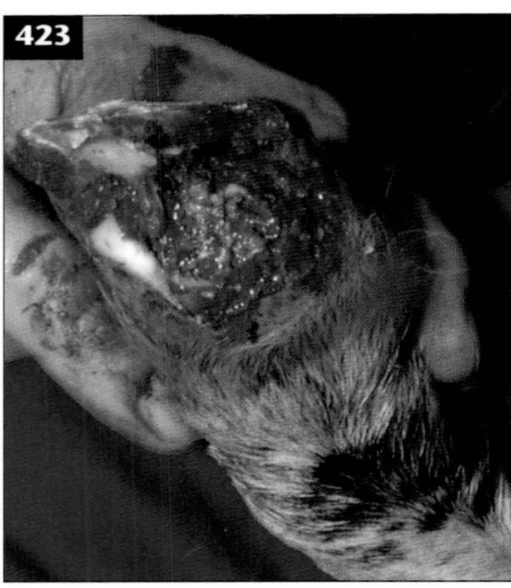

423 Virulent footrot with underrunning of the horn extending up the abaxial wall to the coronary band.

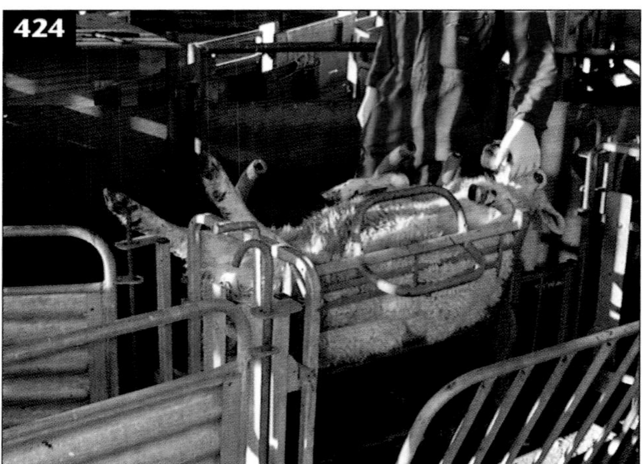

424 Foot turning crates make working conditions easier for stockmen.

horn can be grasped and lifted up, exposing the underlying corium (**422**), which is reddened and granular, and bleeds readily. The infection may extend to underrun the abaxial hoof wall (**423**). Usually, both claws of the foot are affected but not necessarily to the same extent. There is a characteristic grey foul-smelling exudate. At this stage the sheep is severely lame and may not rest the foot on the ground. Lameness affecting two or more feet causes the sheep to spend long periods in sternal recumbency.

Myiasis is not uncommon in cases of virulent footrot.

Differential diagnoses

- In individual sheep the differential diagnosis of severe lameness caused by virulent footrot includes white line abscess and septic pedal arthritis.
- Ovine digital dermatitis may also present as an outbreak of marked lameness affecting a large percentage of sheep in the group, but more commonly it affects growing lambs rather than adult sheep.

Diagnosis

Diagnosis is based on clinical examination with findings of extensive underrunning of hoof horn. A lesion scoring system has been developed in Australia as part of the eradication programme. Strain typing of *D. nodosus* is rarely undertaken in other countries.

Treatment

The standard approach to footrot treatment involves removal of all underrun horn (**424**). Particular attention should be paid to the axial wall. If the feet are severely affected and painful, it is prudent first to treat the sheep with parenteral antibiotics for welfare reasons and then pare the feet several days later. In some studies, single large doses of parenteral oxytetracycline or penicillin have been found useful for treating severely affected sheep. Sheep with considerable exposure of the corium should not enter a formalin footbath; rather the diseased horn should also be sprayed with oxytetracycline aerosol at the time of parenteral antibiotic therapy.

The remaining sheep in the group should then enter a footbath containing either 5% formalin or 10% zinc sulphate solution containing sodium lauryl sulphate (**425**). It is essential to ensure sufficient contact time between the chemical and diseased tissue (2–5 minutes for 5% formalin solutions and up to 60 minutes for 10% zinc sulphate solution). Footbaths can be used at weekly intervals.

Overzealous paring and exposure of the sensitive corium, in combination with frequent formalin footbath treatments, may result in the generation of toe fibromas.

Prevention/control measures

Footrot spreads under wet, warm conditions at pasture, and in housed sheep (**426, 427**). A dense sward is associated with a higher incidence of footrot, with little or no spread during very dry weather. Control programmes are much more likely to be successful during non-transmission stages if prolonged dry environmental conditions exist at some stage in the year. In the UK, for example, foot paring is often undertaken before ewes are turned out to pasture with their lambs (**428**), which may serve only to remove overgrown horn.

Wherever possible, sheep producers should maintain a closed flock in order to prevent purchasing in diseased sheep. If purchases are essential, ewe lambs should be bought from known sources rather than old ewes, which are often chronic carriers. All purchased stock must be quarantined for one month and examined for footrot before introduction into the main flock. Foot bathing should be undertaken regularly during this quarantine period.

Prior infection does not confer any appreciable immunity. There are some reported split-flock trials of footrot vaccines in the UK that have shown beneficial results.

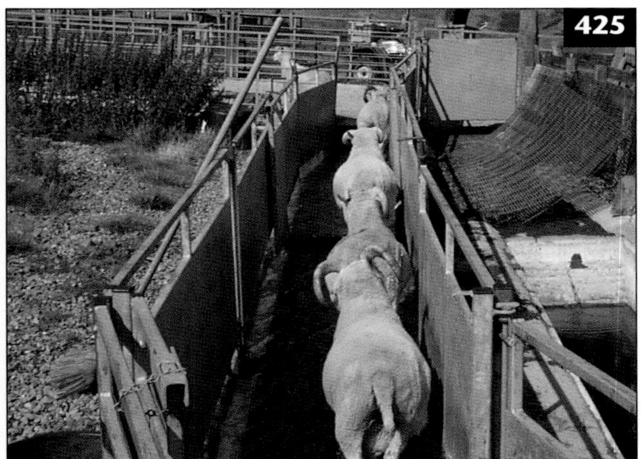

425 Footbaths should be of sufficient length to ensure contact with the chemical used. A dry stand afterwards is essential.

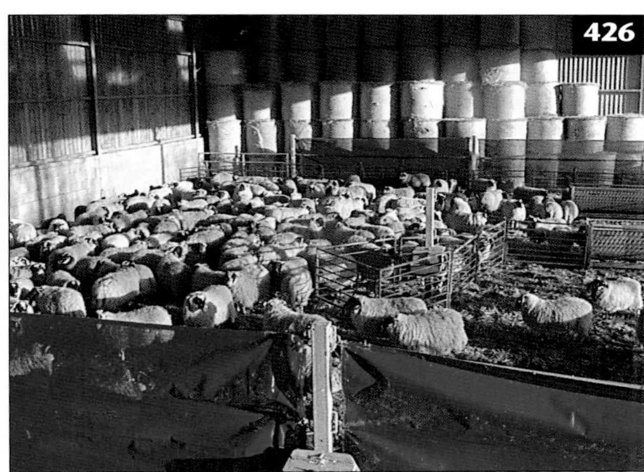

426 Buildings should have adequate drainage, which is not always the case with multi-purpose buildings.

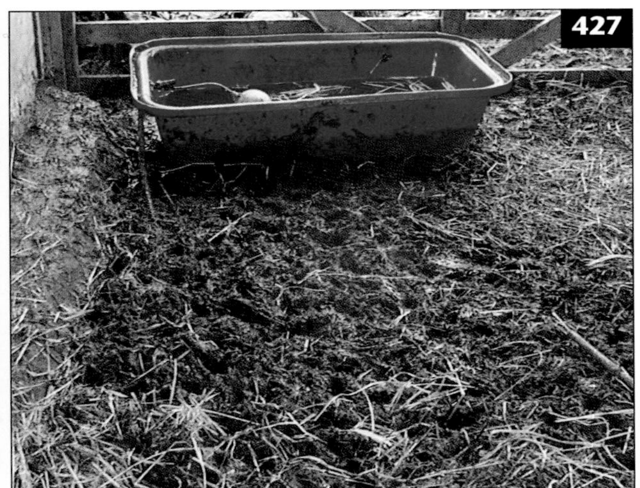

427 Waterlogged bedding from leaking water troughs increases the spread of footrot.

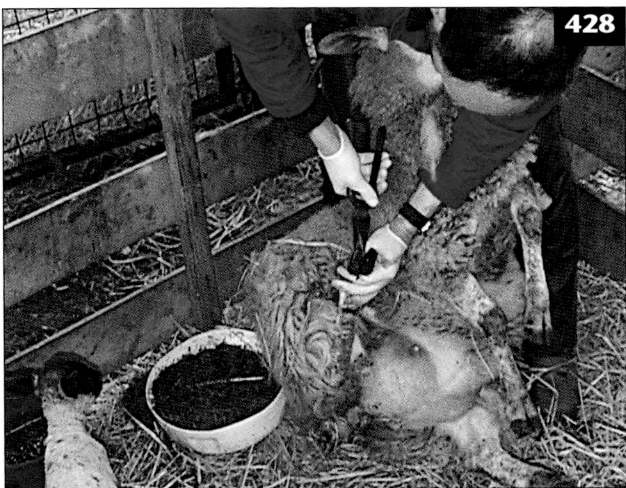

428 Routine foot paring at lambing time.

Disadvantages associated with vaccination, including cost (up to 2% of the value of the sheep), short duration (booster vaccinations required every six months or before the anticipated challenge period) and occasional severe localized reaction at the injection site, have limited their widespread use. Poor injection technique has resulted in infection tracking into the extradural space in the cervical region, causing tetraparesis in a small percentage of sheep. Accidental self-injection is a serious concern and it is recommended that the operator report immediately to the nearest Accident and Emergency Department with the data sheet should this occur.

The vaccine used in the UK contains ten strains of inactivated *D. nodosus* with an oil adjuvant. It is recommended that all sheep are vaccinated, thus limiting future environmental contamination and challenge. A single dose of vaccine is given, which can be boosted 4–6 weeks later if significant levels of disease still remain in the flock. Subsequent doses should be administered according to prevailing conditions or in anticipation of the climatic conditions that favour disease.

All breeds are susceptible to footrot. In the UK, Suffolk sheep are more susceptible than most other breeds when co-grazed. In New Zealand, British breeds are more resistant than Merino sheep. There is variation in susceptibility to footrot within a breed and breeding for resistance to footrot is feasible; however, progress is slow.

While cattle are suitable hosts for *D. nodosus*, these strains are usually benign for sheep, allowing some degree of control by alternate grazing or co-grazing.

Eradication of footrot has been achieved in many areas of Australia but is unlikely to be achieved in the UK due to environmental and climatic conditions.

Economics
The financial impact of footrot varies between farms within a region, between regions and between countries. In many situations, particularly in Australia, footrot is regarded as the single most important disease limiting production of sheep.

Welfare implications
Virulent footrot is a very painful condition. Because of its high prevalence, severity and chronicity, with extended convalescence after treatment, virulent footrot is considered to be an important welfare issue. Welfare problems arise with footrot because:

- High-dose antibiotic therapy is expensive relative to the value of many commercial value sheep, particularly store lambs. The cost of such treatment may be equivalent to half or all of the annual veterinary and medicine fees for a breeding sheep.
- Labour requirements. Foot paring is a skilled, time-consuming procedure. It has been estimated that a shepherd can reasonably be expected to trim the feet of 150 sheep per day. The use of a sheep turning crate greatly facilitates foot paring. Veterinary instruction is essential before a farmer embarks on a control programme to ensure that paring is undertaken correctly. Foot bathing is time-consuming because few farmers have invested in adequate facilities. In particular, few farms have sufficient dry standing areas available after foot bathing. When not undertaken correctly, gathering and inappropriate foot bathing may simply serve to spread infection further.
- Distant grazings. Sheep are often grazed considerable distances away from centralized foot bathing facilities. Sheep are often grazed on more distant pastures during the summer months, a time when transmission of footrot is at its peak. While mobile facilities can be used, again there are rarely dry standing facilities available after foot bathing.
- Inadequate instruction regarding effective control of footrot.

TOE FIBROMA/GRANULOMA

Definition/overview
Toe fibromas most commonly result from overzealous foot paring, with exposure of the corium, and excessive use of formalin footbaths. Toe fibromas can occur in association with virulent footrot where horn lysis results in exposure of the corium. Toe fibromas are in themselves not painful but exposure and infection of the adjacent corium leads to lameness.

Aetiology
Repeated insult to the exposed corium leads to granulation tissue proliferation.

Clinical presentation
Toe fibromas present as a large fibrous growth protruding from the toe (**429**), which may be overlain by overgrown hoof horn. Careful paring of the hoof wall often reveals a narrow stalk attaching the fibroma to the corium (**430**).

Differential diagnoses
- Abscess formation in the white line.
- Virulent footrot.
- Penetrating foreign body.
- Septic pedal arthritis.
- Ovine digital dermatitis.

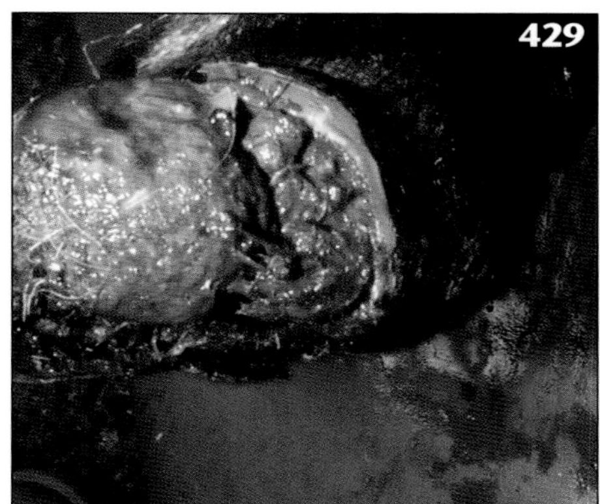
429 Large toe granuloma.

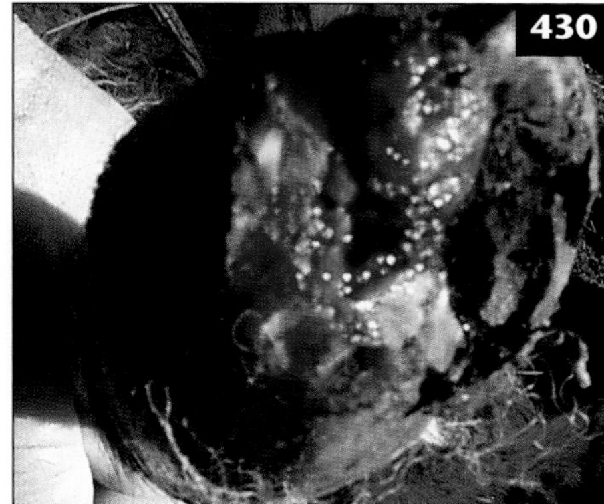
430 Careful foot paring to reveal the origin of a toe fibroma.

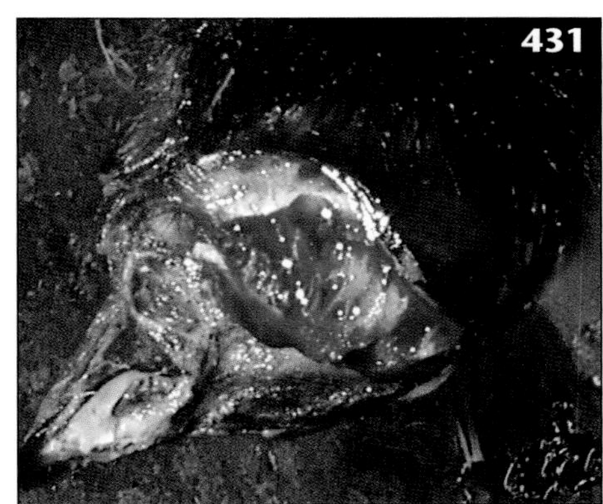
431 Excision of the large toe granuloma in **430**.

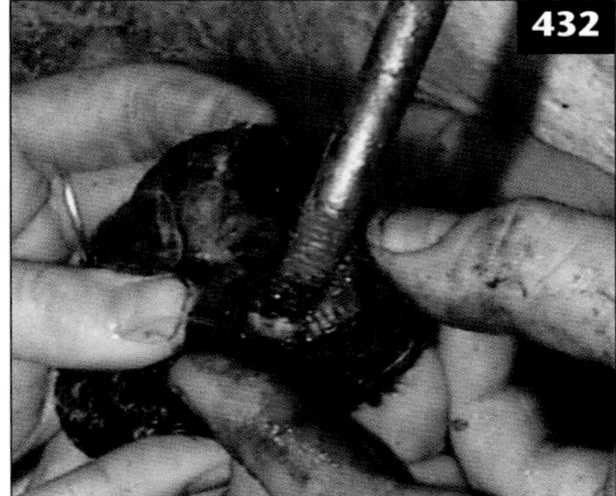
432 Cautery has been recommended for toe fibroma but it merely delays healing by destroying the surrounding corium.

Diagnosis
Diagnosis is confirmed by careful foot paring.

Treatment
This condition can be resolved by careful foot paring (**430**), excision of the growth (**431**) and application of a pressure bandage to the affected area. Toe fibromas are comprised solely of exuberant granulation tissue without a nerve supply; therefore, they can be excised without the need for any analgesia. The fibroma is cut off level with the sole using a scalpel blade (a hoof knife is not sharp enough for this procedure). A pressure bandage is carefully applied over the exposed corium and removed after 3–5 days. While some authors have recommended cautery to prevent re-growth of the fibroma (**432**), such action is counter-productive as it destroys the surrounding healthy corium and thus delays healing. A pressure bandage inhibits granulation tissue formation and achieves more rapid healing.

Deep infection of the third phalynx or distal interphalyngeal joint does not result from toe fibroma.

Prevention/control measures
Careful foot paring may expose but will not damage the sensitive corium. Sheep with damaged (profuse bleeding) or exposed areas of corium must not be put through formalin foot baths. These sheep should be treated with topical oxytetracycline, re-checked 3–5 days later and re-treated. Any toe with granulation tissue present should be bandaged to prevent fibroma formation.

Economics
Toe fibromas can readily be treated by the shepherd and are not a serious economic concern.

Welfare implications
Toe fibromas indicate either neglect of virulent footrot or unskilled and overenthusiastic foot paring.

WHITE LINE ABSCESS

Definition/overview
White line abscesses occur sporadically in sheep in all countries worldwide. The condition is more common in overgrown and misshapen hooves resulting from footrot.

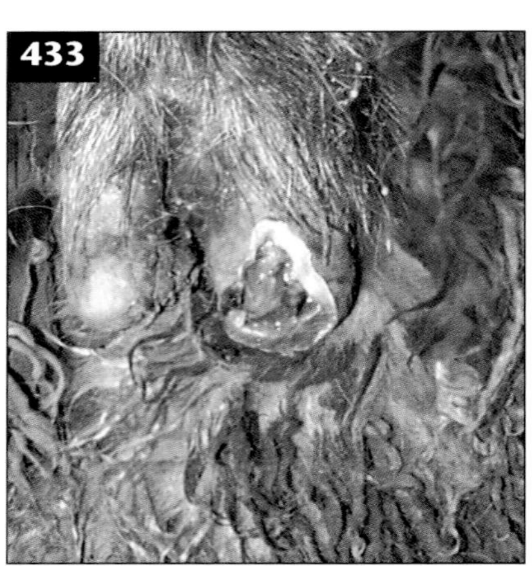

433 Abscess formation, which arises following bacterial entry into the white line area, commonly at the toe.

434 Infection may extend to discharge at the coronary band.

Aetiology
White line abscesses arise following bacterial entry into the white line area, commonly at the toe (**433**), and they may extend to discharge at the coronary band (**434**).

Clinical presentation
Affected sheep often present with sudden severe lameness of the affected limb, with the foot held off the ground. Pressure on the overlying hoof wall will elicit a pain response and immediate foot withdrawal. The lesion is especially painful if it has extended to the coronary band and caused swelling; rupture of the abscess some days later (**434**) often relieves the pain, with a dramatic reduction in lameness.

Careful foot paring reveals separation and impaction of the white line with dirt leading to an abscess, which is under pressure and may spurt pus on release. There is a marked improvement in locomotion within two days. Care must be taken not to expose the sensitive corium, which could lead to granuloma formation and persistence of lameness. Granuloma formation is more common following exposure of the corium at the toe.

Differential diagnoses
White line abscess can be differentiated from septic pedal arthritis by lack of interdigital swelling and swelling localized to a small discrete area of the abaxial coronary band.

Diagnosis
The presence of an abscess is confirmed on release of pus.

Treatment
The abscess is treated by releasing the pus by careful foot paring with removal of all underrun horn. The corium should not be exposed as this results in delayed healing and may result in granuloma formation.

Prevention/control measures
There are no specific control measures for white line abscesses but control measures for footrot should also limit the incidence of white line abscesses.

Economics
Painful foot lesions result in rapid weight loss and resultant delays to marketing. Ram lameness during the mating period can result in failure to mate ewes; this leads to an extended lambing period and more barren ewes than usual.

Welfare implications
White line abscesses can cause marked lameness and necessitate prompt attention.

INTERDIGITAL GROWTHS

Interdigital growths (**435**) are uncommon in sheep. They are best treated by removal of all granulation tissue under intravenous regional anaesthesia, followed by application of a pressure bandage to halt formation/protrusion of granulation tissue. These lesions generally heal well (**436**) but they may require the application of a pressure bandage for up to 14 days. Topical antibiotic aerosol applied to the lesion when the dressing is changed should limit superficial bacterial infection.

SEPTIC PEDAL ARTHRITIS

Definition/overview
Septic pedal arthritis occurs sporadically in adult sheep in many flocks but such lame sheep are often ignored. Ankylosis between P2 and P3 may eventually result after

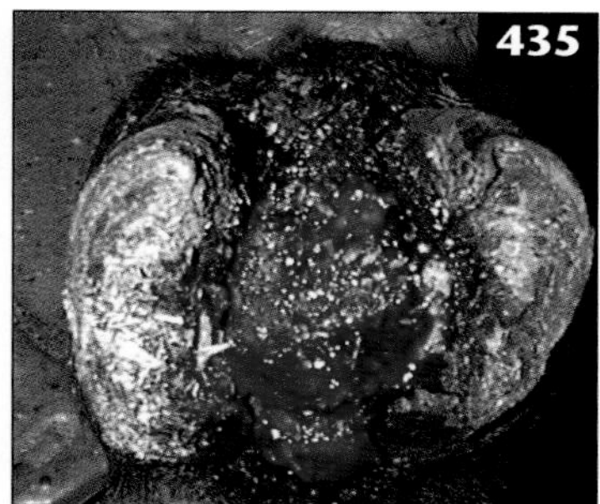
435 Large interdigital growth in a Suffolk ewe.

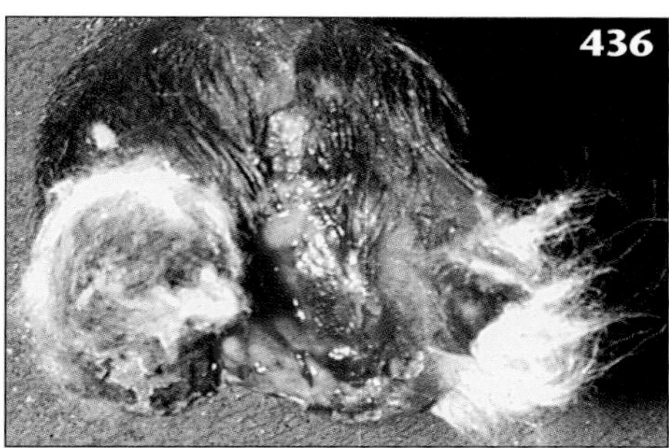
436 Two days after debridement and application pressure bandage to the lesion in **435**.

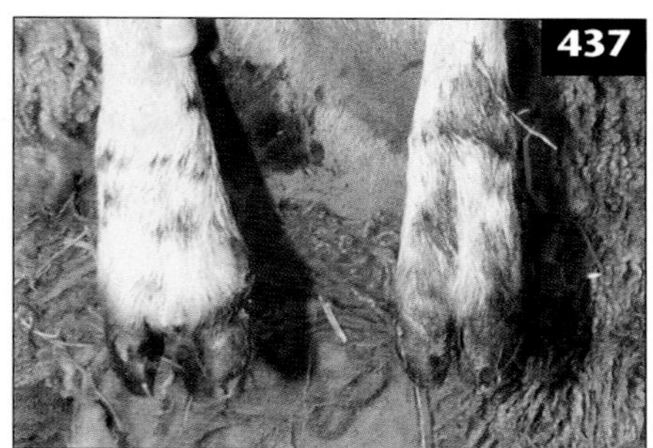
437 Septic pedal arthritis affecting the medial claw of the right forelimb of a Greyface gimmer. There is widening of the interdigital space and a discharging sinus above the coronary band.

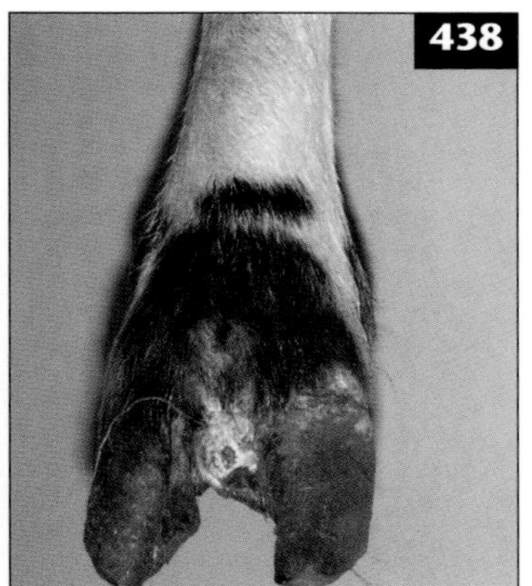
438 Septic pedal arthritis affecting the medial claw. There is widening of the interdigital space and loss of hair around the coronary band.

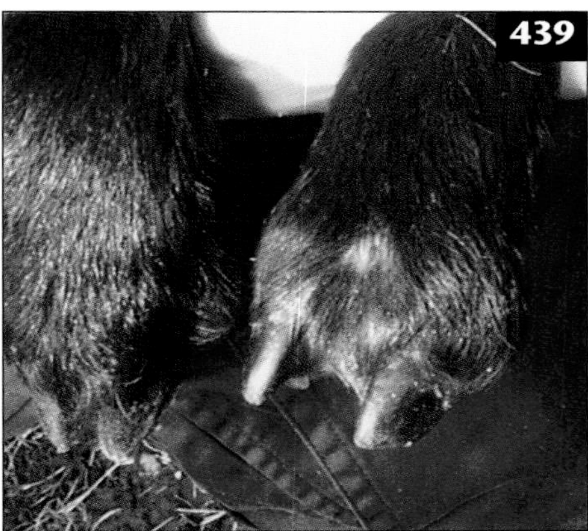
439 Septic pedal arthritis affecting the lateral claw of the left forelimb of a Suffolk lamb. There is widening of the interdigital space and swelling above the coronary band.

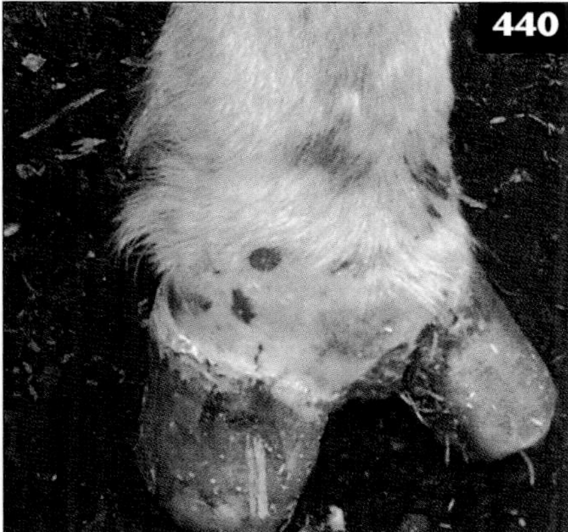
440 Chronic infection of the distal interphalyngeal joint. There is widening of the interdigital space and a broad band of hair loss above the coronary band.

many months of unnecessary pain and lameness. While this condition generally has a very low prevalence, it raises important welfare concerns. There are reports of severe outbreaks of septic pedal arthritis in flocks in Australia and New Zealand caused by prolonged periods of heavy rain leading to interdigital infection, then tracking to the distal interphalangeal joint.

Aetiology

Bacterial infection usually gains entry to the distal interphalangeal (pedal) joint from an interdigital lesion, which then tracks abaxially to discharge above the coronary band (**437**). Septic pedal arthritis is usually preceded by virulent footrot, which extends to involve the interdigital skin. As the distal interphalangeal joint capsule is protected only by skin and a small amount of subcutaneous tissue at its axial margin, it is prone to penetration at this site. Infection of the distal interphalangeal joint rarely arises from sole ulceration as commonly occurs in dairy cattle.

Clinical presentation

Affected sheep show severe lameness (10/10) with marked muscle atrophy of the affected limb. There is general body condition loss due to reduced grazing/feeding. There is marked swelling of the drainage lymph node, which may be 4–5 times its normal size. The foot is swollen, with obvious widening of the interdigital space (**437–439**) and a discharging sinus(es) above the coronary band on the abaxial aspect of the hoof wall. In chronic cases (**440**) there may be considerable widening of the interdigital space and loss of hair around the coronary band, with palpable new bone deposition involving P2 but no evidence of ongoing bacterial infection. Rupture of the axial collateral ligament in some cases leads to increased mobility and abaxial deviation of the toe, and eventual dislocation of the third phalanx.

Differential diagnoses

Differential diagnoses include:

- A neglected white line abscess, which has tracked up the wall of the hoof to discharge at the coronary band.
- Interdigital infection (**441**).

Diagnosis

The combination of widening of the interdigital space and a discharging sinus(es) above the coronary band on the abaxial aspect of the hoof wall is consistent with a diagnosis of septic pedal arthritis. The diagnosis can be confirmed by radiography (**442, 443**) but this is cost prohibitive in most practical situations. Arthrocentesis is rarely useful because only a small amount of inspissated pus is present within the joint. Injection of sterile saline into the distal interphalangeal joint results in discharge via the sinuses at the coronary band and/or interdigital sites, confirming joint involvement.

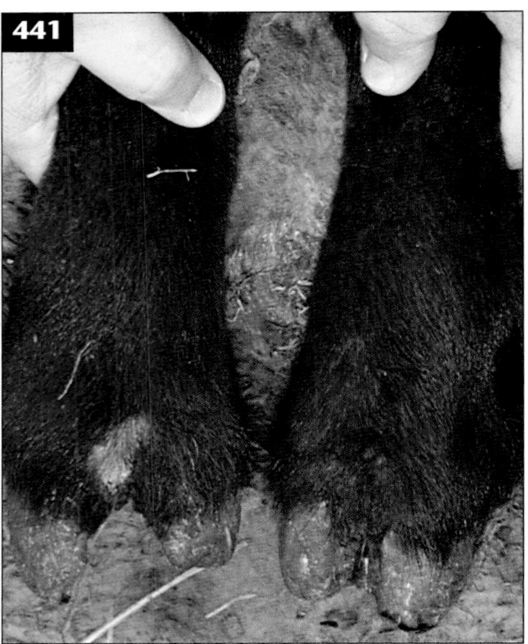

441 Interdigital infection in a Suffolk ram. While there is widening of the interdigital space, there is no evidence of infection tracking across the distal interphalangeal joint to the coronary band.

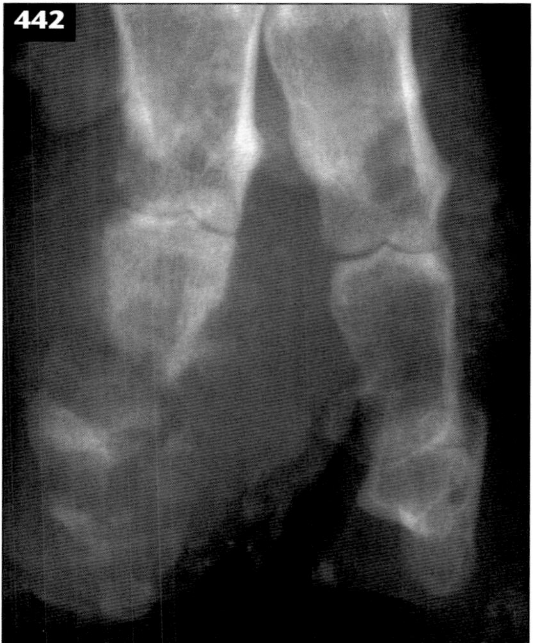

442 Radiograph of an infected distal interphalangeal joint. There is extensive bone destruction of the second phalanx. The third phalanx has been almost obliterated.

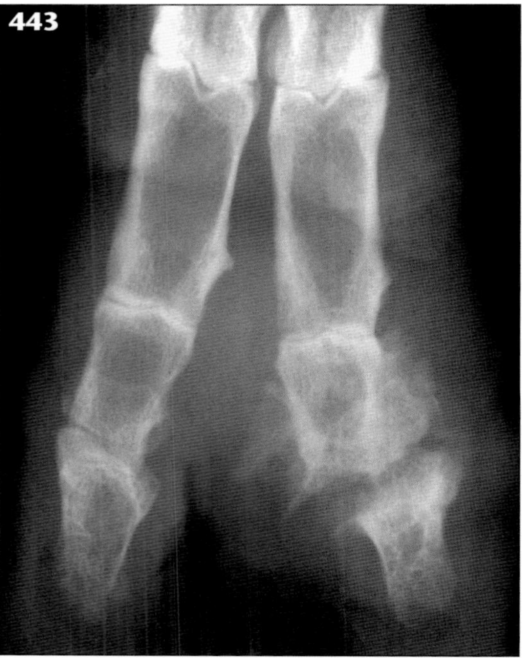

443 Radiograph of the foot in **440**. There is disarticulation of the distal interphalangeal joint; however, the extensive osteophyte proliferation has almost resulted in ankylosis.

Treatment

Antibiotic therapy is useless in these cases. Digit amputation under intravenous regional anaesthesia (**444**) gives excellent results. Intravenous injection with an NSAID such as flunixin is recommended prior to amputation. The procedure can be performed in less than 15 minutes and uses the minimum of drugs and dressings, thus keeping costs reasonable even for non-pedigree sheep. Five to seven ml of 2% lidocaine solution (or equivalent) is injected into a superficial vein after application of a tourniquet either above the hock or below the carpus as appropriate. Rubber flutter valve tubing can be used for this purpose. Insertion of a 19 gauge 25 mm needle into the distended superficial vein releases 5–10 ml of blood under pressure; blood flow then quickly reduces to the occasional drop if the tourniquet is tight enough. Analgesia should be effective within 2–5 minutes and is tested by pricking the coronary band.

The interdigital skin is incised as close to the infected tissue as possible and the incision extended along the full length of the interdigital space. The depth of the incision is approximately 5 mm at the cranial margin extending to 15 mm at the most caudal extent. A length of embryotomy wire is introduced into the incision and the digit removed through the proximal aspect of the second phalanx, and above the discharging sinuses, by rapid sawing action (**445**). Topical antibiotic spray is applied to the wound (**446**). A Melolin dressing (Smith and Nephew) is applied to the wound and pressure applied using a large amount of cotton wool incorporated into the bandage. A course of parenteral antibiotics is not necessary in most cases. The dressing is removed 2–3 days later and the granulating wound sprayed with oxytetracycline aerosol. A light protective bandage is applied for a further 2–3 days, by which time the sheep is much less lame. The sheep should then be turned out on to clean pasture, not a muddy field. The long-term prognosis after digit amputation in ewes and rams, unlike dairy cattle, is excellent.

Prevention/control measures

In most cases prompt attention to interdigital infections should prevent spread to the distal interphalangeal joint. Sheep should not be kept on muddy fields but moved to dry pasture whenever possible.

Economics

Digit amputation for correction of septic pedal arthritis is an effective procedure in sheep and should be undertaken at the first veterinary examination; prolonged courses of antibiotics will not effect a cure in such cases. The cost of surgery is only 15–20% of the value of a ewe plus the cost of dressings (4–5%).

Welfare implications

Septic pedal arthritis is a major welfare concern because many cases are neglected unless the affected sheep is valuable (e.g. a breeding ram). Ankylosis of the distal

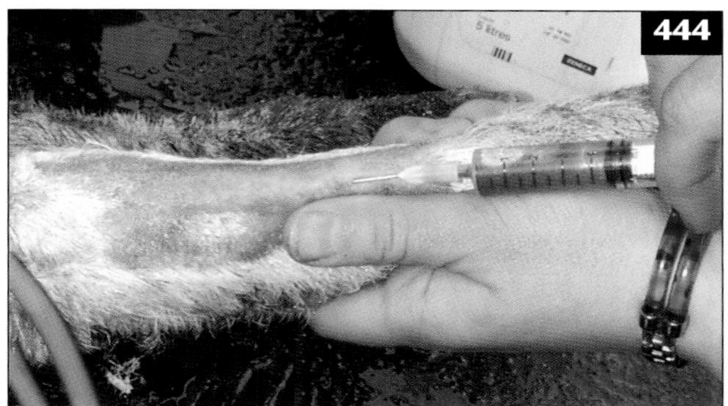

444 Intravenous injection of 2% lidocaine solution prior to digit removal. A rubber tourniquet is applied above the hock joint.

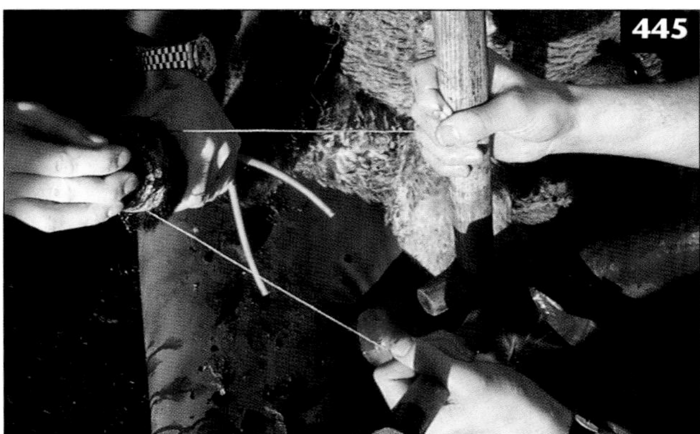

445 Digit removal using embryotomy wire.

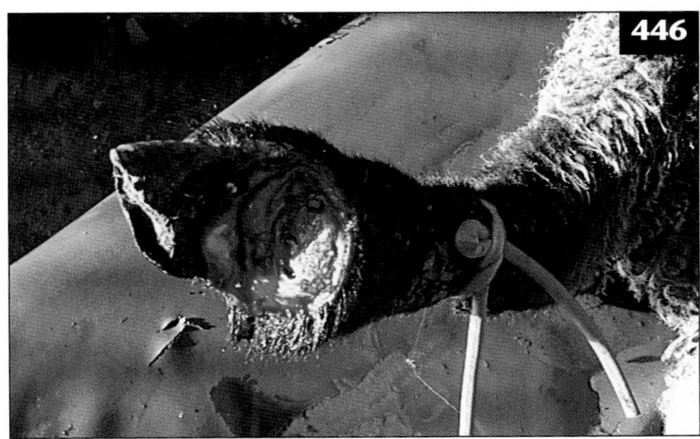

446 Digit removed through proximal P2.

interphalangeal joint may eventually result but only after many months of unnecessary suffering, which is totally unacceptable. Sheep with ankylosed joints still show some residual lameness. Some authors advocate that digit amputation should only be undertaken in exceptional circumstances; however, in some countries such neglected lameness over many months could lead to prosecution under animal welfare legislation. Veterinarians should therefore consider the advice they offer to clients very carefully; the low cost of digit amputation and excellent long-term productive life of these sheep clearly indicate the proper course of action to veterinarians.

INFECTIOUS POLYARTHRITIS (JOINT ILL)

Definition/overview

Localization of bacteria within a joint(s), causing an infectious arthritis with moderate to severe lameness, is a major economic problem and welfare concern in all sheep-producing countries. The problem is greatly increased when lambs are born indoors under unsanitary conditions.

The prophylactic or metaphylactic administration of procaine penicillin to all lambs at 36–48 hours of age is very effective in the face of a disease outbreak of *Streptococcus dysgalactiae* polyarthritis but it raises many concerns about indiscriminate antibiotic usage.

Aetiology

Bacteraemia in neonatal lambs results from entero-invasion or entry via the upper respiratory tract, tonsil or, perhaps, an untreated umbilicus. Bacteraemia occurs in lambs kept under poor sanitary conditions and with delayed or inadequate colostrum intake. Poor husbandry standards, understaffing, adverse weather conditions (**447**) and lack of client education of risk factors all contribute to an increased prevalence of neonatal diseases and compromised sheep health and welfare. Recent bacteriological surveys have identified *S. dysgalactiae* as the most common isolate from infected joints of young lambs in the UK (>85% of isolates), followed by *Escherichia coli* and *Erysipelothrix rhusiopathiae*.

Clinical presentation

S. dysgalactiae infections are acquired during the first few days of life, with lameness ranging from moderate (4/10) to non-weight bearing (10/10) present from 5–10 days of age (**448–450**). The number of infected joints is highly variable; typically, only one joint is affected in approximately 50% of lambs, with 2–4 joints in the remainder. It is not unusual to find both the fetlock and carpus affected in the same limb, with all other joints normal. The rectal temperature may be marginally elevated but it is frequently within the normal range. The umbilicus may be thickened in some lambs but not every lamb with a thickened umbilicus has polyarthritis.

Lame lambs spend long periods in sternal recumbency and appear reluctant to follow their dam, often being found sheltering behind walls and hedgerows. Only the toe of the affected limb points to the ground when walking. Lambs experience great difficulty walking when two or more limbs are affected and they may have a 'crab-like' stance.

The joints most commonly affected, with decreasing frequency, are the carpal, hock, fetlock and stifle joints. Affected joints are swollen, hot and painful.

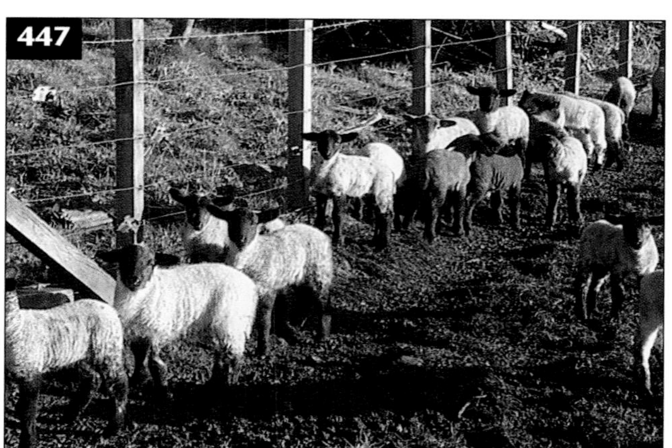

447 Overcrowding and environmental contamination may be important factors in the aetiology of infectious polyarthritis.

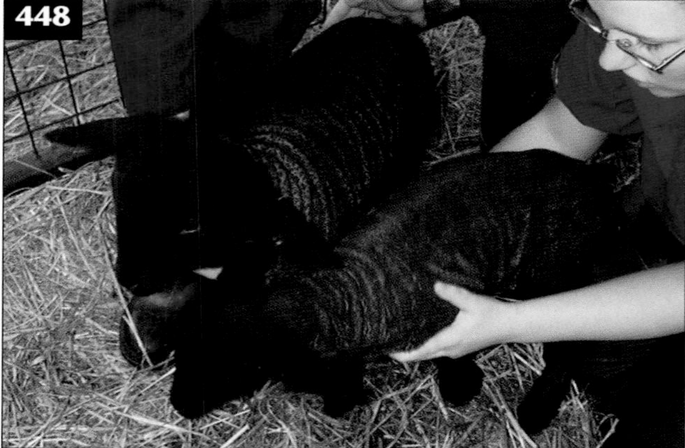

448 Two-week-old Suffolk twin lambs. The lamb with polyarthritis is in poor condition and has a pathetic appearance.

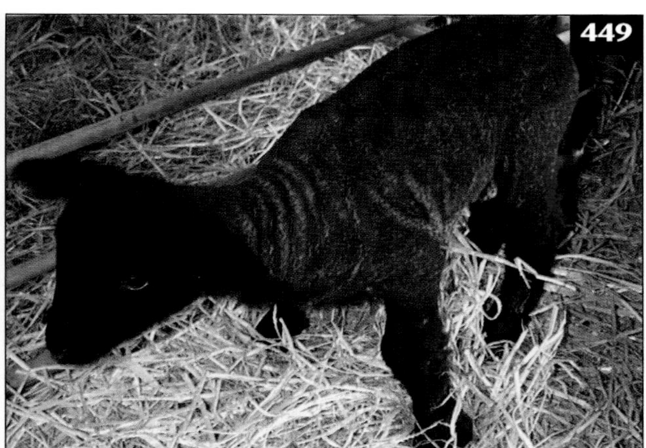

449 Gross swelling of the left elbow and carpal joints in the lamb in **448** with polyarthritis.

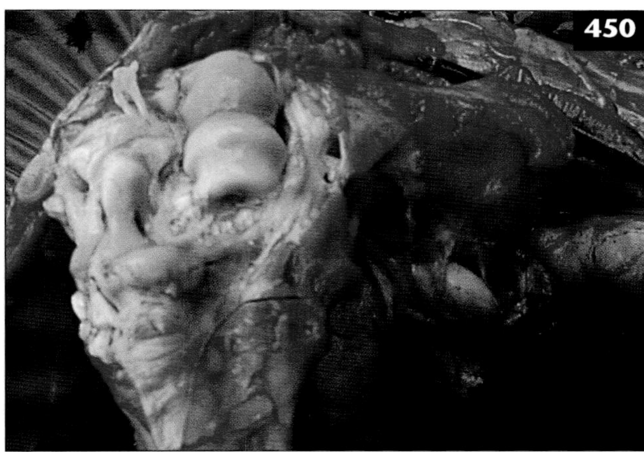

450 Suppurative arthritis of the elbow joint.

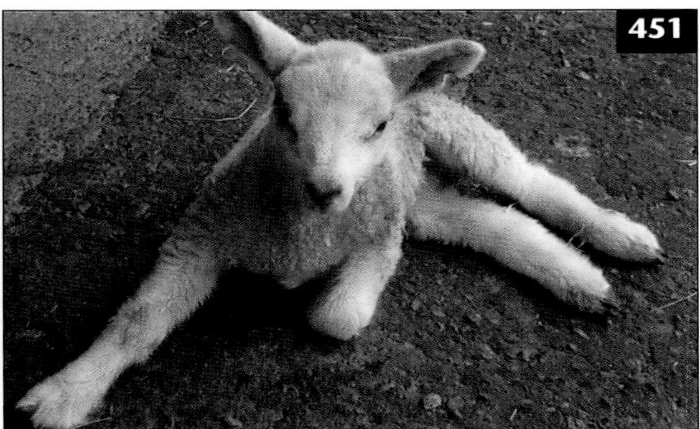

451 Infection of the atlanto-occipital joint is a common manifestation of *S. dysgalactiae* infection, causing sudden-onset tetraparesis.

Initially, the joint swellings result from joint effusion. The lymph nodes (prescapular or popliteal) are typically 2–4 times their normal size, although it is not easy to palpate the popliteal lymph node. Infection causes considerable muscle wastage over the gluteal/shoulder regions. After 2–3 weeks, lambs with polyarthritis are much smaller than their co-twins and in very poor body condition.

Infection of the atlanto-occipital joint is a common manifestation of *S. dysgalactiae* infection, causing sudden-onset tetraparesis and recumbency, although these lambs remain bright and alert (**451**). They do not always show evidence of other joint infection.

As inflammatory changes progress over several weeks, much of the joint fluid is resorbed and there is considerable thickening of the fibrous joint capsule. Affected joints feel enlarged but firm with much reduced joint excursion. Bony changes with osteophyte formation are visible radiographically after 4–6 weeks in chronically inflamed joints. Crepitus can be appreciated in these joints (following euthanasia).

In some cases the contents of the joint become purulent and cause increasing joint distension with thinning of overlying skin and loss of hair, although rupture is uncommon. Lancing such joints releases thick green pus of toothpaste consistency.

Differential diagnoses

- Lameness affecting a single limb may result from a foot abscess or interdigital lesion. Interdigital dermatitis is very common in young growing lambs and can cause marked lameness.
- Cellulitis following dog bites is not uncommon and is noticed several days after gathering by an over-zealous sheepdog.
- Trauma to joints may cause marked lameness; the stifle is the most commonly injured joint.
- Lameness may also result from fracture of a long bone.
- Unlike in calves, osteomyelitis is very uncommon in lambs.
- Endocarditis, with associated multiple joint swellings, is uncommon in growing lambs, although this condition may be encountered in older lambs with erysipelas.
- Recumbency can result from spinal cord compression associated with vertebral empyema, which is a common condition of growing lambs from four weeks old.
- Muscular dystrophy causes paresis leading to recumbency.
- Delayed swayback could be considered in those at-risk flocks that fail to adopt appropriate preventive measures.

Diagnosis

Diagnosis of an infected joint is based on clinical findings, although it may prove difficult to differentiate traumatic lesions from early infective conditions. In lambs less than two months old it has been recommended that all swollen joints should be considered septic until proven otherwise.

During the acute stages of infection there may be sufficient joint effusion to obtain a sample by needle aspiration. A typical arthrocentesis sample from a septic fetlock joint will yield a turbid sample with a protein concentration of 34.8 g/l (normal = <3 g/l) and a white cell concentration of 134×10^9/l, comprised almost exclusively of neutrophils. In most chronically lame lambs there is little joint effusion and arthrocentesis often yields more blood from the punctured synovial membrane than joint fluid.

By the time veterinary attention has been sought, lambs have generally been treated with antibiotics for a number of days and are unsuitable for sampling. If the prevalence of polyarthritis in the flock is high (>5%), swabs of joint fluid, but preferably samples of synovial membrane, should be collected at necropsy from sacrificed lame lambs that have not previously received antibiotic therapy.

Treatment

Sporadic cases of polyarthritis are encountered on most sheep farms but the choice of treatment is most critical when the prevalence exceeds 10–30% of the lamb crop. In the UK, for example, procaine penicillin is the drug of choice for polyarthritis as *S. dysgalactiae* and *E. rhusiopathiae* are the most common joint pathogens, accounting for over 90% of positive joint fluid cultures. High doses of penicillin (44,000 iu/kg q24h for at least 5 consecutive days) administered during the early stages of lameness effect a good cure rate in many *S. dysgalactiae* infections. However, dead bacteria and white blood cells remaining within the joint may induce further inflammatory changes, including proliferation of the synovial membrane and fibrous thickening of the joint capsule, such that some degree of lameness persists.

Penicillin therapy may render the joints sterile in most cases but some infections are not cleared with the result that progressive and degenerative changes occur within the joint. These physical changes in joint structure are not improved by further antibiotic therapy. Therefore, the prognosis is very poor for lambs that remain lame after at least five consecutive days' penicillin therapy, although some temporary improvement may result after another course of antibiotic therapy. Lambs with polyarthritis that continue to show mild to severe lameness after two courses of antibiotic therapy do not grow well. This situation is not uncommon on sheep farms and represents a major welfare concern.

There are no analgesic drugs licensed for use in sheep but there is sufficient published work and clinical experience to indicate that these preparations are safe and effective. Either flunixin or ketoprofen can be administered intravenously or intramuscularly for three consecutive days to alleviate pain.

Joint lavage can be attempted to treat a single infected joint in young lambs but this method requires appropriate analgesia and is therefore expensive and time-consuming. High caudal blocks can be used in the case of hindlimb joints (**452**), and intravenous alphaxalone/alphadolone combination for general anaesthesia for treatment of a forelimb joint. There is variable response to joint lavage depending on which joint is affected and the duration of infection before treatment (**453–456**). The prognosis for fetlock joint lavage is much better than that for stifle, hock or carpal joints.

A single injection of dexamethasone has a dramatic effect in tetraparetic lambs where the cause is infection of the atlanto-occipital joint. They are able to walk within 12 hours of intramuscular injection of penicillin and dexamethasone. The role of corticosteroid therapy in such bacterial infection can be questioned but the treatment response is very good, with no apparent increased relapse rate compared with antibiotic treatment alone.

Prevention/control measures

Every effort must be taken to reduce the risk of bacteraemia by ensuring timely adequate passive antibody transfer and reducing environmental bacterial challenge. The lamb must ingest sufficient colostrum (200 ml/kg) during the first 24 hours of life and 50 ml/kg within the first two hours, if not earlier.

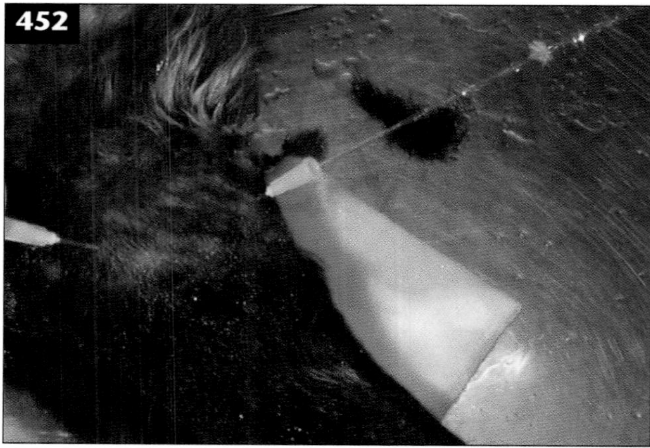

452 Lavage of the hock joint during the early stages of joint infection. Contrast with **453** and **454**, and **455** and **456**.

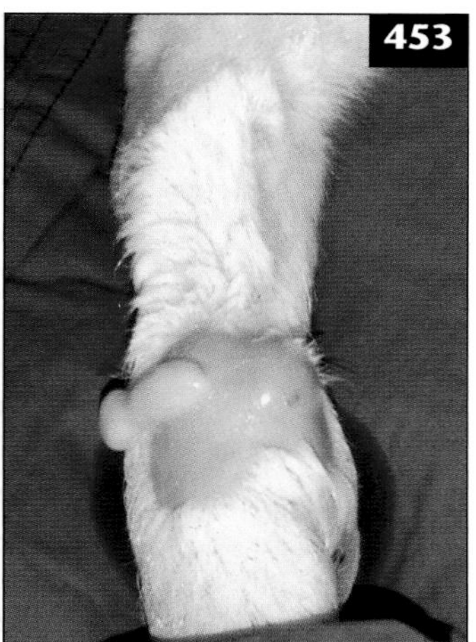

453 Arthrotomy of fetlock joint revealing viscous pus.

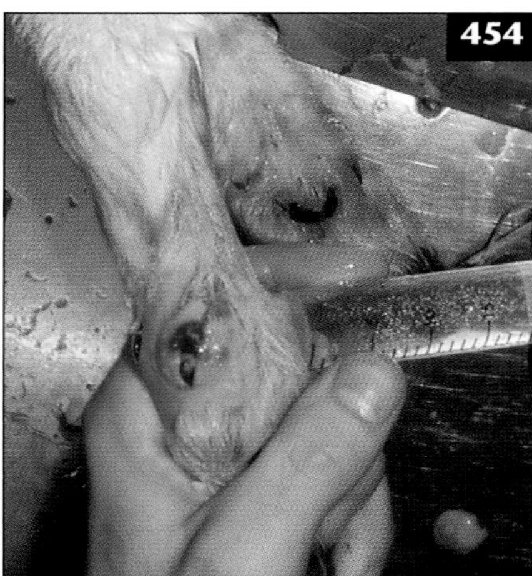

454 Lavage of the fetlock joint in **453**.

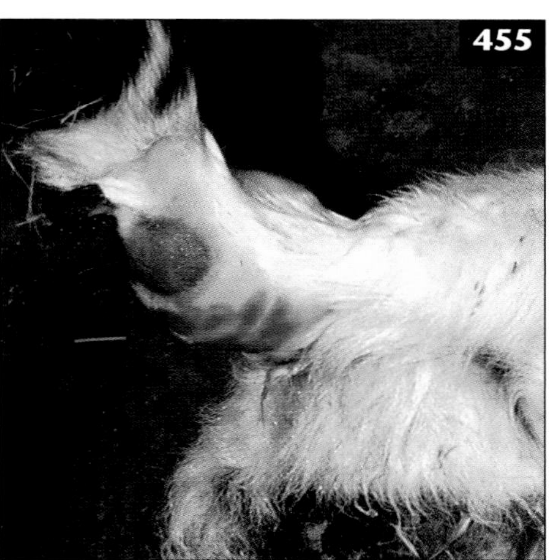

455 Distended hock joint in a three-week-old Scottish Blackface lamb with tick bite pyaemia.

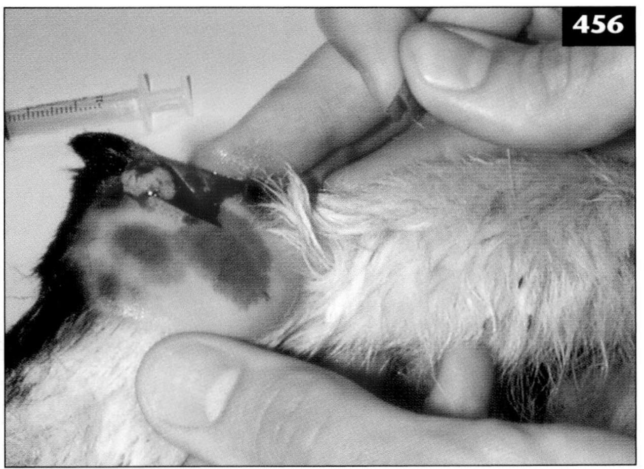

456 Arthrotomy of the hock joint in **455** revealing viscous pus.

The umbilicus (navel) must be fully immersed in strong veterinary iodine BP within the first 15 minutes of life and repeated at least once 2–4 hours later (see Chapter 4: Neonatal lamb diseases, p. 95). Antibiotic aerosol sprays are much inferior to strong veterinary iodine BP for dressing navels, and they are much more expensive.

Ewes should lamb on clean pasture. While this can rarely be achieved under UK farming conditions, it is practised in more favourable climates. Recent research has shown that *S. dysgalactiae* can survive for a number of weeks in bedding material. Unfortunately, most farmers elect to add new straw to the pen after each litter rather than remove all bedding material, disinfect the pen, leave it to dry and then add clean dry straw. Many individual lambing pens are so designed that it can prove impossible to clean them out (e.g. old wooden pallets tied together with baler twine). With such management, the bedding can build up, which may provide an ideal microenvironment for bacterial multiplication, especially when one considers the heat generated by the overlying ewe.

Change of lambing accommodation is rarely an option. Turnout to pasture for the remainder of the lambing period has been reported markedly to reduce morbidity.

Swabs of joint fluid and synovial membrane should be cultured and ewes vaccinated in future years if *E. rhusiopathiae* is isolated.

There are no specific recommendations for the control of *S. dysgalactiae* polyarthritis. A single injection of procaine penicillin to all lambs at 36–48 hours of age is very effective in the face of a disease outbreak but it must be considered as a last resort after all aspects of lamb management and husbandry practices have been reviewed. The use of prophylactic antibiotic injections to control diseases that could be controlled by good husbandry practices will come under ever closer scrutiny by regulatory bodies.

Economics

While antibiotic treatment costs are not high, catching large numbers of young lambs at pasture to administer treatments involves a large amount of staff time.

Lame lambs do not grow well and marketing is delayed by several months. Reaction in the drainage lymph nodes may result in condemnation of lambs that show only mild lameness but have chronic joint swellings caused by fibrosis of the joint capsule.

Welfare implications

Polyarthritis is a major welfare concern in lambs that do not respond to antibiotic therapy. Lame lambs that do not recover after two treatment courses must be euthanased for welfare reasons (457, 458). Further antibiotic therapy will not influence the joint pathology associated with chronic infections, and affected sheep should be destroyed (459, 460). Further examples of compromised sheep welfare are shown (461, 462), with a reminder that clinical examination of swollen joints must be undertaken with great care and empathy.

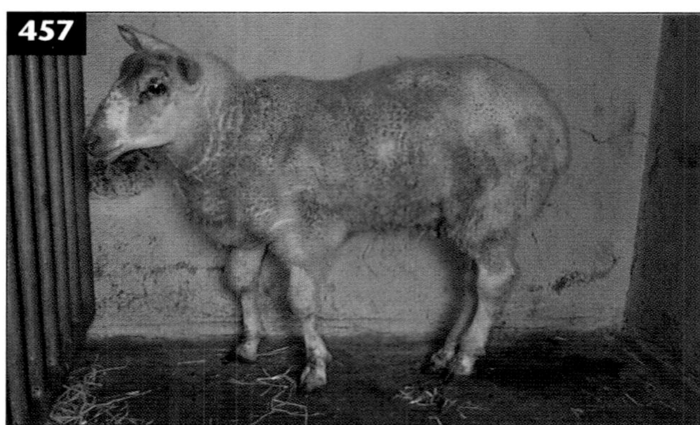

457 Severe polyarthritis in a yearling sheep.

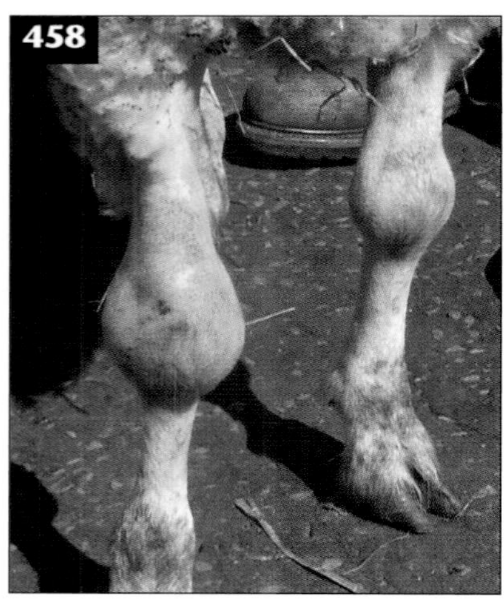

458 Polyarthritis. Marked carpal swelling caused by fibrous tissue proliferation surrounding the capsule and osteophyte formation.

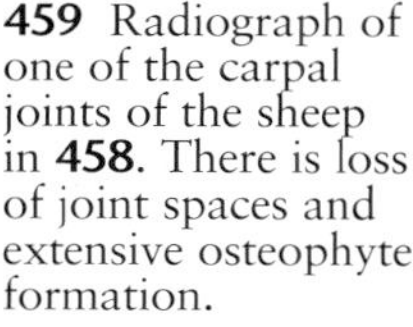

459 Radiograph of one of the carpal joints of the sheep in **458**. There is loss of joint spaces and extensive osteophyte formation.

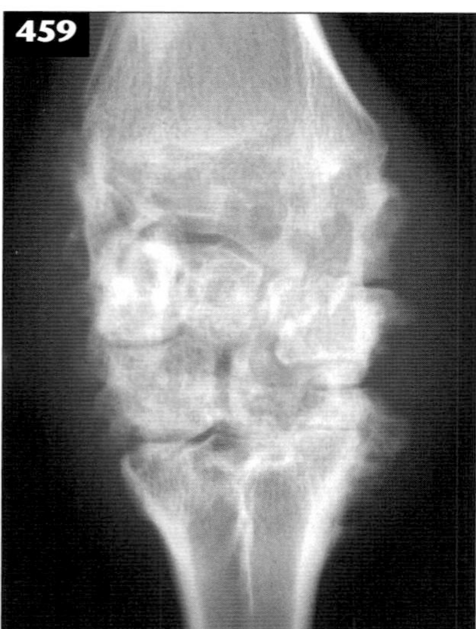

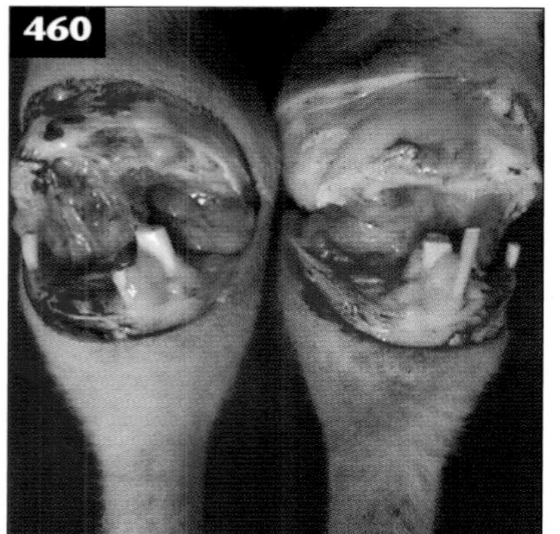

460 Postmortem examination of the hock joints of the sheep in **457**. There is destruction of articular surfaces and proliferation of synovial membrane.

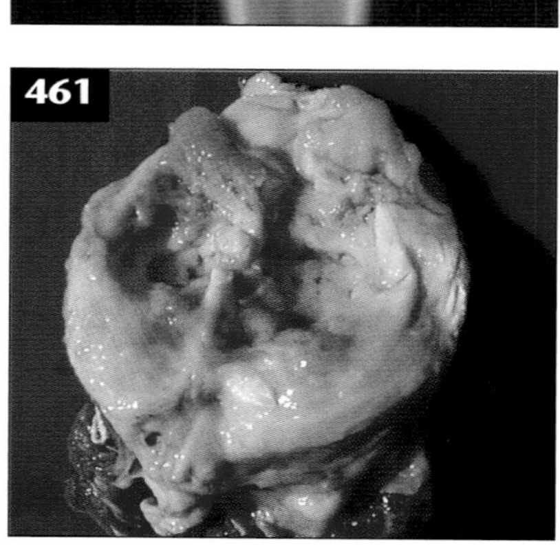

461 Chronic osteoarthritis of the stifle joint. There is erosion and pitting of articular cartilage of both chondyles of the tibia, and marked proliferation of synovial membrane and thickening of the joint capsule.

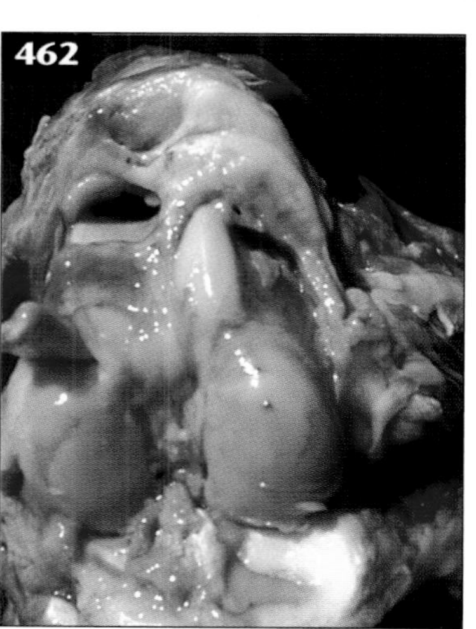

462 Acute septic stifle. There is pus within the joint but no articular cartilage damage and little synovial tissue proliferation or fibrous tissue reaction.

ERYSIPELAS

Definition/overview

Erysipelothrix rhusiopathiae causes an infective arthritis with high morbidity and moderate to severe lameness, typically affecting growing lambs aged six weeks to four months. While erysipelas can be controlled by vaccination, it remains a major economic problem and welfare concern in unvaccinated sheep in many sheep-producing countries.

Aetiology

Erysipelothrix rhusiopathiae causes disease in a wide host range, including pigs and poultry. It is able to survive for many months in the environment. While some texts refer to outbreaks of erysipelas following contamination of castration and docking sites, few farmers use a knife for these procedures, preferring to use elastrator rings, which do not present such a portal for bacteria. Outbreaks of erysipelas are more commonly associated with prolonged periods of wet weather leading to contamination of overcrowded shelter areas.

Clinical presentation

There is sudden-onset moderate to severe lameness affecting a large number of growing lambs. Lame lambs spend long periods in sternal recumbency and do not follow their dam. Lambs are often lame on two or more limbs. The joints most commonly affected are the carpal and hock joints. As the condition progresses over several weeks to months, further inflammatory changes include proliferation of the synovial membrane and fibrous thickening of the joint capsule, such that the joint is swollen and firm; there is little joint effusion (**463–465**). The drainage lymph nodes are enlarged. Erosion of articular cartilage results in lambs neglected for several months. While crepitus can be appreciated in severely affected joints, such painful examination of the joint(s) is neither indicated nor necessary; the more gentle the touch, the greater the sensitivity of, and information gained from, such palpation.

Differential diagnoses

Interdigital dermatitis is common in this age group of lambs and can present as an outbreak of moderate to severe lameness; however, this condition responds dramatically to topical oxytetracycline application.

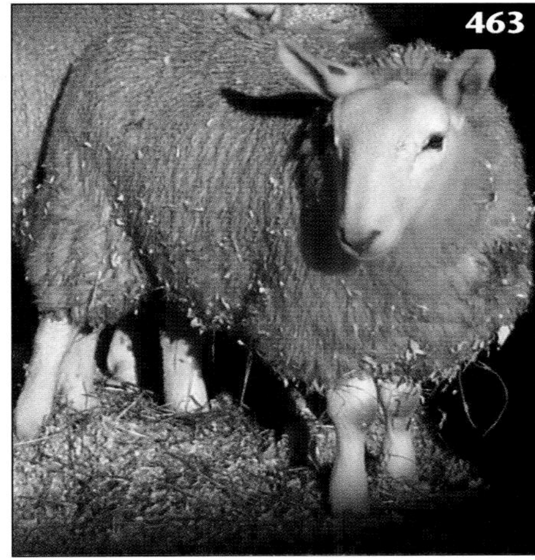

463 Six-month-old lamb suffering from erysipelas. There are obvious carpal swellings.

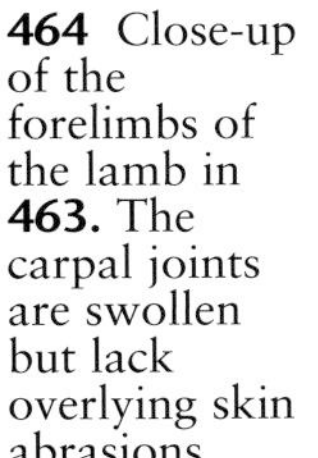

464 Close-up of the forelimbs of the lamb in **463.** The carpal joints are swollen but lack overlying skin abrasions.

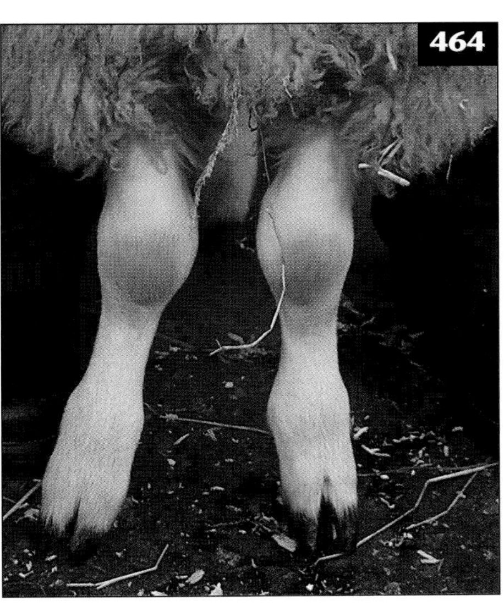

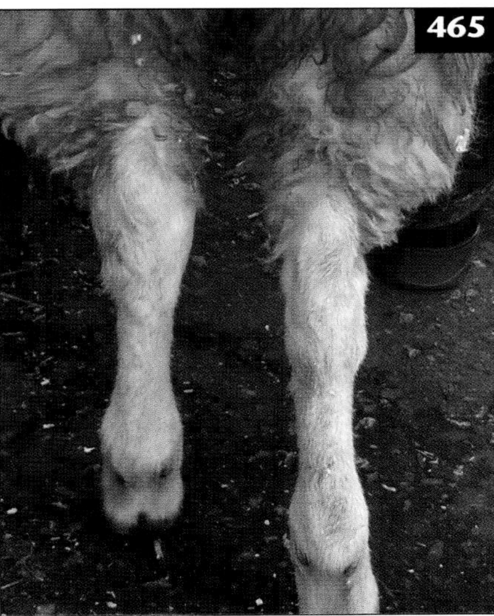

465 Close-up of the hindlimbs of the lamb in **463**. The left hock is swollen.

Diagnosis

The clinical findings and epidemiology of a large number of severely lame growing lambs with joint lesions, in unvaccinated flocks, is highly suggestive of erysipelas. There is little joint effusion and arthrocentesis often yields more blood from synovial membrane traumatized during attempted aspiration than joint fluid.

The best course of action for diagnostic purposes is to collect synovial membrane at necropsy for bacteriological culture from two or three severely lame lambs that have not received any antibiotic therapy.

Serology is not helpful because of the high seroprevalence in clinically normal sheep.

Treatment

Identification and treatment of lame growing lambs present many practical problems. Lame lambs are often distributed throughout all groups of grazing sheep on the farm. This necessitates gathering and identification of the lame lamb, its dam and possibly its co-twin. These sheep must then be isolated to permit easy handling for subsequent antibiotic treatments. During an outbreak of erysipelas, lame lambs continue to be identified within the grazing groups for up to two weeks. For antibiotic treatment to be effective it must be administered during the early stages of disease but is often delayed for 2–3 days because of the logistical problems listed above.

Either flunixin or ketoprofen should be administered intravenously or intramuscularly for three consecutive days to alleviate pain, but attention must be paid to licensing regulations pertaining to such preparations in various countries. Penicillin (44,000 iu/kg q24h for at least 5 consecutive days) during the early stages of lameness effects a good cure rate in many lambs suffering from *E. rhusiopathiae* polyarthritis; however, recurrence of lameness is not uncommon 5–10 days after cessation of the original course of antibiotics.

Prevention/control measures

There are no reports of the usefulness of metaphylactic antibiotic injection during the early stages of an outbreak of erysipelas polyarthritis in sheep.

Vaccination of ewes in flocks that have had a high prevalence of erysipelas in growing lambs achieves very good control of disease following passive antibody transfer. Replacement female breeding stock are vaccinated twice on introduction into the flock, then annually one month before lambing.

Economics

The cost of annual vaccination is very small (approximately 0.25% of the value of a breeding ewe). Chronically lame lambs do not grow well and cannot be presented at livestock markets, which represents considerable loss.

Welfare implications

An outbreak of lameness caused by erysipelas in unvaccinated flocks can result in severe lameness in a large number of growing lambs, with serious welfare concerns. Lame lambs that do not recover after two treatment courses must be euthanased. Farmers are often reluctant to euthanase 4–5-month-old lame lambs because they believe the lameness will somehow eventually resolve; therefore, these lambs suffer further chronic lameness for several months before they are eventually destroyed or die.

POST-DIPPING LAMENESS

Definition/overview

Post-dipping lameness is a severe lameness affecting sheep of all ages but predominantly growing lambs 1–4 days after dipping in contaminated dip solutions.

Aetiology

Post-dipping lameness is caused by *Erysipelothrix rhusiopathiae*, which gains entry from contaminated dip wash through traumatized skin.

Clinical presentation

There is severe lameness leading to recumbency in a large number of sheep in the flock within a few days of dipping. While 90% of lambs can be affected, the prevalence is more usually around 25%. Typically, sheep dipped at the end of the day or on the second day's use of dip wash are affected. The coronary band of the affected limb(s) is swollen, hot and painful, arising from cellulitis after bacterial entry. Bacteraemia and polyarthritis are uncommon sequelae.

Differential diagnoses

Interdigital dermatitis is common in this age group of lambs and can present as an outbreak of moderate to severe lameness.

Diagnosis

Diagnosis is based on clinical findings and a history of recent dipping.

Treatment
Penicillin (44,000 iu/kg q24h for 5 consecutive days) effects a good cure. In New Zealand most affected sheep make a spontaneous recovery without treatment.

Prevention/control measures
The disease can be prevented by using an appropriate bacteriostat in the dip wash as specified in the manufacturer's instructions. Dip washes must be discarded at the end of each working day because dangerous levels of bacterial contamination can build up during this time.

Economics
There is a temptation to re-use the same dip wash for a second day but this is unwise. Treatment of large numbers of lame sheep with post-dipping lameness is time-consuming, expensive and unnecessary. An episode of severe lameness adversely affects lamb growth rate and delays marketing.

Welfare implications
Post-dipping lameness causes severe lameness and obvious pain and suffering.

SEPTIC PHYSITIS

Definition/overview
While localization of bacteria within joint(s), causing an infectious arthritis, is relatively common in lambs, infection of a growth plate or physitis is uncommon.

Aetiology
Bacteraemia in growing lambs can arise from the upper respiratory tract, the tonsils, the gastrointestinal tract, foot lesions and skin wounds.

Clinical presentation
The rectal temperature may be marginally elevated but is frequently within the normal range. Lambs aged 4–12 weeks are most commonly affected but yearling sheep may occasionally present with septic physitis, presumably following puncture wounds (**466–468**). The metacarpal and meta-tarsal physes are most commonly involved. Typically, only one physis is affected, with the lameness ranging from moderate (4/10) to non-weight bearing (10/10). The associated drainage lymph nodes (prescapular or popliteal) are typically 2–4 times their normal size. Chronic

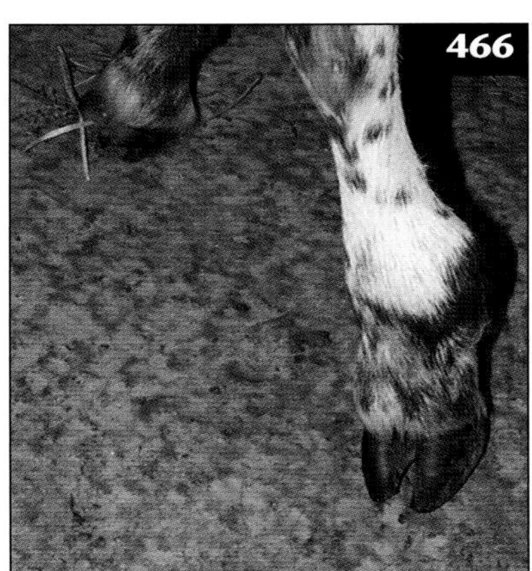

466 Infection of the distal metacarpal growth plate in a Greyface gimmer.

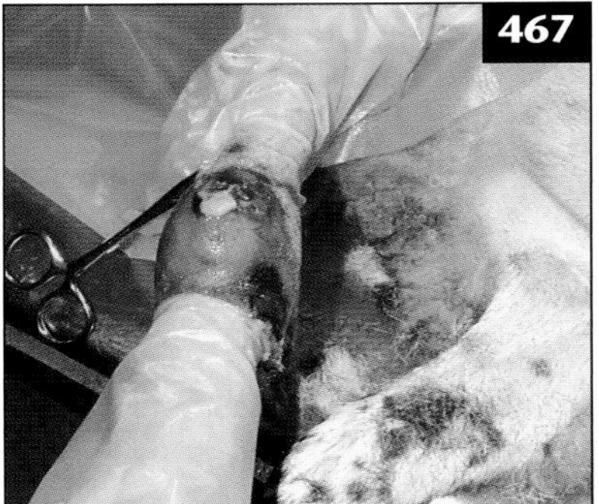

467 Growth plate infection. Discharging sinus on the lateral aspect.

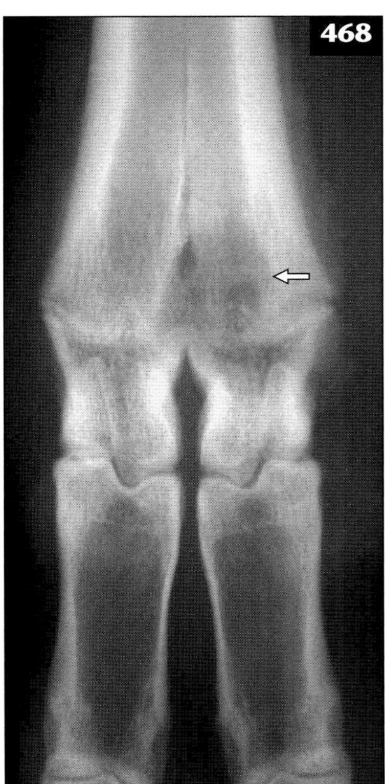

468 Growth plate infection. Radiograph of the infected growth plate. Showing bone lysis (arrow).

infection causes considerable muscle wastage over the gluteal/shoulder regions. There is a uniform firm swelling around the physis, which can readily be differentiated from the adjacent joint.

Differential diagnoses
The cause of the lameness should be differentiated from a physeal fracture and suppurative arthritis. It is not uncommon for physeal fractures to become infected, leading to septic physitis.

Diagnosis
Diagnosis is based on careful clinical examination and confirmed by radiography where possible (**469**).

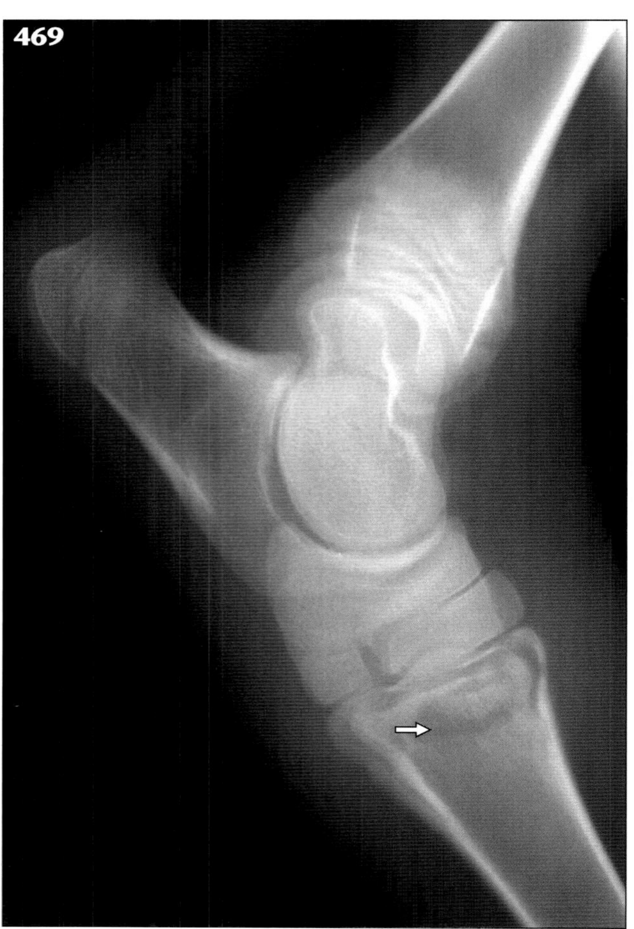

469 Lateral radiograph of the hock region in an eight-week-old Suffolk ram lamb revealing infection of the proximal third metatarsal growth plate (arrow).

Treatment
The prognosis is poor. Procaine penicillin is the drug of choice for septic physitis as the most common isolate from such lesions is *Arcanobacterium pyogenes*. Procaine penicillin (44,000 iu/kg) should be administered intramuscularly once daily for at least three weeks. Unlike cattle, isolation of *Salmonellae* species from such lesions is rare.

Curettage can be attempted in early infections but this proves cost prohibitive in most cases. High caudal blocks can be used in hindlimb lesions, and intravenous alphaxalone/alphadolone combination for general anaesthesia for treatment of a forelimb joint.

Prevention/control measures
The condition occurs sporadically and there are no specific control measures. Lambs with physeal fractures should also be treated with procaine penicillin for the first 10–14 days to reduce the risk of bacteria seeding the fracture site.

Economics
Septic physitis is very uncommon and not an economic concern.

Welfare implications
Lambs with septic physitis should be euthanased if they fail to respond to prolonged antibiotic therapy.

LONG BONE FRACTURES

Definition/overview
Limb fractures, particularly involving the hindlimbs, are not uncommon in young lambs. Correct alignment often cannot be achieved by traction alone, and general anaesthesia may be indicated. In hindlimb fractures, lumbosacral extradural injection (**470, 471**), which causes paralysis of the hindlimbs, allows pain-free alignment for fracture fixation (**472, 473**).

Aetiology
Fractures may result during confinement in lambing pens due to the ewe standing on the lamb's limb, falling wooden pen divisions/gates, etc. Often the cause of the fracture cannot be determined.

Clinical presentation
Long bone fractures present as moderate to severe lameness, with a palpable fracture typically of the third metatarsal/metacarpal bone in growing lambs.

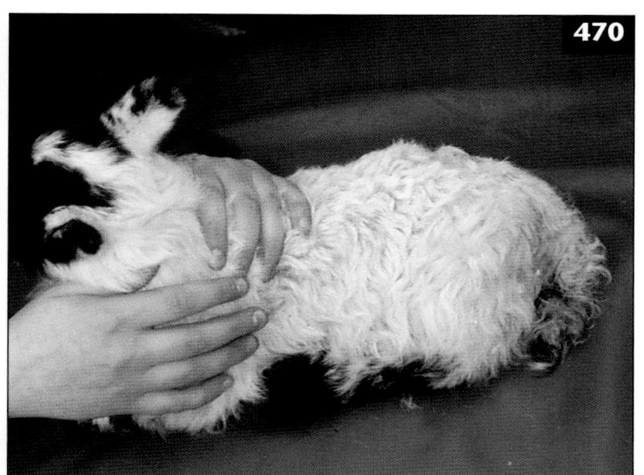

470 Fracture repair. Lamb positioned for lumbosacral extradural injection.

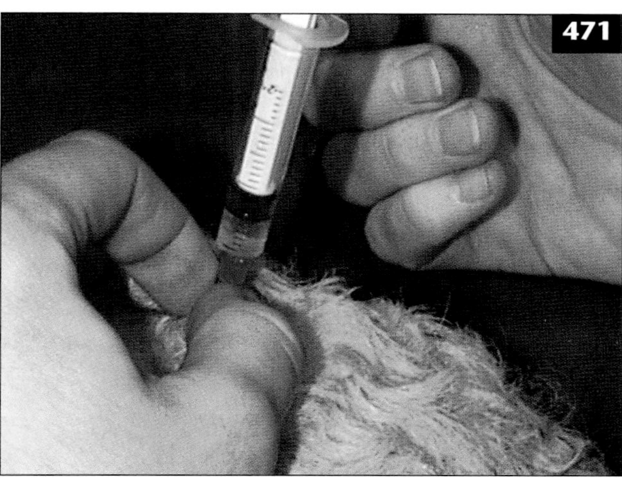

471 Fracture repair. Lumbosacral extradural injection of 2% lidocaine.

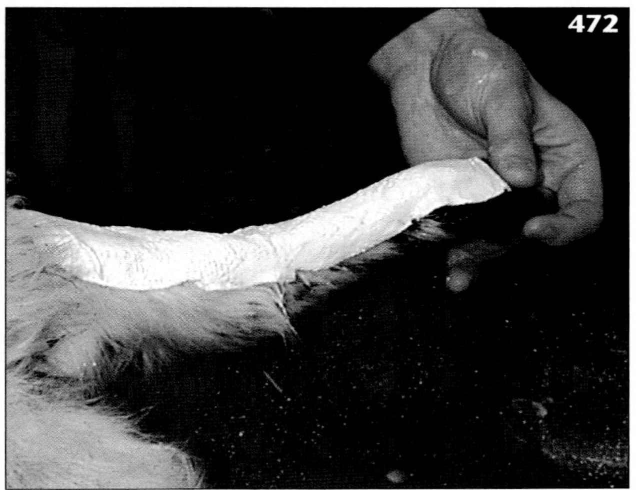

472 Fracture repair. Hindlimb paralysis allowing fracture re-alignment and casting.

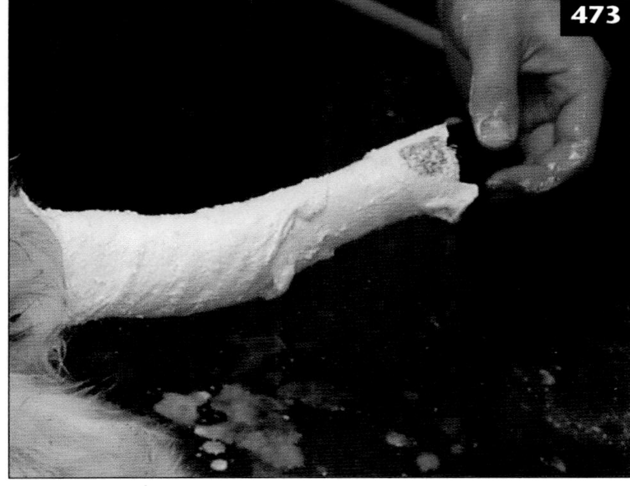

473 Fracture repair. Plaster of Paris-type casts may appear antiquated but they never drop off or cause pressure sores when correctly applied as shown. The casting material is laid along the full length of the proposed (**472**) cast; only then is it wrapped circumferentially.

Differential diagnoses

- Differential diagnoses of moderate to severe lameness include joint trauma and joint sepsis.
- Foot abscess and interdigital infections can be readily excluded on clinical examination.

Diagnosis

Radiographic examination is precluded for economic reasons except for potentially valuable pedigree breeding stock. Evaluation of each case is based on detailed palpation and gentle manipulation of the affected limb. Examination is facilitated by administration of appropriate analgesia.

Treatment

Fractures should be treated by the application of a plaster cast or modern equivalent after appropriate reduction (**472, 473**). Correct fracture alignment hastens recovery and return to full function of the limb. Unless the fracture is stabilized, healing will be delayed or not occur, with formation of a false joint. Newborn lambs can safely be transported to the veterinary surgery 'packed in a cardboard box'. The cast is extended from the foot to the first joint proximal to the fracture site. Typically, fractures of the third metatarsal bone or third metacarpal bone necessitate immobilization of the hock and carpus, respectively.

No cotton wool or other bandaging material should be used with plaster of Paris type casting materials. Excellent results are achieved by first applying folded pre-measured strips of casting tape along the whole length of the proposed cast (**473**). These strips are applied along the limb, usually requiring two 5 cm or 7.5 cm wide strips, depending on the size of the sheep. These longitudinal strips readily conform to the contours of the limb. The remainder of the cast material is then lightly rolled circumferentially onto these strips. This casting technique works extremely well; the cast never falls off and there is no risk of pressure sores developing. Plaster of Paris type casting materials have the added advantages that they are much cheaper than their modern rivals and are more easily removed (**474**). The cast can also be removed with a hacksaw blade by the shepherd. The disadvantage is that the cast material is much heavier but lambs readily adapt to this temporary constraint.

Splints can also be used to stabilize distal limb fractures. Plastic foam-lined splints can be applied to the front and rear of the distal limb and taped in position. Such splints are popular with shepherds as they can be quickly applied in the field without requirement for water, and there is no delay waiting for the cast to harden. Once removed, the plastic casts can be cleaned and re-used.

Fractures of the humerus and femur cannot be satisfactorily stabilized using a cast; they require internal fixation but farmers are only able to pay for such surgery in the case of pedigree breeding stock.

There are no injectable general anaesthetic drugs licensed for use in sheep and those that can be used, such as alphaxalone/alphadolone or propafol, may be considered prohibitively expensive. Furthermore, in older animals with a fully developed rumen, general anaesthesia introduces numerous risks including passive regurgitation of rumen contents in animals that have not been previously starved.

Excellent analgesia of the hindlimbs can be achieved after lumbosacral extradural injection of 3 mg/kg of 2% lidocaine solution (see Chapter 15, p. 319). This regimen allows a pain-free clinical examination, with more effective fracture reduction and alignment than can be achieved by physical restraint alone (**475–477**). It also presents a cheap and readily available alternative to a protocol involving injectable general anaesthetic drugs.

Prevention/control measures

Limb fractures occur sporadically in neonatal and growing lambs. Solid partitions rather than post and rail divisions will reduce the risk of broken limbs when sheep are worked through handling facilities.

Economics

The lidocaine injection for extradural injection is very inexpensive and the cost of casting material typically ranges from 5–10% of the sale value of the lamb.

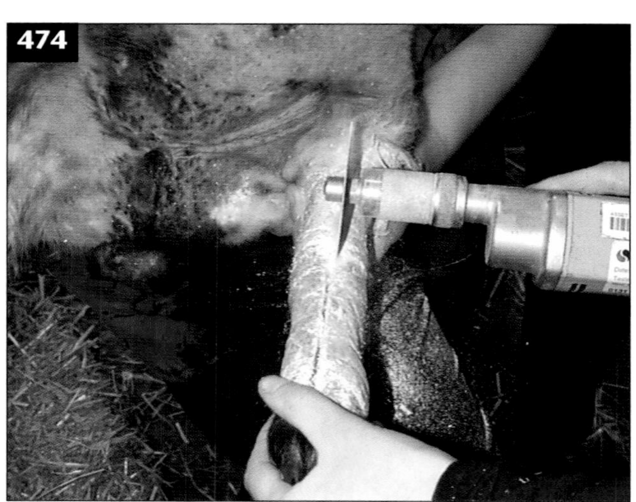

474 Fracture repair. Cast removed after three weeks.

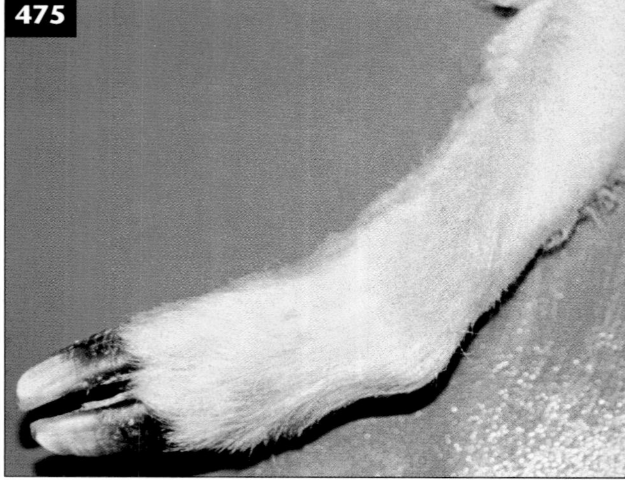

475 Lumbosacral extradural injection is especially useful for reduction of displaced fractures.

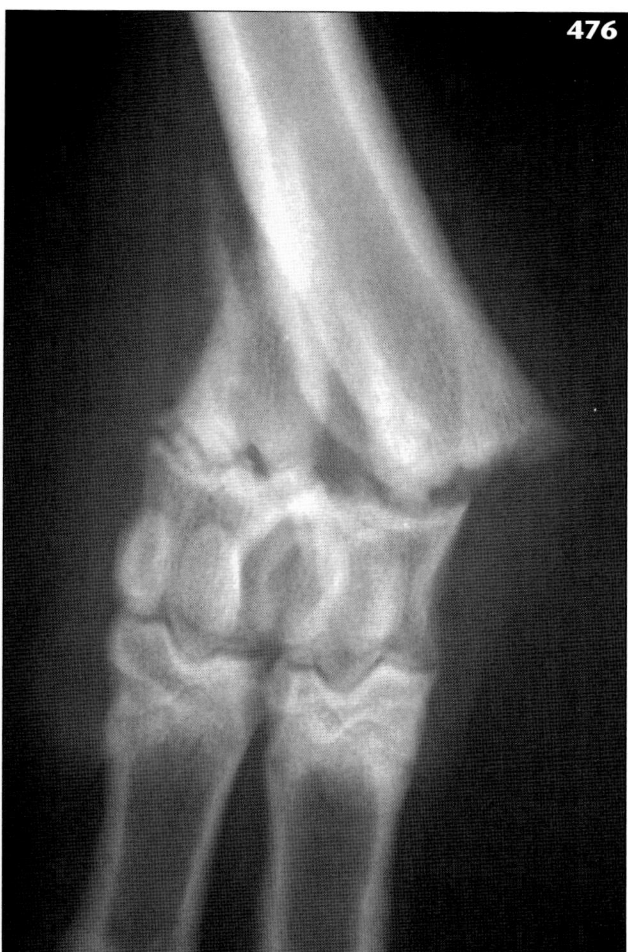

476 Radiograph of the limb of the sheep in **475**.

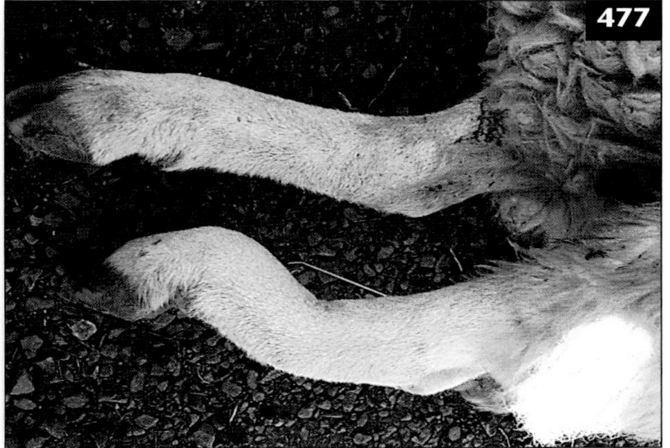

477 Reduction of this type of fracture must never be attempted by force alone. Such force would undoubtedly cause pain and can be simply avoided by lumbosacral extradural injection of 2% lidocaine.

Welfare implications

Correct fracture alignment and fixation hastens recovery and return to full function of the limb. Problems with malalignment and pressure sores often result when farmers attempt to stabilize fractures using wooden splints and electrical insulation tape.

OSTEOARTHRITIS IN ADULT SHEEP

Definition/overview

Osteoarthritis in growing lambs commonly follows joint infection; in adults, degenerative joint disease more commonly results from serious trauma. In sheep the stifle is the most common site for joint trauma, closely followed by the elbow and hip joints. In some countries, degenerative joint disease may be caused by maedi-visna virus infection.

The elbow is the joint most commonly affected by degenerative joint disease in the UK. Unlike in other joints, arthropathy of the elbow joint in adult sheep, following trauma to the mechanism preventing over-extension of the joint, is characterized by osteophytic reaction and extensive enthesophyte formation involving the lateral ligament (*lig. collaterale ulnae*).

Aetiology

Joint trauma may occur during transport, handling and fighting injuries in rams. Enthesitis is a term that has been broadly used to describe a traumatic disease occurring at the insertion of a muscle, tendon, ligament or articular capsule where recurring concentration of stress provokes inflammation with a strong tendency towards fibrosis and calcification. The elbow joint is a typical ginglymus, with movements restricted to flexion and extension. The lateral ligament of the elbow is short and strong and, along with tension in the medial collateral ligament and *biceps brachii* muscle, is largely responsible for limiting the degree of extension of the elbow joint.

Clinical presentation

The clinical presentation of osteoarthritis depends on the number of joints affected and the duration of the condition. Sheep accommodate joint injury reasonably well. This, when coupled with poor supervision, results in advanced changes being present when the sheep is eventually examined by a veterinarian.

Following the initial injury the joint is hot, painful and distended due to effusion. Over a course of some weeks there is muscle atrophy over the affected limb(s) and joint capsule reaction, with palpable thickening due to fibrous tissue reaction. There is reduced joint excursion because of the fibrous tissue reaction such that the sheep may drag the dorsal surface of the hoof along the ground, causing excessive wear at the toe. Elsewhere in the foot, reduced wear of the normal weight-bearing surfaces (abaxial wall) results in horn overgrowth. Affected sheep spend long periods in sternal recumbency. Reduced grazing leads to a gradual loss of body condition.

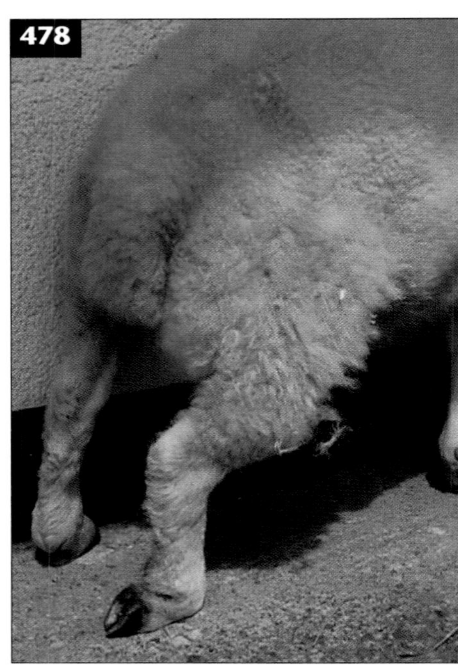

478 Severe stifle trauma with inability to protract the leg causing knuckling of the distal limb.

Stifle arthritis

Trauma to the stifle joint often results in severe lameness due to damage to the cruciate ligament(s) and other joint support structures. Affected sheep typically present 10/10 lame. The stifle and hock joints are more flexed than usual, with the foot often carried free of the ground, but the sheep may bear weight on the dorsal surface of the hoof when at rest (**478**). Careful palpation and ultrasonographic examination reveal marked thickening of the stifle joint capsule (**479, 480**), more easily detected at its distal insertion over the tibial crest where the normal sharp triangular contour feels rounded. Initially, there may be joint effusion but there is scant joint fluid in advanced cases.

Hip arthritis

Sheep with osteoarthritis of the hip joint present similarly to those with stifle joint lesions, with 'knuckling' of the fetlock joint common when at rest (**481**). Diagnosis of a hip lesion (**482**) is based largely on elimination of palpable lesions involving the stifle joint and distal joints.

Elbow arthritis

Sheep with elbow arthritis are typically 2–5 years old with either unilateral, or more commonly bilateral, forelimb lameness of three months' duration or longer. Rams are more commonly presented for veterinary examination but this may simply reflect their higher economic value. Elbow arthritis is also commonly seen in old sheep kept as pets, presumably because of their longer life span, as they are rarely bred, and their excess body weight resulting from overgenerous concentrate allowance and ginger biscuits.

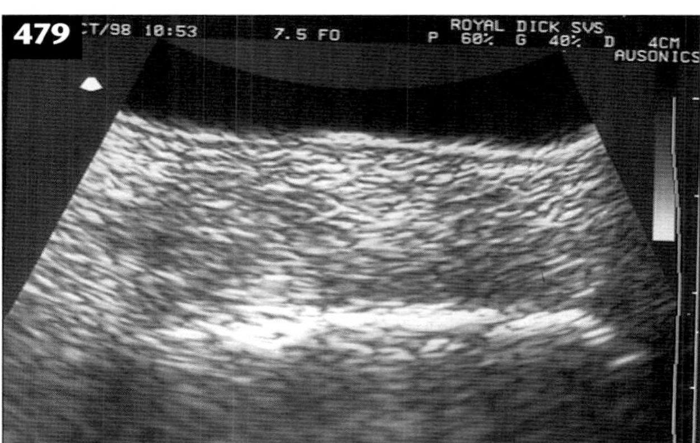

479 Ultrasonogram of the stifle joint capsule of the eight-month-old lamb in **478**. There is marked thickening of the joint capsule evidenced by separation of the probe head from the articular surfaces (bone represented by broad hyperechoic line with shadow beyond).

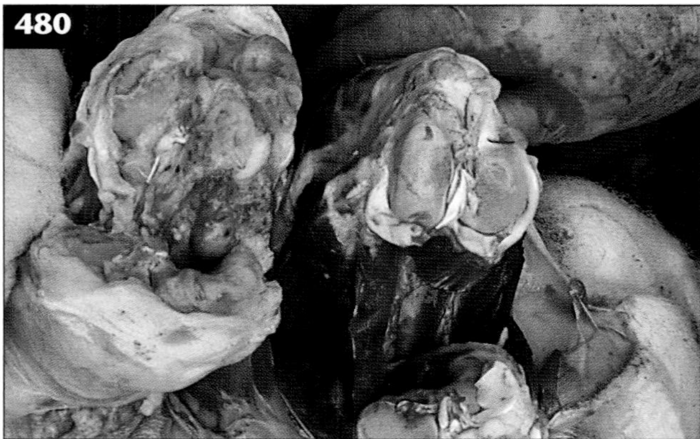

480 Comparison between the damaged (left) and normal (right) stifle joints.

Affected sheep are in poorer bodily condition than other sheep in the group. They spend long periods in sternal recumbency, with extension of the shoulder and carpal joints such that the forelimbs are positioned in front of the animal rather than alongside the chest with the joints flexed. Affected sheep experience considerable difficulty rising. Varying intervals are spent with weight borne by the flexed carpal joints before finally standing. Skin abrasions over the carpal joints, with chronic skin trauma causing callus formation and changes in hair colour in some sheep, indicate that the sheep have spent several months grazing on their knees.

When standing, sheep with unilateral lesions hold the affected forelimb in rigid extension and positioned more caudally and slightly abducted (**483**). There is considerable muscle wastage over the scapula, with a prominent spine and acromion, compared with the contralateral limb. Sheep with bilateral lesions adopt a characteristic stance with the hindlimbs positioned well forward underneath the body. The head is not held upright as normal but level with the thoracolumbar vertebral column. This head posture, with the neck flexed, makes the neck appear shorter than normal because the head is held in towards the shoulders (**484**). The sheep are reluctant to walk and display a characteristic stilted forelimb gait with marked abduction of affected forelimbs. Affected

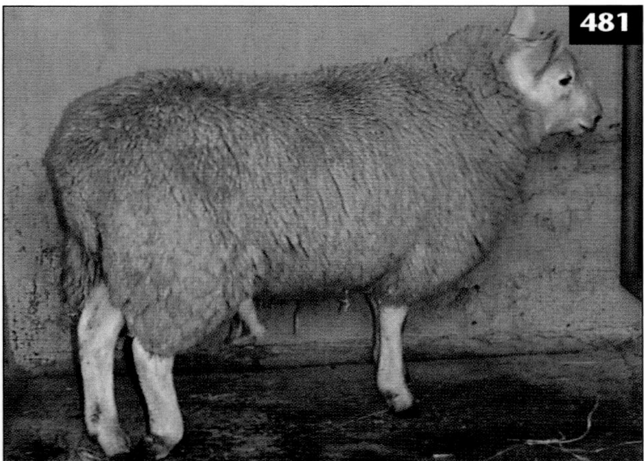

481 Reduced protraction of the limb caused by severe hip damage.

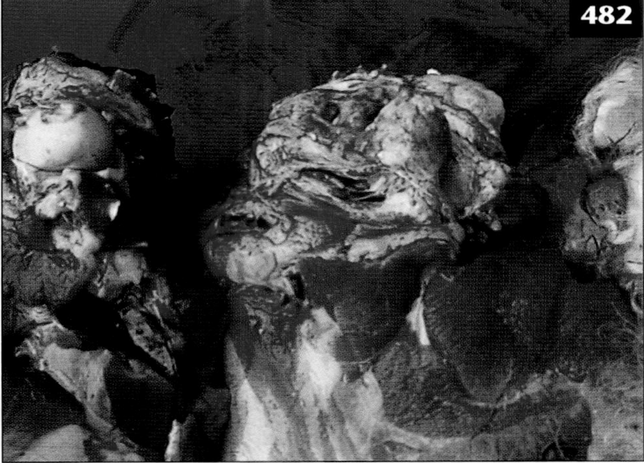

482 Severe arthritis of the hip joint of the sheep in **481**. There is loss of the acetabular rim and fibrous tissue proliferation surrounding the joint capsule.

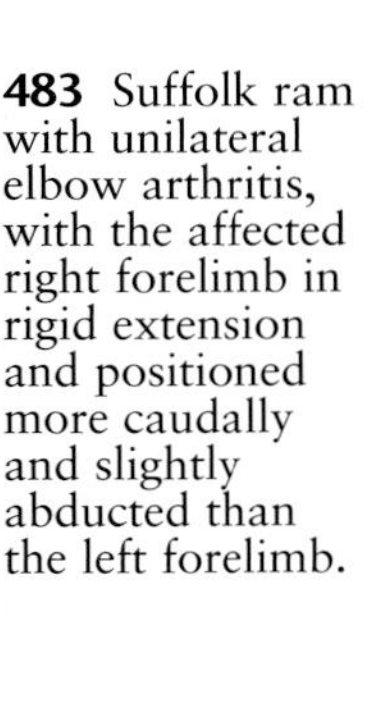

483 Suffolk ram with unilateral elbow arthritis, with the affected right forelimb in rigid extension and positioned more caudally and slightly abducted than the left forelimb.

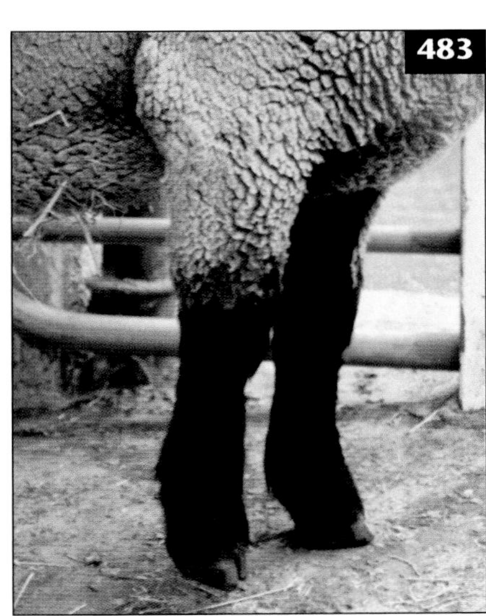

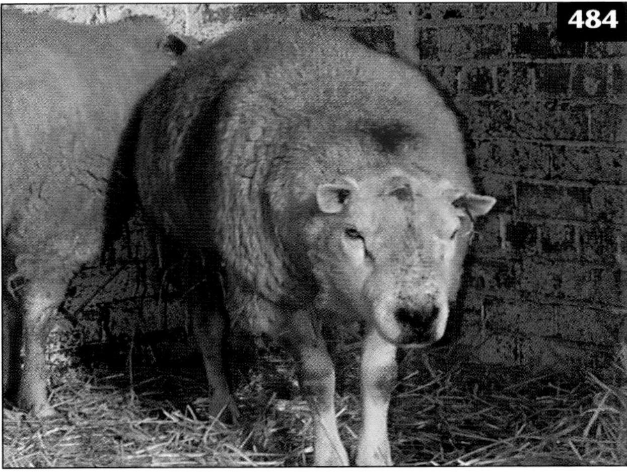

484 Lowered head carriage and abducted elbows in a Texal ram suffering from elbow arthritis.

sheep experience great difficulty turning and this is achieved only by pivoting on their hindlimbs, which are positioned far forward underneath the body (**485, 486**).

There is no enlargement of the prescapular lymph node(s). Affected elbow joints are grossly swollen but the joint capsule does not feel thickened and there is no excess joint effusion. The joint swelling is caused by considerable enthesophytic reaction on the lateral aspect of the elbow. This extends distally from the attachment of the lateral ligament immediately proximal to the lateral epicondyle of the humerus and proximally from the lateral tuberosity of the radius (**487**). There is considerably less bony reaction on the medial aspect of the elbow joint (**488**). Careful palpation of the craniolateral aspect of the affected elbow joints at the level of the articular surfaces in some rams may reveal a 10–15 mm wide depression between the advancing edges of enthesophyte proliferation. In exceptional cases, with an estimated duration of several years, fusion of these advancing bony margins occurs, effectively achieving ankylosis of the elbow joint. Measurement of the forelimb with McLintock callipers across the proximal radius of affected elbow joints, immediately distal to the gap described above, reveals an increased width of 10–30 mm compared with readings for sound sheep of equivalent age, breed and sex. Typically, measurements range from 40–50 mm for normal adult Blackface and Greyface ewes and 50–65 mm for Suffolk rams. In many affected elbow joints, gentle manipulation reveals that excursion is severely restricted to 15–30°.

Differential diagnoses

- Virulent footrot and ovine digital dermatitis are the major causes of lameness in adult sheep.
- Joint infections in adult sheep are relatively uncommon except for infections of the interdigital area, which extend into a distal interphalyngeal joint.

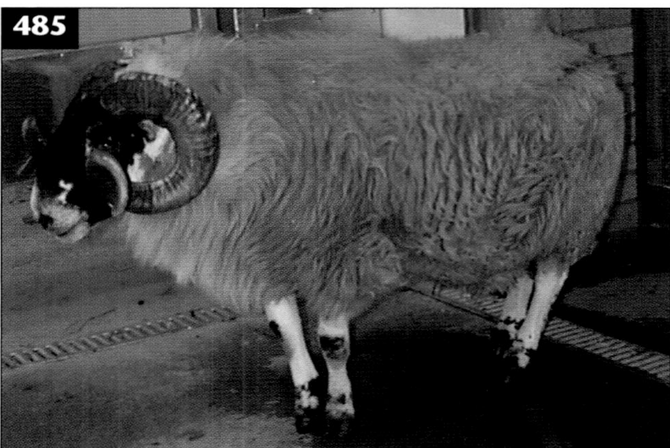

485 Scottish Blackface ram with elbow arthritis. The forelimbs are stilted and the hindlimbs are drawn well forward under the body.

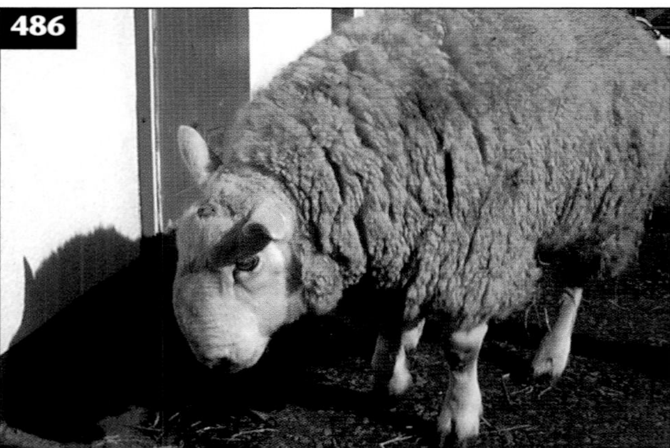

486 Cheviot ram with elbow arthritis. The head carriage is lowered with the hindlimbs drawn well forward under the body.

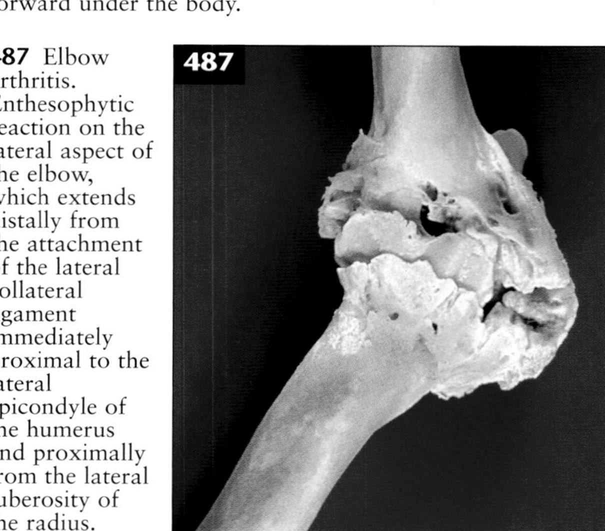

487 Elbow arthritis. Enthesophytic reaction on the lateral aspect of the elbow, which extends distally from the attachment of the lateral collateral ligament immediately proximal to the lateral epicondyle of the humerus and proximally from the lateral tuberosity of the radius.

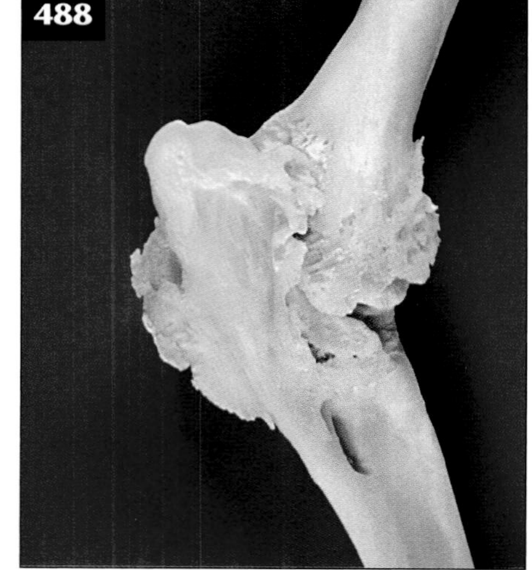

488 Elbow arthritis. There is considerably less bony reaction on the medial aspect of the elbow joint.

- Occasionally, puncture wounds may penetrate into a joint.
- It has been proposed that joint trauma with associated haemorrhage may predispose to joint infection following localization of bacteraemia, but such a postulate is difficult, if not impossible, to prove.
- Endocarditis can present with severe lameness and multiple joint effusion; rarely is there any significant joint capsule thickening.

Diagnosis

In most situations, diagnosis of degenerative joint disease is based on careful clinical examination with gentle palpation of the affected joint(s), appreciating that these joints are painful. Palpation is aimed at determining the extent of any effusion and thickening of the joint capsule.

In general, palpable joint effusion, joint laxity and no appreciable thickening of the joint capsule are consistent with a recent injury. Reduced joint excursion, absence of palpable joint effusion but obvious thickening of the joint capsule (between three and five millimetres) is consistent with an injury of some weeks' to months' duration. Detection of crepitus is not a necessary part of the joint examination and such manipulation only serves to increase allodynia (pain) and aggravate any existing significant lesion. Swollen joints are very painful whatever the aetiology. It is important to appreciate that fact and examine all sheep with compassion.

Arthrocentesis

Arthrocentesis is rarely undertaken in cases of degenerative joint disease because there is scant joint fluid. The technique is painful unless the joint is distended.

Ultrasonography

Ultrasonography using a 7.5 MHz linear scanner with stand-off is very useful for measuring the extent and nature of any joint effusion and the thickness of the joint capsule. The contralateral joint, if normal, can be scanned for direct comparison.

Radiography

Anteroposterior and lateromedial radiographs of affected joints will identify soft tissue swelling and new bone formation. Erosion of articular cartilage can be identified by reduction in the joint space. Radiographic examination is limited, by cost, to valuable breeding sheep.

Stifle arthritis

Proliferation of the fibrous joint capsule in cases of chronic joint trauma can be easily palpated and confirmed on ultrasonographic examination if necessary. Arthrocentesis rarely yields any worthwhile sample unless there is obvious joint effusion.

Elbow arthritis

Radiographic examination using a dorsolateral, palmeromedial oblique view of the elbow joint in the standing sheep reveals osteophyte formation and pronounced enthesophyte formation proximal to the lateral epicondyle of the humerus and immediately distal to the lateral tuberosity of the radius and involving the lateral ligament (**489**). The gap, often palpable, between the leading edges of enthesophyte formation is clearly visible on the radiographs in affected elbow joints. A lateromedial radiograph of the affected elbow joint provides no additional information (**490**) and is not necessary.

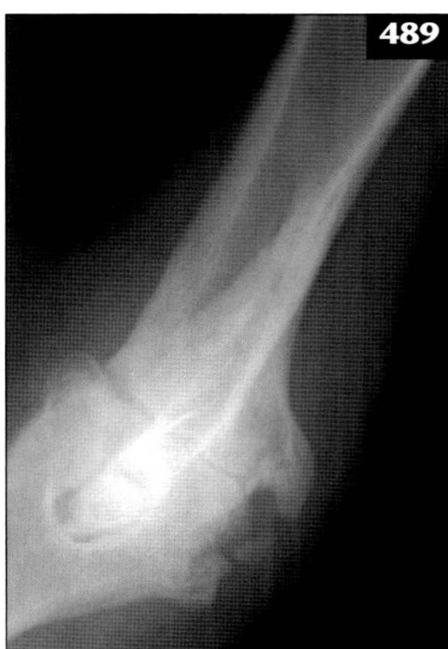

489 Oblique radiograph showing extensive enthesophyte formation associated with the lateral collateral ligament.

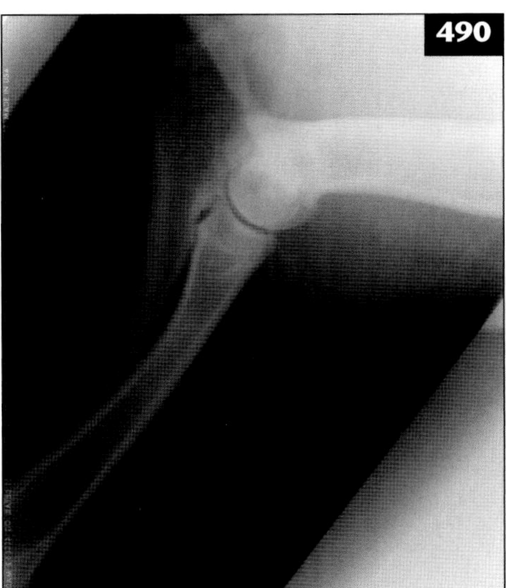

490 A lateral radiograph of the elbow in **489** does not reveal the extent of the bony changes.

Ultrasonographic examination of the lateral aspect of affected elbow joints does not reveal any joint effusion. At the craniolateral extent of the bony swelling there is often sudden disruption to the broad hyperechoic line representing bone surface. These margins of the hyperechoic line observed during ultrasonographic examination correspond to the typical enthesophytic reaction noted during radiographic examination.

Gross postmortem examination of affected elbow joints reveals severe erosion of articular cartilage and extensive osteophyte formation. Enthesophyte formation is best demonstrated by 'boiled-out' preparations (**487, 488**, p. 226).

Treatment

There is no effective treatment for elbow arthritis and affected sheep should be culled. Chondroprotective agents such as chondroitin sulphate or polysulphated glycosaminoglycan are useful in other species for degenerative joint disease but are not licensed for use in sheep. It is probable that these agents would be less effective in sheep because of the advanced pathological state when presented for diagnosis and treatment.

In acute cases, NSAIDs such as ketoprofen or flunixin should be administered for 3–5 days. The sheep should be isolated and confined to a small pen. Long-term pain relief can be attempted by daily administration of phenylbutazone (10 mg/kg).

Prevention/control measures

Joint injuries occur sporadically during handling and transport. Greater care and patience could be exercised when handling stock, especially when herded by overenthusiastic, poorly trained dogs. Care must be taken when introducing new rams into established groups.

The rapid growth and excessive body condition in ram lambs and shearlings demanded for sale purposes may predispose to elbow ligament damage. However, the apparent sex predisposition encountered in the author's practice may be considerably influenced by economic factors, with rams costing a great deal more than ewes. Trauma to the elbow joint may result during management procedures such as shearing and foot trimming, which involve casting the sheep.

Economics

Elbow arthritis necessitates culling of severely affected sheep, thus shortening the sheep's productive life span. This financial loss is greater when culling rams rather than ewes.

Welfare implications

Elbow arthritis represents a considerable welfare concern because of the chronicity and severity of the lesions, and the large number of sheep affected.

ARTHRITIS ASSOCIATED WITH MAEDI-VISNA VIRUS INFECTION

Definition/overview

There is a large variation in the manifestation of clinical disease caused by maedi-visna virus (MVV) infection. In the USA, periarticular lesions caused by MVV infection are a major cause of carcase condemnation in older ewes; such joint-associated lesions are rarely encountered in the UK. In the USA, MVV is more commonly referred to as ovine progressive pneumonia (OPP).

Aetiology

Arthritis caused by infection with MVV.

Clinical presentation

The carpal joints are most commonly enlarged due to fibrous tissue reaction in the joint capsule and periarticular structures. There is little joint effusion. Affected sheep rarely present with severe lameness, although there is restricted joint excursion and they tend to graze on their knees, resulting in the development of callused skin.

Differential diagnoses

- The major differential diagnoses are elbow arthritis and carpal hygromas.
- Chronic footrot and other painful foot lesions can also cause sheep to graze on their knees, leading to abrasions and fibrous tissue reaction.

Diagnosis

MVV infection can be confirmed serologically but it must be remembered that seropositive sheep can also present with elbow arthritis and footrot.

Treatment

There is no treatment for chronic joint lesions in sheep caused by MVV infection.

Prevention/control measures

MVV control strategies are discussed in more detail in Chapter 6 (p. 150).

Economics
MVV arthritis is a significant economic problem only in the USA where it results in the downgrading and possible condemnation of cull ewe carcases.

Welfare implications
Sheep with obvious lameness must not be transported and should be killed for welfare reasons once a definitive diagnosis has been established.

SPIDER SYNDROME

Definition/overview
Spider syndrome is an inherited osteopathy of Suffolk sheep. It is prevalent in Suffolk sheep in the USA, and occurs in those countries that have imported such breeding stock.

Aetiology
Spider syndrome is an inherited autosomal recessive condition.

Clinical presentation
There is pronounced carpal valgus; lateral deviation of the distal hindlimbs is much less pronounced. The long bones are much increased in length and have a thinner cortex than normal. These skeletal abnormalities may be present at birth or develop from 4–6 weeks of age. Problems with locomotion and feeding result in a very high mortality rate amongst spider syndrome lambs within the first month.

Differential diagnoses
The distinct clinical features of spider syndrome rule out other differential diagnoses.

Diagnosis
Diagnosis is based on clinical findings.

Treatment
There is no treatment and affected lambs should be euthanased for welfare reasons.

Prevention/control measures
Accurate recording of breeding data and culling heterozygous sheep can readily control this situation. Unfortunately, stud rams heterozygous for spider syndrome often have desirable characteristics that breeders are loath to lose from their flock. This practice of breeding from heterozygous sheep is remarkably short sighted and ill-judged.

In New Zealand, carrier sheep are detected by a DNA test and this has largely eliminated the problem in that country.

Economics
Culling affected sheep would cause short-term financial losses but greater long-term gains.

Welfare implications
Spider lambs must be euthanased as soon as the condition has been confirmed.

CLINICAL PROBLEM 1

A five-day-old Suffolk-cross lamb is presented with a displaced fracture of the distal tibia (**491**). The lamb weighs approximately 4 kg.

Describe how effective analgesia for fracture re-alignment and repair can be achieved.

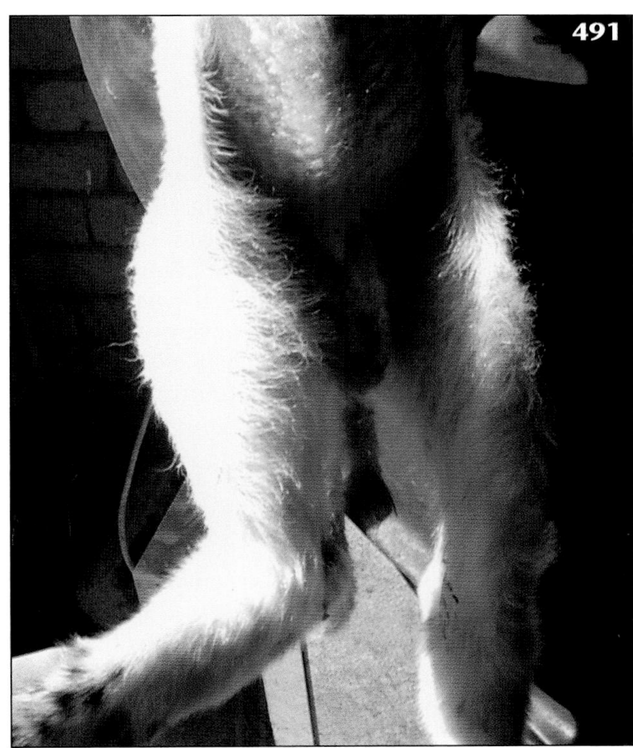

491 Five-day-old Suffolk-cross lamb with a displaced fracture of the distal tibia.

Options to achieve fracture alignment

- Elect simply to restrain the lamb with an assistant applying considerable traction to the distal limb.
- Attempt sedation of the lamb with xylazine.
- Alphaxalone/alphadolone is a very effective and safe general anaesthetic for a variety of surgical procedures in neonatal lambs. Unfortunately, alphaxalone/alphadolone may be considered prohibitively expensive for neonatal lambs.
- Effective analgesia after either lumbosacral or sacrococcygeal extradural injection of 4 mg/kg of 2% lidocaine solution (see Chapter 15: anaesthesia) allows a more detailed and pain-free clinical examination, and more effective fracture reduction and alignment, than can be achieved by physical restraint alone. This technique presents an inexpensive and readily available alternative to a protocol involving injectable general anaesthetic drugs. Brute strength is not acceptable.
- In many situations a simple metatarsal fracture can be splinted by the shepherd. Various materials can be used (**492**) and healing progresses uneventfully. Where the bone fragments are overriding, paralysis of the limb is essential to ensure correct and pain-free alignment.

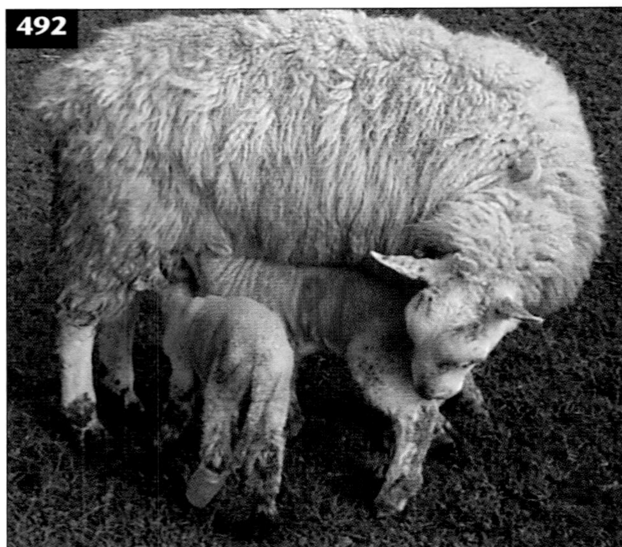

492 Fractures are commonly splinted by the shepherd, using various materials.

Aftercare

Paralysis of the hindlimbs following lumbosacral extradural injection lasts for up to four hours. After casting the leg, the lamb should be confined to a corner of the pen until ambulatory to prevent possible treading injury. Postoperative analgesic drugs (e.g. ketoprofen or flunixin meglumine), whilst not licensed for use in sheep species, should be administered for three consecutive days. As there is always the risk of sepsis in neonatal ruminants, even with closed fractures, a course of procaine penicillin should be administered for at least five consecutive days.

CLINICAL PROBLEM 2

A group of six Charollais-cross lambs, which were weaned three months ago, are presented because they have been lame 'for some time'. The lambs have been housed for the past six weeks and fed 0.6 kg of concentrates daily. Five of the six lambs are in sternal recumbency and appear reluctant to stand. All five lambs experience difficulty in raising themselves to their feet. The lambs have a stilted gait as they walk around the pen and do not run to avoid being caught. The lambs are reasonably well-grown (approximately 30 kg live weight) but in average body condition (BCS 2.0–2.5). The lambs on this farm are sold fat (average 36–42 kg live weight), and there are only 40 from 1,500 lambs remaining. It is estimated that these six lambs are four months behind their peers with respect to live weight gain. The lambs have a poor dry fleece, which lacks crimp.

All six lambs have one or both stifle joints affected. There is little joint effusion but marked thickening of the joint capsule (up to 1 cm), which physically restricts joint excursion. Four of the six lambs have bilateral carpal swellings (**493**) with associated enlargement of the prescapular lymph node. Two of the lambs have only one knee affected with an appreciable amount of wasting of the musculature over the shoulder relative to the unaffected side. Three of the lambs have enlarged hock joints (**494**).

The farmer reports that he treated approximately 60 of the 1,500 lambs for stiffness from approximately five weeks old.

How should this problem be investigated?
What is the prognosis for these lambs?
Comment on possible control measures.

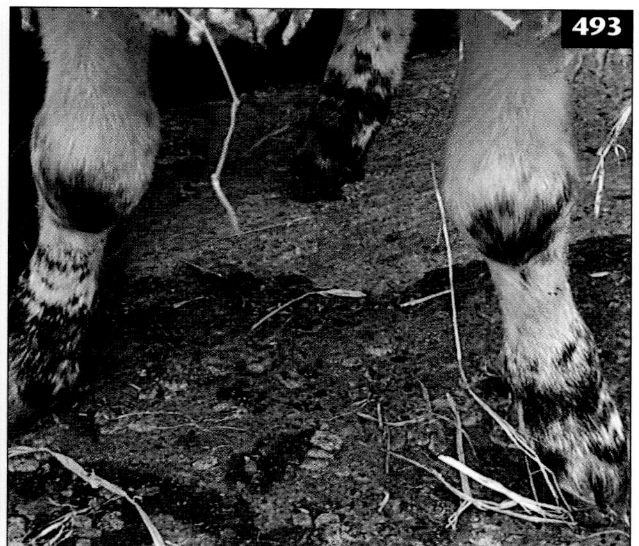

493 Bilateral carpal swellings in an eight-month-old Charollais-cross lamb.

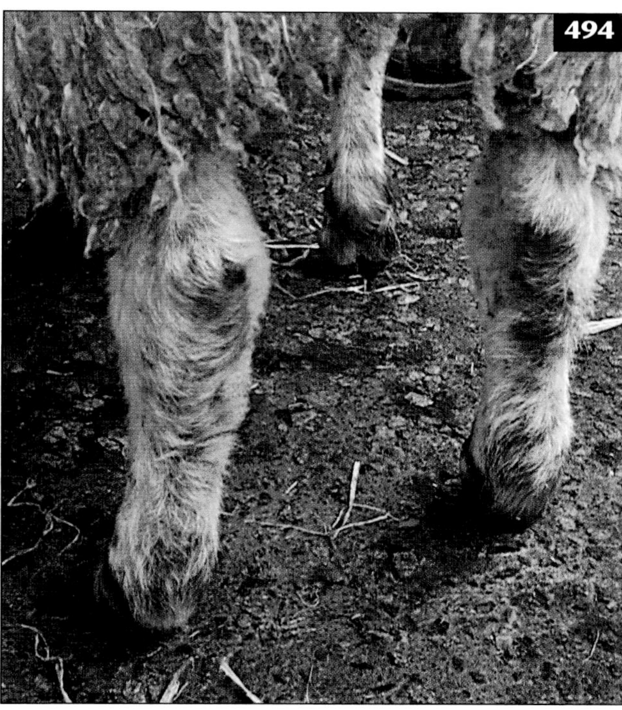

494 Enlarged right hock joint in an eight-month-old Charollais-cross lamb.

Investigations

There is little joint effusion; therefore, arthrocentesis cannot be undertaken.

The best course of action for diagnostic purposes would be to collect synovial membrane at necropsy for bacteriological culture from two or three severely lame lambs that have not received any antibiotic therapy. These lambs had all received antibiotic treatment some months ago but it was decided that such sampling offered the best chance for a positive diagnosis.

Postmortem examination of two lambs revealed that all the superficial carcase lymph nodes were chronically enlarged. The right carpal joint and both stifle joints revealed a severely proliferative synovial membrane thrown into many fronds. There were no gross abnormalities in the articular cartilage. Both stifle joints were very enlarged, with a proliferative synovial membrane. These changes are consistent with chronic polyarthritis, which is likely to have arisen by haematogenous spread of bacteria.

Erysipelothrix rhusiopathiae was grown in pure culture from synovial membrane from both lambs. *E. rhusiopathiae* is an important cause of infective arthritis, with high morbidity and moderate to severe lameness typically affecting growing lambs aged four weeks to four months.

Prognosis

The remaining four lambs were killed because they could not be presented at a slaughterhouse and such a degree of lameness and suffering must not be allowed to continue. Bacterial polyarthritis remains all too common in growing lambs and this has important welfare implications.

Control

Annual vaccination of the dam, affording passive protection of growing lambs, costs approximately 0.5% of the sale value of a lamb.

9 Urinary System

INTRODUCTION

Infections of the urinary system are rare in sheep and are invariably predisposed by either a traumatic event such as dystocia or urethral surgery to correct an obstruction. In contrast, urolithiasis is male sheep is common whenever inappropriate rations leading to calculi formation are fed.

CLINICAL EXAMINATION OF THE URINARY SYSTEM

Knowledge of the diet and the onset and progression of the condition is important. Observation of urination provides valuable information; a steady flow lasting 10–15 seconds is normal in the ram. Tenesmus, with only a few drops of urine voided, is grossly abnormal. Blockage to the free flow of urine leads to bladder distension and abdominal pain, which is expressed as frequent tail swishing, bruxism and periods spent in sternal/lateral recumbency. Affected sheep soon become inappetent and profoundly depressed. Frequent vocalization is common in lambs suffering from obstructive urolithiasis, while bruxism is more common in adults.

Examination of the preputial hairs reveals the presence of a small number of calculi in many normal sheep and is not a reliable indicator of urolithiasis. The penis can readily be exteriorized in sexually mature males; this allows examination of the glans and vermiform appendix. An assistant sits the ram on its rump. The penis is grasped through the sheath at the sigmoid flexure and extended, at the same time retracting the prepuce. A gauze swab is wrapped around the penis just proximal to the glans. Exteriorization of the penis appears painful in urolithiasis cases, presumably due to pressure of abdominal viscera on the distended bladder when the ram is sat on its rump. In such cases the penis should be exteriorized with the ram positioned in lateral recumbency.

URINALYSIS

Sheep rarely develop urinary tract infections. Urine collection can be attempted as part of the laboratory investigation of obstructive urolithiasis but little or no urine is voided. Catheterization of the bladder is possible in females but is rarely indicated. Urine specific gravity ranges from 1.015–1.045 in normal sheep, with pH values from 7.4–8.0. Urine should be checked for the presence of sediment, in particular struvite crystals. Glucose, ketones, protein, blood and bilirubin should be absent from urine. Because ultrasonography provides instant results with respect to urolithiasis diagnosis and gross bladder infection, urinalysis is rarely necessary.

BIOCHEMISTRY

Serum creatinine and blood urea nitrogen (BUN) concentrations are commonly used to determine renal function. Due to its distribution throughout the body, the BUN concentration may fall more slowly than serum creatinine following return to more normal renal function; therefore, BUN affords the more accurate prognosis. Under certain grazing conditions the high dietary nitrogen content may be reflected in an elevated BUN concentration but this rarely exceeds twice the normal level.

BACTERIOLOGY

Bacteriology of a urine sample is rarely undertaken because of the rare occurrence of primary urinary tract infections. Those infections that do arise post urethrostomy surgery are invariably associated with *Corynebacterium renale*.

Bacteraemic spread to the parenchymatous organs from a septic focus elsewhere may result in bacterial shedding into the urine from a renal infarct, but such secondary lesions rarely compromise renal function.

ULTRASONOGRAPHY

Ultrasonography has great practical application in the field investigation of urolithiasis in male sheep. Bladder distension, uroperitoneum and subcutaneous urine accumulation post urethral rupture can readily be determined using both linear array and sector scanners. Examination of the right kidney can be undertaken only with a sector scanner.

RADIOGRAPHY

Unlike in dogs and cats, radiography is rarely used to gather further information of the urinary tract in sheep. Radiography is costly, presents numerous safety concerns and is not readily portable for on-farm use, and it adds no new information to that gathered by ultrasonography.

Renal biopsy

While theoretically it is possible to undertake ultrasound-guided renal biopsy, this technique is not indicated in sheep as they rarely develop glomerulonephritis or similar conditions.

UROLITHIASIS

Definition/overview

Partial or complete urethral obstruction is a common condition of intensively reared entire male and castrated lambs (**495**) fed incorrectly formulated rations, and it also occurs occasionally in mature rams (**496**). Early recognition of clinical signs by the farmer, and prompt veterinary treatment, are essential to ensure a satisfactory outcome, because irreversible hydronephrosis quickly results from urinary back pressure. Early diagnosis is also important to allow rapid implementation of control measures and reduce the occurrence of future cases. Urolithiasis rarely affects pasture-fed lambs, and it is not recorded in ewes.

Aetiology

The most common cause of urolithiasis in male sheep is magnesium ammonium phosphate hexahydrate (struvite) calculi associated with feeding concentrate rations high in phosphate (>0.6%) and magnesium (>0.2%). Proteins within the bladder combine with these minerals to form calculi, which lodge within the urethra just proximal to the sigmoid flexure or within the vermiform appendix.

Clinical presentation

The early clinical signs of urinary tract obstruction in male sheep include separation from other sheep in the group and long periods spent in sternal recumbency. There is frequent tail swishing and foot stomping, especially in lambs. Affected sheep have a wide stance with the hindlimbs held well back, and they stretch frequently (**495**). They are inappetent, have an anxious, painful expression (**496**) and may often dog-sit. There is frequent tenesmus accompanied by painful bleating (lambs) and teeth grinding (adults). The mucous membranes are congested and the heart and respiratory rates are increased. Nil or only a few drops of blood-tinged urine are voided rather than a clear continuous flow. The preputial hairs are often dry compared to the moist/wet appearance in normal sheep. Calculi are frequently present on the preputial hairs of normal male sheep and are not indicative of urolithiasis.

Rarely does the considerable urinary back pressure cause bladder rupture; rather, urine leaks across the taut bladder wall, resulting in uroperitoneum. Rupture of the urethra/penis commonly occurs in

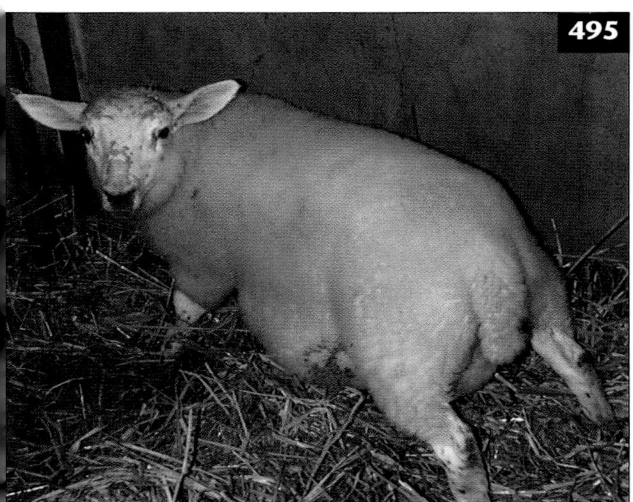

495 Urinary tenesmus in a housed three-month-old lamb. It has a wide-based stance and fluid swelling of the ventral abdominal wall due to urine accumulation.

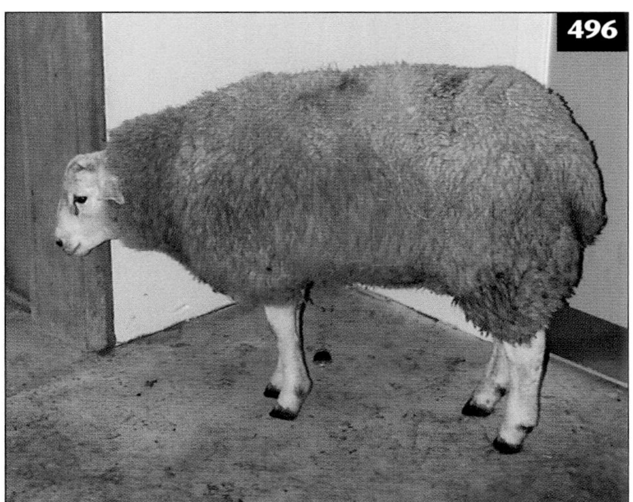

496 Depressed Texel ram suffering from urolithiasis. It has a roached back stance and lowered head carriage.

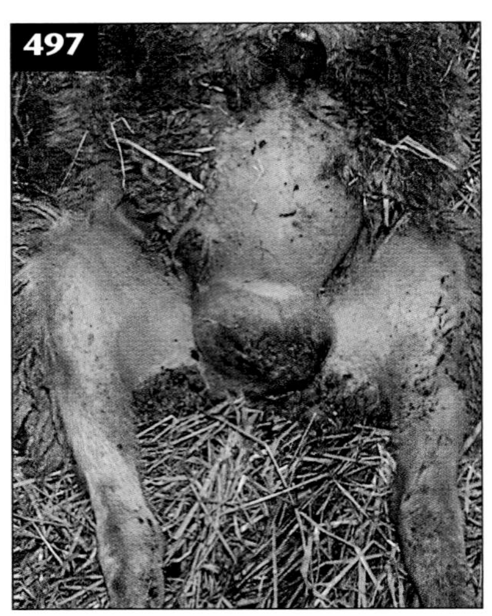

497 Urine accumulation along the prepuce and ventral abdomen of a ram. (See also **504**.)

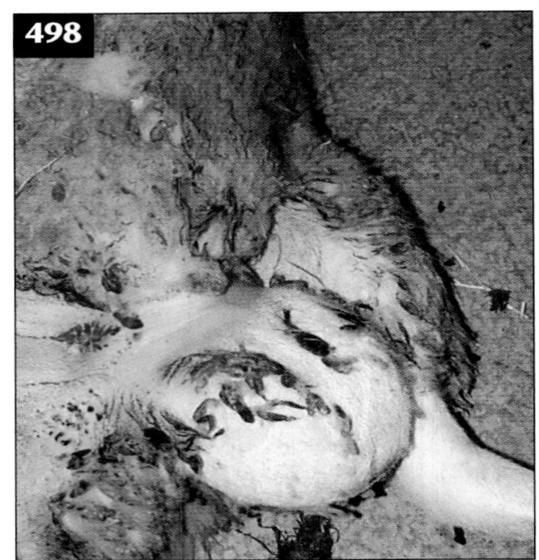

498 Scrotal swelling and fluid accumulation along the ventral abdomen following rupture of the penis caused by urolithiasis. (See also **502** and **503**.)

cases that have been neglected for a few days, with the resultant extensive subcutaneous swelling (up to 6 cm deep) extending from the scrotum cranially to the prepuce (**497**). The scrotum and prepuce are often markedly oedematous (**498**). Large sharply demarcated areas of purple discoloured skin develop along the ventrum overlying the subcutaneous urine accumulation. The discoloured skin becomes cold and, with associated necrotic muscle, will slough after 10–14 days if the animal survives the uraemic state and urinary back pressure/hydronephrosis.

Differential diagnoses

The differential diagnosis list can be restricted by a thorough examination. Abdominal ultrasonography readily identifies the painfully distended urinary bladder.

- The initial signs of colic in young growing lambs can be mistaken for abomasal/small intestinal volvulus but these conditions cause marked abdominal distension and profound toxaemia, with rapid deterioration. Coccidiosis and intussusception in lambs cause frequent tenesmus and abdominal pain.
- The clinical signs are frequently less pronounced in rams (inappetent, lethargic [**496**], long periods in sternal recumbency). Many infectious diseases present with similar clinical signs including painful foot lesions, respiratory disease/pleurisy and peritonitis.

Diagnosis

Excision of the vermiform appendix

Partial/complete urethral obstruction in mature rams occurs most commonly at the vermiform appendix. During the clinical examination the calculus can often be felt within the vermiform appendix when the penis is extruded. The diagnosis is confirmed by excision of the vermiform appendix, which produces a free flow of urine. The portion of the vermiform appendix distal to the calculus is frequently discoloured and often necrotic. While excision confirms the diagnosis of partial or complete urethral obstruction, it is not possible to establish an accurate prognosis based on clinical examination alone. Farmers are often unsure how long the sheep has been ill, and they tend to underestimate the duration of illness lest they are criticized for poor stockmanship.

Laboratory tests

In cases where the urethral obstruction occurs proximal to the vermiform appendix, and where there is no access to ultrasonography, laboratory tests are necessary to confirm the diagnosis. Marked elevations of BUN and creatinine concentrations occur as a result of partial or complete urethral obstruction; however, such increases are not pathognomic and there are no recognized threshold concentrations.

For example, in abdominal catastrophes such as intestinal volvulus, BUN and creatinine concentrations can be increased five-fold due to secondary influences on circulatory function and renal perfusion.

BUN and creatinine concentrations can be increased by many times the normal range (30–60 mmol/l [normal = 2–6 mmol/l] and >500 μmol/l [normal = 110–170 μmol/l], respectively) in male sheep with urolithiasis of less than two days' duration that recover after excision of the vermiform appendix. Such concentrations are not significantly different from those in sheep with a more prolonged urethral obstruction that has resulted in hydronephrosis. Rams in the latter category fail to recover irrespective of the treatment regimen.

Ultrasonographic examination

Diagnostic quality images of the bladder can readily be obtained using a 5.0 MHz sector transducer connected to a real-time, B-mode ultrasound machine. Many farm animal practices own a 5.0 MHz linear array scanner. This is used for early pregnancy diagnosis in cattle but it can also be used to examine the abdomen in sheep, although the depth of field is limited to 10 cm (see **508**, p. 238). Examination using a 5.0 MHz linear array scanner will readily identify uroperitoneum and a distended bladder. However, the true size of the bladder may not be measurable because it may extend to 20 cm in diameter. The bladder in normal male sheep is contained within the pelvis: therefore, the presence of a bladder extending for up to 10 cm or more beyond the pelvic brim is abnormal. Determination of the actual size of the bladder is of secondary importance.

Ultrasonographic examination of the bladder and caudal abdomen are undertaken in the standing animal. The right inguinal region immediately cranial to the pelvis is cleaned using a mild detergent solution diluted in warm tap water to remove superficial grease and debris. Ultrasound gel is applied liberally to the wet skin to ensure good contact. The transducer head is firmly held at right angles against the abdominal wall. There is scant peritoneal fluid in normal sheep and this cannot be visualized during ultrasonographic examination.

The distended bladder is clearly visible as an anechoic (black) area bordered by a bright white (hyperechoic) line (**499**) where the diameter may exceed 18 cm. Urine within the abdominal cavity appears as an anechoic area; the walls of abdominal viscera appear as broad hyperechoic (bright white) lines/circles displaced dorsally by the urine (**500**). Fibrin tags can sometimes be visualized within the uroperitoneum as hyperechoic filaments within the anechoic fluid.

Bladder distension is a very useful indicator of partial or complete urethral obstruction and it can be determined within minutes of an ultrasonographic on-farm investigation. The distended bladder is typically 6–8 cm in diameter in 20–40 kg growing lambs, increasing to 16–20 cm in mature rams (**499**).

The distended bladder and clinical findings confirm the diagnosis of partial or complete urethral obstruction. Prognosis is determined by the duration of the obstruction resulting in hydronephrosis. Examination of the right kidney can be undertaken using a 5.0 MHz sector transducer. The concave nature of the right sublumbar fossae precludes use of a 5.0 MHz linear transducer. The skin overlying the right sublumbar fossa is shaved using a scalpel blade; electric clippers do not afford a sufficiently good contact between the skin and the probe head. The right kidney is juxtaposed to the caudal pole of the liver underlying the dorsal aspect of the right sublumbar fossa. Advanced hydronephrosis is identified by an increased size of the renal pelvis,

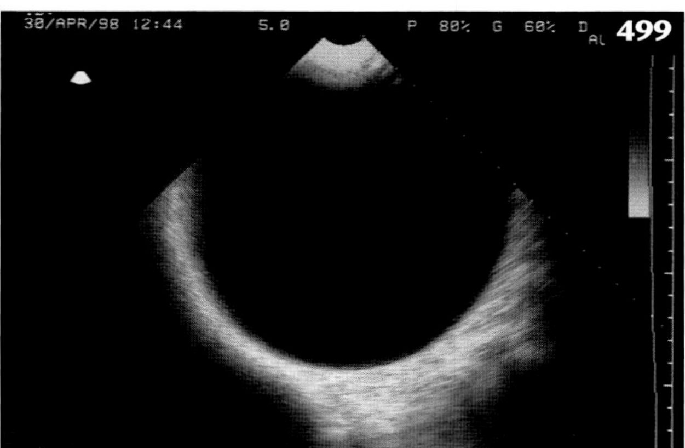

499 Ultrasonogram showing massive distension of the bladder of the Texel ram lamb in **496**. The bladder wall appears as a broad hyperechoic line. The urine appears anechoic. (5 MHz sector scanner.)

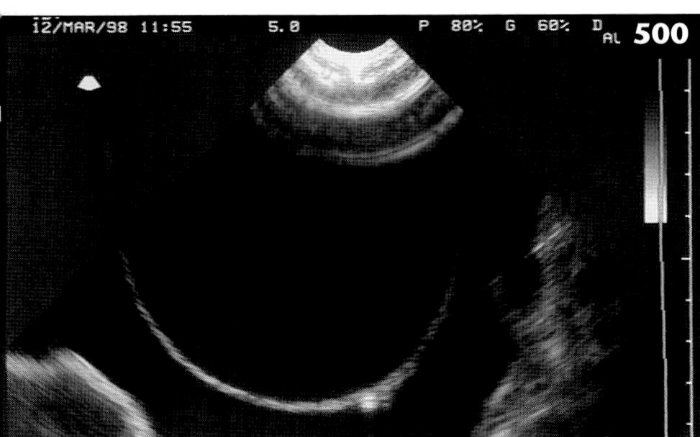

500 Ultrasonogram showing massive distension of the bladder with leakage into the peritoneum (uroperitoneum). The bladder wall and omentum appear as broad hyperechoic lines. The urine appears anechoic. (5 MHz sector scanner.)

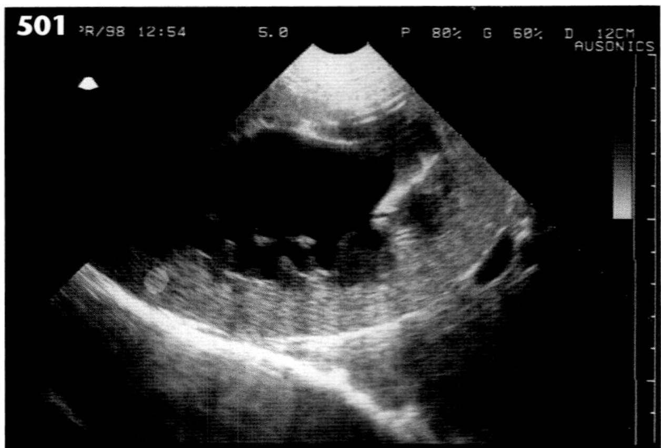

501 Ultrasonographic examination revealing hydronephrosis. There is urine distension of the renal pelvis.

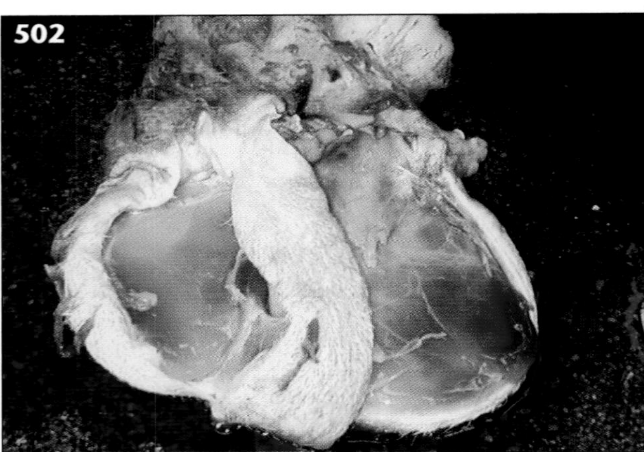

502 Necropsy finding of the scrotal swelling in **498**.

which is represented by the anechoic (fluid-filled) centre of the kidney (**501**). It is not possible to scan the left kidney in sheep but such examination is not necessary because the urinary tract obstruction is distal to the ureter; therefore, the condition is bilateral.

Treatment

In mature rams the blockage is commonly relieved when the penis is extruded and the vermiform appendix excised during clinical examination (see Diagnosis). Subsequent acidification of the urine by daily drenching with ammonium chloride is seldom undertaken and appears not to be necessary, as recurrence is uncommon. Antibiotic therapy is not indicated in such cases.

Surgical correction of urolithiasis caused by blockage proximal to the sigmoid flexure involves a subischial urethrostomy under caudal block; however, this is not a simple procedure. There are a number of important factors to consider prior to this salvage procedure: first, the welfare of the sheep, especially if there are considerable accumulations of urine subcutaneously; second, the likely interval to slaughter; and finally, the cost of surgery relative to the salvage carcase value. It must be remembered that drainage lymph nodes such as the deep inguinal lymph nodes could remain reactive for many weeks, resulting in condemnation of the carcase hindquarters at slaughter. Ascending infection of the sectioned urethra after surgery frequently causes cystitis/pyelonephritis, with clinical signs apparent around 4–6 weeks following surgery. The author recommends that subischial urethrostomy is not undertaken and that affected sheep are humanely destroyed as soon as the condition has been confirmed on clinical examination.

A subischial urethrostomy would not be appropriate in a breeding ram, where the more complicated and costly tube cystotomy procedure has been described. However, this procedure should only be undertaken when the veterinarian is certain of his/her diagnosis and anticipates a probable full recovery after surgery (i.e. no evidence of hydronephrosis).

Urethral rupture

Rupture of the urethra results in a subcutaneous accumulation of urine involving the prepuce and extending caudally along the ventral abdomen to the scrotum (**502**). The extent of this swelling can be difficult to determine during clinical examination, not least because this area is painful. The true extent of any subcutaneous swelling can be readily quantified during ultrasonographic examination (**503, 504**) using a 5.0 MHz linear transducer. It is not uncommon for urine to collect to a depth of 6–8 cm (**504**). In such cases, even if surgery is successful, considerable sloughing occurs. The multiloculated ultrasonographic appearance of the subcutaneous swelling indicates that drainage through a single or multiple skin incisions should not be undertaken.

Pathology

The extent of the bladder distension (**499**) can readily be appreciated at necropsy (**505, 506**) in sheep that are euthanased following a diagnosis of advanced hydronephrosis (**501, 507**).

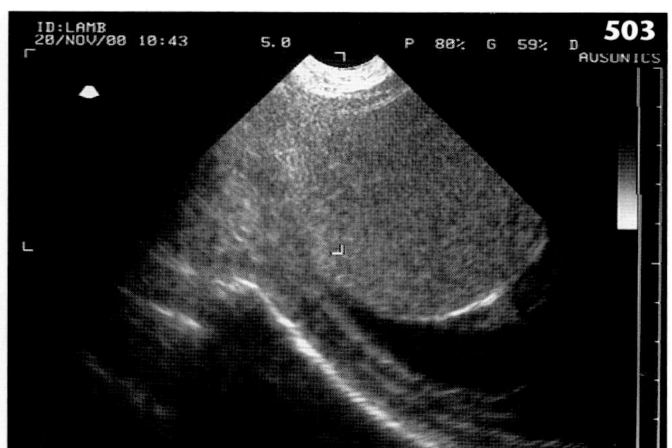

503 Ultrasonographic appearance of the scrotal swelling in **498**.

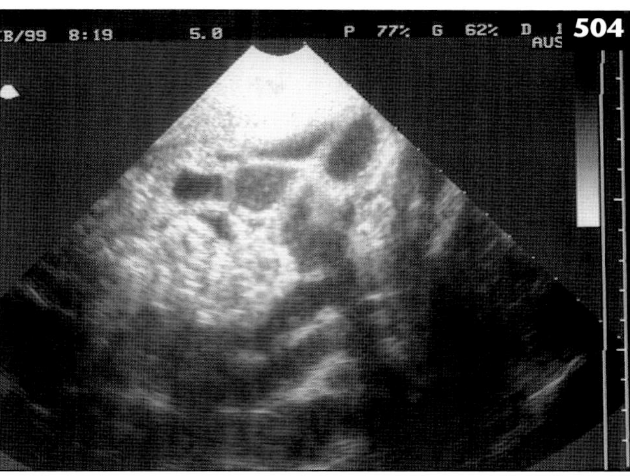

504 Ultrasonographic appearance of the subcutaneous tissue along the prepuce and ventral abdomen of the ram in **497**.

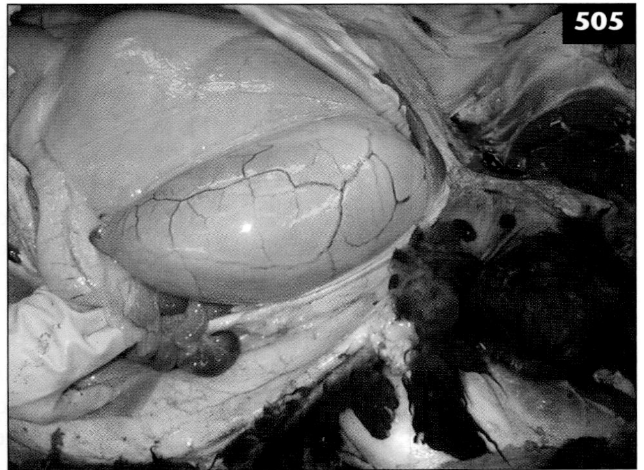

505 Necropsy revealing a massively distended bladder caused by urolithiasis. (See ultrasonogram in **499**.)

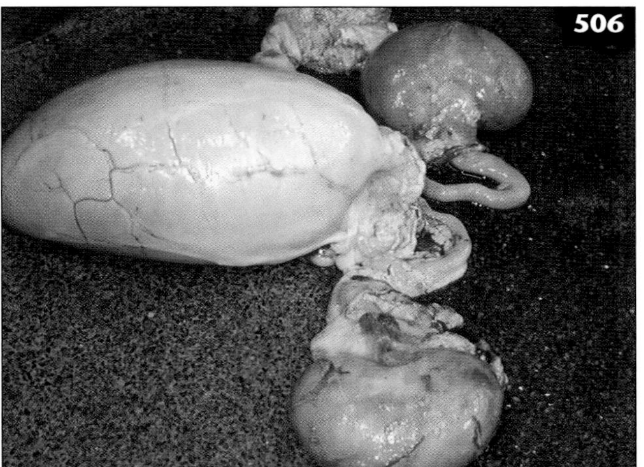

506 Dissection of the urinary tract revealing hydronephrosis, hydroureter and bladder distension. (See ultrasonograms **499** and **501**.)

Prevention/control measures

Correct ration formulation with appropriate mineralization is the basis for prevention of urolithiasis in intensively reared sheep. Urine acidifiers such as ammonium chloride are commonly added to the rations. Sodium chloride has been added to rations to promote water intake. Provision of roughage promotes saliva production and water intake. Fresh clean water must always be available and frequent checks must be made for frozen pipes and water troughs during subzero temperatures.

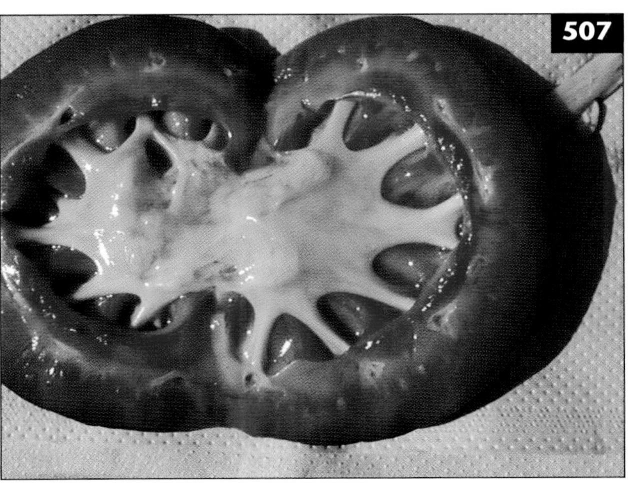

507 Necropsy revealing hydronephrosis of the kidney in **501**.

Economics

Excision of the vermiform appendix soon after obstruction affords an excellent prognosis in adult rams and involves little expense. However, surgical correction of urolithiasis by subischial urethrostomy is a salvage procedure and is not warranted for either welfare or financial reasons.

Welfare implications

With the exception of simple blockage relieved after excision of the vermiform appendix, all sheep with urolithiasis should be euthanased at first presentation. Efforts are more effectively directed at prevention of further cases.

URINARY STRICTURE

Urinary stricture with development of urolithiasis is uncommon in the ewe but the following case report further emphasizes the application of ultrasonography in general practice.

A four-year-old Scottish mule ewe was presented with a cervicovaginal prolapse. The prolapsed tissues were thoroughly cleaned with diluted disinfectant solution, replaced under caudal analgesia and retained with a Buhner suture of 5 mm umbilical tape. Approximately two days later, despite instruction to untie the suture before first stage labour commenced, both lambs were expelled, which tore out the suture and caused a large vaginal tear. The vaginal tear was immediately repaired under caudal analgesia and the ewe injected with oxytetracycline (20 mg/kg i/m for 5 consecutive days). The ewe made a good recovery and nursed both lambs until presented for veterinary exam-ination three months later.

The shepherd observed that the ewe was separated from other sheep in the group and was spending long periods in sternal recumbency. There was frequent tail swishing, tenesmus and bruxism and the shepherd suspected early cutaneous myiasis. On veterinary examination the ewe was dull and in poor body condition (BCS 1.5). The mucous membranes were congested. The heart and respiratory rates were within normal limits. Ruminal movements were absent. The ewe made frequent attempts to urinate but only a very fine jet of blood-tinged urine was voided under great pressure for 2–5 seconds rather than a continuous flow. The vulval orifice was reduced to only 2 mm diameter by fibrous tissue.

On ultrasonographic examination the distended bladder was clearly visible as an anechoic area measuring 9 cm diameter (**508**) bordered by a broad white (hyperechoic) line. The bladder wall appeared much thicker than normal, with many large fibrin tags on the mucosal surface, which appeared as broad hyperechoic strands extending 2–3 cm from the mucosal surface (**509**). Up to five cross-sections of uterine horn, measuring up to 5 cm in diameter, were imaged craniodorsal to the bladder (**509**). The uterine contents appeared anechoic but contained numerous hyperechoic spots. Examination of the right kidney was undertaken using a 5.0 MHz sector transducer. Hydronephrosis was identified by the increased size of the renal pelvis.

The ewe was euthanased immediately the degree of hydronephrosis was established, and a postmortem

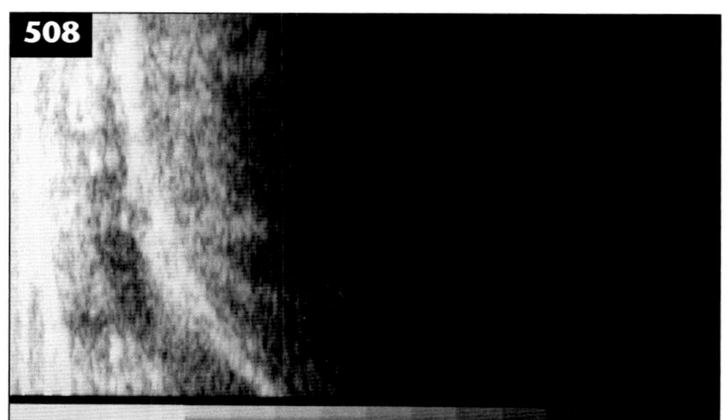

508 Urinary stricture. Ultrasonogram showing a distended bladder in a Scottish mule ewe (5.0 MHz linear array scanner). The probe is at the left of the image. The bladder wall appears as a broad hyperechoic (white) line with numerous fibrin tags on the mucosal surface.

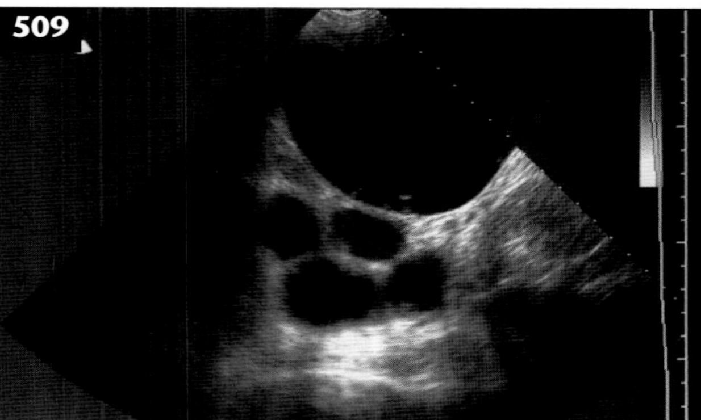

509 Urinary stricture. Fibrin is deposited on the mucosal surface of the distended bladder. The uterine horns are distended with purulent material, which appears as an anechoic (black) area with multiple hyperechoic (white) dots.

examination performed. The vagina was greatly distended with blood-tinged urine and it contained a large 8 cm diameter fibrinous clot. There was a severe purulent cystitis (**510**) with numerous large fibrin tags on the mucosal surface. Both kidneys showed marked hydronephrosis.

ULCERATIVE POSTHITIS (*Syn*: sheath rot)

Definition/overview

Ulcerative posthitis is an ulcerative condition of the sheath commonly associated with high dietary protein intake. Affected sheep often have concurrent lameness. Long periods spent in sternal recumbency may exacerbate the sheath infection.

In Australia and New Zealand ulcerative posthitis is known as pizzle-rot, and the severe form as balano-posthitis. In can be a serious problem in these two countries, particularly in Merino wethers being kept for wool production.

Aetiology

The condition is caused by *Corynebacterium renale*, which contains the enzyme urease. Urease is capable of breaking down urea in the urine to release ammonia, which is caustic to the epithelium of the prepuce.

Clinical presentation

Sheep with ulcerative posthitis have a strong ammoniacal smell from the stained fleece around the prepuce. Typically, the prepuce is swollen and oedematous, with a necrotic circumferential lesion about 1 cm wide at the skin/prepuce margin (**511**). The lesion is often covered by scab material and bleeds profusely if the scab is removed. Secondary cutaneous myiasis may occur in neglected cases.

Differential diagnoses

Urolithiasis.

Diagnosis

Diagnosis is based on the clinical signs and rapid response to antibiotic therapy.

Treatment

Ulcerative posthitis can be treated with penicillin (i/m daily for 5 or more consecutive days). Topical antiseptics can be applied to the lesions. Reducing the protein content in the diet is not possible when rams are at pasture; any concentrate supplementation should have a low protein content. In Australia and New Zealand, early cases have been reported to respond well to reducing feed intake whilst maintaining access to water. This causes urine acidification. Ammonium chloride *per os* may also aid this process. Any lameness should be treated promptly to prevent prolonged sternal recumbency and urine scalding and also to reduce the risk of infectious posthitis. Phimosis is uncommon following infectious posthitis. The farmer should be advised to remove the wool from around the prepuce to reduce the risk of contamination predisposing to cutaneous myiasis.

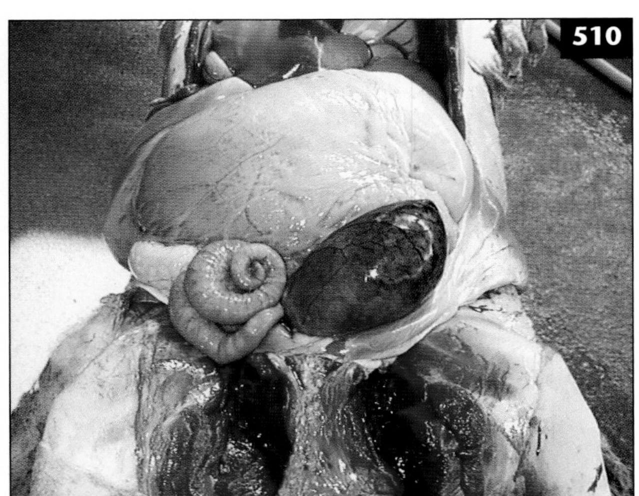

510 Urinary stricture. Necropsy. The bladder is distended and has a severely inflamed wall. The uterine horns are distended with purulent material.

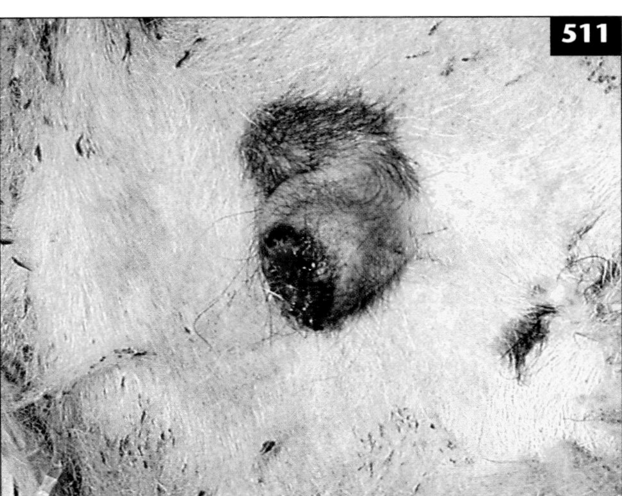

511 Posthitis in a ram suffering from sheath rot. The sheath is oedematous and there is diphtheresis at the preputial orifice.

Prevention/control measures
Appropriate nutrition and prompt attention to lameness should prevent this condition. Testosterone implant treatment is often used in Australia to prevent posthitis in wethers.

Economics
Ulcerative posthitis can be readily treated and is of little or no economic importance.

Welfare implications
The preputial lesions are painful but respond readily to antibiotic therapy.

NEPHROSIS

Definition/overview
Nephrosis occurs sporadically in young lambs between two and four weeks old, and in growing lambs between two and four months old. Cases in the latter age group often appear after an outbreak of coccidiosis and/or nematodirosis.

Aetiology
The aetiology of nephrosis has not been resolved, although a toxic insult is considered the probable aetiology.

Clinical presentation
Affected lambs are very depressed (**512**) and do not suck. They appear thirsty as they frequently stand with their heads over a water trough (**513**) but they drink little. The lambs appear gaunt with little abdominal content and they rapidly become emaciated. The rectal temperature is normal. There is often evidence of faecal staining of the perineum. The faeces are soft and malodorous.

Differential diagnoses
The important differential diagnoses include:
- Coccidiosis.
- Nematodirosis.
- Listeriosis.
- Starvation.

Bacterial infections, including hepatic necrobacillosis, chronic suppurative pneumonia, chronic peritonitis and infected urachus, can also present with many of the clinical signs listed above.

Diagnosis
Diagnosis is based on the clinical findings and biochemical findings of hypoalbuminaemia and markedly elevated BUN concentrations.

For example, a six-week-old lamb with nephrosis revealed a markedly elevated BUN concentration of 58.2 mmol/l (normal = 2–6 mmol/l) and a low serum albumin concentration of 20 g/l (normal = 30–36 g/l). While these biochemical results are also consistent with urolithiasis, there was no bladder enlargement and no urine accumulation within the abdominal cavity or the subcutaneous tissue of the ventral abdomen.

Necropsy of sheep with nephrosis reveals very pale swollen kidneys (**514, 515**).

Treatment
There is no treatment and affected lambs should be euthanased.

Prevention/control measures
The condition occurs sporadically and there are no recognized control measures.

Economics
Nephrosis is not a major economic concern because of its sporadic occurrence.

Welfare implications
Affected lambs appear very gaunt and do not feed, and they eventually die of starvation/uraemia. Such lambs are rarely presented for veterinary examination. Diligent stockmanship will identify affected lambs, which should be euthanased once they have failed to respond to anthelmintic/anticoccidial/antibiotic therapy.

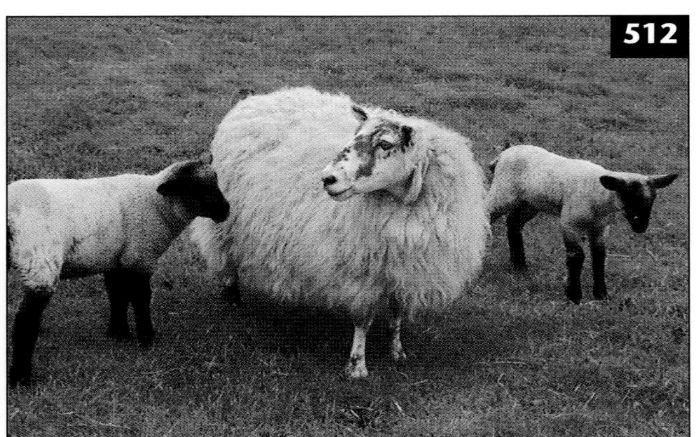

512 Nine-week-old lamb (right side) suffering from nephrosis. Compare this lamb with its normal co-twin.

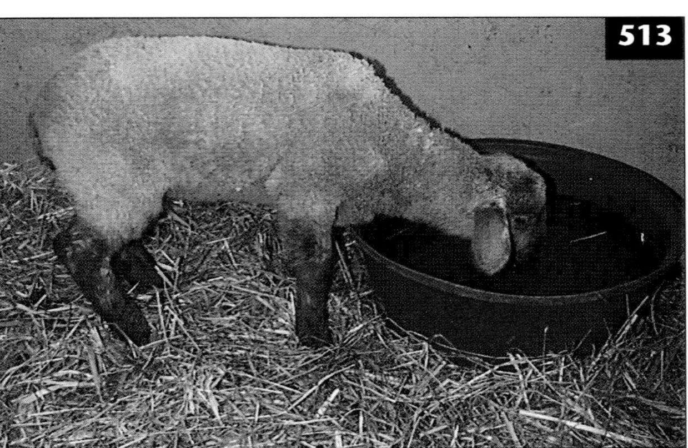

513 Obvious thirst in a lamb suffering from nephrosis.

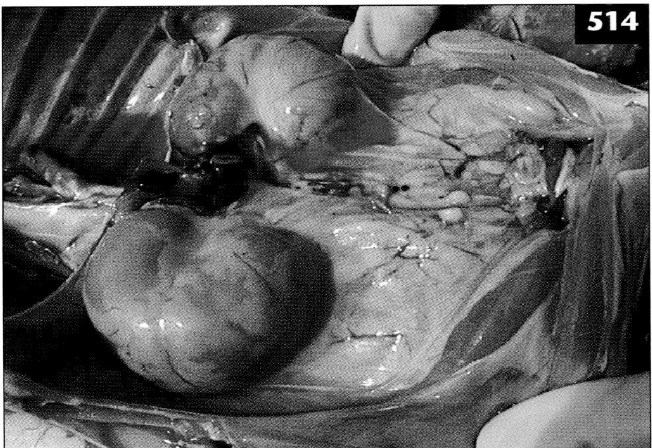

514 Necropsy of the lamb in **513**. The enlarged pale kidneys are typical of nephrosis.

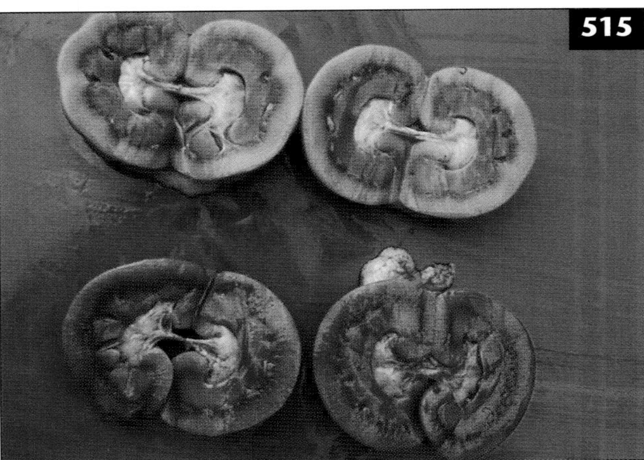

515 Nephrotic kidneys (top) from a six-week-old lamb compared with a normal lamb (bottom).

CLINICAL PROBLEM 1

A yearling pedigree Suffolk ram is presented. It has been dull and inappetent for the past six hours. The farmer reports that the ram had been lying down more than usual and occasionally straining.

Clinical examination

When presented the ram is dull and easily caught and restrained. There is frequent bruxism. The rectal temperature is normal (39.5°C). The heart rate is increased to 90 bpm. The mucous membranes are normal. Auscultation of the chest fails to reveal any abnormalities. There are reduced rumen sounds.

The ram shows abdominal straining but only a few drops of urine rather than a continuous flow are voided. The urine is slightly blood tinged. There are no calculi on the preputial hairs.

What conditions should be considered and what further clinical examination should be undertaken?

Differential diagnoses

Urolithiasis.

Action

The ram was positioned on its hindquarters and the penis was extruded (**516**). A calculus could be felt within the tip of the vermiform appendix. The vermiform appendix was excised with a scalpel blade. The ram was allowed to stand and a continuous flow of approximately 500 ml of urine was produced.

Outcome

The ram was reported to be normal the following morning and no further problems were encountered.

Further tests

BUN and creatinine determinations and ultrasonography of the bladder and kidney could be undertaken but were not necessary in this case because of the short duration of illness and resolution of the problem after amputation of the vermiform appendix.

Early recognition of partial/complete urethral obstruction is essential in sheep because hydronephrosis develops rapidly due to the back pressure within the urinary tract. Invariably, the penis is much easier to exteriorize in cases of urolithiasis than normal, presumably due to the increased pressure within the urinary tract.

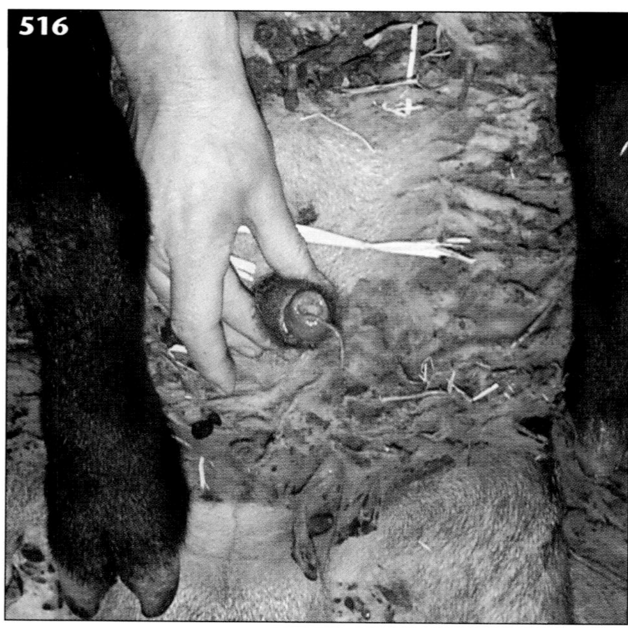

516 A calculus is clearly visible within the distal 2 cm of the vermiform appendix.

10 The Skin

INTRODUCTION

Diseases of the skin are important for numerous reasons. Wool yield and quality are adversely affected, which is the major product of the sheep industry in many countries such as Australia, and generalized infections can lead to debility and possibly death.

Focal bacterial infections of the skin are common in sheep and may become generalized under favourable climatic conditions such as prolonged wet weather after shearing. Viral infections of the mucocutaneous junctions are common in young lambs but may also affect adults. Ectoparasite infestations are very common in sheep, causing severe economic losses and raising serious welfare concerns. Some ectoparasites are also vectors for bacterial, rickettsial and viral infections, which may cause serious disease outbreaks. Therefore, the skin should not be considered in isolation and reference will be made to diseases of other organ systems (e.g. louping ill, which is transmitted by ticks).

CONTAGIOUS PUSTULAR DERMATITIS

(*Syns*: orf, scabby mouth, contagious ecthyma)

Definition/overview

Contagious pustular dermatitis (CPD) is a viral infection of the coronary band and the muco-cutaneous junction of the mouth. Outbreaks of CPD may occur within 10–14 days of pasture change, especially on to pastures that contain thistles, gorse or stubble, which cause superficial trauma to the lips/buccal cavity. CPD has a worldwide distribution and is a major disease problem in many countries. CPD is a zoonosis.

Aetiology

CPD is caused by a pox virus (genus Parapoxvirus), which can remain infective for many months in dried scabs.

Clinical presentation

CPD virus most commonly results in proliferative lesions at the coronary band (**517**) and the mucocutaneous junction of the mouth (**518**). It is particularly severe in artificially reared lambs less than two months old. Morbidity can be high but mortality in uncomplicated cases is low. Lesions persist for 2–4 weeks then slowly regress. Disease in a flock generally persists for 6–8 weeks.

Initial papule and vesicle stages are rarely observed. Scabs progressing to large proliferative wart-like structures, which bleed profusely following trauma to their base, are the more common presentation. Large scabs are often present at the commisures of the lips and along the gum margins surrounding the incisor teeth. Much less commonly, lesions may involve the hard palate and tongue.

The virus can spread rapidly within a group of orphan lambs sharing the same feeding equipment. In sucking lambs, lesions frequently develop on the medial aspect of the ewe's teats due to trauma by the lamb's incisor teeth. This permits entry of the virus. The teat lesions are painful and the ewe will typically not allow its lamb(s) to suck. Mastitis, occasionally gangrenous in nature, may follow the development of teat lesions.

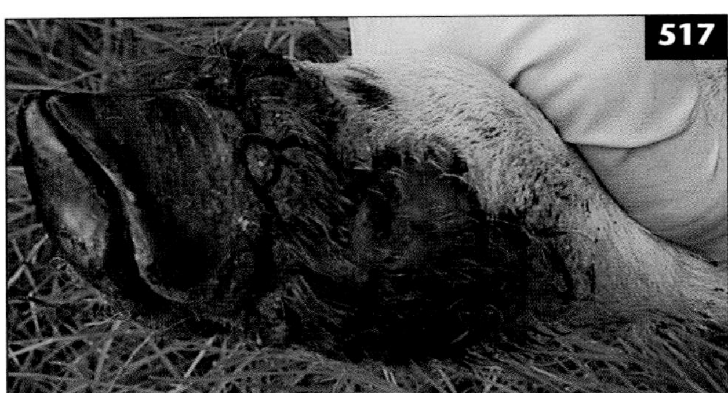

517 CPD virus infection causing proliferative lesions at the coronary band.

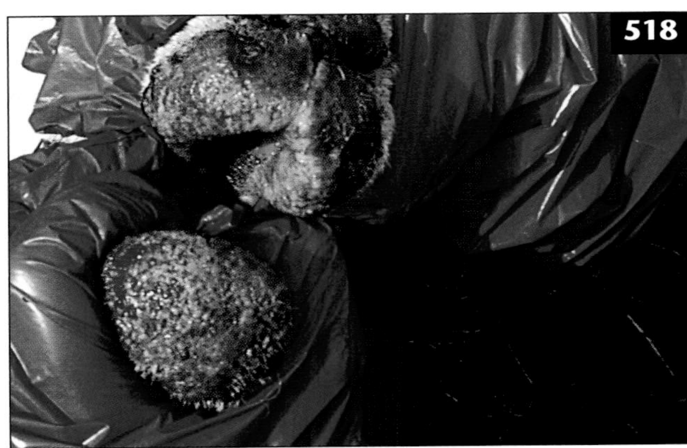

518 CPD virus infection causing proliferative lesions at the mucocutaneous junction of the mouth.

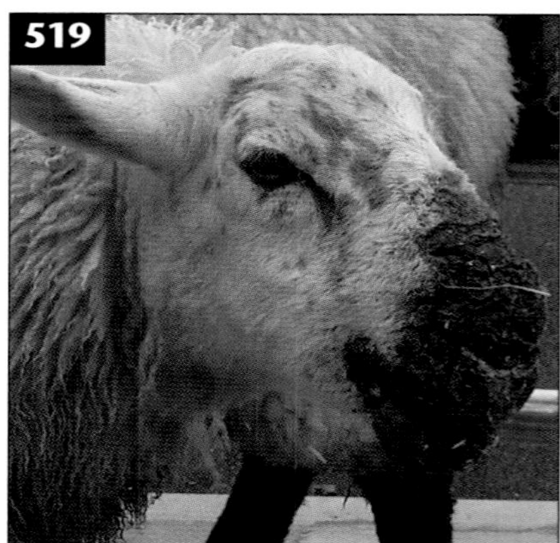

519 CPD virus and *S. aureus* may act synergistically, causing severe facial dermatitis.

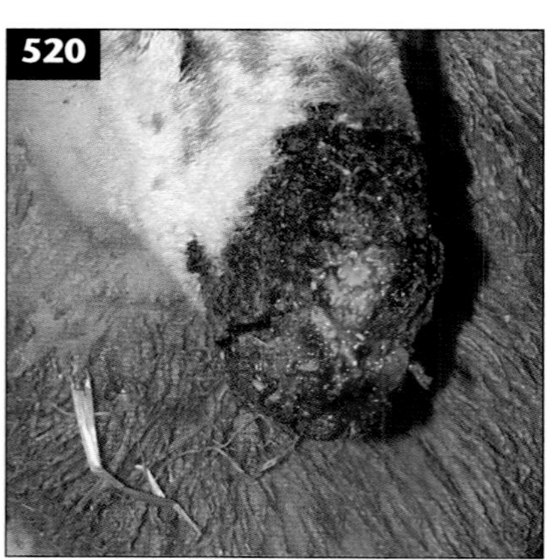

520 CPD virus and *S. aureus* may act synergistically, causing severe facial dermatitis involving the lower lip.

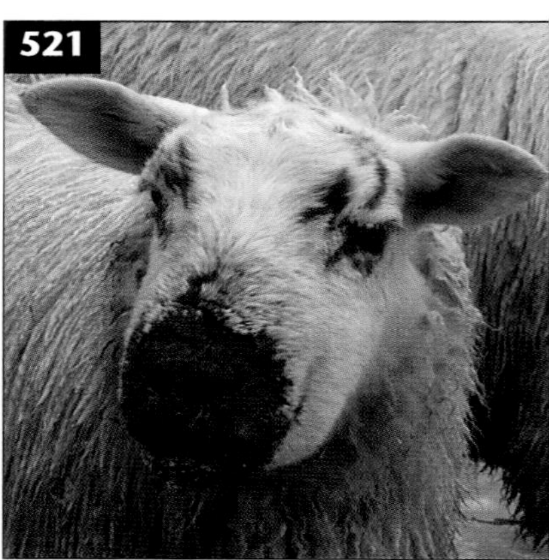

521 Facial lesions become desiccated, forming hard scabs separated by deep fissures.

CPD virus and *Staphylococcus aureus* may act synergistically to cause severe facial dermatitis, which appears as sharply demarcated areas extending up 8 cm from the muzzle (**519**) and involving the lower lip (**520**), with scab material also palpable within the hairs extending for a further 2–3 cm from the periphery of the visible lesions. The skin is oedematous, with serous exudation and superficial pus accumulation and adherent straw and other foreign material, which may become desiccated and form hard scabs separated by deep fissures (**521**). Careful removal of the scabs reveals a deep bed of exuberant granulation tissue. Exuberant granulation tissue and overlying scab material narrowing the nostrils may cause dyspnoea, with stertor and abdominal breathing.

CPD virus and *Dermatophilus congolensis* may act synergistically to produce large granulomatous masses extending 4–8 cm proximally from the coronary band; this is often referred to as 'strawberry footrot'. These lesions bleed profusely when traumatized. Typically, strawberry footrot lesions only affect one limb. They are more commonly seen in weaned lambs recently moved on to stubble. While lesions are severe in individual lambs, the morbidity is generally low. Healing takes many months. Slaughter is delayed because of marked reaction in the drainage lymph nodes.

Differential diagnoses

- The very early stages of CPD with papule and vesicle formation could be mistaken for FMD but the CPD lesions affect the lambs' mouths only and are not seen around the coronary band. Furthermore, not all CPD lesions would be at this early vesicular stage and more typical proliferative crusting lesions would also be present. Sheep affected with FMD are febrile, inappetent and often severely lame for a brief period, with vesicles in the interdigital skin and around the coronary band, although these signs may be easily overlooked.
- Facial dermatitis in growing lambs can be caused by *S. aureus*, *D. congolensis* and photosensitization. *S. aureus* infection of the skin of the head typically causes oedematous painful eyelids with rapid hair loss from adjacent skin (periorbital eczema); these infections are more severe in orphan lambs (**522**). *D. congolensis* infection of haired skin typically results in multiple, small superficial pustules but rarely causes significant skin lesions except in debilitated lambs.
- Sheep pox should also be included in the differential diagnoses in countries where this infection is endemic.

Diagnosis

Diagnosis is based on the finding of large proliferative lesions around the lips and nostrils of growing lambs. Virus can be demonstrated by direct electron microscopy of fresh lesions.

Treatment

Treatment is largely unsuccessful except in lambs with superficial secondary bacterial infection of scabs and associated oedema, which show a good response to intramuscular procaine penicillin injections and topical oxytetracycline for 3–7 consecutive days (**523**).

There is some evidence that levamisole (2.5 mg/kg s/c every 3–4 days) speeds up remission of lesions.

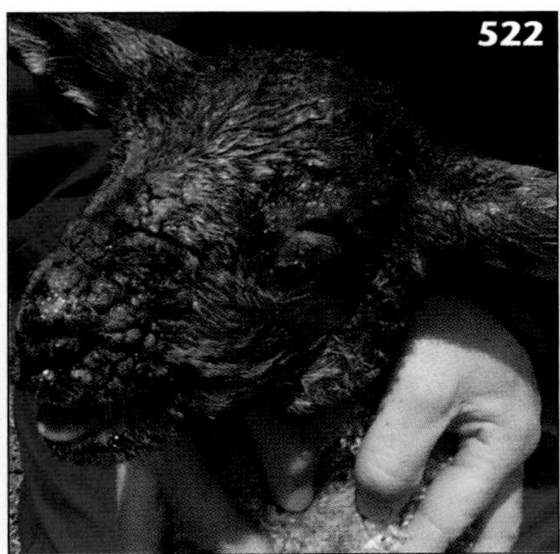

522 Severe staphylococcal folliculitis in an orphan lamb.

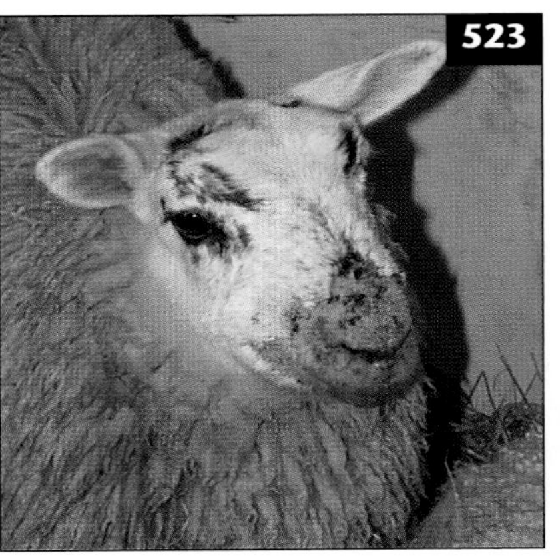

523 A good response achieved for severe facial dermatitis in the lamb in **521** following intramuscular procaine penicillin injections and topical oxytetracycline for five consecutive days.

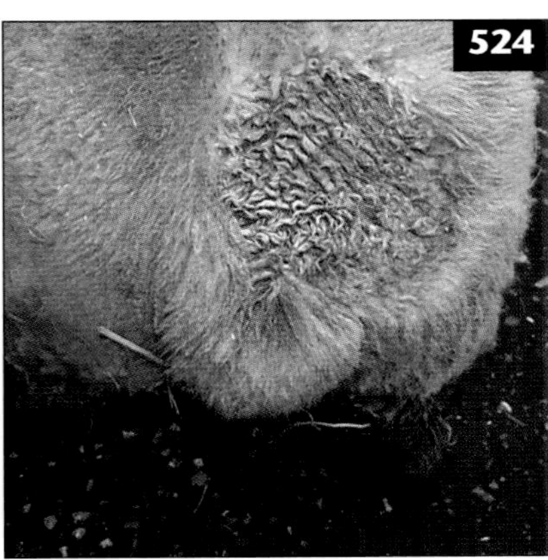

524 Dermatophilosis affecting the tailhead of a Suffolk ewe. Such lesions are commonly struck.

Prevention/control measures
Disease is introduced into a flock by carrier sheep with no obvious skin lesions. Infection can remain viable in dry scab material in buildings for many months and is the likely reason for persistence of infection from year to year on the same premises. Thorough cleaning and disinfection of lambing accommodation may, there- fore, help to break the usual annual appearance of disease.

Control following scarification with a live vaccine proves difficult to quantify but is routinely undertaken in many flocks in the UK. Vaccine must never be used in a clean flock. Vaccination is by scarification of the inner thigh in lambs and the axillary region in ewes. The timing of vaccination is approximately six weeks before the anticipated occurrence of disease. Care must be exercised during handling the live vaccine as it is affected by high temperatures and inactivated by disinfectants.

Economics
CPD is a significant problem in orphan lambs and other ill-thriven lambs. CPD is rarely a major problem in well-fed, well-thriven stock. Vaccination is inexpensive (0.7% of the sale value of a lamb; 0.3% of the value of a ewe) but the procedure is time-consuming and there is a risk of human infection.

Welfare implications
Severe oral and foot lesions cause obvious discomfort and are associated with weight loss and poor body condition, especially in orphan lambs. Unless every effort is undertaken to rear orphan lambs using automated feeders, they should be sold within the first week of life. Many farmers do not rear orphan lambs well and they pose a source of many pathogens, including CPD virus, when they are eventually turned out to pasture with the remainder of the flock.

DERMATOPHILOSIS
(*Syns*: lumpy wool, mycotic dermatitis, rain scald)

Definition/overview
Dermatophilosis is a common skin infection of sheep worldwide. Dermatophilosis is of minor significance in the UK but is a major concern in sheep economies that rely on fine wool production (e.g. Australia and New Zealand).

Aetiology
Dermatophilosis is caused by *Dermatophilus congolensis*. Transmission of infection requires wet conditions and close contact (e.g. during gathering). Prolonged moist skin allows penetration of the bacterium and establishment of infection. It is reported that under certain circumstances infection may cause a severe suppurative inflammation of the skin.

Clinical presentation
In the UK, dermatophilosis is encountered along the dorsum in short-wooled breeds such as the Suffolk (**524**) and the Border Leicester, where it causes serum exudation and scab formation at the base of the wool fibres, which then slowly grow out. Dermatophilosis is

usually encountered in summers when there has been wet weather for 3–6 weeks after shearing. The lesions rarely develop clinical significance (**525**), being restricted to a small number of well-circumscribed scabs up to 5 cm in diameter, which eventually lift off exposing superficial skin infection. The damaged skin re-grows pigmented wool, which appears unsightly in sale rams. Occasionally, the scabs attract blowfly strike. Discrete 3–5 mm diameter 'bottle-brush' lesions are often found around the muzzle (**526**) and on the margins of the ears of poorly-thriven sheep but they are of no clinical significance, being more an indication of debility than a cause thereof.

In New Zealand it is reported that young lambs may suffer extensive skin lesions of dermatophilosis with loss of fleece protection, which may result in death during adverse weather. In addition, lumpy wool lesions attract blowflies, leading to cutaneous myiasis. Such severe infections are rarely encountered in the UK. In Australia it is reported that lumpy wool causes shearing difficulties and downgrading of fine wool.

Differential diagnoses

- Dermatophilosis lesions along the dorsum are readily differentiated from sheep scab on clinical examination.
- Dermatophilosis lesions on the face and muzzle should be distinguished from ringworm.

Diagnosis

Diagnosis of dermatophilosis is based on clinical examination and, if necessary, stained smears from the underside of scabs plucked from the fleece, which reveal coccoid bacteria.

Treatment

Treatment is rarely indicated but rams intended for sale are sometimes treated to prevent skin lesions re-growing black wool, which is considered a defect at sale. Procaine penicillin injected intramuscularly for three consecutive days effects a cure but it may take several weeks for the scabs to be shed from the growing fleece.

Prevention/control measures

A variety of dip solutions have been used in New Zealand and Australia to prevent dermatophilosis following shearing, including 1% potassium aluminium sulphate spray or dip solution. Dermatophilosis is rarely a disease of well-fed sheep; severe disease occurs only in sheep debilitated from another cause.

Economics

Effective control strategies, including antibiotic therapy and sprays/dips, limit production losses in those countries producing fine wools. Dermatophilosis is not an economic concern in the UK.

Welfare implications

Dermatophilosis presents welfare concerns in countries where secondary cutaneous myiasis is common (e.g. Australia and New Zealand) but not in the UK.

CASEOUS LYMPHADENITIS

Definition/overview

Caseous lymphadenitis (CLA) is a chronic contagious disease of sheep, goats and cattle with the incidence of disease increasing with age. The epidemiology of CLA varies between countries, from little within flock transmission in the UK to epizootic proportions in flocks in Australia and the USA.

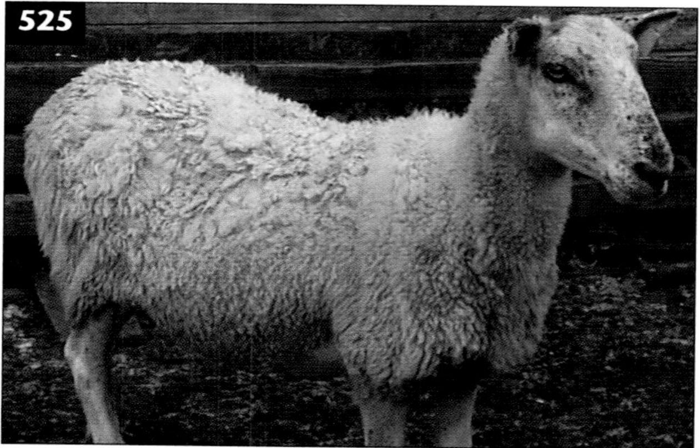

525 Generalized dermatophilosis affecting the dorsum of a Greyface ewe. Compare the affected matted fleece over the dorsum with the fleece on the ventral neck.

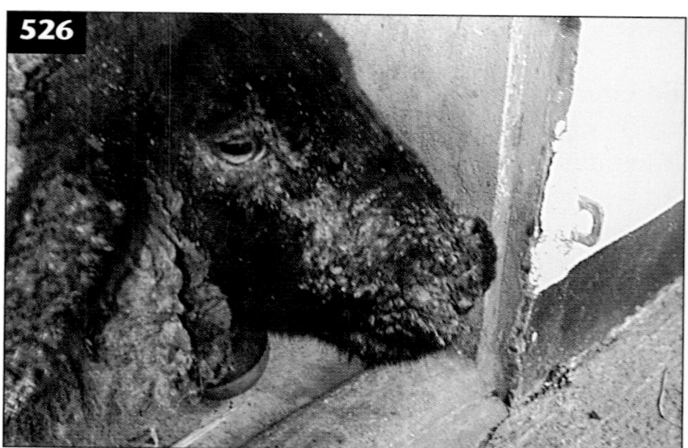

526 Severe dermatophilosis on the ears and around the muzzle of a Suffolk lamb.

Aetiology

CLA is caused by *Corynebacterium pseudotuberculosis*. Transmission occurs either directly between sheep during close confinement or indirectly via shearing equipment contaminated with fomites from sheep with lung lesions or discharging skin lesions. Shearing cuts are believed to be the major portal of entry, although it is reported that the organism can also penetrate intact skin. Fighting resulting in skin lesions to the head has been reported to facilitate disease transmission between rams in the UK. The prevalence of infection increases with age, and in sheep under intensive management conditions.

Clinical presentation

CLA is characterized by suppurative necrotizing inflammation of superficial lymph nodes, partic-ularly the parotid (**527**), submandibular, popliteal, precrural and prescapular lymph nodes. This form of the disease is often referred to as the cutaneous or superficial form of CLA. Spread of infection to the mediastinal and bronchial lymph nodes and internal viscera, including lungs, spleen, kidneys and liver, constitutes the visceral or internal form of CLA. Sheep with the superficial form of CLA may show no clinical signs of illness unless enlargement of the abscess causes compression of either the pharynx or larynx and impairs function.

In Australia, shearing wounds lead to infection of the prescapular and precrural lymph nodes with <1% of lesions affecting lymph nodes of the head region. Carcase lymph nodes may be 15 cm in diameter and are characterized by the lamellar ('onion-ring') appearance of affected lymph nodes containing yellow-green viscous pus, which may become inspissated with a toothpaste-like consistency. Conversely, CLA in the UK is characterized by abscessation of the parotid and submandibular lymph nodes.

The visceral form of CLA is commonly associated with the 'thin ewe syndrome' with lesions in the lungs, mediastinum, liver and kidneys. Less common sites are the vertebral column, udder and scrotum. Large lung and mediastinal lesions may result in dyspnoea and this form of the disease is common in the USA, where affected sheep are referred to as 'lungers'. Spread of infection to cause significant visceral lesions is rare in the UK.

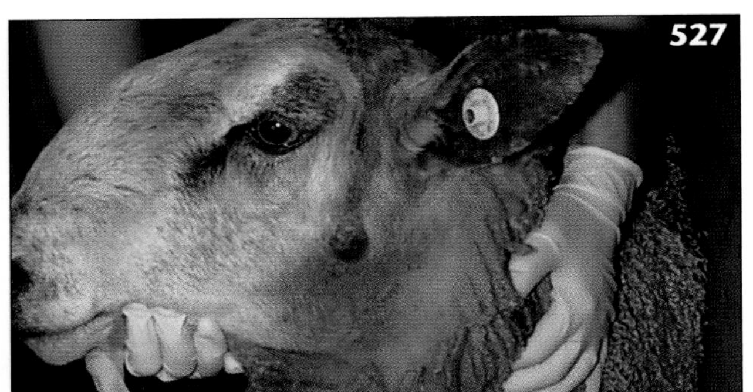

527 CLA lesion affecting the parotid lymph node.

Differential diagnoses

- Flock history may be important in forming a provisional diagnosis. The characteristic location of superficial lesions within drainage lymph nodes differentiates CLA infection from abscesses and cellulitis lesions. Skin tumours and lymphosarcoma are rare in sheep.
- The differential diagnosis list should also include actinobacillosis and tuberculosis.
- Common differential diagnoses for the visceral form of CLA affecting the chest include chronic suppurative pneumonia, pleural or mediastinal abscesses, and SPA.
- In more general terms, common causes of chronic ill-thrift in adult sheep include restricted nutrition, poor dentition, chronic parasitism, paratuberculosis, maedi-visna virus infection, chronic suppurative processes and tumours of the gastrointestinal tract.

Diagnosis

Definitive diagnosis of the cutaneous form of CLA is based on careful clinical examination of suspected cases and culture of *C. pseudotuberculosis* from discharging lymph nodes.

CLA lesions in the liver and superficial lesions involving the visceral pleura may be imaged using ultrasonography, and those within the lung and mediastinum by radiography. Liver-specific enzymes will only identify the occurrence of an hepatic insult, not the cause. Surprisingly, in many cases of liver abscessation, liver-specific enzyme concentrations are not significantly elevated. Samples for bacteriology can be collected at necropsy from suspicious lesions.

There is a humoral response to the *C. pseudotuberculosis* exotoxin and this forms the basis for serological testing. A seropositive result indicates exposure to the exotoxin and may indicate active infection; however, severely debilitated animals may yield a false-negative result (low sensitivity). Vaccinated animals will be seropositive and this may lead to an erroneous conclusion, especially in purchased sheep with an unknown vaccination history. Diagnosis is confirmed at necropsy with culture of *C. pseudotuberculosis*.

Treatment

Despite the sensitivity of *C. pseudotuberculosis* to a number of antibiotics *in vitro*, therapy is unsuccessful due the intracellular site of the bacteria and the fibrous capsule surrounding the lesions. Lancing lesions only results in contamination of the environment, increasing the potential for disease spread. Abscesses frequently recur after drainage and lavage with antiseptics.

Prevention/control measures

Disease prevention in clean flocks can be maintained by effective biosecurity measures. The role of shearing equipment and handling facilities (e.g. mobile plunge dippers and feeders) as vectors for disease must be carefully considered. However, disease risks are highest from purchased animals, which must be inspected before purchase and quarantined for at least two months. Replacement breeding stock must be purchased from disease-free flocks whenever possible. Alternatively, unvaccinated sheep should be purchased and serological testing undertaken before admission of seronegative stock to the flock.

In endemically infected flocks the control programme must involve reducing exposure to possibly contaminated fomites, culling sheep with unexplained ill-thrift, and vaccination. Young animals should be raised separately from older infected animals. Shearing equipment, particularly the combs and blades, must be regularly disinfected, especially after contact with a discharging lesion. Sheep should be shorn in age groups; the youngest first and those with skin lesions last. Skin wounds inflicted during shearing should be treated with topical iodine spray. Shower dipping for ectoparasite control and keeping sheep under cover for one hour or more after shearing increased the likelihood of high CLA incidence in Western Australian flocks.

Commercial vaccines have reduced the incidence of CLA within flocks but they do not prevent all new infections or cure sheep already infected. Commercial vaccines are used in many countries with a high CLA prevalence (e.g. the USA and Australia) but presently they are not used in many countries within Europe. All commercial vaccines contain the phospholipase D (PLD) toxoid and some also contain killed whole bacterial cells. Clostridial antigens may also be included in the vaccine. Care must be exercised not to challenge heavily pregnant sheep with too many vaccine antigens at the same time, as reduced feed intake may precipitate OPT.

Eradication of CLA is difficult and involves culling all infected sheep from vaccinated flocks. Thereafter, once clinical disease is at a low level, vaccination can be stopped and unvaccinated seropositive animals removed. In unvaccinated flocks, all seropositive animals must be culled and testing repeated until disease is eliminated.

Economics

Economic losses result from poor performance including reduced milk and wool production, weight loss, carcase condemnation and restricted trade.

Welfare implications

The superficial form of CLA may increase the risk of cutaneous myiasis. The visceral form of disease can result in debility and emaciated sheep should be destroyed during routine flock inspections.

CELLULITIS/SUBCUTANEOUS ABSCESSES

Definition/overview

Cellulitis lesions, which develop into large abscesses tracking along fascial planes, are not uncommon in sheep following puncture wounds to the skin but they are not of economic importance.

Aetiology

Dog bites or sharp objects can introduce infection through the skin and cause cellulitis/abscesses. *Arcanobacterium pyogenes* is the most common isolate from such lesions.

Clinical presentation

The clinical signs depend on the site and extent of the lesion(s). Large swellings adjacent to or involving the limbs result in mechanical lameness. In many cases the abscess does not result in illness but it is recognized some weeks after the event as a large subcutaneous swelling (528).

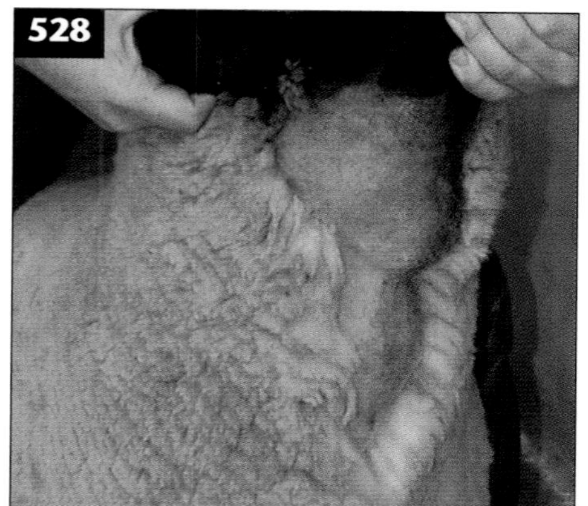

528 Large subcutaneous abscesses in the neck region of a Suffolk ram.

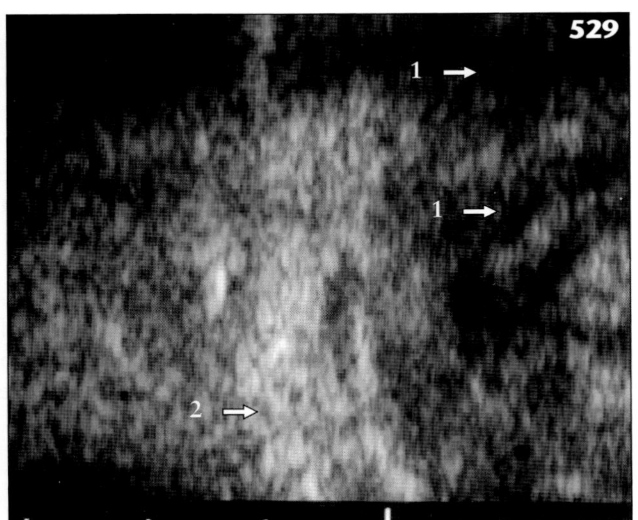

529 Ultrasonogram of a cellulitis lesion (**1**). The linear probe head is to the left of image. The adjacent skin and subcutaneous tissue measure approximately 2 cm, followed by the abscess capsule (**2**) represented by a broad hyper-echoic (white) line. The abscess appears as an anechoic area with multiple bright white dots extending for at least 4 cm.

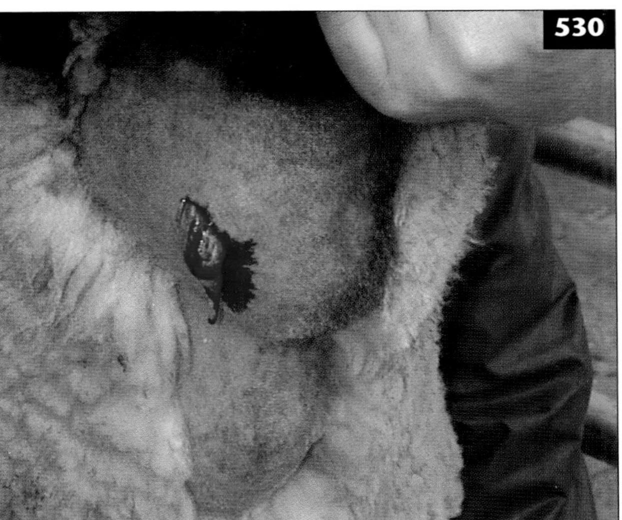

530 Lancing the lesion.

Differential diagnoses

CLA is the most common differential diagnosis but CLA lesions involve lymph nodes.

Diagnosis

Investigations could include ultrasonography (**529**) and fine needle aspirate. The abscess is confirmed following aspiration of pus.

Treatment

Abscesses should be lanced (**530**) provided there is no risk of CLA.

Prevention/control measures

Cellulitis/subcutaneous abscesses can be prevented by ensuring that there are no sharp protruding objects in the handling facilities and that sheepdogs are trained not to bite sheep.

Economics

Subcutaneous abscesses are of no economic importance.

Welfare implications

Early cellulitis lesions are painful but many large subcutaneous abscesses are only detected because of their size and not because the sheep is ill. These lesions are prevented by sound husbandry and management practices.

PHOTOSENSITIZATION (*Syns*: yellowses, plochteach, alveld, facial eczema)

Definition/overview

Photosensitization occurs sporadically worldwide but severe outbreaks are occasionally reported in southern hemisphere countries and in Norway. Typically, lambs 2–6 months old are affected during the summer months. In New Zealand, and in areas of Australia and South Africa, facial eczema is one of the most important diseases of sheep.

Aetiology

In sheep, photosensitization occurs either as a primary condition or secondary to hepatotoxic damage resulting in retention of the photosensitizing agent phylloerythrin.

Primary photosensitization follows ingestion of photodynamic agents (e.g. hypericin from St. John's Wort [*Hypericum perforatum*]). In Norway, ingestion of bog asphodel (*Narthecium ossifragum*) is reported to cause photosensitization in large numbers of lambs. In New Zealand, facial eczema is caused by ingestion of the toxin sporidesmin, which is produced by the saprophytic fungus *Pithomyces chartarum*, which proliferates in vegetation during the autumn months. Sporidesmin is absorbed and accumulates in the liver and bile where metabolic changes result in the release of free radicals, with consequent damage to the biliary tree and reduced excretion of phylloerythrin. The clinical signs depend on the amount of sporidesmin ingested and the amount and intensity of direct sunlight.

Clinical presentation

Typical cases of ovine photosensitization occur in white-faced breeds (**531**). Initially, affected animals are dull and attempt to seek shade. Lambs are often separated from their dam. The ears in particular are affected and become swollen, oedematous and droopy (**532**). The face, eyelids, lips and lower limbs may also become oedematous. The vulva may be affected in sheep where the tail is docked unnecessarily short. There is frequent head shaking and there is often self-trauma to the head by rubbing against fence posts or kicking at the head with the hindfeet. Affected skin may ooze serum, with development of superficial secondary bacterial infection. Necrosis of the ear tips develops within a few days, which gives them a 'curled-up' appearance.

Severely affected sheep may die if neglected but the response to protection from sunlight and corticosteroid and antibiotic therapy is generally good. In most cases the skin overlying the affected area dries, cracks and is sloughed. The ears may be lost.

In New Zealand it is reported that recovered sheep may develop cirrhosis, which may not be evident clinically until periods of increased metabolic demand such as late gestation.

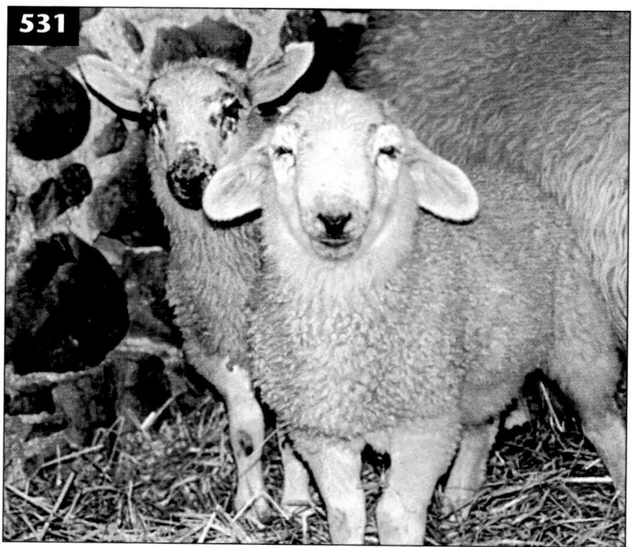

531 Typical cases of ovine photosensitization. There is depression and swollen face and ears.

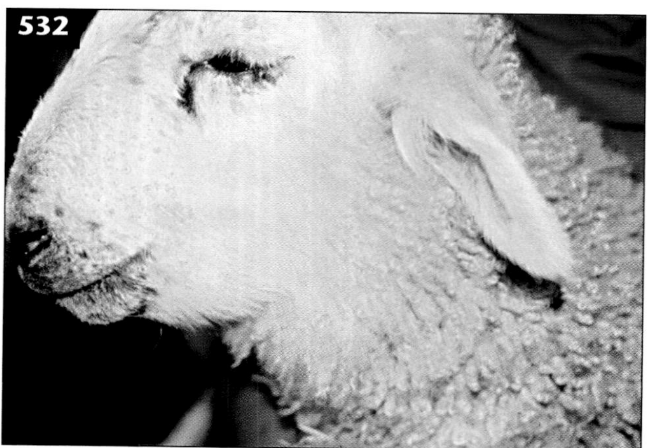

532 Close-up of one of the sheep in **531**. The face is very swollen and the ears are pendulous.

Differential diagnoses

- Bighead.
- Cellulitis (e.g. dog bite).
- Submandibular oedema associated with many protein-losing conditions including haemonchosis and fasciolosis and, much less commonly, paratuberculosis.

Diagnosis

Diagnosis is based on the clinical signs and exposure to plants known to cause primary or hepatogenous photosensitization. In secondary photosensitization, liver enzyme concentrations indicating both acute (AST) and chronic hepatocellular damage (GGT) are elevated.

Treatment

Affected sheep must be removed from pasture and confined in dark buildings to prevent further exposure. Corticosteroids are helpful during the early stages to reduce the associated oedema. Other symptomatic treatments include topical antibiotic powders and fly control preparations.

Prevention/control measures

Primary photosensitization occurs sporadically and the cause is often not determined. It would be prudent to avoid those pastures where outbreaks of photosensitization have occurred in previous years.

There is considerable variation in breed susceptibility to photosensitization, and in New Zealand the individual variation within a breed is used to commercial advantage in breeding programmes. Growth of *P. chatarum* in New Zealand has well-recognized weather influences, and spore counting on pasture is employed to recognize high-risk grazings. Challenge with small doses of sporedesmin, combined with monitoring of serum GGT, has been used to identify resistant rams.

Economics
Facial eczema is a major commercial concern in New Zealand. Economic loss from sporadic cases is very low in northern Europe.

Welfare implications
Affected sheep must be housed and given symptomatic treatment as necessary.

PERIORBITAL ECZEMA

Definition/overview
Periorbital eczema is a common skin condition in the UK, often resulting when sheep have too little space allowance at feed troughs. The cornea is unaffected.

Aetiology
Trauma to the skin allows entry of *Staphylococcus aureus*, which causes severe local infection.

Clinical presentation
Affected sheep have markedly swollen eyelids, which may close the palpebral fissure and effectively block vision. The eyelids are oedematous and painful (**533**). Ewes with both eyes affected are blind, wander aimlessly and frequently become caught in objects such as fences. Sheep with healing lesions have sharply demarcated hair loss extending for 2–3 cm around their eyes (**534**).

Differential diagnoses
- Photosensitization.
- Infectious keratoconjuctivitis (pink eye).
- Anterior uveitis.

Diagnosis
Diagnosis is based on the clinical signs and rapid response to antibiotic therapy.

Treatment
A single intramuscular injection of procaine penicillin affects a rapid response within 24 hours. Ewes with impaired vision in both eyes should be housed to ensure adequate feeding and prevent death by misadventure.

Prevention/control measures
Periorbital eczema can be prevented by appropriate space requirements at the troughs (450 mm per sheep). An alternative regimen involves feeding the grain ration as cobs on a clean area of pasture using a feed dispenser pulled by a quad bike.

Economics
Periorbital eczema is not a major economic concern to the sheep industry unless blindness leads to losses from misadventure or increased susceptibility to ovine pregnancy toxaemia because of reduced feeding patterns.

Welfare implications
The condition is obviously painful and must be treated promptly.

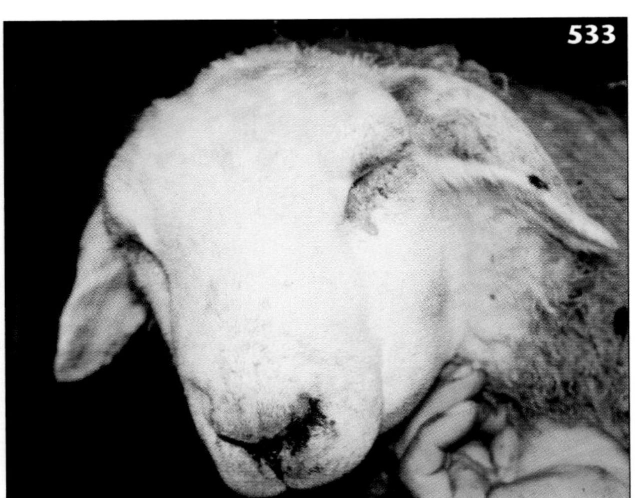

533 Oedematous and painful eyelids in a sheep with periorbital eczema.

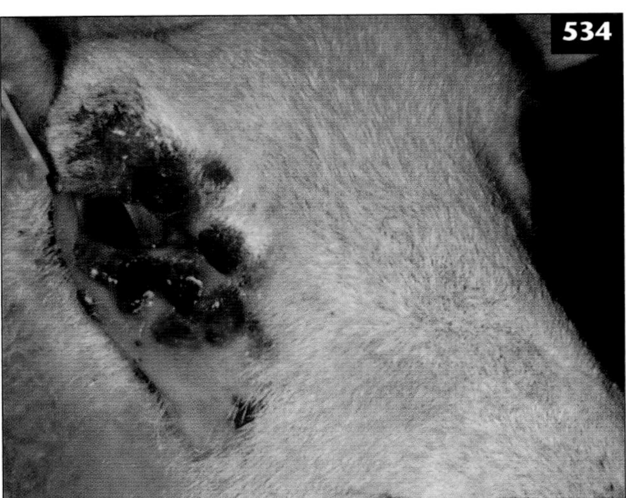

534 Sharply demarcated hair loss extending to 2–3 cm around the eyes in healing lesions of periorbital eczema.

RINGWORM

Definition/overview
Ringworm is uncommon in sheep; however, it has recently been reported more commonly in UK flocks. It is a zoonosis.

Aetiology
Most outbreaks of ringworm are caused by *Trichophyton verrucosum*. Outbreaks may appear some 4–8 weeks after shearing.

Clinical presentation
The lesions are well-circumscribed, extending up to 10 cm in diameter. They are more common on the head and neck (**535, 536**) but may involve the wooled areas.

Differential diagnoses
Differential diagnoses include dermatophilosis and sheep scab.

Diagnosis
Diagnosis is based on demonstration of ectothrix spores on microscopic examination of plucks of hair surroundings the lesions. Culture of *T. verrucosum* requires selective media.

Treatment
Topical natamycin is commonly used (**537, 538**) but may not be effective in all outbreaks. Griseofulvin is more effective than natamycin but is not licensed for use in sheep in many countries.

Prevention/control measures
Sheep should not have access to cattle with active lesions or to their immediate environment. Prompt recognition of clinical cases and their isolation is essential to try to limit spread within the flock. Biosecurity measures are vital to prevent introduction of infected sheep into the flock.

535 Ringworm infection on the face of a Blueface Leicester ram.

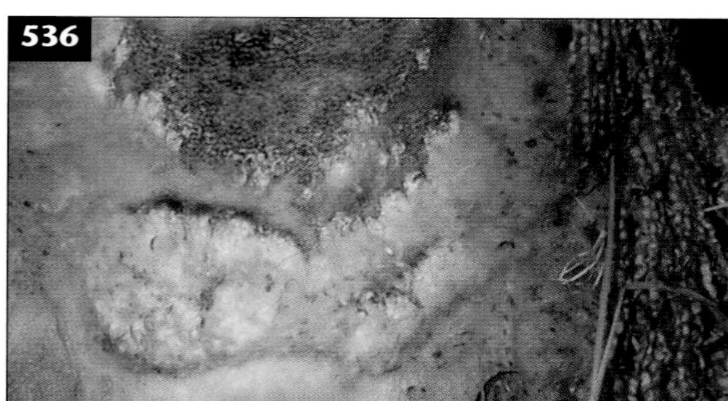

536 Ringworm infection extending down the neck of the ram.

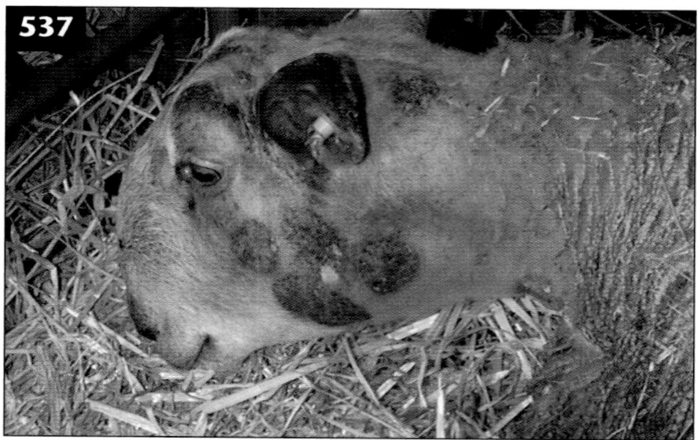

537 The ram in **535** two weeks after natamycin treatment.

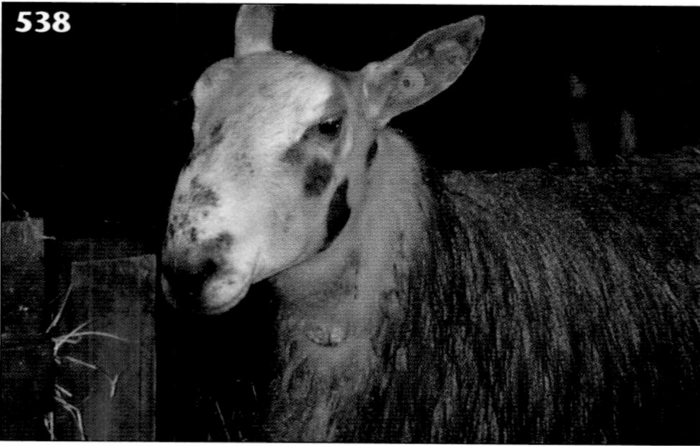

538 Pigmentation at the site of healed ringworm lesions. There is an active lesion on the ventral neck.

Economics
Ringworm lesions are unsightly and prevent the sale of pedigree sheep; therefore, infection could have a major impact in a pedigree flock.

Welfare implications
There are no specific welfare concerns.

SQUAMOUS CELL CARCINOMAS

Definition/overview
Squamous cell carcinomas (SCCs) are commonly reported affecting middle-aged to old sheep in many subtropical countries worldwide, especially Australia. They are very uncommon in northern Europe.

Aetiology
SCCs occur following prolonged exposure of areas of epidermis to ultraviolet radiation. The frequency of these tumours increases at high altitudes.

Clinical presentation
Numerous tumours occur at one or more sites including the eyelids, the dorsal surface of the ears, the muzzle and the musculocutaneous junctions of the vulva and anus. They also occur at sites of Mules mutilation. (**NB**: Mules 'operation' suggests some degree of professional care, but it is in fact a mutilation.) The proliferative lesions are readily traumatized and become secondarily infected. Metastases to drainage lymph nodes do occur but can be difficult to appreciate during clinical examination because bacterial infection of lesions will also increase local lymph nodes. Fly strike of lesions is very common.

Differential diagnoses
- Ocular lesions should be differentiated from periorbital eczema.
- Lesions around the face/muzzle should be distinguished from CPD, although age prevalence differs significantly.

Diagnosis
Diagnosis is based on clinical examination and elimination of other common differential diagnoses. The epidemiology of SCC will likely be well known on the farm.

Treatment
Treatment in the first instance is symptomatic, with antibiotic therapy to limit bacterial involvement and removal of maggots in fly struck lesions. Surgical removal is not an option for commercial value sheep; these must be culled for welfare reasons.

Prevention/control measures
Provision of shade is not a practical option on extensive grazing systems. Ewes must have sufficient tail length to at least cover the vulva. There is no justification for Mules mutilation.

Economics
Culling of ewes with significant lesions will increase the replacement rate.

Welfare implications
Superficial bacterial infection of SCCs will cause pain and discomfort but it can be treated with antibiotics. Of greater concern is the risk of cutaneous myiasis. Culling of ewes with early SCC lesions should reduce the risk of such complications.

SHEEP SCAB (*Syn*: psoroptic mange)

Definition/overview
Sheep scab is found in many sheep-producing areas of the world with the notable exceptions of North America, Australia and New Zealand, where the infestation was eradicated in the 1890s. If left untreated, infestations cause rapid loss of body condition, debility and eventually death in severe cases, although there appears to be considerable variation in breed susceptibility.

Aetiology
Sheep scab is caused by the host-specific mite *Psoroptes ovis*. Sheep scab can be transmitted by direct contact when sheep are gathered and held tightly together (e.g. during sales) or by contact with infested scab material on fenceposts or vehicles used for animal transport.

Clinical presentation
Disease is typically encountered during the autumn/winter months. During the early stages of infestation some sheep in the group have disturbed grazing patterns and are observed kicking at their flanks with their hindfeet and/or rubbing themselves against fence

posts or other similar structures, which leads to loss of wool and a dirty ragged appearance to the fleece (**539–541**). There is serum exudation, which gives the fleece overlying the skin lesions a moist yellow appearance (**542**). Some infested sheep have low mite numbers and show few clinical signs.

The skin lesions are most commonly observed on the flanks and over the back of the sheep but, in neglected situations, may extend to involve the whole body (**543, 544**). As the condition progresses over several weeks the sheep appear increasingly uncomfortable and nibble at their flanks and rub themselves against the pen divisions with greater frequency, causing excoriation. Some ewes appear in considerable distress and kick at themselves with their hindfeet. The fleece is wet, sticky and yellow and frequently contaminated with dirt from the hindfeet. It may prove difficult to part the wool fibres overlying the lesions due to serum exudation, which has formed a thick layer within the fleece.

Typically, after about eight weeks infestation the hair loss on the flanks may extend to 20 cm in diameter, surrounded by an area of hyperaemia and serum exudation at the periphery. The skin at the denuded centre of the lesions shows keratinization (**544**). The skin is thrown into thickened corrugations in many advanced cases. There is often marked enlargement of the drainage lymph nodes, the prescapular lymph nodes being the easiest to palpate. The lymph node enlargement is not dependent on

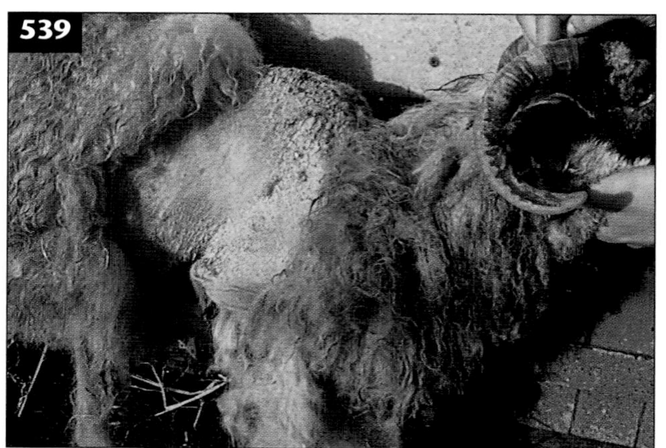

539 Scottish Blackface ewe with severe sheep scab infestation. There is fleece loss, wet and ragged 'sticky' fleece surrounding the lesion, and hyperaemic skin with serum exudation and excoriation from self-inflicted trauma. The affected skin is thickened and thrown into numerous folds.

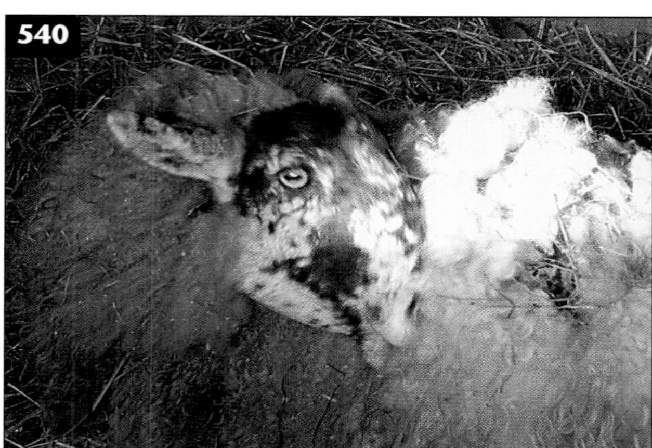

540 Chewing and nibbling at wool in a ewe infested with sheep scab.

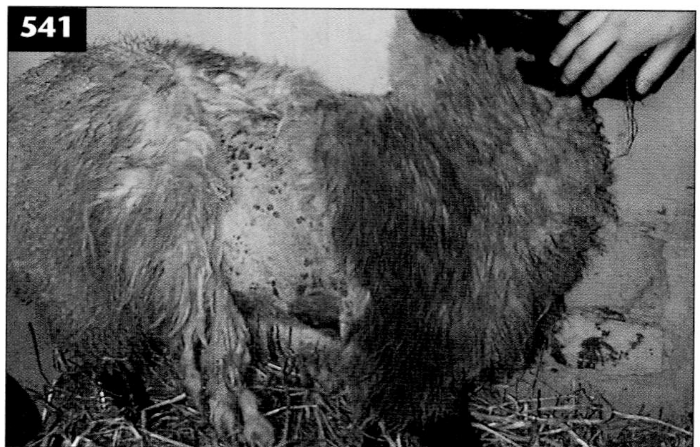

541 Suffolk-cross fattening lamb with sheep scab infestation. There is fleece loss and also dirty fleece over the shoulder region caused by kicking at the lesion with the hindfeet.

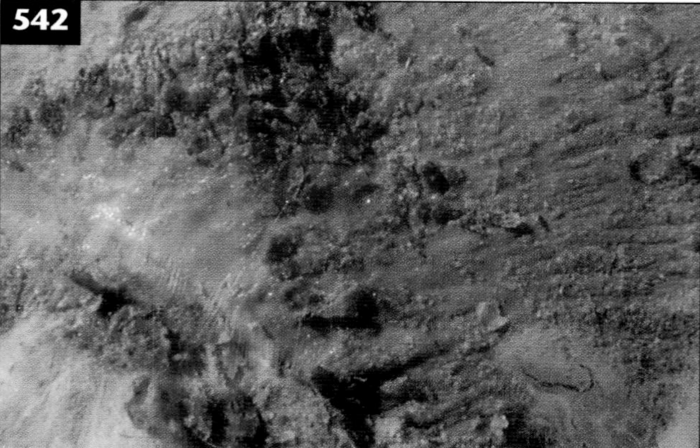

542 Serum exudation and crusting at the periphery of the skin lesions in the lamb in **541**. The denuded skin is thickened and thrown into folds.

puncture wounds to the skin. By this stage, infested sheep have lost considerable body condition and are frequently emaciated. Death may result in some sheep.

In particularly severe cases, cutaneous stimulation during handling procedures may precipitate seizure activity, which lasts for 2–5 minutes before the animals recover fully. This is particularly distressing for the sheep and should be treated immediately with dexamethasone (see Treatment).

Eventually, once the whole body has been infested and the fleece lost, there is no longer an active periphery of the lesion and the sheep may recover without treatment, although the healing process may only start some 4–6 months after initial infestation. The fleece begins to regrow and mite isolations may be restricted to cryptic sites such as the external auditory canal, inguinal area and infraorbital fossae.

Aural haematomas have been reported in flocks with chronic sheep scab but they were mainly attributed to reaction with *Psoroptes cuniculi* infestation.

Differential diagnoses

- Louse infestation.
- Keds.
- Severe dermatophilosis.
- Cutaneous myiasis.
- Severe photosensitization.
- Scrapie should be considered in individual sheep showing emaciation, seizure activity and fleece loss.

Diagnosis

While the exudative skin lesions involving areas of alopecia over the flanks in many sheep in the group have the typical field presentation and appearance of sheep scab mite infestation, confirmation is essential by demonstration of live mites. Skin scrapings taken using a scalpel drawn at right angle over the skin surface at the periphery of active lesions demonstrate large numbers of mites under ×100 magnification. Prior digestion in potassium hydroxide is not usually necessary. Liquid paraffin can be applied to the skin to aid collection of the scrapings.

Lice and keds can be visualized on careful examination of the fleece/skin.

Treatment

Systemic endectocides: avermectins and milbemycins

The avermectins (ivermectin and doramectin) and the milbemycins (including moxidectin) have a wide range of activity against immature and mature arthropods and nematode species when administered by injection. One injection of doramectin is effective against sheep scab mite infestation but two injections of ivermectin, one week apart, are needed for scab control. Ivermectin provides no significant residual protection against reinfestation from a contaminated environment; therefore, it is essential that sheep are not returned to the same pastures/buildings for at least 17 days post treatment. Although doramectin and moxidectin do have some residual action against re-infestation, it would be prudent to apply this rule to all systemic endectocide treatments.

Plunge dips

Dimpylate (diazinon), flumethrin and propetamphos-containing dips treat and prevent sheep scab, while high *cis* cypermethrin-containing dips are effective for

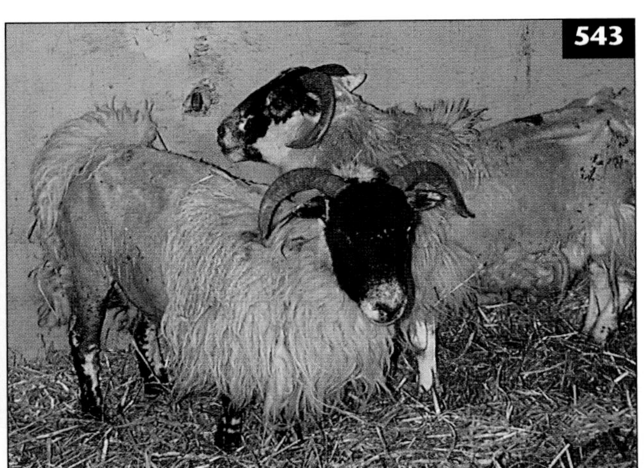

543 Two ewes with sheep scab. There is fleece loss and hyperaemic skin.

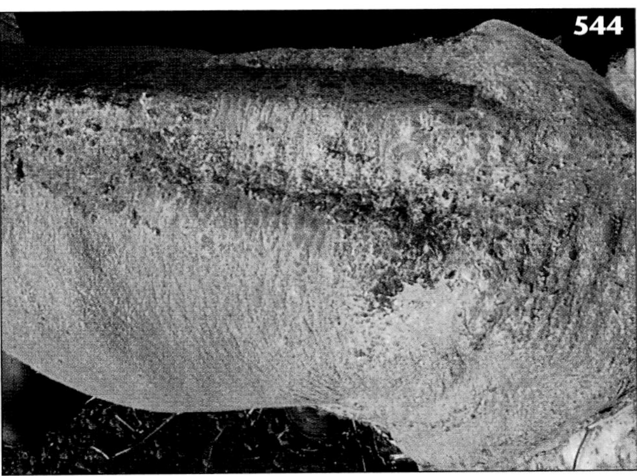

544 Skin corrugations associated with chronic scab infestation.

treatment only unless used for a second time after 14 days. Treatment for sheep scab necessitates that sheep are immersed in the dip wash for 60 seconds with the head submerged twice. Sheep dipped in high *cis* cypermethrin-containing dips must not be returned to infested pastures after dipping because of the limited residual action against scab mites.

In addition to scab treatment, severely affected animals should be treated with dexamethasone (i/m) in an attempt to reduce the anaphylactic reaction occasionally encountered in severely infested sheep.

Following treatment sheep may still appear distressed and nibble at their flanks for a couple of days. Thereafter, they appear more settled with no rubbing or scratching noted. Two weeks after treatment the skin appears normal and the fleeces less 'sticky'. Re-growth of the fleece is often apparent after 2–3 weeks (**545**, **546**), with black pigmentation in those areas where there had been considerable skin trauma.

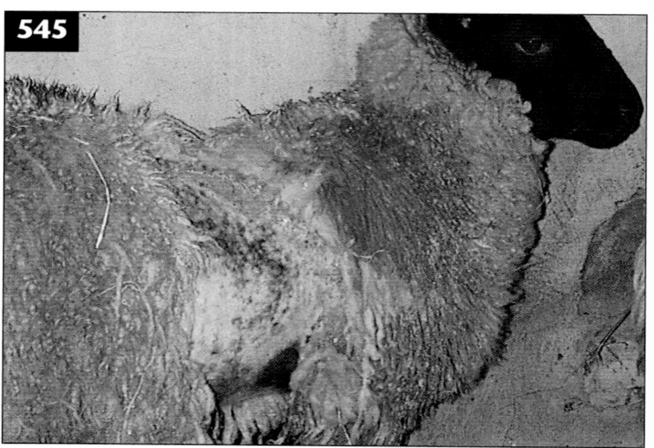

545 Suffolk-cross fattening lamb in **541** two weeks after treatment for scab.

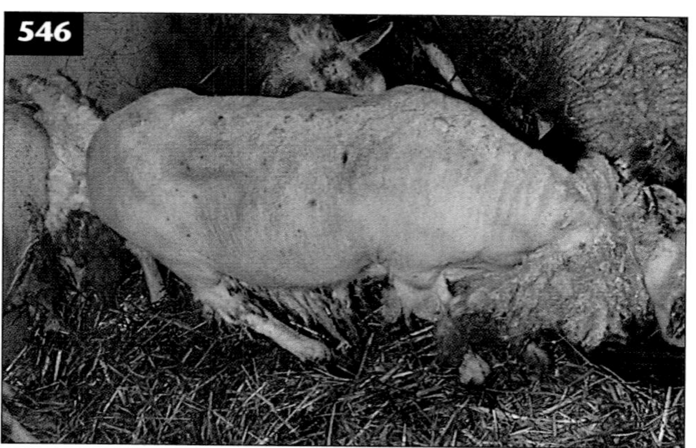

546 One of the ewes in **543** two weeks after treatment for scab. While almost all the fleece has been lost, the skin appears normal with early signs of fleece re-growth.

Prevention/control measures

Effective ring fencing with proper treatment of all sheep moved on to the farm are essential measures to prevent introduction of sheep scab.

There are individual reports of mite resistance to flumethrin and propetamphos in the UK, but no reports of avermectin or milbemycin resistance. Potential mite resistance problems only serve to emphasize the urgent need to eradicate this problem before it becomes even more widespread.

Economics

Sheep scab is a major economic concern despite the existence of many effective treatment and control strategies. Financial losses result from damage/loss of wool, poor growth, considerable weight loss in significant infestations and death of neglected cases. Lambs born to ewes with significant scab lesions have lower birth weights and experience increased neonatal mortality.

Welfare implications

Sheep scab is one of the most important welfare concerns affecting the sheep industry but there is neither the political will nor the desire by the farming industry to eradicate this scourge despite the availability of numerous highly efficacious treatment options. Infested sheep show obvious discomfort even with early infestations, leading to self-excoriation/trauma while the condition remains neglected. Seizure activity, while temporary, is particularly distressing for the sheep. Damage to the fleece and eventual loss renders the sheep highly susceptible to adverse weather conditions until significant wool regrowth occurs.

CUTANEOUS MYIASIS

(*Syns*: fly strike, blowfly)

Definition/overview

Cutaneous myiasis causes major economic losses worldwide and is a most serious welfare concern (**547**).

Aetiology

Cutaneous myiasis is caused by the larval stages of flies of the order Diptera. In the UK, three species parasitise sheep: *Lucilia sericata*, which is the most important, *Phormia terrae-novae* and *Calliphora erythrocephala*. The obligate blowfly *L. sericata* is an important species in southern hemisphere countries. The primary fly, *L. cuprina*, often referred to as the 'little green fly', is the most important fly in Australia and it has now migrated to New Zealand. It is a very tenacious fly and it strikes

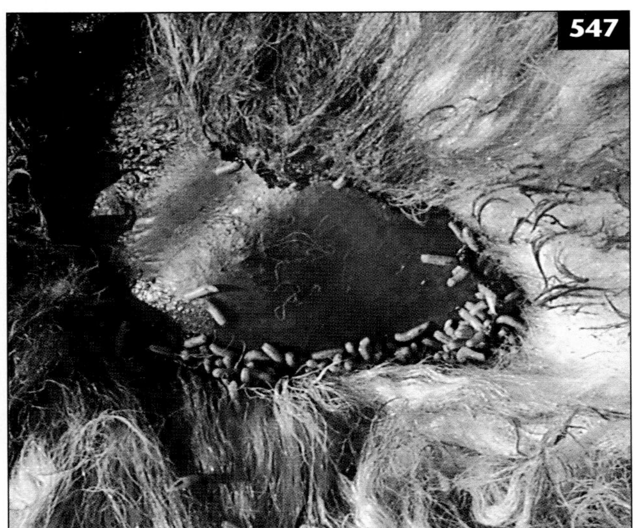

547 Lesion on the lumbar region of a toxaemic ewe resulting from severe cutaneous myiasis. Cutaneous myiasis is a serious welfare concern.

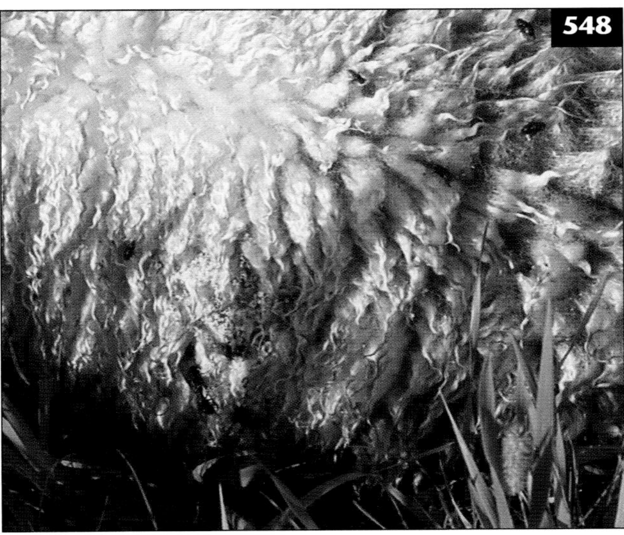

548 Adult flies on fleece and large numbers of deposited eggs.

very quickly and prolifically. Eggs are deposited on soiled areas of the fleece (**548**) or adjacent to traumatized skin. The larvae attack the skin surface with a combination of anterior hooks and proteolytic enzymes.

Clinical presentation

Fly strike more commonly affects growing lambs but on occasion ewes and rams can also be infested. Fly strike is most common during hot humid weather with little wind. The severity of cutaneous myiasis depends on numerous factors including flock husbandry, the degree of supervision and the diligence of the shepherd. Lesions may range from 1 cm diameter areas of skin hyperaemia with a small number of maggots when detected during the first days of infestation, to extensive areas of traumatized/devitalized skin covering up to one third of the skin area and causing death of the sheep.

Adult flies are attracted to areas of faecal staining surrounding the perineum; less commonly to virulent footrot lesions with exposed corium/exuberant granulation tissue; to dermatophilosis lesions on the skin; and to urine scalding around the prepuce. Urine scalding is aggravated by prolonged sternal recumbency in lame sheep. Granulating wounds in growing lambs caused by delayed rubber ring castration and tail docking also attract blowflies. Occasionally, head wounds acquired by rams during fighting become infested with maggots, and frequent head shaking and lowered head carriage are common in this situation.

During the early stages, affected sheep frequently turn their head and attempt to nibble at the affected area, usually the tailhead. Grazing behaviour is disrupted as sheep nibble at pasture for 5–10 seconds then suddenly trot away with frequent tail swishing before re-commencing grazing. This cycle of abnormal behaviour is repeated many times. The fleece surrounding the lesion becomes wet and discoloured. As the infestation progresses the sheep may rub against fences and hedges, causing a ragged appearance with fleece loss.

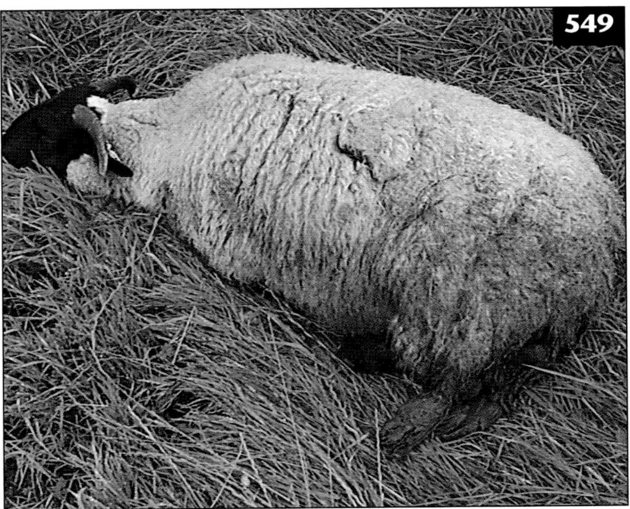

549 Profound toxaemia in a Scottish Blackface lamb with severe myiasis. The fleece is wet and stained around the perineum and extending on to the flanks.

In severe infestations the sheep are depressed and isolated from the flock (**549**). Large numbers of adult

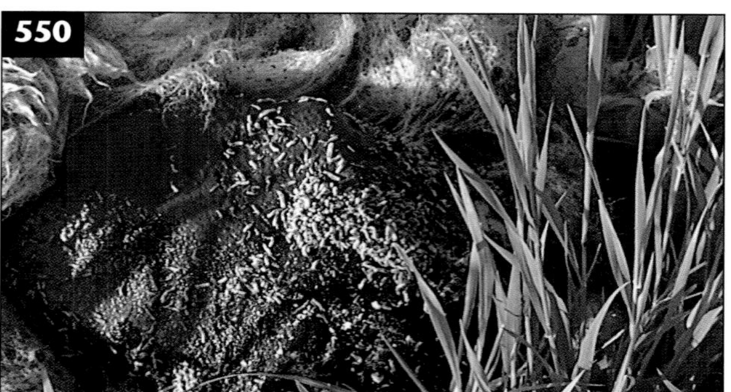

550 Severe myiasis in the lamb in **549**. Half of the lamb's skin is affected and it has a brown/black leather-like appearance. The lamb died 30 minutes later.

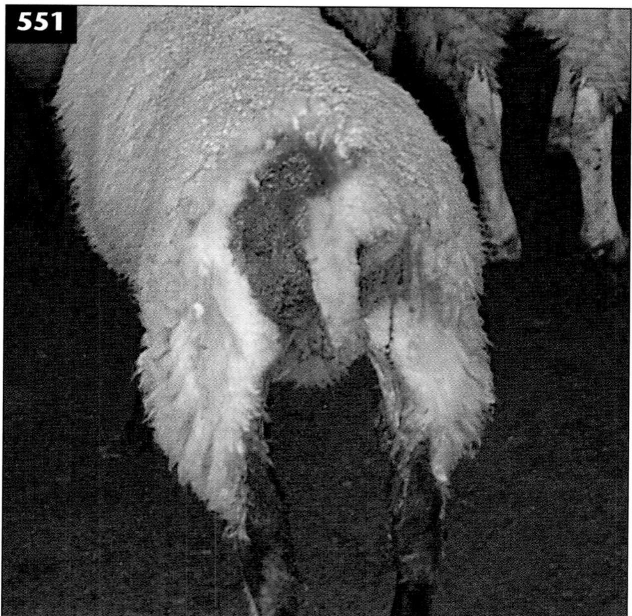

551 Treatment of fly strike. Removal of overlying fleece followed by application of an acaricide. Antibiotic can be applied topically after the maggots have been removed.

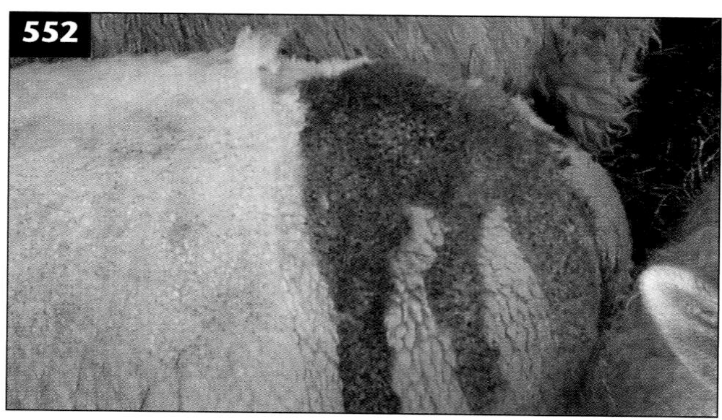

552 Pigmented wool re-growth on skin damaged by fly strike.

flies are seen on the fleece, with maggots on the blackened skin once the surrounding fleece has been lifted clear. There is an associated putrid smell. Clinical examination reveals toxic mucous membranes and dehydration. Severely affected sheep have a drawn-up appearance due to poor rumen fill, and have lost considerable condition. Death soon follows in severely affected sheep (**550**).

Differential diagnoses

Clinical inspection (**550**) eliminates other possible diagnoses.

Diagnosis

Diagnosis is confirmed by gathering and close inspection of the skin.

Treatment

Affected sheep can be treated by plunge dipping using a synthetic pyrethroid or organophosphate preparation, but it is more usual to treat infested sheep with dip wash applied directly to the struck area after first clipping away overlying wool (**551**). Affected skin grows pigmented wool (**552**).

Prevention/control measures

Before preventive measures using various chemicals are considered, much can be done to reduce the attraction of blowflies. In the UK, for example, a grazing programme to prevent the massive build-up of infective helminth larvae on permanent pasture during July and August (mid-summer rise) reduces diarrhoea caused by high parasite burdens. It should be possible to turn weaned lambs on to silage or hay aftermaths to further reduce larval challenge and diarrhoea during the fly season.

In the absence of a clean grazing system, control of parasitic gastroenteritis relies on strategically timed anthelmintic treatments, which should be part of the veterinary-supervised flock health programme. In many situations, parasitic gastroenteritis can be largely controlled by a programme that includes prophylaxis for *Nematodirus battus* followed by treatments at 3–4-week intervals. Using the UK as an example, treatments during mid-May (*N. battus*), early and late June and at weaning in mid-July will largely control parasitic gastroenteritis and faecal staining of the perineum. Thereafter, turnout of weaned lambs on to aftermaths should avoid high pasture larval burdens and reduce the need for further regular anthelmintic treatments.

Where faecal staining of the perineum occurs, contaminated wool must be removed (**553**) ('dagging' or 'crutching'). This is an unpleasant task for the shepherd but just reward for poor pasture management and ineffective parasite control.

In adult sheep, removal of the fleece and any faecal contamination by shearing removes this attraction well before the peak of the blowfly season (554). Problems of fly strike in ewes only arise when shearing is delayed either due to poor ewe nutrition during lactation and lack of 'rise' in the fleece or to poor management. Shearing time is very important because it also determines the timing of summer dipping some three weeks later. If shearing of ewes is delayed (e.g. until mid-July in the UK), dipping cannot be undertaken until there is sufficient fleece growth to hold the dip chemicals, usually some three weeks later (early August in the UK). In the UK this is too late because the high-risk blowfly period occurs from early July onwards.

All sheep carcases must be disposed of immediately as they provide a site for rapid fly multiplication (555).

Human health concerns and environmental controls have reduced the use of organophosphorus dips, which provide good protection against blowfly strike for up to six weeks. Dimpylate (diazinon) and propetamphos are effective against blowfly strike and the data sheet instructions must be read carefully before use, with particular attention paid to the protection of operators. In some countries, proficiency tests with proof of competence are necessary before farmers can use organophosphorus dips. These compounds are strongly lipophilic and replenishment of dips is important to maintain effective concentrations within the bath. The synthetic pyrethroids, including high *cis* cypermethrin, have a much higher human safety margin than the organophosphorus compounds and persist in the fleece for up to eight weeks.

While plunge dips are commonly used in the UK, shower dips are more popular in New Zealand. Specific recommendations for shower times in relation to the interval since shearing must be followed. Jetting wands can be used as an alternative to plunge or shower dipping for applying dip wash to target areas. The wand is combed through the fleece, applying the correct volume of dip wash at skin level. The advantages of jetting wands are that they apply clean dip wash to the target areas and use less concentrate dip, therefore reducing costs, but the process is time consuming and hard work. Handguns can be used to apply dip wash to the target areas along the back and crutch areas.

While topical application of high *cis* cypermethrin pour-on preparations provides protection against fly strike, these preparations only persist for 6–8 weeks and require re-application in most situations.

The insect growth regulator, cyromazine, applied before the risk period, is very effective against blowfly

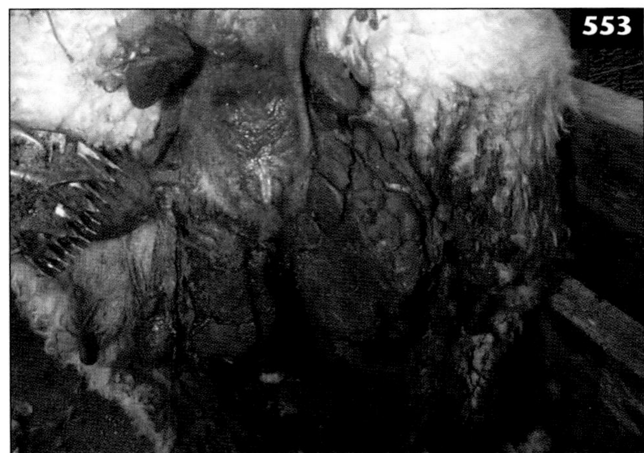

553 Removal of faeces from around the tail and perineum.

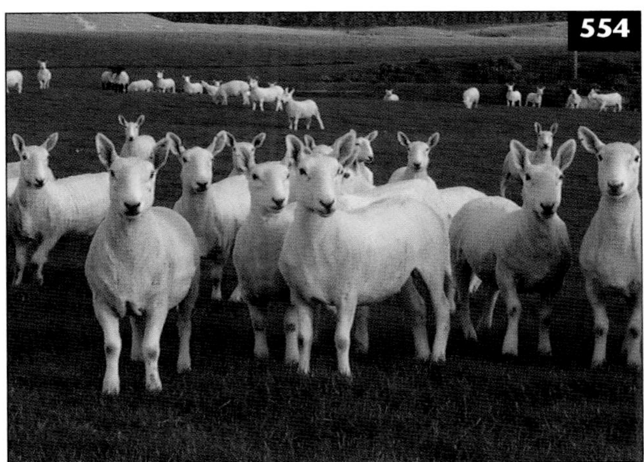

554 Shorn ewes are rarely struck.

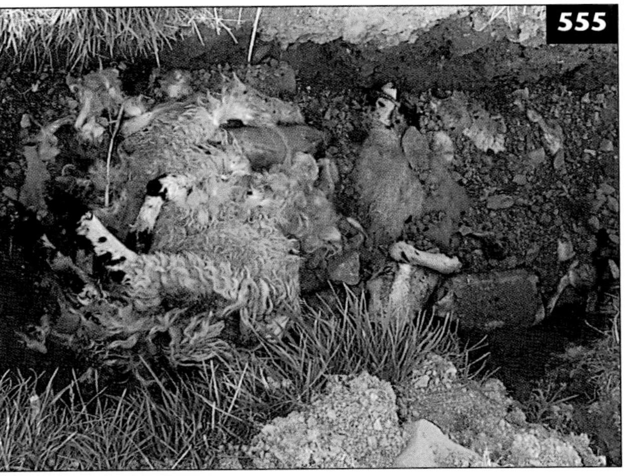

555 Burial pits must always be covered by sufficient soil to prevent scavenging and access by flies.

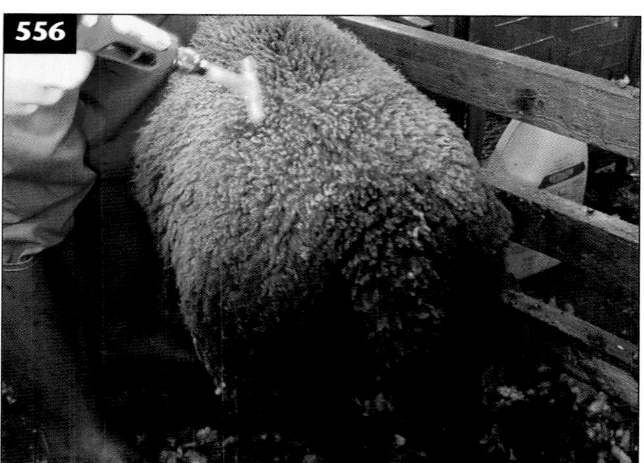
556 Topical application of acaricide or insect growth regulator.

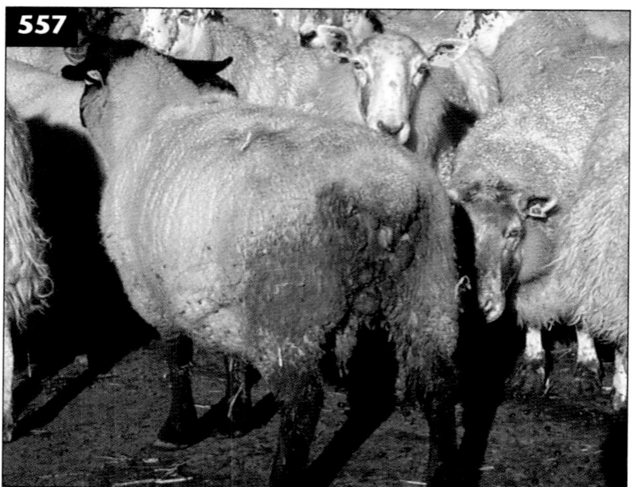
557 Tail docking does not eliminate faecal staining of the perineum.

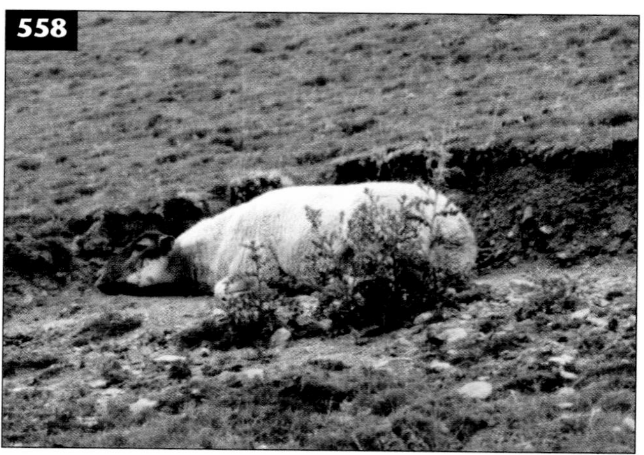
558 Greyface ewe 'demented' by headflies. Affected sheep often attempt to bury their head into the hillside.

strike for up to ten weeks after topical application (**556**). More recently, the introduction of dicyclanil affords 16 weeks' full body protection against cutaneous myiasis. Dicyclanil acts specifically on larvae, interfering with moulting and pupation and therefore preventing larval development. No resistance has been reported to these insect growth regulators, which are very safe; however, they are considerably more expensive than other control measures and this may limit their use.

Docking tails beyond the legal limit (**557**) has little effect on faecal contamination of the perineum. Fly traps have been developed in Australia but have limited application in Europe.

Economics

Cutaneous myiasis is of major economic concern worldwide, with considerable prevention and treatment costs. Pour-on products containing high *cis* cypermethrin to prevent blowfly strike typically cost 0.8% of the value of a growing lamb and 0.6% of the value of an adult sheep. Insect growth regulators are approximately twice the cost of these pour-on products.

Welfare implications

Where falling income from sheep farming has resulted in farmers attempting to reduce costs, this has resulted in the cessation of prophylactic measures, with adverse consequences in terms of both sheep welfare and profitability.

HEADFLY

Definition/overview

Headflies can present a major problem during the summer months in horned sheep grazed near woodland.

Aetiology

The muscid fly *Hydrotea irritans* causes considerable irritation around the horn base during feeding, which may result in self-trauma. The flies may also feed on lachrymal secretions.

Clinical presentation

Grazing patterns are disturbed and affected sheep often isolate themselves and remain in shade where available. They may stand with their head held lowered and with frequent head shaking and ear movements. Alternatively, sheep adopt a submissive posture in sternal recumbency with the neck extended and the head held on the ground (**558**). Kicking at the head often greatly exacerbates the damage caused by headflies to the horn base (**559**), and it may also traumatize the skin of the neck and ears (**560**). Head rubbing also causes considerable self-trauma. Bleeding and serum exudation attract other flies, which aggravates the problem. There is rapid loss of condition in severely affected sheep.

Differential diagnoses
Inspection of affected sheep confirms the cause of the head (and superficial skin) wounds.

Diagnosis
Diagnosis is confirmed by gathering the sheep and close inspection of the skin.

Treatment
Housing is essential for sheep with large skin lesions to allow time for complete healing. Parenteral antibiotic administration may be indicated if there is localized reaction but this is unusual. Topical emollients and antibiotic preparations are not usually necessary, and skin wounds heal well provided the flies are denied access to these areas, which is best achieved by housing. Affected sheep must never be turned out on to the top of an open hill in the expectation that there are no flies there, as tradition dictates.

Prevention/control measures
Control of headflies proves more difficult once a lesion is present on the head; prevention is much more important than cure. Pour-on fly control preparations, such as high *cis* cypermethrin or deltamethrin, must be applied before the anticipated headfly season and especially to horned sheep. Treatments should be repeated every 3–4 weeks during the fly season or as directed by the data sheet instructions.

Economics
Lesions resulting from headfly activity in mid-summer cause sheep great distress (**561**) and result in considerable weight loss and poor lactation, with consequent poor lamb weaning weights. Disruption to grazing continuing throughout the late summer leads to poor condition of lambs at sale and ewes at the prebreeding check, which may result in premature culling.

Welfare implications
Headfly lesions present a serious welfare issue because they cause great distress to affected sheep. Lesions may become large because horned mountain breeds often graze extensive pastures and are infrequently shepherded. It is essential that horned sheep, especially

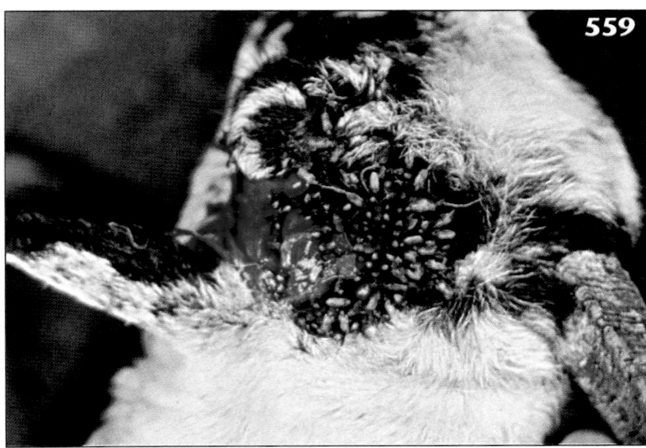

559 Headflies feeding at the horn base after horn had become detached.

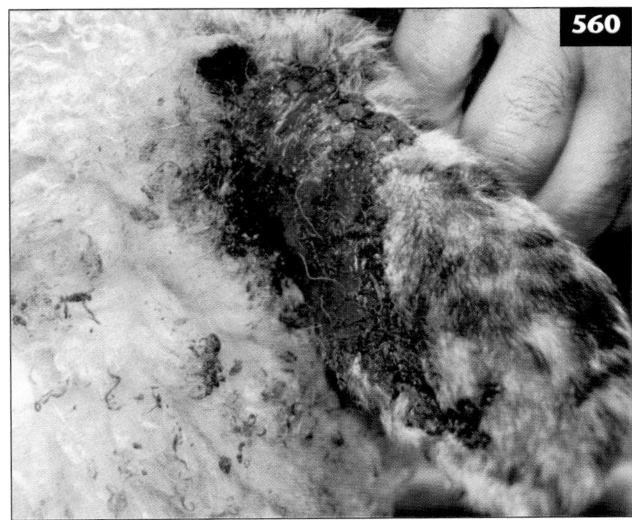

560 Self-inflicted trauma to ear caused by kicking at the head with a hindfoot.

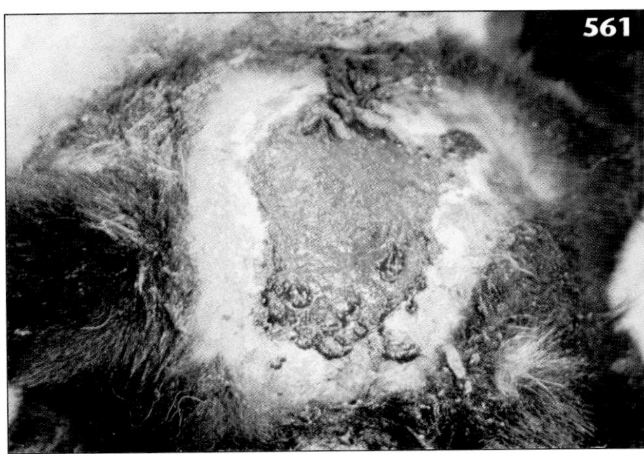

561 Headfly lesions can take many weeks to heal.

lambs, are handled correctly and never caught by the horns. Damage or loss of a horn during handling readily attracts headflies, causing a major problem from self-inflicted trauma.

LICE (*Syn*: pediculosis)

Definition/overview

Infestations with lice probably affect all sheep-producing countries but they cause production concerns only in Australia and New Zealand, where the body louse *Bovicola ovis* reduces fleece quality. Louse populations are highest in sheep in poor body condition kept under unhygienic conditions, rather than the reverse situation where lice cause debility.

Aetiology

Three species of louse infest sheep: the chewing louse *Bovicola ovis* and the bloodsucking lice *Linognathus ovillus* and *Linognathus pedalis*. Infestation with *B. ovis* may cause disrupted feeding patterns, fleece damage/loss and self-inflicted trauma. Spread is by close contact and it occurs more quickly in hot climates than in temperate climates, with increases in population size during cooler weather. The whole life cycle of the louse (egg, three nymph stages and adult) is spent on the sheep. The slow reproductive capacity of *B. ovis* results in a gradual build-up of louse numbers over several months. Shearing removes many lice and exposes the remaining population to desiccation, with rain further reducing numbers.

Clinical presentation

Many louse infestations are asymptomatic but heavy infestations during cooler weather cause irritation, leading to rubbing against structures such as fences and fleece damage/loss. Sheep may abruptly stop grazing and nibble at the fleece overlying the dorsal midline. Lice congregate in colonies on the fleece; therefore, a minimum of 10–20 fleece partings to a depth of 10 cm should be examined per sheep, with a minimum of ten sheep examined per group. An average count of more than five lice per fleece parting is generally considered a heavy infestation with *B. ovis*.

Differential diagnoses

- The important differential diagnosis for flock problems of pruritus and fleece loss is sheep scab.
- Other differential diagnoses include cutaneous myiasis and, in individual sheep, scrapie.

Diagnosis

Careful inspection of the fleece using a magnifying glass will identify significant *B. ovis* populations. Further investigation involves microscopic examination of fleece samples.

Treatment

Infested sheep can be treated by plunge dipping using a synthetic pyrethroid or organophosphate preparation. Plunge dipping for other reasons (e.g. control of sheep scab, cutaneous myiasis and headfly problems) also effectively eliminates any louse infestation.

Prevention/control measures

Reliance on systemic endectocides to control sheep scab has resulted in an upsurge of louse infestations in sheep flocks (in the UK). Maintenance of a closed flock and effective biosecurity measures will prevent introduction of louse infestations. Plunge dipping for other reasons and topical application of high *cis* cypermethrin or deltamethrin also controls louse infestations.

Economics

Louse infestations do not present a significant financial concern apart from in Australia, where wool rather than meat is the more significant sheep product. There are presently no data in the UK to show a significant production loss from louse infestations.

Welfare implications

Heavy louse infestations cause irritation and disrupted grazing patterns and therefore warrant treatment for welfare reasons. The cause of any underlying debilitating condition/disease should be investigated and corrected.

SHEEP KEDS

Definition/overview

Infestation with the sheep ked *Melophagus ovinus* occurs in many temperate countries but it is unimportant compared with cutaneous myiasis and sheep scab, where control programmes also remove keds.

Aetiology

Keds spend their entire life on the sheep, with a life cycle of approximately five weeks. The rate of multiplication is relatively slow, with a female producing approximately 15 larvae in its lifetime.

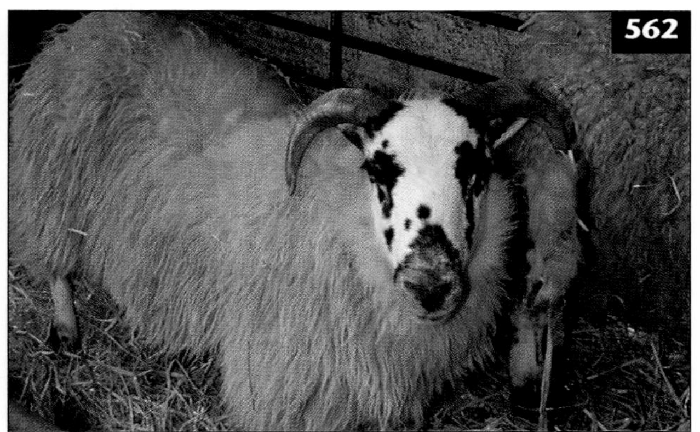

562 The ewes have been noticed nibbling at their flanks and rubbing themselves with their horns.

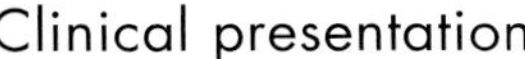

Clinical presentation
Clinical signs only occur in heavily infested sheep and include restlessness and kicking/rubbing at the fleece. Anaemia may result where there is heavy infestation but this is very uncommon except in otherwise debilitated sheep.

Differential diagnoses
The common differential diagnoses include cutaneous myiasis, sheep scab and lice; however, keds are readily visible to the naked eye.

Diagnosis
Adult keds are 4–6 mm long, dark red and readily visible on the neck and forelimbs.

Treatment
Sheep keds are controlled as part of a more general programme of ectoparasite control (e.g. for cutaneous myiasis and sheep scab). Infestations can be controlled by plunge dipping in organophosphate and synthetic pyrethroid dips, use of pour-on synthetic pyrethroid preparations, and the use of systemic endectocides.

Prevention/control measures
Routine annual ectoparasite treatments will control sheep keds. Biosecurity measures, including secure boundary fences, are important in preventing introduction of infested sheep.

Economics
Sheep keds are not an important ectoparasite of sheep.

Welfare implications
Heavy infestations can lead to disrupted grazing patterns, excoriation and, in severe cases, debility associated with anaemia.

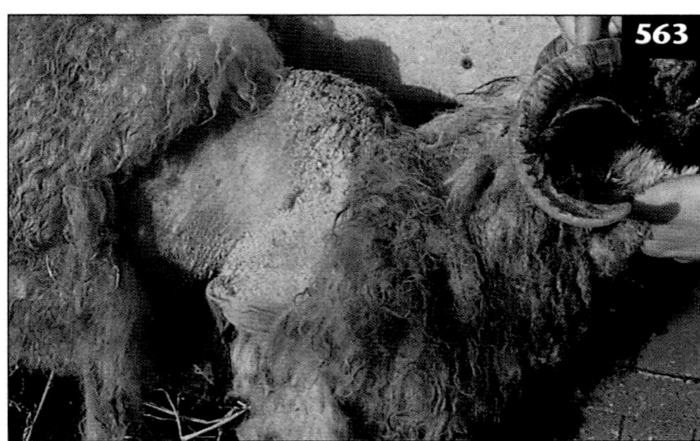

563 The fleece is wet, sticky and yellow.

CLINICAL PROBLEM

During the winter a small group of Blackface ewes is presented with moist, discoloured fleeces. The sheep have been collected from numerous markets at bargain prices. The ewes are housed and fed almost *ad libitum* concentrates to gain condition quickly, although many are in poor bodily condition. Some of the ewes have been noticed nibbling at their flanks and rubbing themselves with their horns (562) and against feed racks.

Clinical examination
The ewes are in poor body condition (BCS 1.5) with considerable fleece loss. They appear uncomfortable and nibble at their flanks and rub themselves against the pen divisions. Some ewes appear in considerable distress and kick at themselves with their hindfeet. The fleece is sticky, yellow and closely adherent to the skin in some areas (563). It proves difficult to part the fleece and the wool fibres have to be gently teased apart due to serum exudation, which has formed a thick layer in the fleece. In other ewes in the group, rubbing has lead to the loss of fleece and a ragged appearance with considerable serum exudation.

What conditions should be considered and how would the diagnosis be confirmed?
What treatment should be administered?

Differential diagnosis
- Sheep scab mite infestation (*Psoroptes ovis*).
- Louse infestation.
- Keds.
- Severe dermatophilosis.

Lice and keds can be visualized on careful examination of the skin (not in these sheep).

Confirmation

Skin scrapings taken from the periphery of the lesion demonstrate large numbers of mites under ×100 magnification.

Treatment for sheep scab

Possible treatments include:

- Avermectins and milbemycins.
- Organophosphorus dips.
- Dimpylate (diazinon), flumethrin and propetamphos-containing dips treat and prevent sheep scab, while cypermethrin-containing dips are effective for treatment only.

One injection of doramectin is effective against sheep scab mite infestation but two injections of ivermectin, one week apart, are needed for scab control.

The ewes were treated with doramectin (s/c) and moved to a clean building. In addition, the worst affected ewes were treated with dexamethasone (i/m) in an attempt to reduce the anaphylactic reaction occasionally encountered in severely infested sheep.

Outcome

The ewes did not appear any better the following day and the farmer complained that despite treatment a large number of ewes were still distressed and nibbling at their flanks. Two days after injection the ewes appeared more settled; thereafter, no rubbing or scratching was noted. Two weeks after treatment the ewes' skins appeared normal and the fleeces were less sticky. Re-growth of the fleece, but with black wool, was beginning in a number of ewes where there had been considerable skin trauma.

11 Eye Diseases

INFECTIOUS KERATOCONJUNCTIVITIS

(*Syns*: contagious ophthalmia, 'pink eye')

Definition/overview

Infectious keratoconjunctivitis (IKC) is often associated with high winds and driving snow during the winter months (**564**), which gives rise to the colloquial term 'snow blindness'. Large numbers of sheep can be affected during these weather conditions. Competition at feed troughs and hayracks also increases the rate of spread of infection. IKC is more commonly seen in adults, presumably because some of the risk factors, such as severe winter weather, do not apply to growing lambs during the summer months. IKC is seen in sheep worldwide.

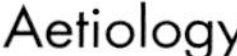

Aetiology

Chlamydophila psittaci and *Mycoplasma conjunctivae* are the only organisms that have been associated with IKC. The disease in the UK is associated with adverse weather conditions but, in New Zealand, IKC is associated with dust and indirect spread by flies.

Clinical presentation

The condition can be either unilateral or bilateral. Most cases are selected for treatment on the basis of obvious epiphora with tear staining of the face (**565**, **566**).

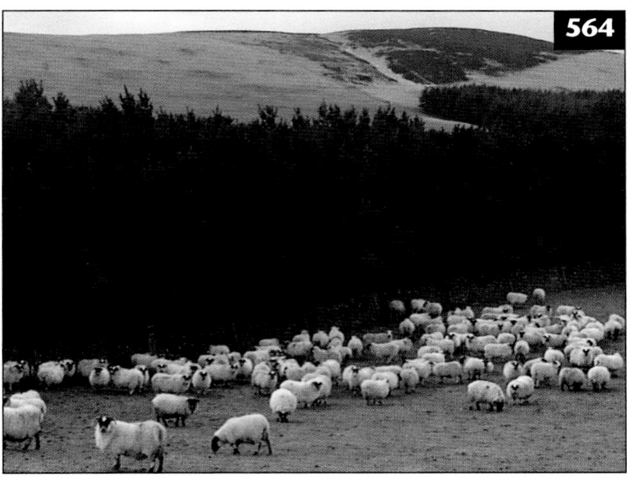

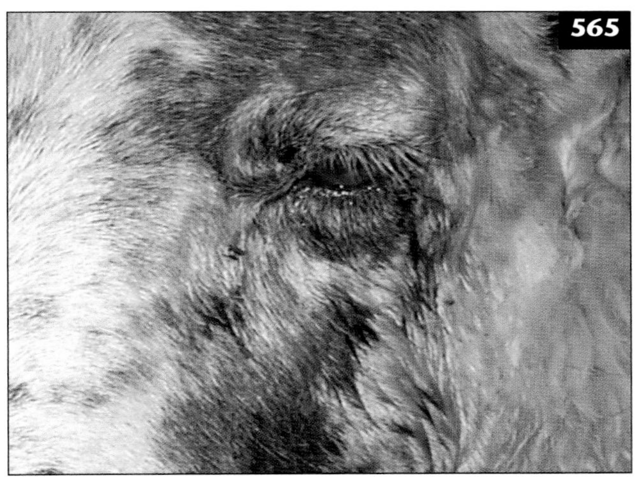

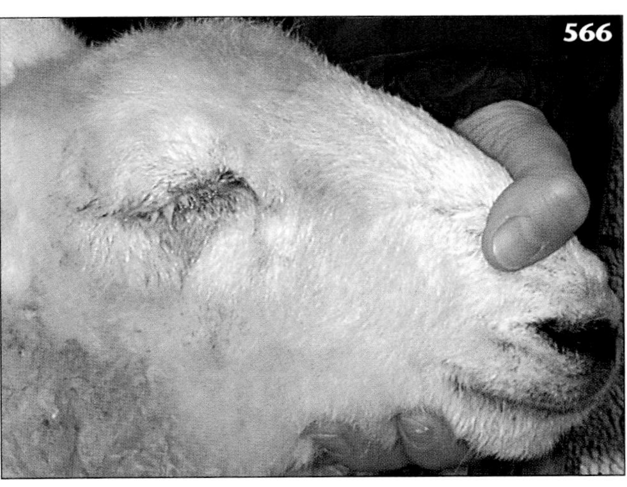

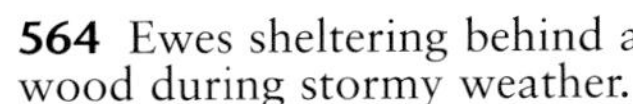

564 Ewes sheltering behind a wood during stormy weather.

565 Epiphora and slight corneal opacity during the early stages of IKC.

566 Blepharospasm and slight purulent ocular discharge in a weaned lamb with IKC.

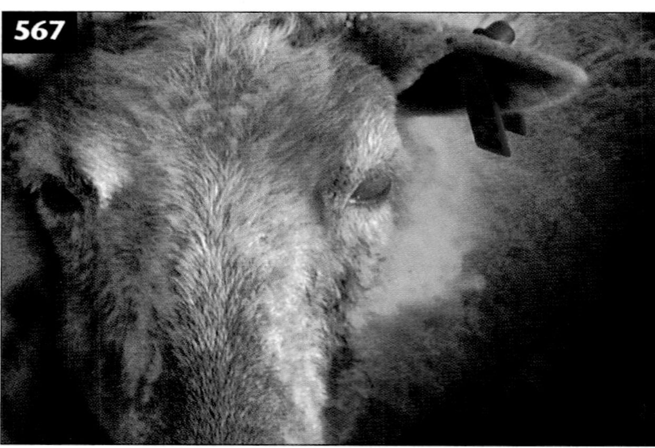
567 Epiphora and corneal opacity in a ewe with IKC.

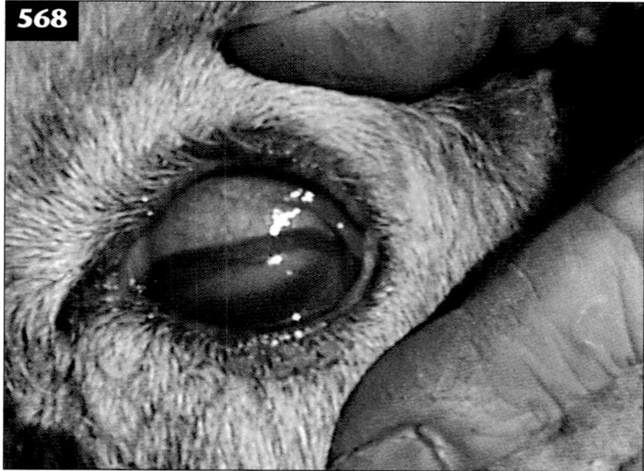
568 Conjunctivitis with scleral injection in a ewe with IKC.

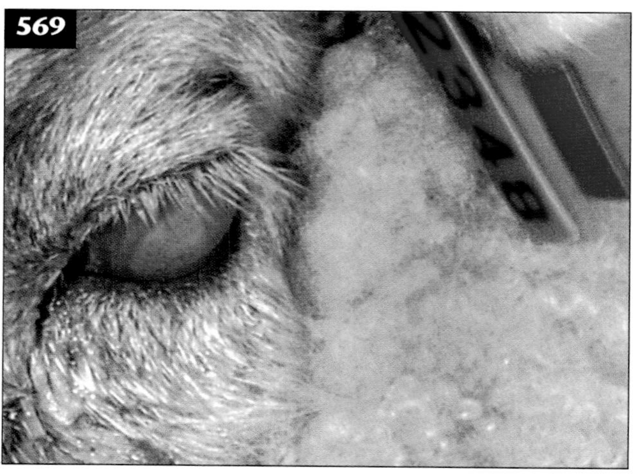
569 Corneal opacity and early ulceration in a ewe with IKC. There is a purulent discharge at the medial canthus.

On closer examination of the affected eye(s) there is marked conjunctivitis (**567**) with injected tortuous scleral vessels and hyperaemic conjuncivae (**568**). There is marked photophobia, with blepharospasm when sheep are exposed to bright sunlight. More advanced cases show ker-atitis (**569**) and, possibly, corneal ulceration, which is readily identified after application of fluorescein-impregnated strips to the surface of the eye. By this stage, lymphoid hyperplasia gives the bulbar conjunctiva and third eyelid a granular appearance. Neovascularization is also evident in severe cases.

Spontaneous recovery starts in most cases 3–5 days after clinical signs are first observed, and is completed by two weeks later. In severe cases, ulceration may progress to rupture of the anterior chamber but this is uncommon.

Sheep may die from misadventure if the condition causes temporary blindness. During late pregnancy, ovine pregnancy toxaemia may result in multigravid ewes as a consequence of blindness and inability to find sufficient food.

Differential diagnoses

Differential diagnoses include:
- Foreign bodies within the conjunctival sac.
- Anterior uveitis.
- Periorbital eczema.

Diagnosis

Diagnosis is based on clinical examination and response to antibiotic therapy. Bacteriological isolation is rarely undertaken. (**NB**: The bacteria are fragile and transport media are required for despatch to the laboratory.) Conjunctival swabs should be taken from early clinical cases with serous, non-purulent ocular discharge.

Treatment

Affected sheep should be housed with ready access to food and water. Sheep must be approached carefully, announcing one's presence to prevent panic in those sheep rendered temporarily blind by the condition. The treatment response to topical oxytetracycline is good. A single intramuscular injection of long-acting oxytetra-cycline is economically justifiable and very effective in sheep, and is the treatment method of choice. Twice daily topical antibiotic therapy is recommended but cannot always be accomplished under farm conditions because of other commitments on staff time. Subconjunctival antibiotic injection can be difficult to achieve in sheep because the conjunctivae are very inflamed and painful, and restraint is not easy with only one operator. This technique has no advantage over intramuscular injection apart from the lower cost because of the smaller antibiotic dose. In severe outbreaks in pregnant ewes, metaphylactic injection of all at-risk sheep with a single intramuscular injection of long-acting oxytetracycline should be carefully considered. Immunity following infection is poor, and lesions recur within weeks in many sheep.

Prevention/control measures

Provision of care can prove very time-consuming because sheep are often grazing large areas and may have strayed from the main group and be difficult to find in poor weather conditions. While affected sheep should be housed with ready access to food and water, it may prove difficult to move these sheep from remote hill pastures. Provision of shelter from storms is good husbandry practice on hill/mountain pastures. Adequate trough space and feeding concentrates on the ground may limit spread of infection throughout a group.

Outbreaks of IKC may occur after the introduction of purchased stock; therefore, whenever possible, all new stock should be managed separately as one group away from the main flock.

Economics

Secondary losses may result from sheep walking into rivers or over ridges, and to secondary ovine pregnancy toxaemia.

Welfare implications

Temporary bilateral blindness must be very traumatic and sheep should be managed quietly indoors in small groups. Individual penning causes considerable distress to blind sheep as evidenced by their frequent vocalization. Pens should have solid walls, as horned sheep may become entangled in wire fences.

ANTERIOR UVEITIS

(*Syns*: ovine iritis, silage eye)

Definition/overview

Anterior uveitis, also referred to as ovine iritis, is occasionally seen in sheep of all ages being fed big bale silage.

Aetiology

Anterior uveitis probably follows conjunctival infection with *Listeria monocytogenes*. There are no reports of sheep developing signs of meningoen-cephalitis following primary anterior uveal listerial infection.

Clinical presentation

The initial presenting signs are excessive lachrymation, blepharospasm, photophobia, miosis and iridocyclitis, either unilaterally or bilaterally. The iris may be thrown into a series of radial folds extending from the ciliary border to the pupillary edge. Within 2–3 days, more severe inflammatory changes develop, with bluish-white corneal opacity starting at the limbic border and spreading centripetally. Focal aggregations of fibrin accumulate in the anterior chamber, attached to the inner surface of the cornea, and they are seen as accumulations of white material beneath the cornea. Regression of ocular lesions takes some weeks without treatment.

Differential diagnoses

Differential diagnoses include:

- Foreign bodies within the conjunctival sac.
- Keratoconjunctivitis.
- Periorbital eczema.

Diagnosis

Diagnosis is based on clinical signs and a history of silage feeding. The significance of isolation of *L. monocytogenes* from conjunctival swabs is equivocal.

Treatment

There is a marked response to a combined subconjunctival injection of oxytetracycline and dexamethasone (1 mg). The dose of dexamethasone is not sufficient to effect abortion. Without treatment, regression of ocular lesions takes several weeks.

Prevention/control measures

It is difficult to feed big-bale silage in another way to sheep. Attention to detail when baling and wrapping silage, and ensuring appropriate fermentation conditions, should limit contamination with *L. monocytogenes*. However, exposure to air for many days before the large bale is eventually eaten provides an ideal environment for *L. monocytogenes* multiplication.

Economics

Anterior uveitis is not a major concern as ocular lesions regress spontaneously. As a consequence, many farmers elect not to treat sheep with anterior uveitis.

Welfare implications

While ocular lesions do regress spontaneously, there is a dramatic response to combined subconjunctival injection of oxytetracycline and dexamethasone.

ENTROPION

Definition/overview

Entropion is a very common hereditary problem of many breeds and their crossbred progeny. In the UK, entropion affects many newborn lambs of the Border Leicester breed and their progeny; thus, many Scottish Halfbred lambs and the progeny of Scottish Halfbred ewes are born with entropion or develop this condition soon after birth. The problem is also often seen in Suffolk-sired lambs and may affect almost all the progeny of a particular ram.

Aetiology

Entropion is an inherited condition, probably transmitted as a dominant allele. This form of entropion is sometimes referred to as primary entropion and is much more common than secondary entropion, which may develop in association with dehydration and loss of retrobulbar fat in debilitating diseases.

Clinical presentation

With primary entropion, inversion of the lower eyelid is either present at birth (570) or appears soon afterwards (571). There is epiphora, blepharospasm (572) and photophobia. The ocular discharge quickly becomes purulent. Direct contact between the

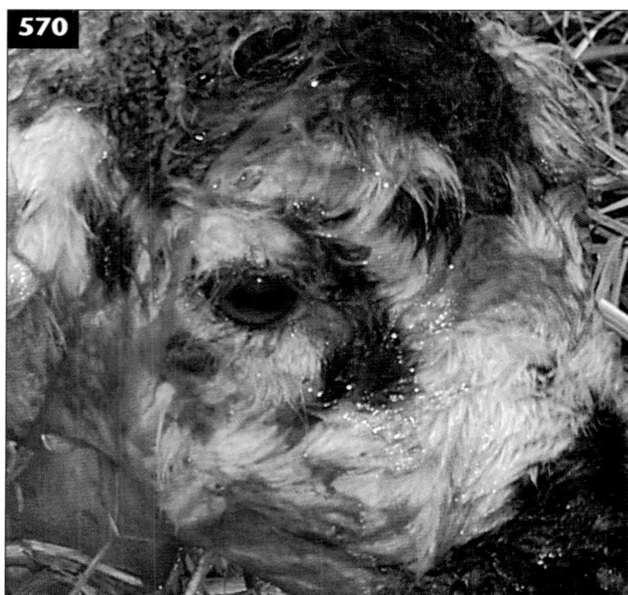

570 Entropion in a newborn lamb.

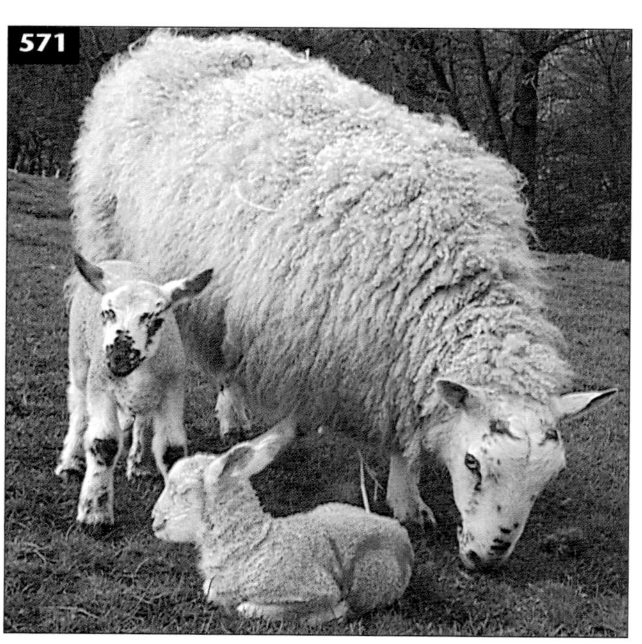

571 Entropion with epiphora in a day-old lamb.

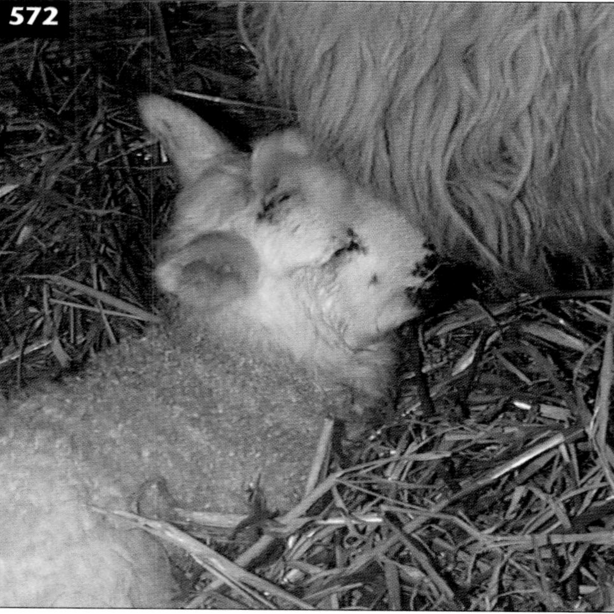

572 Blepharospasm with epiphora in a two-day-old lamb caused by entropion.

eyelashes and cornea causes a severe keratitis, with ulceration in more advanced cases (**573**) resulting in temporary blindness. The condition is frequently bilateral. Hypopyon develops in neglected lambs.

Differential diagnoses

- Infectious keratoconjunctivitis.
- Anterior uveitis.
- Hypopyon following bacteraemia.

Diagnosis

Diagnosis is based on the routine supervision of all newborn lambs and, at regular intervals within the first few days of life, of those lambs with epiphora.

Treatment

In simple cases of entropion of short duration the lower eyelid is everted by rolling down the skin immediately below the lower eyelid. Topical antibiotic is then applied to the cornea to control potential secondary bacterial infection. In addition, the oily presentation lubricates movement of the lower eyelid, thus reducing the likelihood of inversion.

If eyelid inversion recurs after rolling out the lower eyelid, 0.5 ml of procaine penicillin is injected into the lower eyelid. The lamb is held securely by an assistant and a 21 gauge, 15 mm needle introduced through the skin of the lower eyelid parallel to, and approximately 10 mm below, the palpebral fissure (**574**). This volume of antibiotic effectively everts the lower eyelid and forms a depot to control possible secondary bacterial infection. This technique is effective in almost all cases of primary entropion.

Thin metal clips, which are placed at a right angle to the palpebral fissure and closed using fine pliers (Eales clips), can also be used to evert the lower eyelid. These clips have the advantage that they can be inserted quickly by one person.

Excision of an elliptical strip of skin and drawing the cut edges together with sutures can be used to evert the lower eyelid but is rarely necessary.

Prevention/control measures

Entropion is managed by regular inspection of all newborn lambs to ensure that the lower eyelids are normally everted.

The genetic component of entropion should be carefully investigated and, when the condition can be attributed to certain rams, they should be culled; in reality this never happens.

Economics

While almost all of the progeny of a certain ram may be affected by entropion, the ram, and his sire, are rarely culled. Many farmers accept entropion as a 'breed characteristic'.

Welfare implications

Keratitis is a painful condition, especially when the condition is not detected early. The high morbidity rate adds to welfare concerns. Sadly, farmers have not, and will not, select rams on absence of entropion in their progeny.

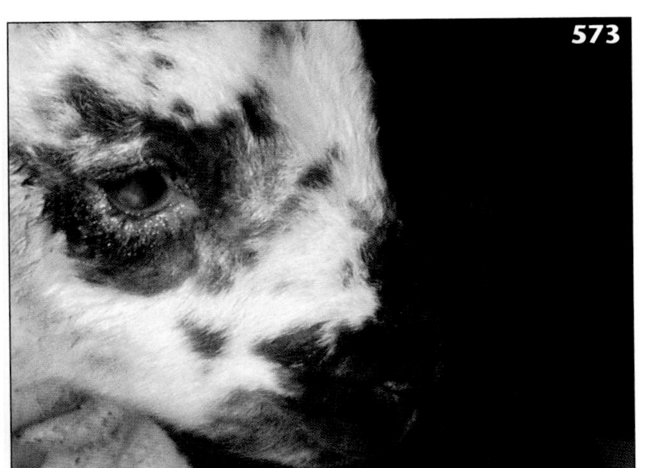

573 Entropion of some days' duration causing severe keratitis and corneal ulceration.

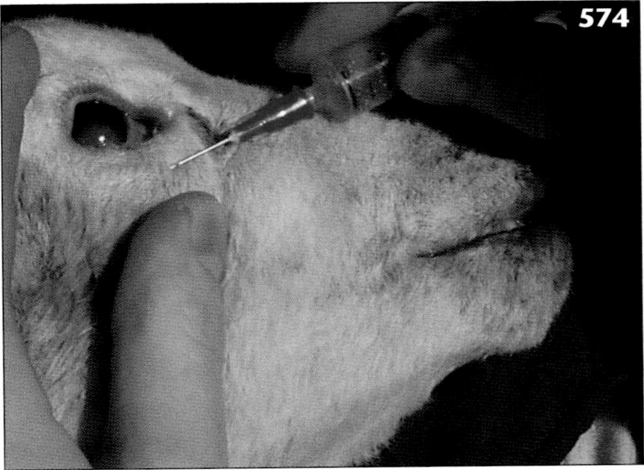

574 Antibiotic injection into the lower eyelid to correct entropion.

CLINICAL PROBLEM

A shepherd complains in late winter that a large number of recently housed Greyface ewes have firmly closed eyelids with tear staining of the face. The ewes avoid bright sunlight and the shepherd is concerned that a number of ewes with bilateral lesions are not coming forward for their concentrate feed.

Clinical examination

The ewes are markedly photophobic and there is obvious blepharospasm. There is marked epiphora with tear staining of the cheek(s). Blind ewes often stand quietly but are hyperaesthetic to sound and touch. Clinical examination reveals pronounced conjunctivitis and keratitis (575).

What conditions should be considered?
What actions/treatments should be recommended?

Differential diagnoses

- Infectious keratoconjuctivitis (pink eye).
- Anterior uveitis (silage eye).

Diagnosis

IKC (pink eye) is common in sheep on exposed ground after severe weather conditions, especially driving snow and high winds, but it can spread rapidly from individual ewes following housing. The condition is diagnosed on clinical examination. Bacteriological examinations are rarely undertaken. Blindness caused by IKC in multigravid ewes during late gestation may lead to ovine pregnancy toxaemia.

Treatment

The two common causal organisms, *Mycoplasma conjunctivae* and *Chlamydophila psittaci,* are susceptible to oxytetracycline. Topical oxytetracycline powder is commonly used because it adheres to the moist conjunctivae, whereas ointments tend to slip off, especially when the contents of the tube are cold. Ewes with bilateral corneal lesions should be injected with long-acting oxytetracycline.

Affected ewes must be isolated, thereby ensuring adequate feeding to prevent ovine pregnancy toxaemia.

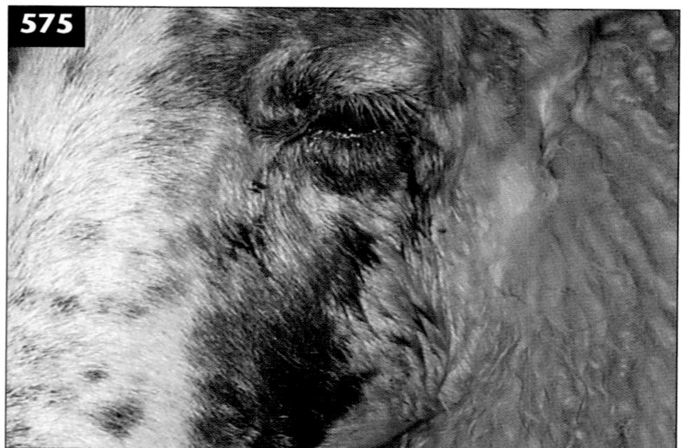

575 Conjunctivitis and keratitis affecting the eyes of a housed Greyface ewe.

12 Mammary Gland

INTRODUCTION

The mammary system has two distinct glands, supported by the median suspensory ligament, each with its own teat, nerve and blood supplies, and lymphatic drainage. The supramammary lymph nodes are only detected by deep palpation and their enlargement is often masked by oedema and swelling of the infected gland. Except for the first few weeks of lactation, it may prove difficult to express more than a few millilitres of milk from the normal glands because of frequent sucking by the lambs.

EXAMINATION OF THE MAMMARY GLAND

Clinical examination of the mammary gland involves palpation for the presence of heat, pain and swelling, and examination of secretions. The normal gland is firm, without obvious swellings and pain, although the ewe may fidget during gland palpation. Inspection of the teats involves casting the ewe on to her hindquarters. Palpation of the gland and examination of mammary secretions are the most informative aspect of clinical examination. Gland secretions can be submitted for standard bacteriological culture and antibiotic sensitivity after aseptic collection.

ULTRASONOGRAPHY

Ultrasound examination of the udder can be undertaken using either 5 MHz linear array or sector scanners to identify deep-seated abscesses, haematomas and fibrosis. Tumours of the mammary gland in sheep are rare. Ultrasonography adds little additional information to that gathered by careful palpation.

BIOPSY

Mammary gland biopsy is rarely undertaken.

MASTITIS

Mastitis is a major disease problem in all intensive sheep production systems worldwide. The clinical manifestations of mastitis in ewes range from peracute gangrenous mastitis with severe illness and toxaemia to chronic mastitis and abscess formation without premonitory signs. Severe illness during the first month of lactation may result in death of the lamb(s) unless they are fed supplementary milk. Chronic mastitis is an important cause of culling in meat-producing sheep and reduced lactation in milking sheep.

Clinical cases of mastitis in sheep occur sporadically and most are predisposed by teat lesions. Unlike in dairy cattle, the California mastitis test is infrequently used to detect increases in bulk milk somatic cell counts, although it may have some application in dairy sheep. Similarly, individual somatic cell counts are not commonly used in sheep to detect subclinical mastitis.

GANGRENOUS MASTITIS

Definition/overview

Gangrenous mastitis occurs sporadically during the first eight weeks of lactation, often preceded by trauma to and/or superficial infection of the teat(s).

Aetiology

Gangrenous mastitis, caused by either *Mannheimia haemolytica* or *Staphylococcus aureus*, occurs sporadically during the first two months of lactation and is associated with poor milk supply related to ewe undernutrition and overvigorous sucking by the lambs. Many sheep farmers believe that gangrenous mastitis is associated with cold weather but this may simply be an association with reduced grass growth during a cold spell and poorer nutrient supply. The condition is more commonly reported in ewes nursing triplets rather than twins, and is rarely seen in ewes rearing singletons. Outbreaks of gangrenous mastitis are often preceded by either staphylococcal skin lesions or CPD infection of the ewe's teat(s).

M. haemolytica is present in the oropharynx of young lambs and can be isolated from the teat skin of lactating ewes. As few as ten colony-forming units of *M. haemolytica* can produce mastitis; therefore, these sites present a constant risk of intramammary infection. *S. aureus* can be isolated from the healthy teat skin of many ewes but especially those with teat skin lesions such as abrasions and CPD infection.

Clinical presentation

The condition is sudden in onset, ewes being healthy 12 hours previously. Affected ewes are separated from the remainder of the flock (**576**) and show no interest or concern over their lambs. They are profoundly depressed (**577**) and have a gaunt appearance with sunken sublumbar fossae due to a poor appetite (**576**). Affected ewes drag the hindlimb ipsilateral to the gangrenous quarter. The udder is visibly swollen and discoloured, first red but quickly turning purple, then black. The lambs are hungry and attempt to suck but the ewe will not stand and walks away. Clinical examination reveals toxic mucous membranes and injected scleral vessels. The rectal temperature is elevated, often >41.0°C. The pulse is greatly increased, often exceeding 120 bpm. The respiratory rate is also increased. There are no ruminal sounds. Examination of the udder reveals marked swelling of one gland, with sharply demarcated purple/black discoloration of the skin (**578, 579**) extending to involve the ventral abdominal wall (**580**). The gangrenous skin lesions result from thrombus formation. While only one gland is affected, the discoloration often extends over two thirds or more of the udder skin. There is marked subcutaneous oedema of the affected gland, extending cranially along the ventral abdomen. The gangrenous areas of skin on the udder and ventral abdomen are cold. There are almost invariably traumatic lesions on the medial aspect of the teats caused by the lambs' incisor teeth. These superficial lesions may be infected with either *S. aureus* (**581**) or CPD virus. Expression of the associated oedematous teat is resented by the ewe and releases a very small quantity (10–20 ml) of yellow/red serum-like fluid.

Differential diagnoses

Clinical examination reveals the extent of the udder infection. The severe mechanical lameness observed during the early stages of gangrenous mastitis must not be mistaken for a toe abscess or joint injury.

Diagnosis

Diagnosis is confirmed during clinical examination, although bacteriological examination is necessary to determine the causal organism.

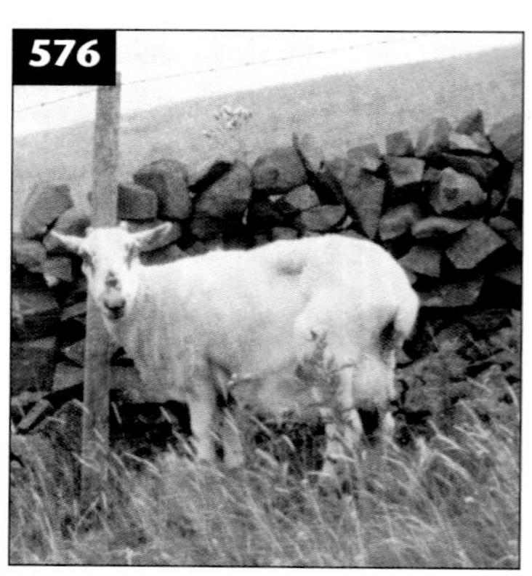

576 Affected ewe separated from the remainder of the flock. The ewe has a gaunt appearance and a ventral swelling.

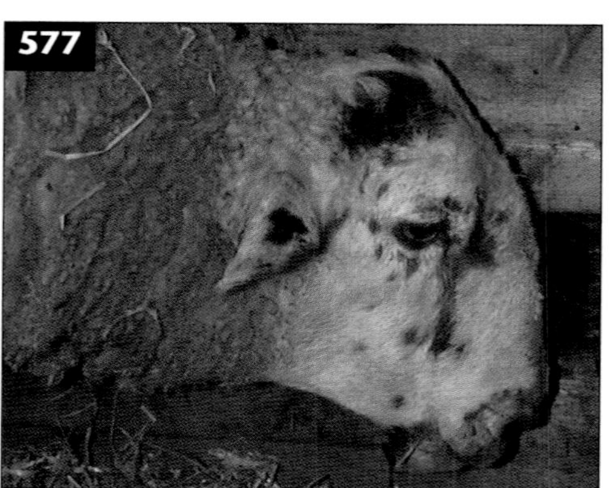

577 Toxaemic ewe suffering from gangrenous mastitis.

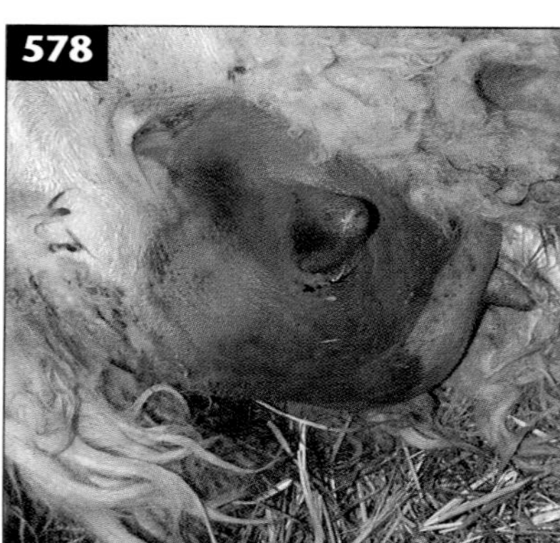

578 Gangrenous mastitis affecting the right gland. The gangrenous lesion is sharply demarcated.

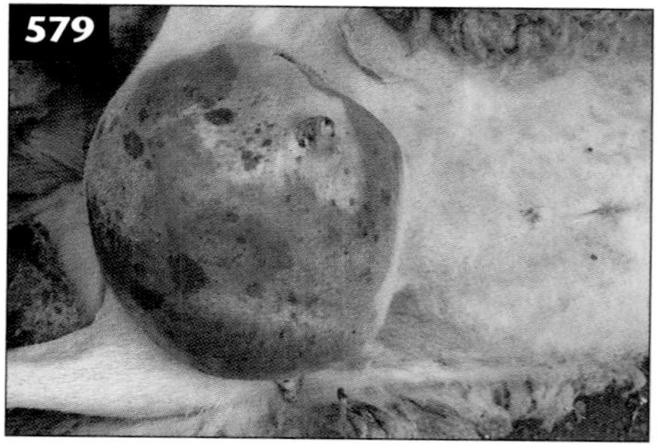

579 Gangrenous mastitis affecting the right gland. Staphylococcal teat lesions are present on the medial aspect of both teats.

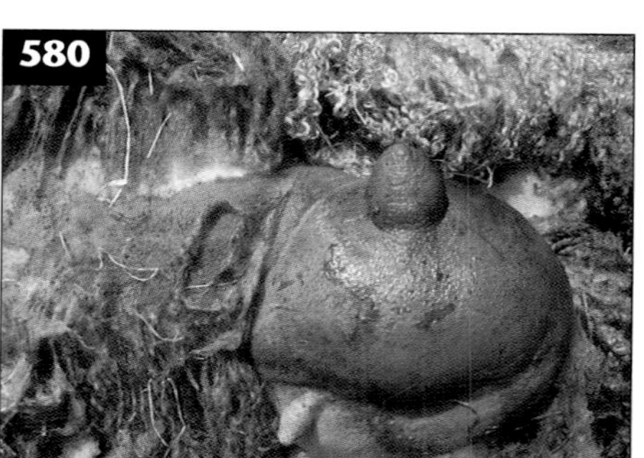

592 Gangrenous mastitis extending along the ventral body wall.

Treatment

Affected ewes should be housed and lambs offered supplementary feeding commensurate with their age. While intravenous antibiotic and NSAID injections will assist the ewe's survival of the initial phase of profound toxaemia, the long-term future for these ewes is hopeless and they must be euthanased before they suffer any further.

Prevention/control measures

With some notable breed exceptions, ewes must not be expected to rear triplets under commercial farming conditions. Appropriate ewe body con-dition score at lambing time and an appropriate level of nutrition during lactation should prevent teat skin abrasions caused by overvigorous sucking by hungry twin lambs. Outbreaks of CPD in lambs may precede gangrenous mastitis in ewes but it should be noted that CPD is most severe in poor lambs on a low plane of nutrition. Staphylococcal teat skin infections have been associated with outbreaks of gangrenous mastitis in housed sheep (**581**). Prompt treatment of these teat skin lesions with procaine penicillin and topical antibiotic, plus supplementary lamb feeding, has prevented further cases of gangrenous mastitis.

Economics

Gangrenous mastitis is a sporadic cause of ewe loss, rarely exceeding 2% of sheep at risk, but loss of lambs may also occur in those ewes affected within the first month of lactation.

In the UK, for example, 100 ewes could be fed an extra 250 g of barley per head per day (3 MJ per head per day) for six weeks for the loss of one ewe with twin lambs at foot. While extra feeding may not prevent all cases of gangrenous mastitis, there are benefits from supplementary feeding (e.g. improved lactation and lamb growth rate). Supplementary feeding will also help restore ewe body condition so that they are in good condition when weaned. Sale of lambs at or before weaning eliminates diseases associated with this stressful period (e.g. systemic pasteurellosis) and avoids the mid-summer challenge from nematode larvae on pasture, cutaneous myiasis and headflies.

Welfare implications

Gangrenous mastitis is a major welfare concern in lactating ewes and is a subject that requires urgent review. Despite antibiotic and supportive therapy during the peracute phase of disease, affected sheep endure an initial phase of profound toxaemia, with resultant marked loss of body condition. After several weeks the gangrenous udder tissue sloughs, leaving a large granulating wound with superficial bacterial infection. The granulation tissue continues to proliferate over the coming months (**582, 583**) and affected ewes cannot be presented at market. They are also unsuitable for breeding stock. There is no market for such sheep and affected ewes must be euthanased during the peracute phase of disease once the diagnosis of gangrenous mastitis has been established.

Acute mastitis

Definition/overview

Acute mastitis occurs sporadically in grazing sheep and causes systemic illness but does not extend to gangrene of mammary tissue. Acute mastitis is a major concern in southern European countries with large populations of milking sheep.

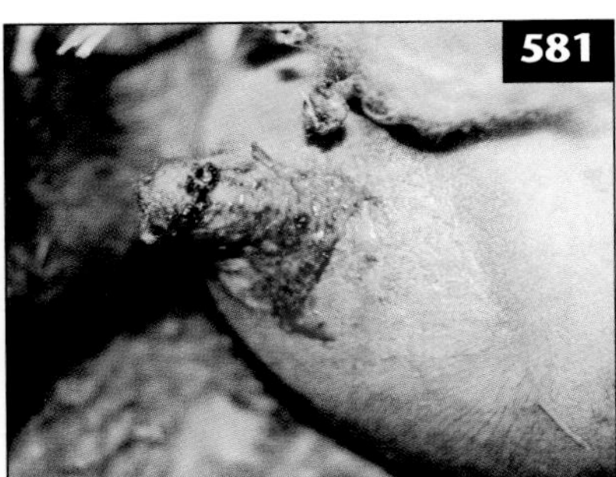

581 Infected lesion on the medial aspect of the teat caused by the lambs' incisor teeth, which may have been a factor in the gangrenous mastitis.

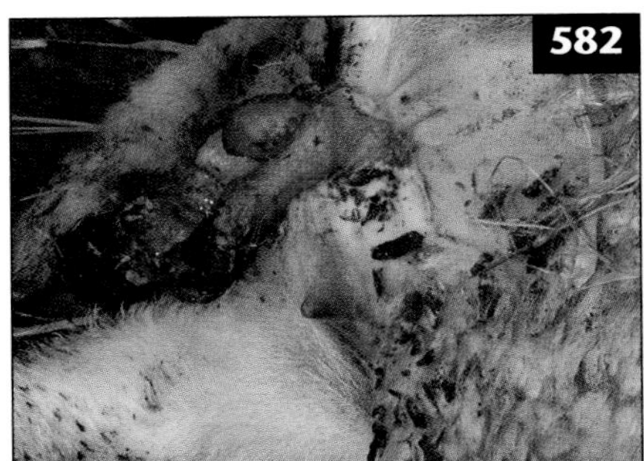

582 Proliferation of granulation tissue over several months following sloughing of the right mammary gland.

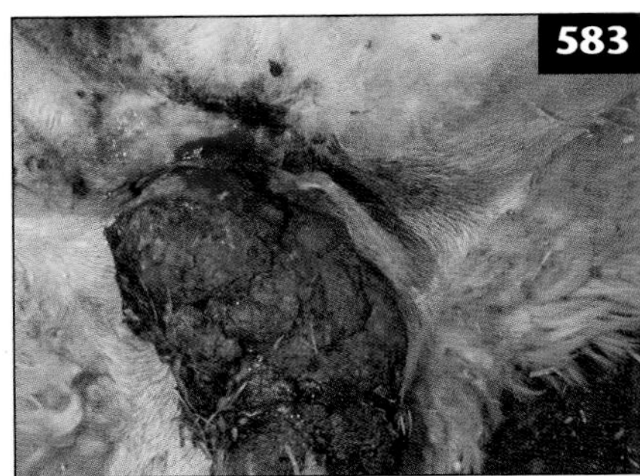

583 Proliferation of granulation tissue over several months following sloughing of the right mammary gland. The farmer has made an unsuccessful attempt at applying a twine tourniquet.

Aetiology
A wide range of bacteria, including *Streptococcus* species and *Escherichia coli*, can gain entry through the streak canal and cause acute mastitis.

Clinical presentation
The initial clinical signs are broadly similar, although less severe, than those for gangrenous mastitis. Affected ewes are separated from the remainder of the flock and are depressed and have a gaunt appearance. The rectal temperature is elevated. There is marked swelling and oedema of the affected gland (**584**), which rarely extends cranially along the ventral abdomen. There may be traumatic lesions on the medial aspect of the teats caused by the lambs' incisor teeth. The udder secretion varies from 'normal' milk containing large white clots to serum-like, depending on the causal organism.

Differential diagnoses
The major differential diagnosis of sudden onset illness in grazing sheep is acute respiratory disease caused by *Pasteurella* (*Mannheimia*) species.

Diagnosis
Diagnosis is confirmed during clinical examination, although bacteriological examination is necessary to determine the causal organism.

Treatment
Treatment involves parenteral antibiotic therapy, typically oxytetracycline or penicillin, with an equivalent intramammary preparation, although there may not be a licensed intramammary formulation in many countries. Tilmicosin is licensed for the treatment of ovine mastitis in many countries; it has the advantages of activity against mycoplasmas and a single injection formulation. Regular stripping of the mastitic gland will remove toxins. Flunixin or ketoprofen will assist treatment of the toxaemia.

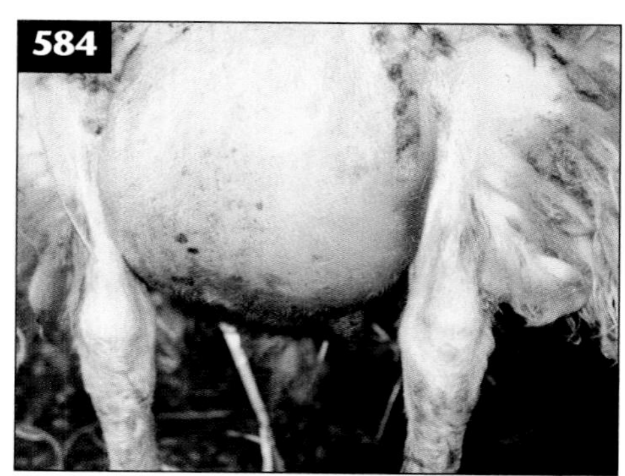

584 Swollen right mammary gland caused by acute mastitis in a lactating Greyface ewe.

Prevention/control measures
The sporadic nature of the condition in grazing meat-producing sheep makes prevention difficult. In milk-producing sheep, control is aimed at hygiene during the milking process and maintenance of the milking plant with regular servicing. Sampling of mastitis cases and bacteriological culture will give some indication of the important epidemiological factors contributing to a high disease incidence in milking sheep.

Economics
Acute mastitis is a major problem of milking sheep in many countries. In meat breeds, losses result from reduced lamb growth rates due to reduced milk supply and the increased culling rate subsequent to the development of chronic mastitis in these ewes.

Welfare implications
There is a considerable body of evidence indicating significant pain associated with both acute and chronic mastitis in cattle. The administration of NSAIDs during the acute phase should reduce pain in sheep with mastitis and it may reduce pain as the condition becomes more chronic.

CHRONIC MASTITIS
Definition/overview
Chronic mastitis develops from an acute episode of disease during lactation, few new mammary infections become established following weaning. Chronic mastitis is a major cause of culling in both meat-producing and milk-producing sheep.

Aetiology
Incomplete resolution of acute mastitis results in the establishment of chronic infection, which manifests as abscess formation within the mammary parenchyma. *Arcanobacterium pyogenes* is almost invariably cultured from udder abscesses, although it may not have been the original pathogen.

Clinical presentation
The teat is often thickened with a fibrous cord blocking the streak canal. Abscesses range in both number and diameter within the udder. Some abscesses may be detected at weaning but they are often masked at this time by milk within the udder. The best time routinely to detect chronic mastitis is the pre-breeding check undertaken some 2–3 months later, when mammary gland involution makes palpation much more accurate. Deep-seated abscesses

(585) have a thick fibrous capsule, which may extend to several centimetres thick, with a core of green viscous pus (586). Superficial abscesses have a thin wall, often only a few millimetres thick, which may rupture and discharge pus. Development and growth of abscesses with proliferation of surrounding fibrous tissue leads to gross enlargement of the associated gland and udder over 3–6 months, and this can measure up to 20 cm in diameter in neglected sheep.

Chronic mastitis cases not detected during the pre-breeding check are subsequently identified post lambing when the first sign is a hungry lamb(s). The teat of the affected gland is thickened and no milk, or only a small amount of inspissated pus, can be expressed from the teat.

Bacteraemic spread to the lungs is not uncommon and results in numerous abscesses, typically distributed in the dorsal areas of the diaphragmatic lobe(s). These abscesses rarely result in signs of respiratory disease but contribute to general malaise in some sheep. Bacteraemic spread to the endocardium and joints from the udder is much less common.

Differential diagnoses

- It may prove difficult to differentiate whether a small deep-seated firm swelling in the udder is an abscess or simply involuted mammary tissue.
- Maedi-visna virus infection can result in chronic fibrosis of the mammary gland, although this manifestation of infection varies between countries, and is uncommon in the UK.

Diagnosis

Diagnosis of a mammary abscess, particularly a deep-seated lesion, can be confirmed by ultrasonographic examination (587, 588) and/or fine needle aspirate.

Treatment

Encouraging results have been reported for the treatment of mild cases of chronic mastitis using tilmicosin (s/c) at weaning. Treatment of chronic mastitis that has progressed to abscessation within the gland is not usually undertaken because of the hopeless prognosis and associated loss of normal mammary tissue and lactogenesis.

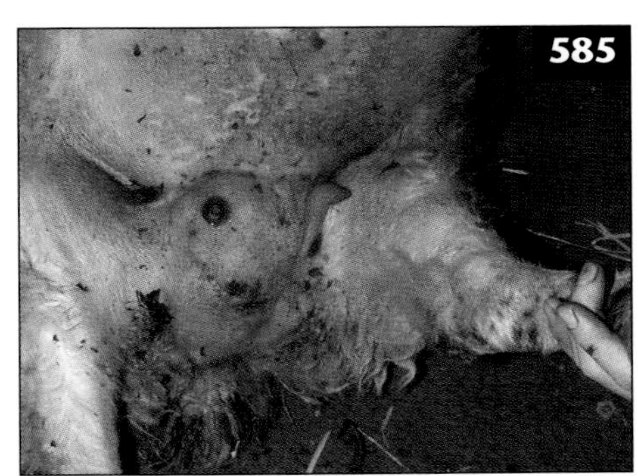

585 Swollen right gland containing numerous abscesses.

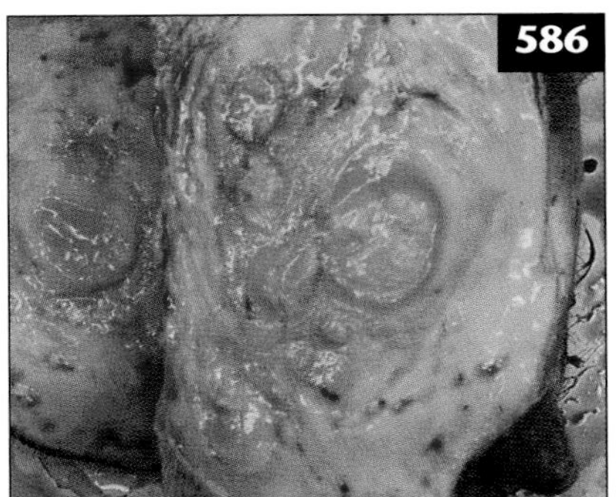

586 Cross-section of mammary gland containing numerous thick-walled abscesses. (See also ultrasonograms **587** and **588**.)

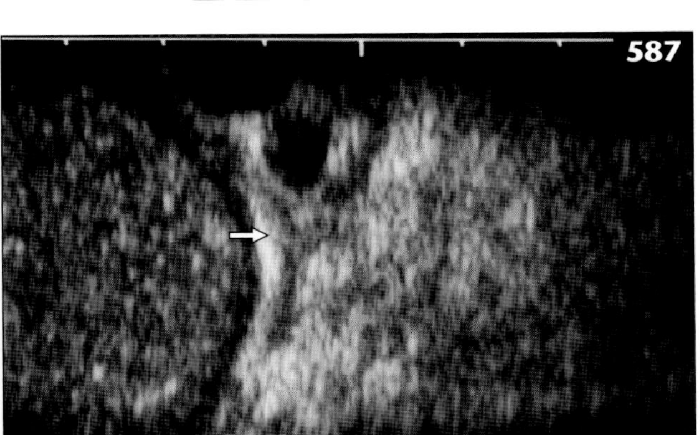

587 Encapsulated abscess 6 cm deep within the mammary gland. The linear probe head is to the right of the image. The abscess appears as an anechoic area containing multiple bright dots, with the capsule represented by the broad hyperechoic (white) line (arrow).

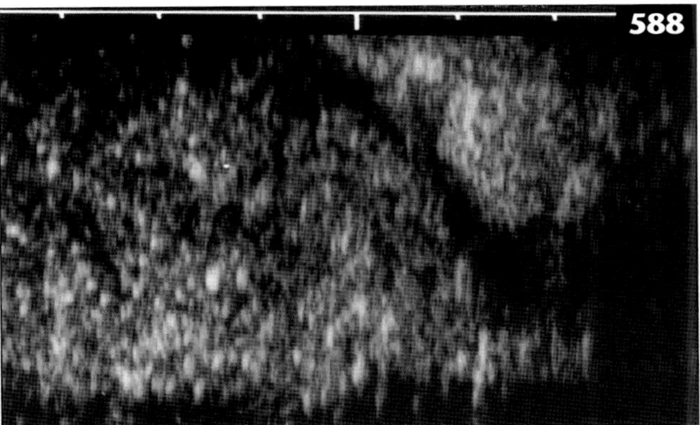

588 Abscess 3 cm deep within the mammary gland. The linear probe head is to the right of the image. The abscess appears as an anechoic area containing multiple bright dots.

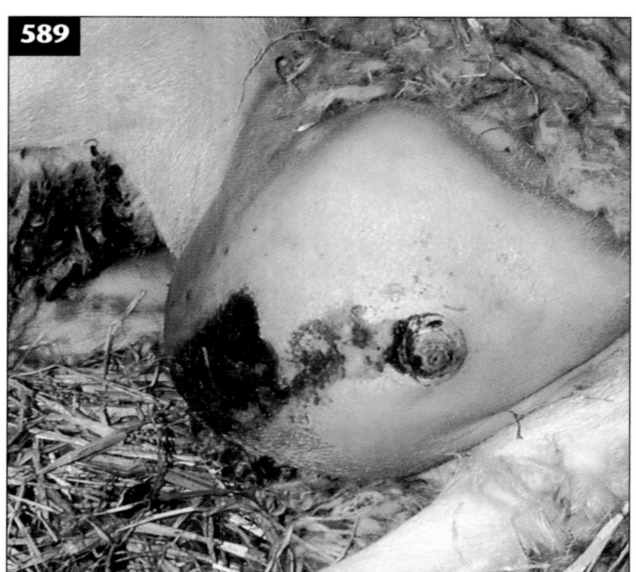

589 Staphylococcal lesion on the medial aspect of the left gland, with mastitis and obvious swelling and oedema. The large 6 cm x 6 cm necrotic skin lesion has been caused by a thrombus.

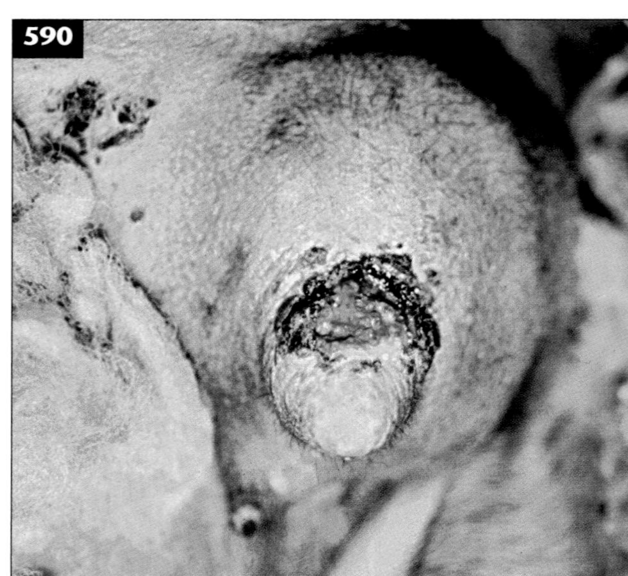

590 Superficial skin lesion infected with *S. aureus*. The teat is oedematous and there is a likelihood of mastitis.

Prevention/control measures

Ewes with chronic mastitis and abscesses should be culled following identification at weaning or at the pre-breeding check.

There are no licensed long-acting intramammary antibiotic preparations in many countries, although preparations for cattle are used 'off-label' at weaning to control/prevent chronic mastitis. Care must be exercised with intramammary infusion in sheep because iatrogenic infections are common when the procedure is undertaken in wet or unhygienic conditions. Appropriate teat disinfection before antibiotic infusion is essential. The intramammary syringe nozzle is held against the teat orifice; it must not be forced into the streak canal.

Economics

Chronic mastitis is an important cause of premature culling in sheep flocks worldwide and as such represents an important economic loss, although there are few recent reliable data. Carcase condemnation may result if there is reaction in the deep inguinal lymph nodes draining the udder. Chronic mastitis also results in reduced lactation and subsequent lower growth rate in lambs.

The use of tilmicosin in all ewes at weaning to treat existing subclinical udder infections and prevent post-weaning mastitis is expensive (approximately 2.5% of the value of a ewe) and restricted to valuable milking sheep and pedigree meat breed ewes.

Welfare implications

Udder abscessation is painful and presents a welfare concern when there are numerous large abscesses, although the extent of the surrounding fibrous capsule may limit the impact of external stimuli such as hindlimb movements.

Teat lesions

In gangrenous and acute mastitis cases there are almost invariably traumatic lesions to the skin on the medial aspect of the teats caused by the lambs' incisor teeth (**589**). They are more common in ewes nursing triplets and may, in part, explain the much higher incidence of mastitis in these ewes. These superficial skin lesions may become infected with *S. aureus*, or with CPD virus if it is present in the flock at that time.

Treatment of staphylococcal teat lesions may become necessary (**590**) and a good response is achieved with procaine penicillin (44,000 iu/kg i/m for 3–5 consecutive days) and topical antibiotic cream/aerosol spray. Supplementary feeding of lambs may be necessary but few nursing lambs will suck from a bottle and teat; therefore, concentrates may offer a better and easier option.

CONTAGIOUS AGALACTIA

Definition/overview
Contagious agalactia affects sheep and goats in many parts of the world, particularly in southern Europe and the Middle East. The disease is not recognized in the UK, Australia and New Zealand.

Aetiology
Contagious agalactia is caused by *Mycoplasma agalactiae* but the role of other mycoplasmas is under discussion.

Clinical presentation
Affected sheep are dull, inappetent and pyrexic. Abortion may result in pregnant sheep in the flock. There is severe bilateral mastitis in lactating ewes, with clots present in the much reduced udder secretions. Nursing lambs are hungry, have a gaunt appearance and die if not given appropriate supplementary feeding. Commonly, there is marked lameness resulting from involvement of the carpal and hock joints, characterized by considerable joint effusion. There may be epiphora and blepharospasm associated with keratoconjunctivitis.

Diagnosis
Diagnosis is based on the clinical findings in a large number of sheep and isolation of *M. agalactiae* from mammary secretions and arthrocentesis samples.

Treatment
Tylosin and tilmicosin are especially effective *in vitro* against mycoplasmas but they may not be licensed for use in sheep in some countries. Problems arise with achieving sufficient antibiotic penetration into joints. Even prolonged antibiotic therapy is unlikely to effect a cure in sheep with numerous infected joints.

Prevention/control measures
Vaccines appear to afford little protection against contagious agalactia.

Economics
Contagious agalactia can result in serious financial loss due to the refractory nature of the condition and consequent high culling rate.

Welfare implications
The prognosis for polyarthritis associated with *M. agalactiae* infection is poor and affected sheep should be euthanased.

MAEDI-VISNA VIRUS

Definition/overview
The clinical manifestations of maedi-visna virus (MVV) infection vary considerably between countries. In the USA, MVV infection is more commonly referred to as ovine progressive pneumonia when affecting the lungs and 'hardbag' when affecting the mammary gland. Such pathology is rarely identified in the UK, where maedi and visna are the more common clinical presentations of MVV infection.

Aetiology
Infection with MVV may cause a lymphocytic mastitis ('hardbag'), as well as joint, brain (visna) and lung (maedi) lesions.

Clinical presentation
Reports describe an indurative mastitis without changes in the milk. The udder is smaller and more fibrous than normal but this proves difficult to detect in the lactating ewe and is better appreciated during the pre-breeding check some 2–3 months after weaning. The shepherd is alerted to these ewes by the unexplained poor growth rate of their lambs.

Differential diagnoses
Chronic mastitis of bacterial origin causes more focal swellings, often resulting in abscessation, which can be identified during ultrasonographic examination.

Diagnosis
Sheep infected with MVV can be detected serologically by CFT or ELISA tests.

Treatment
There is no treatment and affected sheep should be culled.

Prevention/control measures
Control measures depend on the flock MVV seroprevalence and other factors (see Chapter 6, Part 1: p. 150.)

Economics
It is reported that indurative mastitis caused by MVV infection is a major cause of starvation of lambs in western range flocks in the USA.

Welfare implications

Indurative mastitis is not painful but concerns arise when lambs die of starvation caused by poor lactation.

CLINICAL PROBLEM

A depressed ewe is presented during early summer (**591**). The ewe had lambed approximately six weeks previously and was nursing triplets. The shepherd noted the ewe separated from the remainder of the group that morning.

Clinical examination

The ewe is in poor bodily condition (BCS 1.5) and depressed with toxic mucous membranes. The rectal temperature is raised (40.6°C). The pulse is increased to 120 bpm, the respiratory rate is normal (25 breaths per minute) and there are reduced ruminal sounds. Examination of the udder reveals extensive gangrenous mastitis of the left gland with associated marked subcutaneous oedema extending to involve the ventral abdominal wall (**592**). The sharply demarcated purple areas are cold and firm. There are numerous skin lesions on the medial aspect of both teats.

What pathogens could be involved?
What is the prognosis?
What action should be recommended?

Aetiology

Gangrenous mastitis caused by *Pasteurella* (*Mannheimia*) species and *S. aureus* occurs sporadically during the first two months of lactation and is associated with poor milk supply related to ewe undernutrition and overvigorous sucking by the lambs. The condition is commonly reported in ewes nursing triplets and this practice must be actively discouraged unless farmers are prepared to feed the ewes very well (up to 2 kg per head daily) and offer good quality creep feed for the lambs. Gangrenous mastitis may be preceded by either staphylococcal skin lesions or CPD virus infection of the ewe's teat(s).

Prognosis

The prognosis is hopeless.

Recommended action

The ewe should (and was) be euthanased for welfare reasons. It would be unacceptable to keep this ewe because, despite antibiotic and supportive therapy, the gangrenous udder tissue will eventually slough and leave a large wound. The granulation tissue will continue to proliferate over the coming months. Ewes cannot be presented at market because the carcase would be condemned at meat inspection.

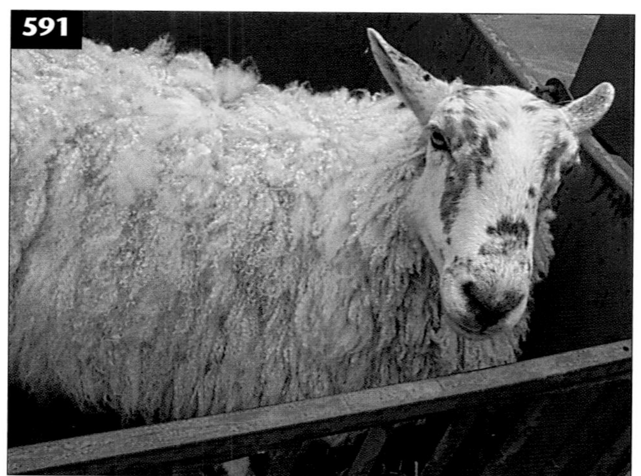

591 Dull ewe that had lambed approximately six weeks previously and was nursing triplets.

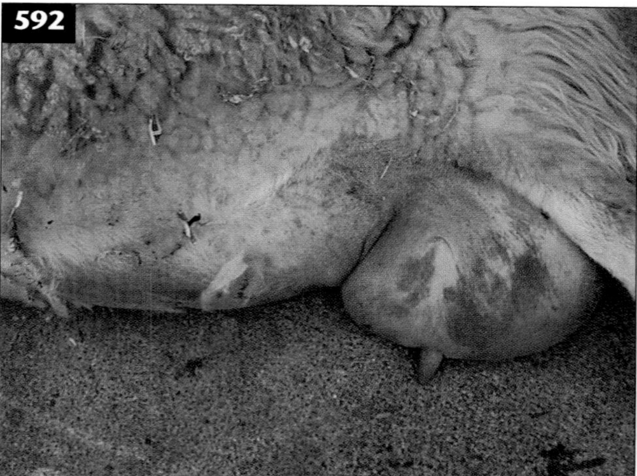

592 Extensive gangrenous mastitis of the left gland with associated marked subcutaneous oedema extending to involve the ventral abdominal wall.

13 Metabolic Disorders and Trace Element Deficiencies

OVINE PREGNANCY TOXAEMIA

(*Syn*: twin lamb disease)

Definition/overview

Ovine pregnancy toxaemia (OPT) occurs in all countries worldwide. In the UK, OPT is most commonly encountered in lowland flocks, affecting multiparous ewes carrying three or more lambs during the last month of gestation. A recent UK survey reported a prevalence of OPT of 0.5%. In countries that rely almost exclusively on pasture-based systems with little supplementary feeding, OPT is seen in severely underfed twin-bearing ewes. Whilst certain unique factors may precipitate disease in individual ewes, the appearance of OPT indicates a severe energy underfeeding problem in the flock and the likely occurrence in other high risk ewes.

Aetiology

Flock factors

OPT occurs following a period of severe energy shortage (e.g. poor roughage quality, inadequate concentrate allowance or high fetal demand) but clinical signs can be precipitated by a sudden stressful event such as adverse weather conditions, handling, vaccination or housing. Parasitism, in particular liver fluke infestation, causing depletion of body reserves may be an important factor leading to OPT, although such chronic conditions more commonly result in chronic intrauterine growth retardation with consequent reduced energy demands of a small fetus(es).

Individual ewe factors

Individual ewe factors such as obesity, severe lameness or vaginal prolapse, or other disturbances such as rumenal acidosis or hypocalcaemia, which cause a temporary lack of appetite, may also predispose to OPT.

Pathophysiology

Severe energy deficiency, whether primary due to management errors or secondary due to reduced appetite, results in excess fat mobilization and fatty infiltration of the parenchymatous organs.

Clinical presentation

The early clinical signs of OPT include disorientation, which leads to isolation from the remainder of the flock. When driven to the feed troughs affected ewes stand amongst the other ewes but do not eat. Occasional bleating may be heard from ewes during the early stages and this is associated with blindness and separation from the remainder of the group (**593**). Over the next 24–48 hours affected ewes become increasingly dull and depressed (**594**) and are easily caught, but they are often difficult to restrain in order to administer treatments because they are hyperaesthetic to tactile and auditory stimuli. Affected ewes are usually in poorer bodily condition, have poorer mammary development and have a more distended abdomen relative to other sheep in the group at a similar stage of pregnancy.

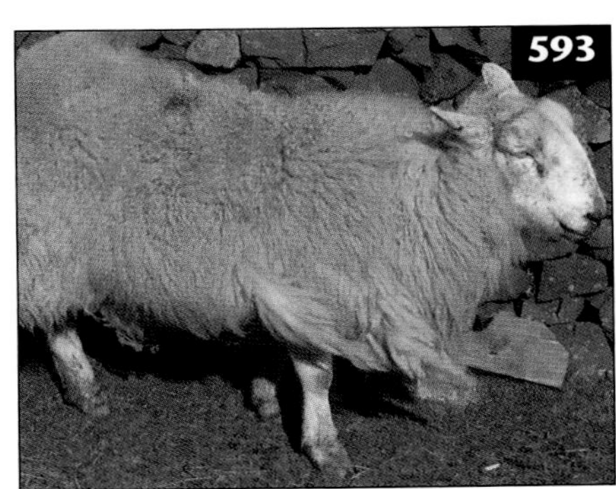

593 Depressed, blind Greyface ewe, which is separated from the remainder of the flock. Lambing starts in three weeks.

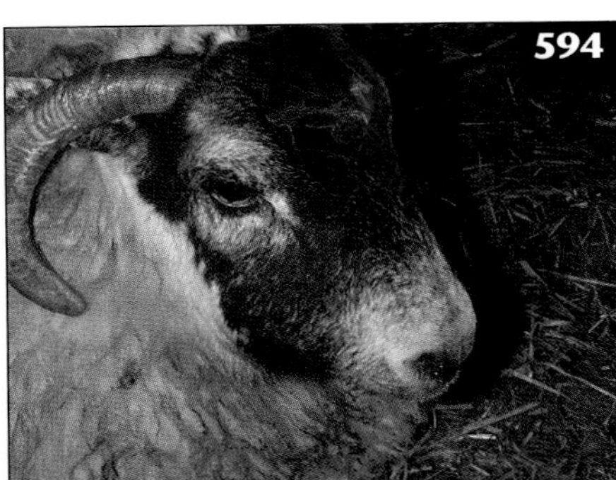

594 Depressed, blind Scottish Blackface ewe, which did not respond to an approaching person.

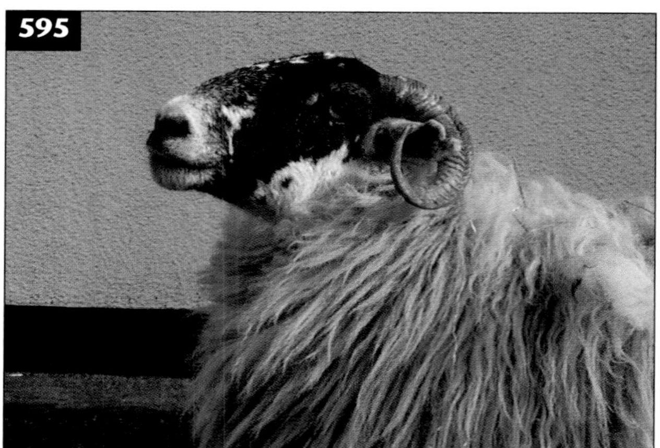

595 Blindness and star-gazing behaviour in a heavily pregnant Scottish Blackface ewe.

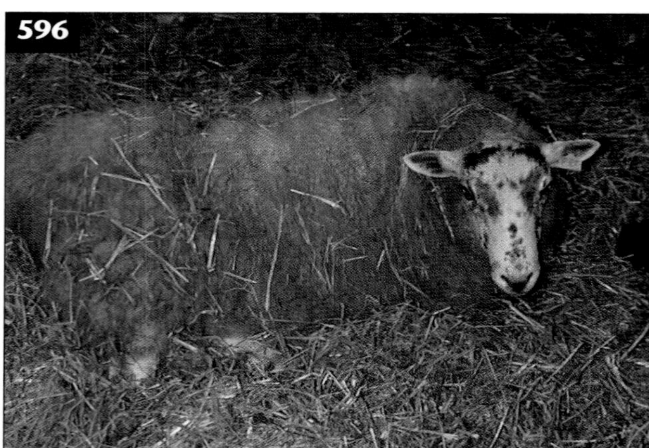

596 Blind, four-crop Greyface ewe that had been scanned for triplets and did not feed this morning. Lambing starts in two weeks.

There is a lack of menace response but pupillary light reflexes are normal. Abnormal behaviour including head pressing, dorsiflexion of the neck (**595**), often termed 'star gazing', and frequent teeth grinding (bruxism) usually develop. Head pressing into the corner of a pen is a common finding. Continuous fine muscle fasciculations causing movement of the overlying skin may be observed around the muzzle and affecting the ears.

Ewes may become recumbent (**596**) with the hips extended caudally and the hindlimbs held out behind the ewe. There is loss of tone in the abdominal wall musculature and the abdomen appears flattened dorsoventrally and 'spread out'. The fetuses can be balloted easily through both sides of the abdomen. Inability to stand leads to urine scalding of the hindlimbs, udder and ventral abdomen and the development of pressure sores despite good nursing. Ewes that become recumbent have a poor prognosis. Abortion as a consequence of OPT is uncommon. In unsuccessful cases, death occurs 5–10 days after the first appearance of clinical signs.

Differential diagnoses

Several ewes affected:

- Acidosis resulting from carbohydrate overfeed.
- Listeriosis.
- Hypocalcaemia.
- Impending abortion.
- Polioencephalomalacia.
- Copper poisoning.

Individual ewes:

- Peripheral vestibular lesion (middle ear infection).
- Space-occupying brain lesions such as coenurosis or abscess.
- Sarcocystosis.

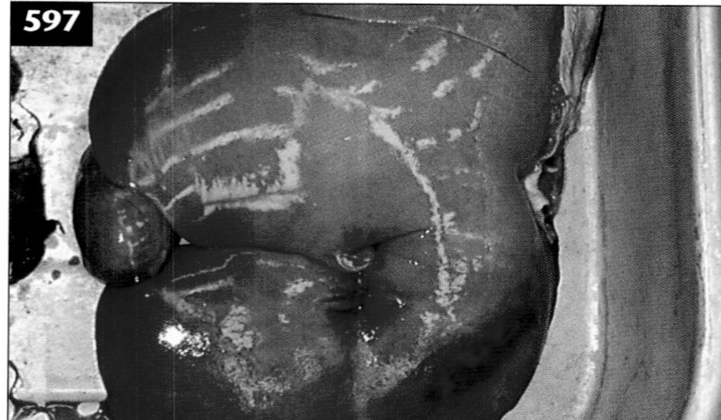

597 Fatty liver from a ewe that died from OPT.

Diagnosis

Each of the conditions listed above can lead to isolation, reduced appetite, emaciation and/or recumbency during late gestation. Diagnosis of OPT is based on the history and clinical findings in a multigravid, multiparous ewe. While serum 3-OH butyrate concentrations >3.0 mmol/l are suggestive of OPT, such values are not pathognomic, because concentrations can rise in sheep when there is high fetal demand for glucose and insufficient energy intake resulting from inappetence of relatively short duration.

Postmortem findings, which include fatty infiltration of the parenchymatous organs, especially the liver (**597**), and the presence of two or more well-developed fetuses *in utero*, are suggestive of, but not pathognomic for, OPT. These necropsy findings can be supported by an aqueous humor 3-OH butyrate concentration >2.5 mmol/l or a CSF value >0.6 mmol/l, which correspond to antemortem serum concentrations >3.0 mmol/l, and absence of significant lesions.

Treatment

The response of OPT to treatment is generally poor even when clinical signs are detected early. Housed ewes should be penned separately and offered palatable feeds, to promote appetite, and fresh water. If ewes are housed, turnout to good pasture may promote appetite, although such grazing is seldom available. Treatment with either a concentrated oral electrolyte and dextrose solution or propylene glycol, intravenous glucose injection and glucocorticoid injection is successful in approximately 30% of OPT cases that are still ambulatory when treatments commence.

It is recommended that 60–100 ml of 40% dextrose is injected intravenously twice daily but this is seldom practical. Ten to 15 litres of fluids containing rumen stimulants can be easily administered by orogastric tube twice daily. Transfaunation can be undertaken in valuable ewes. Injection of 16 mg dexamethasone, administered as part of the treatment regimen, may result in abortion in ewes more than 136 days pregnant. The administration of a long-acting glucocorticoid injection is claimed to have similar glucogenic effects as dexamethasone but not to result in abortion. Some practitioners routinely administer calcium borogluconate to recumbent ewes suffering from OPT because blood analysis often reveals marginal hypocalcaemia. However, there is no convincing field evidence that calcium administration improves the recovery rate. Clinical hypocalcaemia can readily be differentiated from OPT during the clinical examination.

Ewes with OPT must be checked at least twice daily for signs of abortion/lambing because they may be too weak to expel the fetuses/lambs. Failure to expel dead fetuses leads to autolysis, with rapid development of toxaemia causing death of the ewe.

The decision to perform a caesarean section must be made during the early clinical stages of disease to achieve best results from this salvage procedure. However, caesarean section performed to save the life of the ewe has a poor success rate due to the emaciated state of the ewe and fatty infiltration of her liver, kidneys and heart. In addition, retention of the fetal membranes commonly leads to septic metritis.

Ewes that do recover from OPT are rarely able to nurse a single lamb and are generally culled once they have regained body condition.

Prevention/control measures

Multigravid ewes must be fed appropriate levels of high quality roughage and supplementary concentrate feeding during the last six weeks of pregnancy. Liquid molasses (**598**) helps promote appetite but is not a substitute for appropriate concentrate allowance. Fetal number can be determined by ultrasonography 45–90 days post mating, allowing grouping based on energy demands. Dietary energy sufficiency can be accurately determined by measuring ewes' serum concentrations of 3-OH butyrate 4–6 weeks prior to lambing (see Chapter 2, Veterinary visit to assess late gestation nutrition, p. 17).

Economics

Farmers rarely present sheep with suspected metabolic disease to their veterinary surgeon. Shepherds remark that they do not have sufficient time to nurse individual sick ewes so the treatment response is often much lower than the 30% figure quoted earlier. The cost of three days' treatment with concentrated oral electrolyte and dextrose solution is approximately 10% of the value of the ewe, further limiting appropriate therapy. Many veterinarians will not dispense dexamethasone to sheep clients because of concerns relating to inappropriate off-label use, thereby removing this treatment option.

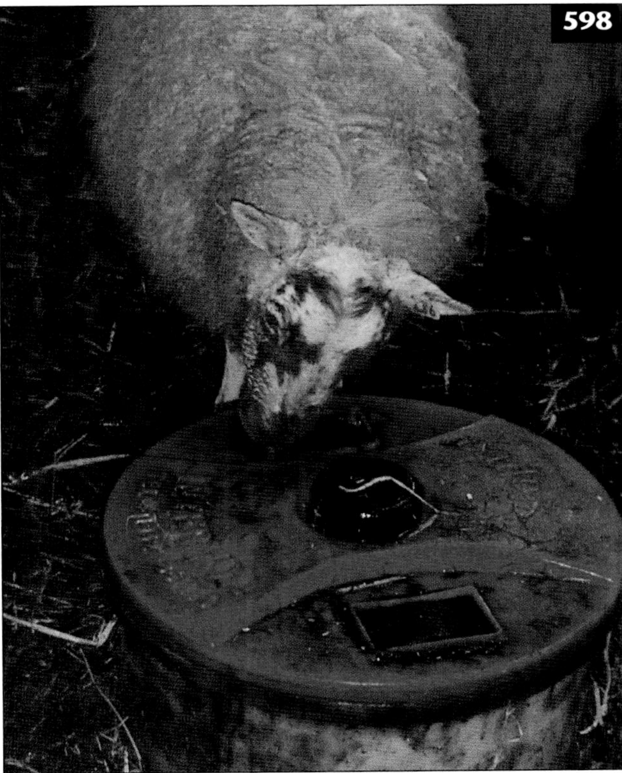

598 Palatable molasses licks may increase energy intake during the last few weeks of gestation.

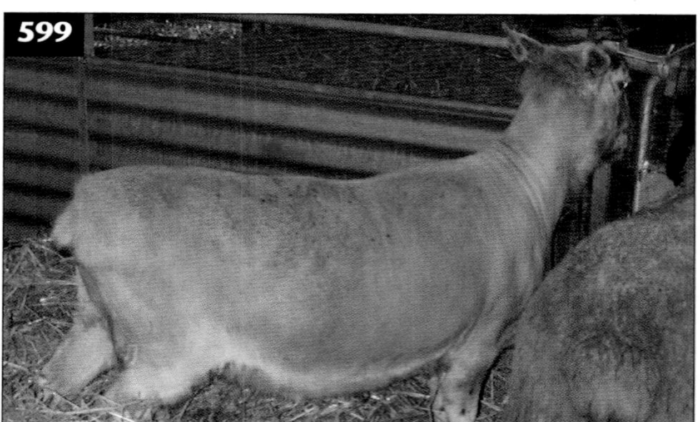
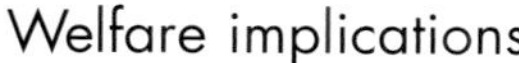

599 Wool slip occurs commonly in recovered ewes.

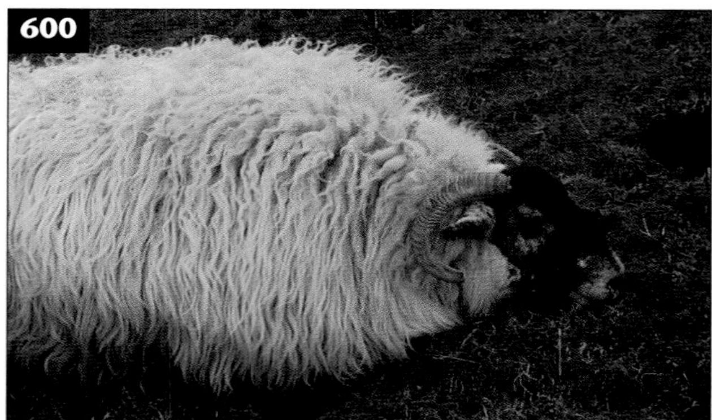

600 Depressed, sternally recumbent Scottish Blackface ewe suffering from hypocalcaemia the day following movement.

Welfare implications

Recovery is very unlikely once the ewe is unable to stand, and euthanasia is indicated for welfare reasons. Wool slip occurs commonly in recovered ewes 4–6 weeks after abortion/lambing (**599**), which may present problems during adverse weather conditions at pasture.

HYPOCALCAEMIA

Definition/overview

Hypocalcaemia is reported in all countries worldwide when sheep are managed intensively. A recent UK survey reported a 0.4% prevalence of hypocalcaemia. Hypocalcaemia is not uncommon in three-crop or older ewes maintained at pasture during late gestation, but it can also occur sporadically during early lactation. Hypocalcaemia is often observed when ewes are brought down off hill grazing on to improved pasture prior to lambing (**600**). 'Outbreaks' of hypocalcaemia can result from errors in formulating home-mix rations, incorrect mineral supplementation, stress-related events such as dog-worrying, movement on to good pastures prior to lambing, or following housing.

Aetiology

The highest demand for calcium in non-milking sheep occurs 3–4 weeks prior to parturition due to calcification of fetal bones. Mobilization of calcium from bone stores takes more than 24 hours; therefore, periods of transient hypocalcaemia may result.

Clinical presentation

During the early stages of hypocalcaemia affected ewes become isolated from the flock (**600**) and, although able to extend their hindlimbs, are unable to raise themselves from their knees and assume sternal recumbency again within 10–30 seconds. A small percentage of sheep appears disoriented and hyperaesthetic and may have a rapid respiratory rate ('panting'). Over the next 2–6 hours the ewe becomes depressed (**601**), weak (**602**) and unable to stand even when supported. There is rumen stasis with development of bloat. The rectum is flaccid and may contain pellets of dried faeces, which are not voided (**603**). Passive reflux of rumen contents may occur, with green fluid present at the external nares and around the lower jaw. These findings, together with the presence of stridor, often result in the shepherd treating the ewe for respiratory disease, with a consequent delay in the request for veterinary assistance. There may be partial prolapse of the rectum/vagina. Unlike cattle, sheep do not assume lateral recumbency in the advanced stages of hypocalcaemia (**602**). Without appropriate therapy the condition develops to coma, and death follows 24–48 hours after onset of recumbency.

Differential diagnoses

- Ovine pregnancy toxaemia.
- Acidosis resulting from carbohydrate overfeed.
- Listeriosis.
- Copper poisoning.
- Rhododendron poisoning.
- Polioencephalomalacia.

Diagnosis

In sheep recumbent due to hypocalcaemia, serum calcium concentrations are $<$1.4 mmol/l. (**NB:** Serum 3-OH butyrate concentrations can be elevated, especially if the ewe had been inappetent for more than 12 hours.) The rapid response of hypocalcaemic ewes to intravenous calcium infusion differentiates this condition from OPT and the other differential diagnoses listed.

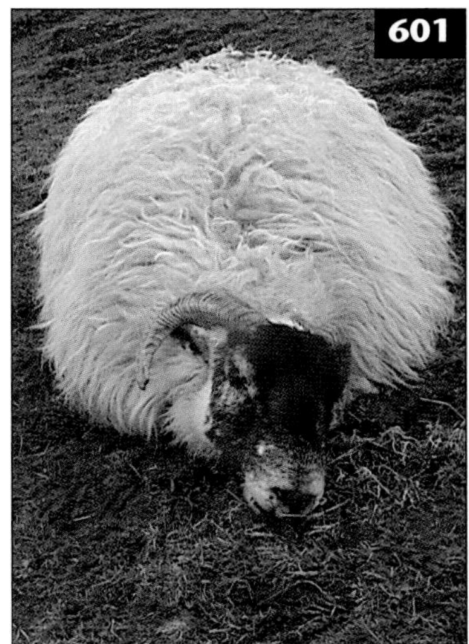

601 This ewe with hypocalcaemia was unresponsive to the observer. Its behaviour is markedly abnormal for the Scottish Blackface breed.

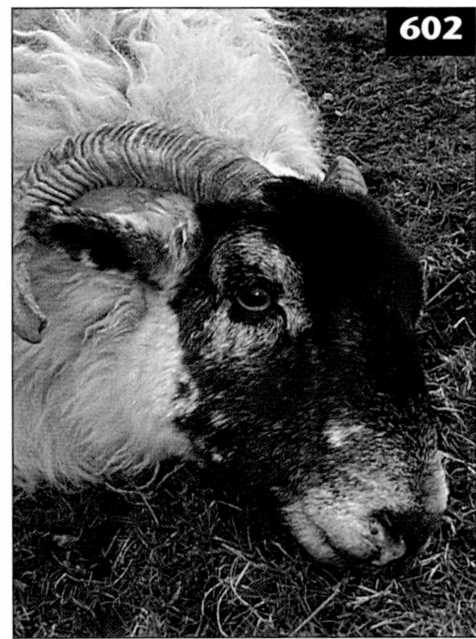

602 Hypocalcaemia. Depression progressing to stupor. There is a mucopurulent nasal discharge.

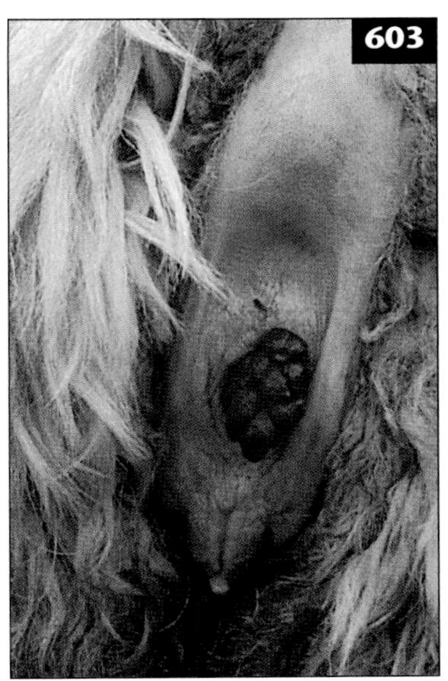

603 Constipation in a ewe suffering from hypocalcaemia.

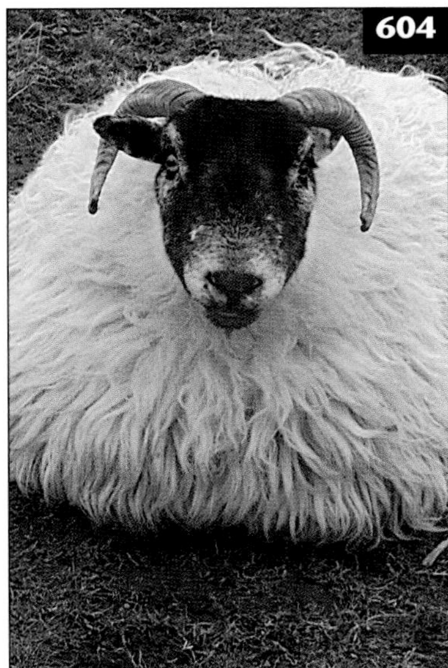

604 Hypocalcaemia. Two minutes after intravenous calcium administration.

Treatment

There is a rapid response to slow intravenous administration of 20–40 ml of a 40% calcium borogluconate solution given over 30–60 seconds (45–80 kg ewes). Eructation is observed 1–2 minutes after intravenous calcium administration. Characteristically, ewes will stand within five minutes of intravenous injection (**604, 605**), then urinate and wander off to rejoin the rest of the flock.

The response to subcutaneous administration of 60–80 ml of 40% calcium borogluconate solution injected over the thoracic wall behind the shoulder may take up to four hours, especially if the solution had not been warmed to body temperature and was injected at one site.

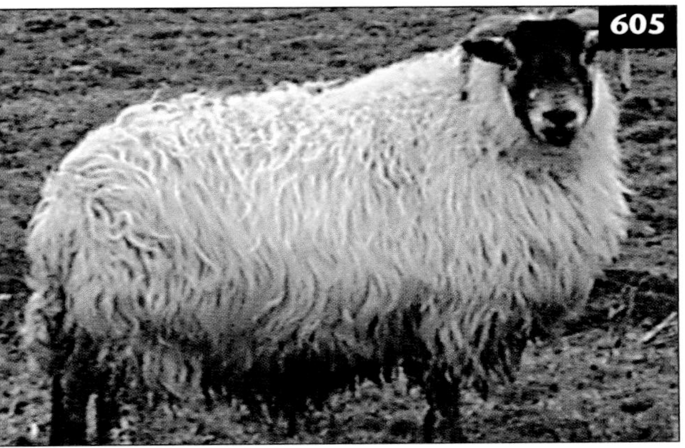

605 Hypocalcaemia. Five minutes after intravenous calcium administration.

Prevention/control measures

Addition of appropriate minerals to the ration during pregnancy and thorough mixing are essential (**606**). Outbreaks of hypocalcaemia occurring over 2–3 days may still result after stressful events such as movement or housing, but these sheep respond promptly to appropriate therapy. At present, sheep rations are not formulated on the basis of cation/anion balance because hypocalcaemia has a sporadic occurrence with excellent treatment response, providing the sheep are treated by a veterinarian.

Economics

Calcium borogluconate is not expensive and one 400 ml bottle is sufficient to treat 5–10 ewes. Incorrect diagnosis will result in death of the ewe. This may total up to 5% of the flock in situations where the condition results from incorrect feed mineralization/ mixing and veterinary attention is not sought.

Welfare implications

Incorrect diagnosis and/or inappropriate treatment will result in unnecessary loss from a disease that should have a 100% treatment response rate. Subcutaneous calcium injection is painful and much less effective than intravenous administration.

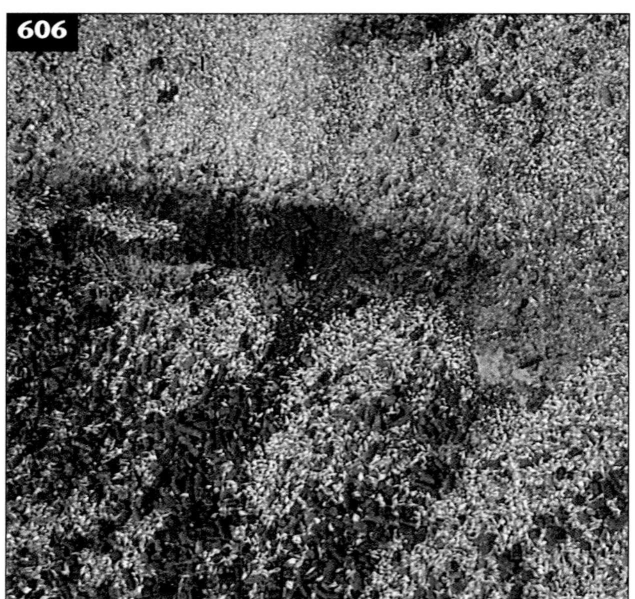

606 Incomplete mixing of mineral mix. Note the minerals in the middle of the pile of rolled barley.

HYPOMAGNESAEMIA

Definition/overview

Hypomagnesaemia is reported as an occasional cause of sudden death in lactating ewes but there are no detailed clinical reports of hypomagnesaemia in sheep. Shepherds' reports of hypomagnesaemia, or 'staggers', usually refer to hypocalcaemia. Sudden death in ewes nursing twins on recently fertilized lush pasture is not sufficient evidence for a diagnosis of hypomagnesaemia unless the postmortem findings are supported by the absence of significant findings of other potential causes of death (e.g. neurological disorders such as listeriosis, PEM, vestibular disease and acute coenurosis) and an aqueous humor or CSF magnesium concentration <0.2 mmol/l.

Aetiology

Hypomagnesaemia has been reported in ewes nursing twin lambs 4–8 weeks after parturition and managed on lush pastures that had received large applications of artificial fertilizers containing high levels of nitrogen and potassium.

Clinical presentation

There are reports of ewes suspected of suffering from hypomagnesaemia being recumbent. They have low serum magnesium and calcium concentrations that do not respond to intravenous calcium alone, but recover following injection of subcutaneous magnesium sulphate.

Other reports detail initial depression but muscle tremors, seizure activity and opisthotonus occur once these sheep are disturbed. Spontaneous horizontal nystagmus, tachycardia and tachypnoea are also reported. Death ensues within 4–6 hours.

Differential diagnoses

Common differential diagnoses for recumbency/seizure activity include:

- Polioencephalomalacia.
- Listeriosis.
- Vestibular disease.

Common differential diagnoses for sudden death in lactating ewes grazing lush pasture include:

- Bloat following lateral or dorsal recumbency.
- Focal symmetrical encephalomalacia (FSE) in unvaccinated stock.
- Pasteurellosis (*Mannheimia haemolytica*).
- Clostridial enterotoxaemia.
- Peracute gangrenous mastitis (*Pasteurella* [*Mannheimia*] species and *Staphylococcus aureus*).

Diagnosis
Careful clinical examination must exclude the common diseases listed under differential diagnoses. Diagnosis of hypomagnesaemia is based on finding a hyperaesthetic, frequently laterally recumbent ewe 4–8 weeks post lambing, grazing lush pasture and with a serum magnesium concentration <0.2 mmol/l.

Treatment
Because making an accurate diagnosis of hypomagnesaemia is difficult, the assessment of treatment protocols is problematic. Twenty to 40 ml of 25% magnesium sulphate should be injected subcutaneously in addition to 40 ml of 40% calcium borogluconate. Unlike in cattle, there are no reports of sedation as part of the treatment protocol for hypomagnesaemia in sheep, and there are no published reports of slow intravenous injection of magnesium/calcium combination products.

Prevention/control measures
Losses from hypomagnesaemia in sheep are very uncommon and no special control measures are undertaken. It is recommended that early season fertilizer applications do not contain potash, thus reducing potassium interference with magnesium absorption.

Economics
Hypomagnesaemia is not an important economic factor in sheep production.

Welfare implications
There are no specific welfare concerns related to hypomagnesaemia, especially with such a low incidence in many countries.

CLINICAL PROBLEM 1

A four-crop Greyface ewe is presented. She had been scanned for triplets and was noted head pressing this morning (**607**). Isolation, inappetence, depression and frequent teeth grinding (bruxism) were noted the previous day. The ewe is afebrile and depressed but hyperaesthetic to tactile and auditory stimuli. There is bilateral lack of menace response (**608**) but the pupillary light reflexes are normal. There are no cranial nerve deficits. Continuous fine muscle fasciculations causing movement of the overlying skin are observed around the muzzle and affecting the ears, with occasional jerking movements of the head. The ewe has a BCS of 2.0.

The ewe is one of a group of 80 cast ewes that are fed *ad libitum* big bale silage plus 0.2 kg/head once daily of a 16% crude protein concentrate. They are due to start lambing in approximately two weeks. Another ewe in the group, which presented with similar clinical signs, died this morning after two days' illness despite antibiotic injection administered by the farmer.

What is a likely diagnosis and what other conditions should be considered?
How would the diagnosis be confirmed?
What treatment(s) should be administered?
What postmortem findings would be expected in the dead ewe?
What advice should be offered?

Differential diagnoses
- Ovine pregnancy toxaemia (twin lamb disease).
- Listeriosis.
- Acidosis resulting from carbohydrate overfeed.

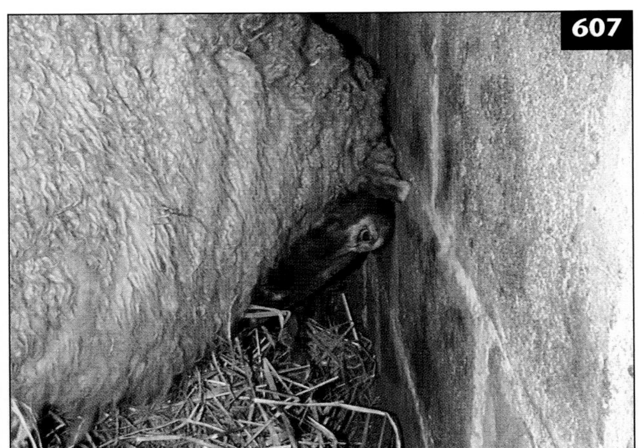

607 Head-pressing in a four-crop Greyface ewe.

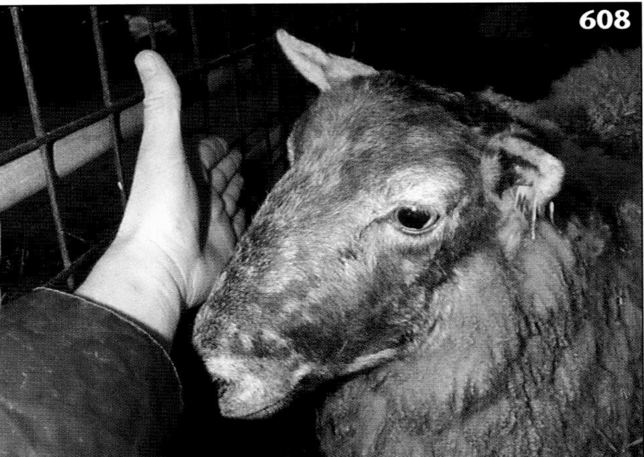

608 Depression and bilateral absence of menace response in the ewe in **607**.

- Early stages of hypocalcaemia.
- Impending abortion.
- Polioencephalomalacia.
- Copper poisoning.

Each of the conditions above can lead to isolation, depression, reduced appetite and/or recumbency during late gestation. Less common conditions to consider could include:
- Acute coenurosis.
- Space-occupying brain lesions such as an abscess.
- Scrapie.

Diagnosis

A presumptive diagnosis of OPT can be made on clinical examination and investigation of current flock management, and this is supported by the finding of a serum 3-OH butyrate concentration >3.0 mmol/l (commonly >5.0 mmol/l). Samples collected from other sheep in the group often show evidence of severe energy underfeeding (concentrations >1.6 mmol/l). Serum 3-OH butyrate concentration is a useful guide to energy supply; however, it must be accompanied by typical clinical signs to constitute a diagnosis of OPT because occasionally, clinically normal ewes that do not develop OPT may present with a serum 3-OH butyrate concentration >3.0 mmol/l during late pregnancy. Plasma glucose and non-esterified fatty acid (NEFA) concentrations are too variable in cases of OPT to confirm the presumptive clinical diagnosis. For example, plasma glucose concentrations can be elevated in the agonal stage of OPT.

Treatment

The ewe was treated with a concentrated oral electrolyte and dextrose solution three times daily (as an alternative one could use propylene glycol) and a multivitamin injection given intravenously. The ewe deteriorated over the next day and the decision was taken to attempt to abort the ewe with dexamethasone (16 mg i/m). Usually, dexamethasone only results in abortion in ewes that are more than 136 days pregnant. Abortion as a consequence of OPT is uncommon. The ewe produced three lambs 24 hours after injection with dexamethasone but only one lamb was viable. The ewe made a slow recovery (**609**). Wool-slip commonly occurs some weeks after the period of illness, presumably because of the high dose corticosteroid injection in addition to the period of debility. An alternative strategy would involve treatment with a long-acting corticosteroid at first presentation, which might result in clinical improvement in some cases without causing abortion.

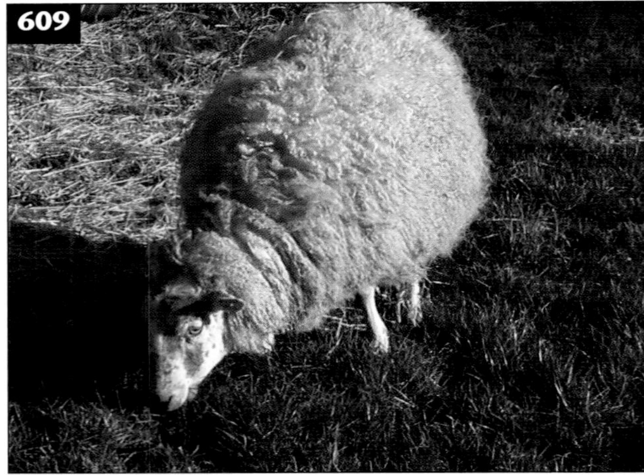

609 Turnout to pasture with improved appetite of ewe with suspected OPT after premature birth of her lambs.

Advice

Correct nutrition during gestation is essential for multigravid ewes that are at most risk from energy deficiency due to high fetal demands. Routine monitoring of late gestation nutrition 4–6 weeks before lambing by sampling 6–10 ewes for 3-OH butyrate concentration is the cornerstone of flock preventive medicine programmes. The mean serum 3-OH butyrate concentration of ten ewes sampled at random on this farm was 1.5 mmol/l. This necessitated an extra 4 MJ ME/day(0.3 kg of concentrates) fed as an extra feed to return the ewes to a satisfactory level of energy supply[1]. Such appropriate late gestation ewe nutrition ensures high birth weight lambs and sufficient colostrum accumulation in the udder, thereby reducing neonatal losses. Access to molasses during late gestation may help to provide an additional palatable source of energy to ewes.

CLINICAL PROBLEM 2

A five-crop Greyface ewe is presented that is due to lamb in one week and has been scanned for twin lambs. The ewe is at pasture with 60 other sheep. They are being fed 1 kg of 18% crude protein concentrate per head per day plus access to poor quality hay. The ewes have been brought into the lambing field for closer supervision.

Clinical findings

On presentation the ewe's head is on the ground and she does not respond to the veterinarian's approach (**610**). The ewe appears very depressed and weak. The menace

610 Depressed weak ewe with reduced menace response but no cranial nerve deficits.

611 The ewe stood within five minutes of intravenous calcium injection.

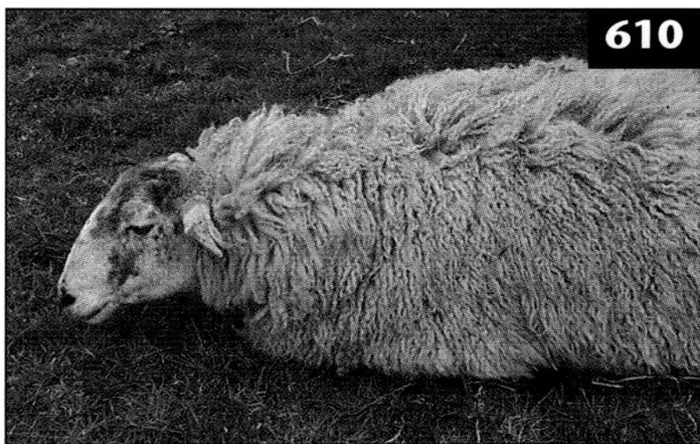

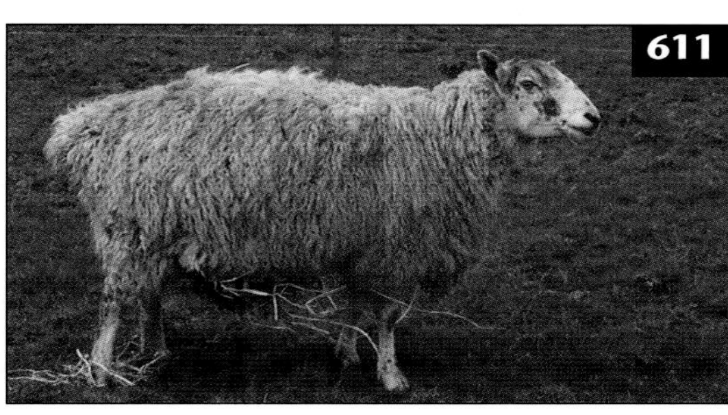

response is present but slow. There are no cranial nerve deficits but the ewe drools saliva continuously. The rectal temperature is 39.5°C. The rectum is flaccid and contains a ball of pelleted faeces. The mucous membranes appear normal. The heart rate is 60 bpm and the respiratory rate 18 breaths per minute. No abnormal sounds can be detected during auscultation of the chest. There is reduced rumen fill and reduced ruminal movement with mainly gaseous sounds. There is no mastitis and no vulval discharge or swelling.

What conditions should be considered?
What is a possible provisional diagnosis?

Differential diagnoses

- Hypocalcaemia.
- Ovine pregnancy toxaemia.
- Mastitis.
- Acidosis resulting from carbohydrate overfeed.
- Impending abortion.
- Copper poisoning.

Diagnosis

The provisional diagnosis of hypocalcaemia was proven correct after the rapid response to slow intravenous administration of 40 ml of a 40% calcium borogluconate solution. Eructation was observed during the administration of the calcium. Characteristically, the ewe stood within five minutes of the injection, urinated and rejoined her flock mates (**611**).

Laboratory diagnosis of hypocalcaemia

In sheep recumbent due to hypocalcaemia, serum calcium concentrations are <1.4 mmol/l. Hypocalcaemia is not uncommon in three-crop or older ewes maintained at pasture during late gestation but it can also occur sporadically during early lactation. Hypocalcaemia should always be considered in ewes that show depression/recumbency during late gestation and early lactation. No ewe should die without first being given the benefit of treatment with calcium borogluconate.

TRACE ELEMENT DEFICIENCIES

Introduction

The clinical signs associated with trace element deficiency in sheep are often insidious in onset and usually present as poorly thriven lambs during late summer/early autumn with few specific clinical features. There is considerable interplay between chronic parasitism, malnutrition and trace element deficiencies to the extent that it may not be possible, or desirable, to ascertain which is the most important condition. While veterinarians will have some knowledge of their clients' sheep farming enterprise, the problem of diagnosing trace element deficiency is often further compounded when purchased sheep are presented as ill thriven.

The trace element deficiency states generally considered are: cobalt, copper, vitamin E and selenium, and iodine, although in certain areas of the world manganese, iron and zinc may be limiting elements.

Vitamin B_1 (thiamine) deficiency may occur under certain circumstances and is detailed in Chapter 7 (Polioencephalomalacia, p. 174).

COBALT DEFICIENCY

Definition/overview

Cobalt deficiency ('pine') occurs in many counties worldwide where there are low soil concentrations. This may be further complicated by dietary factors and parasitic gastroenteritis, which may interfere with absorption of vitamin B_{12}.

Aetiology
Cobalt has its only biological role as a constituent of vitamin B_{12}, which is manufactured by rumen microflora.

Clinical presentation
Clinical signs of cobalt deficiency are most commonly observed in grazing lambs after weaning. Signs are non-specific and include lethargy, poor appetite, poor quality wool with an open fleece, small size and very poor body condition despite adequate nutrition, and epiphora with staining of the cheeks. Pale mucous membranes, especially of the conjunctivae, develop late in the deficiency state, possibly due to the four months' lifespan of erythrocytes.

Ovine white liver syndrome has been described in grazing lambs in many countries and is attributed to cobalt deficiency. In extreme cases a secondary hepatic encephalopathy develops, with a variety of neurological signs including depression extending to stupor, head pressing and aimless wandering.

It is reported that cobalt-deficient sheep suffer from a non-specific immunosuppression and are more susceptible to infectious diseases, including the clostridial diseases and pasteurellosis.

Cobalt deficiency is less common in adults but is reported to cause reduced fertility and poor mothering ability, but these signs may be related to a more generalized poor body condition.

Differential diagnoses
Diagnosis is often compounded by the fact that lambs may have been recently treated with an anthelmintic and moved on to better pasture immediately before veterinary examination. The main differential diagnoses for cobalt deficiency are conditions that affect a large proportion of the lamb crop and include:

- Poor ewe nutrition/overstocked pasture means that lambs do not have a good start to life.
- Poor grazing/overstocked pasture after weaning.
- Coccidiosis and/or severe nematodirosis can cause a serious growth check, often around 6–8 weeks old, with protracted convalescence.
- Parasitic gastroenteritis is a very common cause of poor lamb growth. There are resistant nematode species, especially to the benzimadazole anthelmintics (Group 1 BZ), in many countries worldwide. A faecal egg reduction test may be indicated to discount a nematode problem despite recent anthelmintic treatment.

Cases of ovine white liver disease showing neurological signs should be distinguished from coenurosis, polioencephalomalacia, sulphur toxicity and focal symmetrical encephalomalacia.

Diagnosis
Diagnosis is based on clinical signs in areas with known cobalt-deficient soils, supported by low plasma and/or liver vitamin B_{12} concentrations. As a general guide, a growth response is expected when the mean plasma vitamin B_{12} concentration falls to <500 pmol/l, and is likely to be significant at <250 pmol/l. A minimum of ten blood samples is recommended to determine the mean plasma vitamin B_{12} concentration but this number is likely to be limited by cost considerations in small flocks. The blood samples must be collected as soon as possible after the sheep have been gathered, as values increase significantly during confinement. Liver vitamin B_{12} concentration can be determined following collection by biopsy, which, while recommended by certain authors, is not regularly undertaken in general practice. A growth response is expected in sheep with a mean liver vitamin B_{12} concentration <280 nmol/kg net weight; concentrations between 280 nmol/kg and 375 nmol/kg are considered marginal.

Perhaps the best, and most cost-effective, method for determining any growth retardation resulting from cobalt deficiency is to undertake a supplementation trial over 8–10 weeks and compare supplemented and control lambs' performance. Typically, a 4–6 kg improvement in growth rate over controls would be expected over 8–10 weeks of supplementation. Where cobalt deficiency is suspected, 10–12 lambs could be left untreated until such time as a demonstrable difference can be appreciated, thus reducing the impact of leaving some lambs unsupplemented.

Methylmalonic acid (MMA) accumulates in plasma in cobalt deficiency and has been used as a diagnostic tool; concentrations higher than 5 μmol/l are considered abnormal.

PCV can readily be determined in the practice laboratory by microhaematocrit, but anaemia may also result from infestations such as haemonchosis and chronic fasciolosis, and in association with many chronic bacterial infections.

Gross postmortem examination is non-specific, revealing an emaciated carcase with serous atrophy of fat. There is bone marrow hypoplasia. In severe cases of cobalt deficiency the liver is enlarged, pale and friable.

Treatment

Treatment is more quickly effected by a combination of intramuscular vitamin B_{12} and drenching with cobalt sulphate (up to 1 mg/kg body weight) than by oral supplementation alone. Thereafter, monthly drenching with cobalt sulphate, often in combination with an anthelmintic preparation, should ensure live weight gain.

Prevention/control measures

Oral cobalt supplementation is very cheap and, with many anthelmintics belonging to Group 1-BZ and Group 2-LM, the cobalt supplement can be added to the drench. Monthly dosing from around three months old with proprietary cobalt-supplemented anthelmintic drench should supply sufficient cobalt to growing lambs in most situations.

Cobalt oxide-containing boluses, which lodge in the reticulum, provide a continuous supply of cobalt but are expensive in those lambs that require a short supplementation period of only 2–3 months.

Soluble glass boluses containing cobalt, selenium and copper are available in some countries but are a very expensive means of supplying cobalt and are only indicated in situations where all three deficiency conditions are considered to exert a negative influence on health.

Economics

Oral cobalt supplementation is very cheap. Labour costs are the major factor in drenching sheep. Conversely, soluble glass boluses containing cobalt, selenium and copper cost 3.5% of the sale value of a lamb, with considerable care required for administration *per os*. The high cost of cobalt-containing fertilizers has curtailed their use as a means of increasing soil and herbage cobalt content.

Welfare implications

Welfare problems arise from reduced growth rate and poor fleece quality, with consequent increased exposure to the effects of adverse winter weather. These welfare concerns are unacceptable considering the negligible costs of oral cobalt supplementation.

COPPER DEFICIENCY

Definition/overview

Copper deficiency is common where sheep graze pasture in certain geographic areas, often as a consequence of antagonists present in the soil, such as iron, molybdenum and sulphur, and management practices, such as lime application, which increase soil pH. The clinical manifestation of copper deficiency varies worldwide, with swayback more common in the UK, poor wool quality and anaemia in Australia and osteoporosis in New Zealand.

As well as being susceptible to copper deficiency, sheep are also prone to copper accumulation and toxicity. There is considerable breed variation with respect to copper absorption and, therefore, to copper deficiency and toxicity.

Aetiology

Copper forms an integral part of numerous enzyme systems in the body.

Clinical presentation

Copper deficiency during mid-gestation may lead to swayback (Chapter 7, p. 170).

In growing lambs, copper deficiency may result in a poor fleece without its natural ‘crimp’, which has been described as ‘steely wool’. Other reports describe poor live weight gain, anaemia and increased susceptibility to bacterial infections.

Osteoporosis leading to long bone fractures, often during handling procedures, has been reported in New Zealand as a result of copper deficiency.

Differential diagnoses

The differential diagnoses of swayback are described in Chapter 7 (p. 170). Long bone fractures occur sporadically in growing lambs during handling procedures in poorly designed facilities.

Diagnosis

Swayback is provisionally diagnosed on clinical examination and confirmed following histopathological examination of the CNS.

Copper deficiency is most reliably diagnosed in growing lambs based on a dose/response study but this is rarely practicable under most farm conditions and farmers are generally reluctant to leave some sheep unsupplemented.

In situations where copper absorption is inadequate, depletion of liver reserves occurs first followed by depletion at non-essential sites; clinical disease follows depletion at essential sites. In a deficiency situation, copper stores are mobilized from the liver to maintain plasma concentrations; low plasma concentration therefore indicates depletion of liver reserves. Plasma samples are most commonly submitted for analysis, with concentrations <9.4 mol/l considered to be indicatative of depletion of liver reserves, but this may not yet have exerted an adverse effect on growth. It is reported that hypocuprosis does not limit lamb performance until plasma concentrations fall to <3 mol/l. The copper-dependent enzyme superoxide dismutase declines more slowly in a copper deficit situation; therefore, low concentrations are considered more likely to reflect negative influences on health and growth (normal concentrations >0.4 and >0.3 U/ml haemoglobin for lambs and adult sheep, respectively).

Liver copper concentrations <157 µmol/kg dry matter (DM) are considered to indicate exhaustion of liver reserves, although biopsy specimens are rarely taken. The liver can be readily imaged using trans-abdominal ultrasonography, which may assist biopsy.

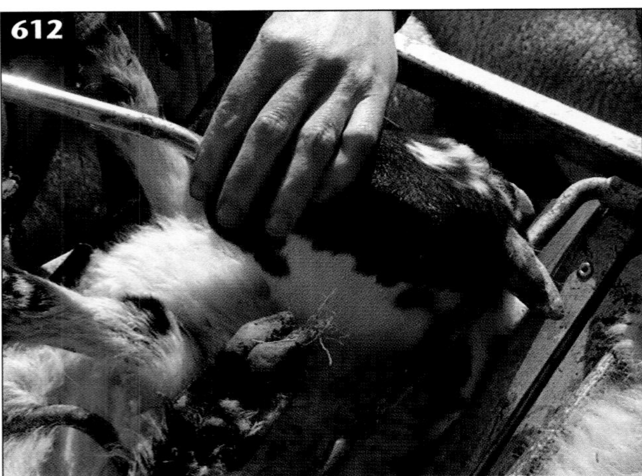

612 Copper supplementation can be effected with copper oxide needles administered orally.

Treatment

Treatment of delayed swayback is described in Chapter 7 (p. 171).

Prevention/control measures

Prevention of copper deficiency in growing lambs is much more important than treatment, because irreversible changes have often taken place in the fleece and full compensatory growth may not result after supplementation. Furthermore, treatment of swayback is hopeless and emphasis must be placed on preventive measures.

While copper deficiency is often a perennial problem on certain farms, farmers must always be made aware of the risks of copper toxicity. Therefore, the timing and type of copper supplementation should be specified in the veterinary flock plan, with specific notes made regarding no other source of extra copper. Sheep must not be given a copper supplement prior to, or during, housing. Toxicity could result from a number of sources, including using more than one method of copper supplementation and the use of feeds with high copper content; typically, such feeds are by-products. Change of sheep breed may result in an incident of copper poisoning because certain breeds are particularly susceptible to copper toxicity (e.g. if the same supplementation method is used, but Texel lambs are purchased one year rather than the usual Scottish Blackface lambs).

Copper is usually given by injection as copper heptonate; copper salts such as calcium copper edetate and cuproxiline are rapidly absorbed from the site of injection and may be toxic to sheep. Certain copper injections are irritant and may cause a large local reaction. Care must be exercised that the injection is given correctly because abscessation, and in some cases tracking of infection to the cervical spinal canal, have been observed after incorrect injection technique.

Supplementation can be effected with copper oxide needles administered orally in a gelatin capsule (0.1 g copper oxide per kg live weight) (**612**). Sheep should not be re-treated for 12 months unless signs of copper deficiency recur.

Appropriate supplementation of ewes during mid-gestation will prevent the development of swayback in their progeny. Weather conditions, in particular snow cover, determines a low risk year in the UK because of reduced intake of inhibitor substances from the soil. Solutions containing copper, administered twice during late gestation to prevent swayback, have been largely replaced by other forms of supplementation so as to reduce handling requirements during late gestation.

The contribution of copper-containing fertilizers is dependent on soil type and is too variable in most practical situations.

Economics

Copper supplementation costs between 0.4% and 0.6% of the value of a ewe for injectable preparations and gelatin capsules containing copper oxide needles.

Welfare implications

Poor fleece quality could lead to increased susceptibility to adverse weather in hill sheep. Predation and death of delayed swayback lambs may occur in extensive management systems.

SELENIUM AND VITAMIN E DEFICIENCY

(*Syns*: white muscle disease, nutritional muscular dystrophy, stiff lamb disease)

Definition/overview

Selenium deficiency occurs in soils of certain geographic areas worldwide, leading to a pasture/crop deficiency. Vitamin E concentrations are high in green crops but fall rapidly under drought conditions. Certain root crops are known to be low in both selenium and vitamin E. Feeding grain treated with propionic acid may increase the risk of white muscle disease.

White muscle disease occurs in the UK, with recognized risk factors such as feeding home-grown cereals and root crops, and incorrectly mineralized rations; however, the disease prevalence is generally low. It is reported that 20–30% of the flock can be affected with white muscle disease in certain areas of New Zealand, where low selenium concentrations in the soil results in low selenium concentrations in plants.

Resistance to bacterial pathogens is reported to be lower in selenium-deficient animals and they show increased disease levels.

Aetiology

Selenium and vitamin E act as cellular antioxidants, protecting cells against free radicals and lipid peroxides. These, if unchecked, cause membrane damage and tissue necrosis. Skeletal, cardiac and respiratory muscle cells and blood cells are especially susceptible to oxidative stress, and selenium and vitamin E deficiency may lead to disease of these body systems.

Clinical presentation

Congenital white muscle disease has been reported in lambs that are stillborn or die soon after birth, often from starvation.

In the UK, white muscle disease typically affects rapidly growing 2–6-week-old lambs, often ram lambs of meat breeds such as the Suffolk and Texel. There is sudden-onset stiffness, with affected lambs reluctant to move such that they are easily caught while others in the group gallop around. Affected lambs are bright, alert and suck well but have a painful expression with the head held lowered. After one or two days, affected lambs are unable to rise and remain in sternal recumbency (**613**), with the ewe searching out the lamb at feeding times rather than *vice versa*. During the early stages the major skeletal muscle groups may be swollen and they are painful under digital pressure. Stress factors such as recent handling or turnout to pasture may precipitate white muscle disease. It is reported that older lambs may suffer respiratory distress, which is often accompanied by secondary pneumonia.

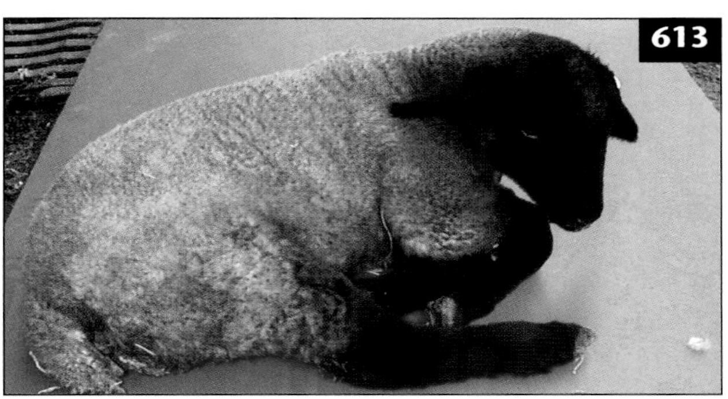

613 Recumbent five-week-old Suffolk ram lamb suffering from white muscle disease.

Selenium-responsive ill thrift in growing lambs has been reported in certain geographic areas of Australia and New Zealand, where dramatic improvements have resulted after supplementation.

Early embryonic loss/failure to implant has been attributed to selenium deficiency. In ewes, an increased lamb crop with fewer barren ewes has been reported after selenium supplementation before the mating period but these responses were highly variable.

Differential diagnoses

- The main differential diagnosis (in the UK) for stiffness leading to recumbency is bacterial polyarthritis, particularly *S. dysgalactiae* affecting the atlanto-occipital joint.
- Erysipelas polyarthritis is common in this age group of lambs but presents with obvious lameness.
- Vertebral empyema of a cervical vertebra will cause recumbency but is uncommon in lambs less than four weeks old.
- Chronic debilitating infections may result in weakness and eventual recumbency but these signs contrast with the previous rapid growth and excellent condition of lambs before they show signs of white muscle disease.
- There are many causes of ill thrift in groups of growing lambs including cobalt deficiency, poor pasture management and parasitic gastroenteritis.
- Likewise there are many causes of returns to service including infertile rams (ewes returning at 17 day intervals) and toxoplasmosis and border disease (ewes returning at intervals greater than 17 days).

Diagnosis
Histopathological examination of myocardium is often necessary to detect the congenital form of white muscle disease.

A provisional diagnosis of white muscle disease in young lambs is based on clinical signs in rapidly growing healthy lambs, with the presence of some of the risk factors listed above. The serum creatine kinase concentration is massively increased during the acute phase of disease, typically to 10,000–20,000 U/l but it can be as high as 100,000 U/l (normal = <500 U/l). White striations may be visible in the gluteal and psoas muscles during gross postmortem examination.

Most laboratories measure glutathione peroxidase as the indicator of selenium status. Ewes with concentrations <20 U/l packed RBCs assayed at 30°C are deemed to be at increased risk, although reference ranges may vary between laboratories. With respect to vitamin E, plasma α-tocopherol concentrations <1 μmol/l are regarded as carrying increased risk of disease even if the selenium status is normal (as determined by glutathione peroxidase concentration).

Soil analysis can be undertaken; however, it is more usual to determine selenium concentrations in tissues such as liver (tissue samples collected by biopsy) or kidney. There is little variation between animals, and 3–5 samples afford an accurate assessment of selenium status.

Treatment
Young lambs should be treated with selenium (as potassium selenate) (0.75–1.5 mg i/m or s/c) and vitamin E (dl α-tocopherol acetate) (34–68 mg i/m or s/c). This results in return to full mobility within 2–3 days.

Prevention/control measures
It is generally accepted that free access licks/minerals are unreliable because of highly variable intakes.

As white muscle disease is seen most commonly in young lambs, prevention can be achieved either by correct supplementation of the dam's ration during late gestation or injection of all newborn lambs with a selenium and vitamin E preparation. The presence of feeds that increase the likelihood of white muscle disease (e.g. root crops, weathered hay and propionic acid-treated grain) necessitates higher levels of dietary supplementation.

Supplementation of growing lambs is best achieved by drenching, often in combination with anthelmintic treatment. This provides adequate selenium for 1–3 months. The standard inclusion in an anthelmintic preparation is 0.4 mg/ml of elemental selenium, with the anthelmintic combination product given at 1 ml per 5 kg body weight. Great care must be exercised when formulating a supplementation programme because selenium toxicity can occur following overdosage, especially in young lambs. The preparation must be shaken vigorously prior to use to ensure thorough mixing. In breeding sheep, selenium supplementation via drenching with sodium selenate is given 1–2 months before the start of the breeding season.

Intraruminal glass boluses are a very expensive means of supplementing with selenium but they are useful where other trace element deficiency states occur concurrently.

Top dressing using slow-release selenium prills (0.5 kg per hectare annually), as used in New Zealand, is an economical means of selenium supplementation.

Economics
Selenium supply via regular anthelmintic drenching (often monthly) is a cheap and reliable means of supplementation for growing lambs but not all anthelmintic preparations are suitable for combined drenching. This latter point must be stressed to farmers who follow an annual rotation between the three anthelmintic groups.

In the absence of a split flock trial, it is very difficult to calculate the cost benefit of selenium supplementation with respect to reproductive wastage. If doubts exist regarding poor reproductive performance, ewes should be drenched at regular intervals prior to mating. The low cost of selenium supplementation may result in more flocks receiving selenium preparations than is necessary, rather than the converse situation.

Welfare implications
White muscle disease is a painful condition that can be readily prevented by correct dietary management/dam supplementation. Ill thriven lambs often present as pitiful individuals with increased exposure to adverse weather due to a poor fleece.

IODINE DEFICIENCY

Definition/overview
Iodine deficiency can arise from a primary lack in the soil or, more commonly, secondarily to the action of goitrogens in leguminous crops, which interfere with iodine metabolism. In New Zealand, feeding brassicas for long periods during pregnancy is related to iodine deficiency and manifests as poor survival of newborn lambs, especially during unfavourable weather conditions. The prevalence and severity of iodine deficiency may vary between years because of differing

grazing and management conditions. Clinical signs are more severe in the Merino than in other breeds.

Iodine is used in the synthesis of the thyroid hormones thyroxine (T4) and tri-iodothyronine (T3).

Clinical presentation

Iodine deficiency may be related to poor embryo survival. Iodine deficiency during pregnancy typically results in late abortion or the birth of weakly lambs with markedly swollen thyroid glands (goitre). In severe cases lambs are born with little fleece, rendering them highly susceptible to hypothermia. Goitre is also recognized in adult sheep associated with goitrogen intake from fodder.

Differential diagnoses

There are many causes of perinatal lamb mortality in extensively managed sheep. Determination of thyroid gland to live weight ratio would be only part of the lamb necropsy investigation.

Diagnosis

Diagnosis of iodine deficiency during pregnancy can be attempted by determining thyroid gland weight from a minimum of 15 lambs, with deficiency indicated by thyroid gland weights >0.4 g/kg live weight. Histopathology can also be performed on the thyroid glands. Determination of plasma thyroid hormone concentration prior to, and during, pregnancy is an unreliable guide to reproductive performance and the appearance of goitre in lambs.

Treatment

Clinical goitre has been successfully treated with oral potassium iodide (20 mg per lamb).

Prevention/control measures

Ewes can be supplemented prior to mating with an intramuscular injection of iodized oil, which is claimed to last for two years. Alternatively, ewes can be drenched twice during pregnancy with potassium iodide.

Economics

It may prove difficult to determine the true cost of iodine deficiency in commercial flocks because losses vary from one year to another depending on nutrition during gestation. A split flock supplementation study offers the most accurate and practical means of determining the real costs of iodine deficiency.

Welfare implications

Increased perinatal mortality has an obvious welfare cost.

COPPER TOXICITY

Definition/overview

Chronic copper toxicity is common in intensively managed sheep. The prognosis is grave once signs of jaundice appear in sheep.

Aetiology

Acute poisoning may occur after accidental overdose with excessive quantities of soluble copper salts when treating suspected deficiency states with drenches or certain injectable preparations.

Chronic copper toxicity results from ingestion of relatively high levels of copper over a prolonged period; the term 'relatively high levels' is important, as dietary factors such as molybdenum and sulphur exert considerable influences on copper availability. During periods of high copper intake, liver copper storage increases until critical levels are exceeded. This results in a sudden massive release of copper into the circulation, causing lipid peroxidation and intravascular haemolysis. This haemolytic crisis may be precipitated by numerous stressors including advancing pregnancy, adverse weather, transportation, housing and sudden reduction in feeding, which may occur during winter storms. The precipitation of chronic copper toxicity may occur some days to weeks after removal of the copper source from the ration.

AST concentrations are markedly raised for several days to weeks before the haemolytic crisis, with values commonly >400 U/l (normal = 45–134 U/l).

There is a wide variation in susceptibility to copper toxicity; UK native breeds, such as the North Ronaldsay (**614**) and Soay, and the Texel are especially prone whilst Scottish Blackface sheep are much less so when fed equivalent rations.

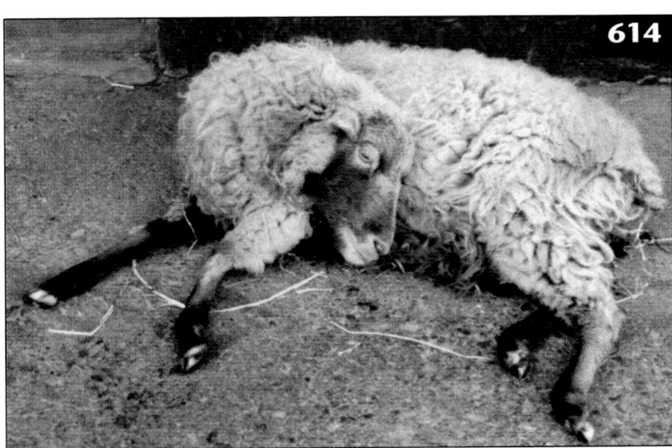

614 Moribund North Ronaldsay ewe suffering from chronic copper toxicity.

Hepatogenous copper toxicity, which occurs after the liver has been damaged by plant toxins causing an increased avidity for copper, is uncommon in sheep.

Clinical presentation

Acute copper toxicity causes severe gastroenteritis with colic signs, diarrhoea and rapid dehydration. Affected sheep are very depressed and anorexic and death usually ensues within three days. Haemolysis and haemoglobinuria may be seen if the sheep survives this peracute phase.

In cases of chronic copper toxicity the appearance of clinical signs is associated with the haemolytic crisis, which may be precipitated by the variety of stressors listed above. Affected sheep are weak, very dull and depressed and are separate from others in the group, and the rectal temperature is normal to slightly increased (<40.2°C). They have a poor appetite and often a fetid diarrhoea with considerable mucus present in the faeces. There is evidence of dehydration and obvious jaundice of mucous membranes, most noticeably affecting the conjunctivae (**615**). The heart and respiratory rates are increased, and an increased abdominal effort may be noted. There is no ruminal activity. The urine is dark red due to the presence of haemoglobin. Affected animals have a grave prognosis despite specific treatment with ammonium tetrathiomolybdate and supportive therapy; careful consideration must be given to humane destruction of sheep with these clinical signs.

Differential diagnoses

Differential diagnoses of sudden onset depression, weakness and anorexia may include:

- Pneumonic pasteurellosis.
- Acute fasciolosis.
- Clostridial diseases such as blackleg and bighead.
- Urolithiasis in rams.
- Ovine pregnancy toxaemia in ewes.

Diagnosis

Diagnosis is based on history, with a source of excess copper, and on clinical findings of jaundice in chronic toxicity. The diagnosis is supported by laboratory findings of a massively increased serum AST concentration, commonly >1,000 U/l and a serum GGT concentration more than ten times normal (normal = 0–44 U/l). The serum total bilirubin concentration is greatly increased (more than ten times normal). There is evidence of anaemia, which worsens during the haemolytic crisis, with PCV values falling as low as 0.10 l/l. RBCs typically show anisocytosis, and very large numbers of normoblasts are observed in blood smears. Surprisingly, serum copper concentrations measured during the haemolytic crisis are frequently only marginally increased and prove of little diagnostic significance.

Necropsy findings

Acute copper poisoning produces severe gastroenteritis with erosion of the abomasal mucosa. In chronic copper toxicity there is jaundice of the carcase, most noticeable in the omentum. The kidneys are swollen and dark grey, and there is dark red urine in the bladder. The liver is enlarged and friable (**616**). The spleen is enlarged and appears dark brown/black on cut section.

Kidney copper concentrations are massively elevated, often exceeding 3,000 μmol/kg DM (normal = <314 μmol/kg DM). Liver copper concentrations are usually also elevated but such determinations are not as reliable as kidney copper determination.

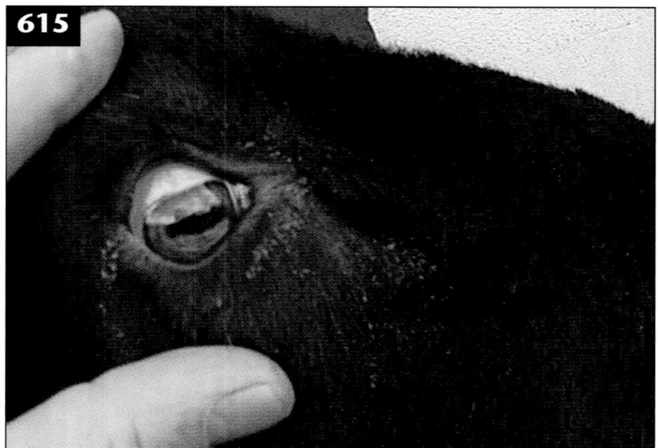

615 Obvious jaundice of the conjunctivae in a Suffolk ram suffering from chronic copper toxicity.

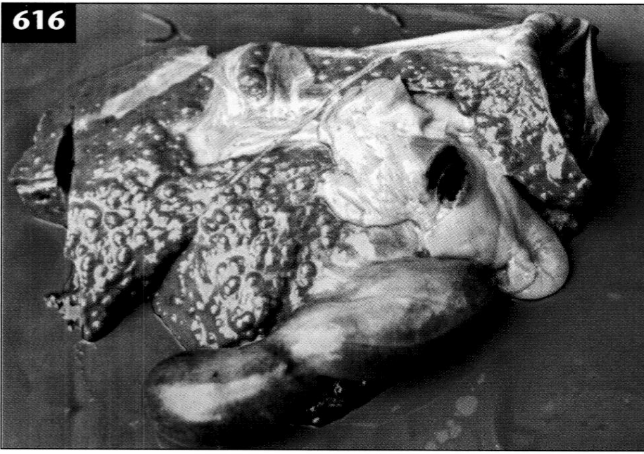

616 The liver is enlarged and friable in chronic copper toxicity.

Treatment

The suspected copper source must be removed immediately but this has often already taken place before clinical signs of illness are first noted. Treatment of severely affected sheep is rarely successful and euthanasia for welfare reasons should be carefully considered. The best results are achieved by selecting the sheep most at risk by determining serum AST concentrations and treating these animals with ammonium tetrathiomolybdate (either 1.7 mg/kg i/v or 3.4 mg/kg s/c on 2–3 occasions 2 days apart). Alternatively, all at-risk sheep can be treated using this regimen but this can prove very expensive.

There is no ammonium tetrathiomolybdate preparation licensed for use in food-producing animals and its use in suspected cases of chronic copper toxicity is poorly defined from a regulatory standpoint. A meat withdrawal period of at least six months has been recommended, thus preventing its use in fattening lambs.

Treatment of sick individuals should be carefully monitored and failure to observe improvement by the second ammonium tetrathiomolybdate treatment indicates a grave prognosis.

Renal failure often develops in animals that survive the initial acute haemolytic crisis and monitoring BUN and creatinine concentrations is strongly recommended. BUN and creatinine concentrations more than five times normal indicate a hopeless prognosis and euthanasia is indicated. Concentrations of BUN and creatinine more than 10–20 times normal are not uncommon during the agonal stages.

Prevention/control measures

Copper supplementation must be carefully considered and the reader is directed to the section detailing management and prevention of copper deficiency (p. 290).

Copper toxicity may arise following feeding cattle feed to sheep. This situation is more common in hobby farmers with small numbers of sheep.

Incorrect mineral supplementation of proprietary concentrates may occur. However, in the UK, copper concentrations are strictly regulated to levels

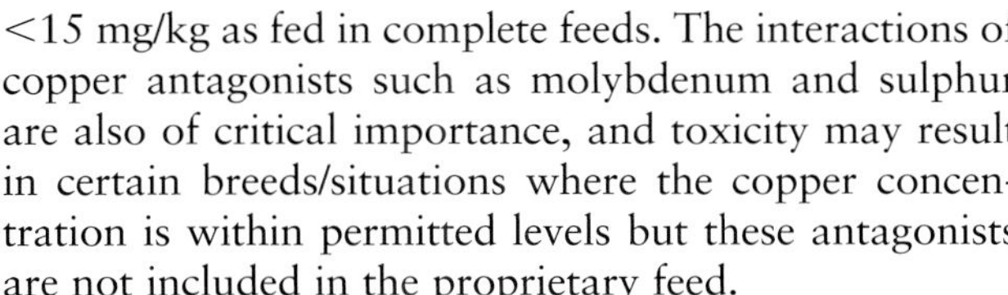

<15 mg/kg as fed in complete feeds. The interactions of copper antagonists such as molybdenum and sulphur are also of critical importance, and toxicity may result in certain breeds/situations where the copper concentration is within permitted levels but these antagonists are not included in the proprietary feed.

Economics

An outbreak of copper toxicity rarely results in the death of more than 5% of the sheep at risk provided the source of copper is removed immediately. The longer-term consequences of copper toxicity, defined as those sheep with elevated serum AST concentrations that are not treated with ammonium tetrathiomolybdate, are much more difficult to quantify. It is claimed that nursing ewes do not lactate well, with resultant poor lamb growth rates, although there are no specific data.

Welfare implications

The welfare of sheep showing severe depression and jaundice is of particular concern. Euthanasia is indicated if there is no improvement after treatment with ammonium tetrathiomolybdate.

CLINICAL PROBLEM

A yearling Suffolk ram is presented in good condition (BCS 3.5) with a two-day history of profound depression (**617**) and inappetence. Prior to veterinary examination the ram had been injected intramuscularly with procaine penicillin for two consecutive days without improvement. The ram has been housed with 20 others and fed 2.5 kg of concentrates daily for the past seven months but had been turned out to pasture one week ago.

Clinical examination

The ram is profoundly dull and depressed with a gaunt appearance. The ram appears weak and stands with its head held lowered. The rectal temperature is 40.2°C. The mucous membranes are yellow (**618**). The eyes

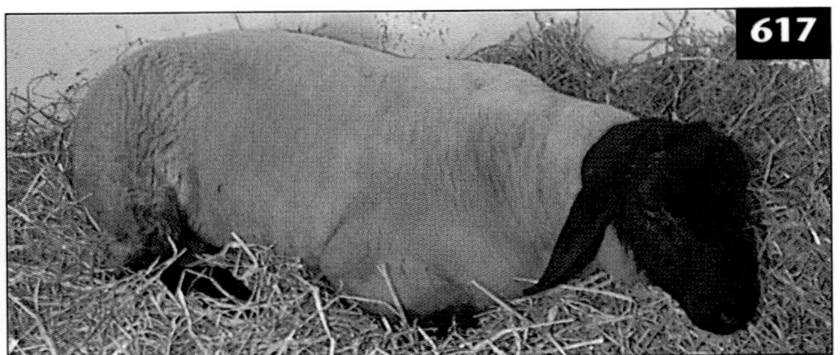

617 Depressed Suffolk ram.

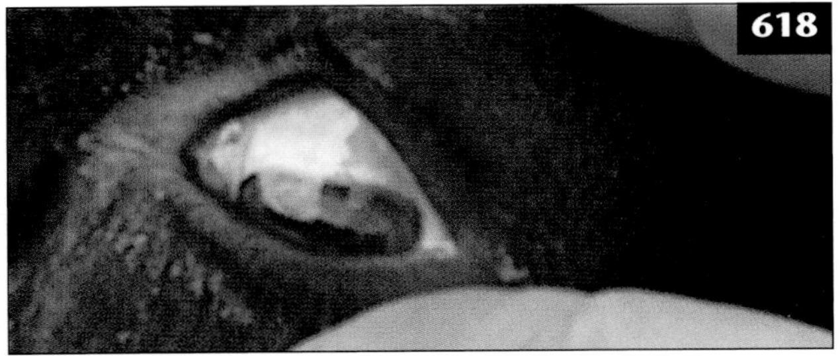

618 Jaundiced ocular mucous membranes.

appear slightly sunken and the skin tent is increased consistent with moderate dehydration. The heart rate is increased to 100 bpm and the respiratory rate to 30 breaths per minute. No abnormal lung sounds are detected. No rumen movements are audible and the abdominal fill is greatly reduced. The ram shows occasional tenesmus with the passage of fetid melaenic faeces, which contain considerable mucus. A free flow of dark red urine is voided.

What conditions should be considered?
What tests should be undertaken?
What treatments should be recommended?

Differential diagnoses

- Chronic copper toxicity.
- Urolithiasis.
- Pneumonic pasteurellosis.
- Pyelonephritis.
- Abdominal catastrophe such as redgut.
- Nitrate poisoning.

Further examination

Ultrasonographic examination of the bladder, caudal abdomen and right kidney are undertaken in the standing animal using a 5.0 MHz sector scanner. There is no increased peritoneal fluid and the bladder is of normal diameter (4 cm), appearing as an anechoic (black) area bordered by a bright hyperechoic (white) line at the pelvic inlet. The kidney appears normal.

Haematological examination reveals a mild anaemia (PCV 0.16 l/l [normal = 0.26–0.36 l/l]; total RBC count 4.6 × 10^{12}/l [normal = 5–9 × 10^{12}/l]; Hb 68 g/l [normal = 80–140 g/dl]). The RBCs show anisocytosis. Normoblasts comprise 33% of the WBCs (total count 13.0 × 10^{9}/l [normal = 4–10 × 10^{9}/l]).

The serum copper concentration is 22.3 μmol/l (normal = 9.4–18.8 μmol/l). The total bilirubin concentration is 45.9 mol/l (normal = $<$6.8 mol/l). The serum AST concentration is 950 U/l (normal = 45–134 U/l) and the GGT concentration is 140 U/l (normal = 0–44 U/l).

Diagnosis

The laboratory results of liver damage and anaemia indirectly support a provisional diagnosis of copper toxicity. The serum copper concentration is not significantly elevated.

Treatment

The ram was treated with ammonium tetrathiomolybdate (1.7 mg/kg i/v twice with a two-day interval).

Progress of case

The ram ate a small amount of concentrates but remained dull and depressed. Further blood samples were taken the day following the second ammonium tetrathiomolybdate injection.

Hematological examination revealed a marked anaemia (PCV 0.12 l/l; total RBC count 2.8 × 10^{12}/l; Hb 4.2 g/dl). The RBCs showed anisocytosis. Normoblasts comprised 23% of the WBCs (total count 7.2 × 10^{9}/l).

The plasma BUN and creatinine determinations revealed very high concentrations: 86.5 mmol/l (normal = 2–6 mmol/l) and 1,819 mol/l (normal = 110–170 mol/l), respectively. The serum copper concentration was 29.4 μmol/l. The total bilirubin concentration was 5.1 μmol/l. The serum AST concentration was 300 U/l and the GGT concentration was 144 U/l.

The failure of the ram to respond to treatment and evidence of renal failure indicated a hopeless prognosis and the ram was euthanased for welfare reasons.

Postmortem examination

The carcase showed obvious signs of jaundice, most noticeable in the omentum. The kidneys were grossly swollen and 'gun-metal grey', with small quantities of dark red urine in the bladder. The liver was enlarged and friable. The spleen was enlarged and appeared dark brown/black on cut section.

Management of other rams in the group

The remaining rams in the group were treated with ammonium tetrathiomolybdate (3.4 mg/kg s/c twice with a two-day interval). No further losses were reported.

Discussion

The rams had been fed 2.5 kg of concentrates daily for the past seven months. The concentrate contained 15 mg/kg of copper in the concentrate but no added copper antagonist. It was thought the high level of concentrate feeding over a prolonged period was the source of the accumulated copper in the liver. The farmer was strongly advised to feed a concentrate specifically designed for intensive ram rearing (i.e. one which contained a copper antagonist such as molybdenum).

REFERENCE

1 Russel A (1985) Nutrition of the pregnant ewe. *In Practice* 7, 23–28.

14 Parasitic Diseases

GASTROINTESTINAL NEMATODE INFESTATIONS

Gastrointestinal nematode infestations are the most important group of conditions limiting intensive sheep production worldwide. Infestations range from acute disease with sudden death to chronic disease, often with reduced performance and extending to considerable weight loss and emaciation. Nematode infestations are especially important with respect of their morbidity and considerable control costs. The appearance of resistance to members of the various anthelmintic groups poses serious challenges to nematode control in many countries worldwide. In many developed countries the growth of the organic food sector has highlighted the need for alternative methods of parasite control.

In the UK (the example country in this particular section) the important nematode infestations are:

- Nematodirosis in young lambs during the late spring/early summer.
- Parasitic gastroenteritis of growing lambs from mid-summer onwards, plus older sheep when control measures fail to be implemented correctly.

NEMATODIROSIS IN YOUNG LAMBS

Definition/overview

Nematodirosis is an important disease affecting young lambs, particularly during the late spring/early summer months when losses can be high.

Aetiology

Sudden death and outbreaks of diarrhoea can occur in young lambs grazing pastures contaminated with large numbers of larvae, which develop from eggs deposited by lambs during the previous grazing season. *Nematodirus battus* is much more pathogenic than *Nematodirus fillicolis* because of the more concentrated hatching period.

Clinical presentation

Only lambs are affected; ewes do not show disease. There is acute onset of profuse watery diarrhoea in young lambs, with faecal staining of the wool of the tail and perineum. The lambs are dull and depressed and rapidly develop a gaunt appearance with obvious dehydration and condition loss. Grazing activity ceases and lambs stop 'mobbing' and playing in groups. Deaths occur from dehydration if lambs are left untreated during the early stages of disease, and there is considerable weight loss in the remaining lambs. It is not unusual with severe larval challenge for 5% of lambs to die within a few days. Convalescence following anthelmintic treatment is protracted, with affected lambs having a greatly extended period to market.

Differential diagnoses

- The initial clinical presentation of severe larval challenge may be one of sudden death of young lambs without diarrhoea. In this situation the important differential diagnoses include pasteurellosis and pulpy kidney disease.
- More characteristically, the appearance of large numbers of lambs with profuse diarrhoea would suggest coccidiosis.

Diagnosis

Faecal worm egg counts are not helpful because acute disease is caused by developing larvae and adults before egg laying (pre-patent infestation).

Postmortem examination may reveal very large numbers of developing larval stages and adults within the lumen of the small intestine but often they have been expelled during the diarrhoeic phase. Confirmation of disease may necessitate microscopic examination of small intestine.

Treatment

Sheep should be moved from infested pastures whenever possible. Anthelmintic resistance is not a problem with *N. battus*. Administration of oral fluid therapy is possible but time-consuming for large numbers of lambs; intravenous fluid is not an option for logistical/cost reasons.

Prevention/control measures

Prevention is based on avoidance of pastures grazed by lambs during the previous grazing season, because adult sheep are highly resistant to infection and only lambs produce significant numbers of eggs.

The infective third stage larva (L3) is very resistant to desiccation and low temperatures and overwinters readily on pasture still within the egg. After a period of cold exposure the L3 hatches once the maximum environmental temperature exceeds 10°C over a period of days. While this simultaneous hatch occurs every year on permanent pasture, nematodirosis only results when the mass hatch coincides with grazing activity of young susceptible lambs. Warm spring weather results in L3 larvae hatching en mass before lambs start grazing, while in cold spring weather hatching is delayed and lambs are becoming age-immune from three months old when they ingest larvae. While it has been demonstrated experimentally that young dairy calves can also act as hosts to *N. battus*, this epidemiology is very uncommon in practice.

Preventing the establishment of patent *N. battus* infestations in lambs during the previous grazing season by regular anthelmintic treatments can reduce the build-up of larval infection on pasture. This programme will not eliminate all egg deposition on pasture and anthelmintic prophylaxis is necessary to avoid overt disease. The timing of anthelmintic prophylaxis is guided by environmental temperatures and disease forecasts. Typically, for lambs born from mid-March onwards (UK) in 'normal risk' years, anthelmintic treatments are given three weeks apart during May. In 'high risk' years, three anthelmintic treatments are given, extending the drenching period into June.

Economics

Chemical prophylaxis is relatively inexpensive (0.1–0.5% of the sale value of a lamb depending on the class of anthelmintic chosen) but drenching is time-consuming, especially when attempting to gather large numbers of sheep from a semi-extensive grazing system. Such reliance on chemical control raises certain environmental issues.

Welfare implications

Profuse diarrhoea in severe infestations may cause death and severe condition loss. While blowflies are not normally active in May in the UK, fleece contamination can persist and can attract flies later in the grazing season.

Parasitic gastroenteritis of growing lambs

Definition/overview

Gastrointestinal nematode infestations are a major problem in many sheep-producing countries but especially in Australia and other southern hemisphere countries where resistance to members of all three major anthelmintic groups poses serious challenges. Diarrhoea with faecal contamination of the fleece attracts blowflies, which leads to myiasis. Many countries have developed integrated nematode control programmes that are specific to their grazing and climatic conditions. This section deals in general terms with parasite control in the UK and may not be applicable to other situations where different host/parasite relationships exist.

Aetiology

In the UK the important genera causing parasitic gastroenteritis are *Teladosagia* (formerly *Ostertagia*) and *Trichostrongylus* (nematodirosis has been described above). In many countries, *Haemonchus contortus* is a serious threat to intensive sheep production.

Clinical presentation

Infestations usually cause profuse diarrhoea, leading to dehydration and reduced performance and extending to considerable weight loss (**619, 620**) and emaciation.

619 Group of lambs with profuse diarrhoea caused by high internal parasite burdens.

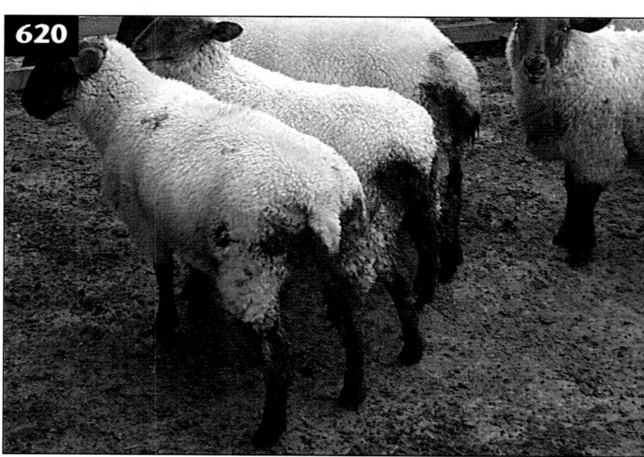

620 Group of lambs with chronic parasitism. Note the poor fleeces.

In haemonchosis (**621**) the most important clinical sign is anaemia (**622**). The severity of clinical signs of parasitism depends on the age of the host, the current nutritional status (especially protein intake), the immune status of the animal, the trace element status and the breed. The classical signs of parasitic gastroenteritis are observed in growing lambs exposed to large numbers of infective larvae during warm summer months.

Teladosagiosis
Disease (type I) is typically seen in growing lambs, with profuse watery diarrhoea, dehydration and reduced weight gain/condition loss. Weight loss results from a number of factors including reduced appetite, changes in the abomasal wall with loss of mature functional cells, and protein loss across the compromised mucosa.

Another form of the disease has been described (type II) but its importance has not been fully investigated on commercial sheep farms. Type II disease occurs during late winter when large numbers of hypobiotic larvae emerge simultaneously from the gastric glands.

Haemonchosis
As a consequence of *H. contortos* feeding on blood, haemonchosis presents with anaemia, submandibular oedema and increased heart and respiratory rates; diarrhoea is not a feature of this nematode infestation (**621**).

Ingestion of large numbers of larvae over a short period of time causes acute disease with lethargy, weakness and rapid loss of condition. This form of the disease is more commonly seen in growing lambs. Ingestion of smaller numbers of infective stages over several weeks to months causes a more general loss of condition, which progresses to emaciation.

Trichostrongylosis
Trichostrongylosis is normally seen during early winter and affects 8–10-month-old lambs but also yearling and adult sheep. The most prominent clinical feature is profuse dark-coloured, foul-smelling diarrhoea with copious mucus present in the worst affected sheep. Other sheep in the group are less severely affected but they all have lost weight and present in poor condition.

Differential diagnoses

Teladosagiosis and trichostrongylosis

- On a group/flock basis the common causes of poor growth/weight loss include poor grazing conditions and overgrazing, especially during adverse weather.
- Trace elements act synergistically with chronic parasitism to cause poor growth and it may prove difficult to determine the primary cause.
- Cobalt (vitamin B_{12}) status should be monitored in the group.
- Selenium status should be investigated in deficient geographic areas.
- Virulent footrot can exert a severe adverse effect on growth rate in store lambs.
- Salmonellosis and yersiniosis should be considered in the differential diagnosis of trichostrongylosis.

Haemonchosis

- On a group/flock basis the common presenting features of peripheral oedema, anaemia and chronic weight loss must be differentiated from chronic fasciolosis, although the seasonal occurrence of these infestations differs markedly (summer versus winter, respectively).

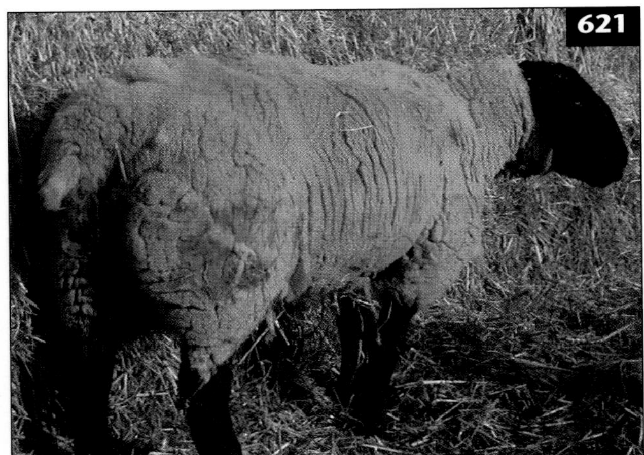

621 Adult ram suffering from haemonchosis.

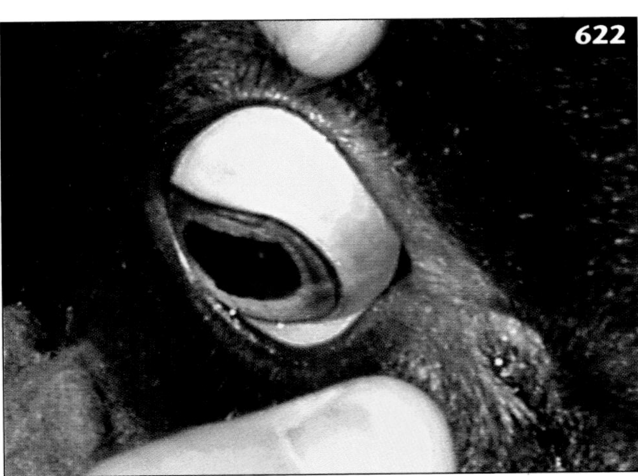

622 Anaemia in the ram in **621** caused by haemonchosis.

- Other chronic nematode infestations can also cause weight loss but with diarrhoea.
- On an individual basis, adult sheep with paratuberculosis typically present with chronic weight loss, mild anaemia, absence of diarrhoea and submandibular oedema in advanced cases.
- Numerous chronic bacterial infections result in weight loss extending to emaciation.

Diagnosis

Teladosagiosis and trichostrongylosis

Faecal egg counts are routinely used to aid diagnosis of nematode infestations but they have certain inherent limitations. Due to numerous factors the faecal egg count may not accurately indicate the adult nematode population present within the gastrointestinal tract at that time. Pathology can be caused by developing stages before infestations become patent, and also by hypobiotic stages.

By identifying only strongyle eggs, it is possible for less pathogenic species to make a disproportionate contribution to the total egg count. As a general rule, a strongyle egg count of >400 epg is considered moderate while >1,000 epg is considered high and worthy of treatment.

Haemonchosis

Identification of anaemia is taken as a reliable indicator of haemonchosis in countries with endemic disease. Egg counts are often very high in patent infestations, with counts >10,000 epg not uncommon. At necropsy, very large numbers of adults are visible on the surface of the abomasum of untreated sheep.

Treatment

Treatment involves the use of an effective anthelmintic (see also Anthelmintic resistance). The three major anthelmintic groups, defined by the active chemical, comprise:

- 1-BZ benzimidazoles, probenzimidazoles. Benzimidazoles such as albendazole and fenbendazole have a similar mode of action. Febantel, netobimin and thiophanate are probenzimidazoles, which are converted to benzimidazoles in the body.
- 2-LM imidazothiazoles, tetrahydropyrimidines. Levamisole and tetramisole are imidazothiazoles. Morantel and pyrantel are tetrahydropyrimidines.
- 3-AV avermectins, milbemycins. Preparations that contain avermectins include doramectin and ivermectin, and milbemycins such as moxidectin.

Closantel and nitroxynil can be used in situations where *H. contortus* is the major parasite. It is essential that a representative number of sheep are weighed before treatment (**623**) and that treatment is based on the heaviest sheep in the group (**624**).

Prevention/control measures

Prevention

With traditional management of sheep on permanent pasture in the UK, parasitic gastroenteritis in growing lambs results from ingestion of very large

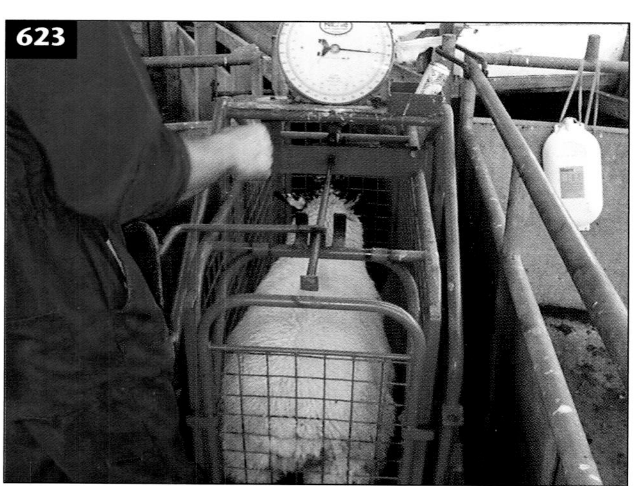

623 Weighing of the group to determine dose rate.

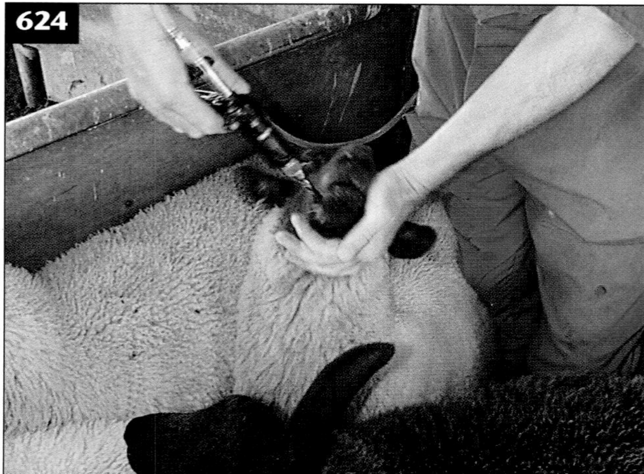

624 Anthelmintic drenching of lambs based on the heaviest sheep in the group.

numbers of infective larvae from the pasture during mid-summer. *Teladosagia circumcincta*, and in warmer areas *H. contortus*, larvae appear first with *Trichostrongylus* species appearing during late summer/autumn.

Pasture larvae arise from two sources:

- Eggs passed by ewes during the periparturient period. The reduction in host immunity permits a significant increase in egg production during the last two weeks of gestation, which may persist until eight weeks post lambing. The reduction in host immunity is influenced by numerous factors including ewe nutritional status, particularly dietary protein intake. Under suitable environmental conditions eggs develop to infective larvae within three weeks but maximum levels may not be present on the pasture for up to six weeks. These infective larvae are the major source of infestations in young lambs.
- Young lambs may also ingest overwintered infective larvae from pasture and these develop to adults. The large numbers of eggs produced by adult nematodes resident in the gastrointestinal tract of young lambs results in the appearance of significant numbers of infective larvae on pasture during mid-summer. Clinical parasitism results unless appropriate action is taken.

Control

Control is based on not grazing potentially heavily infested pastures with susceptible lambs. Avoidance of infested pastures from July onwards can be integrated into some farm management systems (**625**) by moving sheep on to hay or silage aftermaths from mid-June onwards. On some mixed farms it may be possible to rotate pastures annually between cattle and sheep and operate a 'modified' two-year clean grazing system.

Alternatively, anthelmintics can be administered to both ewes and lambs to prevent the build-up of critical larval populations on continually grazed pasture.

Use of prophylactic anthelmintics

Anthelmintic treatment to prevent the periparturient rise in egg output by ewes can be given at various times depending on the farm management system (e.g. when housing ewes during mid-gestation, at the same time as vaccination against the clostridial diseases 4–6 weeks prior to lambing, or immediately prior to turnout to pasture when lambs are 1–2 days old).

It is important that the anthelmintic chosen to counter the periparturient rise is effective against hypobiotic larval stages. To gain maximum benefit from the residual activity of moxidectin, ewes should be drenched/injected at turnout to pasture with their lambs rather than at housing; this affords up to 7–11 weeks' residual action. The importance of good ewe nutrition during early lactation should not be underestimated with respect to parasitic gastroenteritis. In addition, ewes that are well fed also produce more milk, so the lambs reach market weight before the peak of the mid-summer pasture larval challenge.

The timing of early season prophylactic anthelmintic administration to control nematodirosis has been discussed earlier but essentially it comprises a strategic anthelmintic drench depending on disease forecasts. While disease forecasts are reasonably accurate, local factors may operate with the result that two drenches are given two weeks apart from early May. Where lambs graze permanent grassland, anthelmintic treatments should be repeated every month until the autumn but the interval will depend upon the persistence of the particular anthelmintic. Grazing heavily contaminated pasture with reliance on chemical prophylaxis/treatment is undesirable, and lambs fail to grow to their potential under such mismanagement. A more integrated pasture management policy is overdue on most intensive sheep farms in the UK.

Economics

The major cost of nematode infestations is lost production in terms of lower fleece weight and poorer quality wool, and poor live weight gain with an extended interval to marketing.

Nematode control is expensive in terms of drugs and labour. The appearance of resistance to certain anthelmintics in many countries has placed almost total reliance on newer, more expensive anthelmintics.

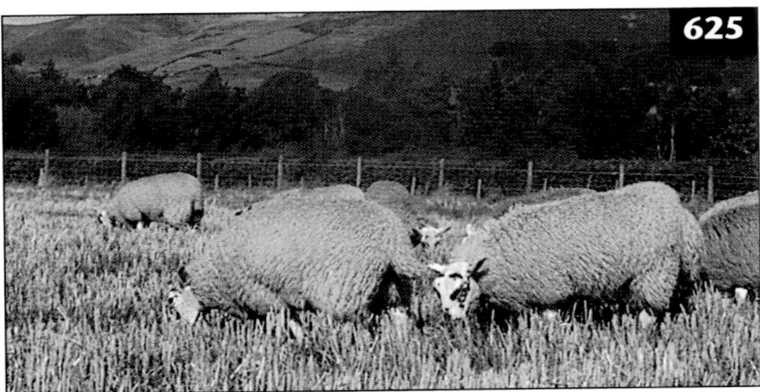

625 Clean grazing on barley stubble undersown with grass.

Welfare implications
Nematode infestations can lead to severe loss of body condition and emaciation with obvious welfare concerns.

TAPEWORM INFESTATIONS

Definition/overview
Tapeworms occur in all major sheep-producing areas but they are of no clinical concern. Segments of tapeworms are often seen in the faeces of growing lambs in the UK but they exert no adverse effects on growth rate.

Aetiology
Only the genus *Monezia* occurs in the UK. Free-living oribatid mites act as an intermediate stage.

Clinical presentation
Tapeworm segments are readily recognized in faeces as white ribbon-like structures up to 10 mm wide.

Diagnosis
Diagnosis is based on the finding of tapeworm segments in the faeces.

Treatment
Treatment is not considered necessary because tapeworms are non pathogenic. Only members of the benzimadazole group (1-BZ) are effective against adult tapeworms.

Prevention/control measures
No control measures are necessary for tapeworms.

Economics
None.

Welfare implications
None.

ANTHELMINTIC RESISTANCE

Since the mid 1980s, anthelmintic resistance has become a very important issue in many intensive sheep production systems, particularly in southern hemisphere countries such as Australia, many South American countries and South Africa. This demographic emergence of anthelmintic resistance is related to intensive management practices, often using irrigated pastures, and climatic conditions that permit a greater number of nematode generations per annum compared with western European countries. Resistance to benzimidazoles has been recognized as widespread in the UK over the past five years or so and, more recently, resistance to members of all three anthelmintic groups has been identified in *Teladosagia* on a Scottish sheep farm.

Gene(s) conferring resistance to an anthelmintic may be present at a very low frequency within a nematode population. Utilization of that anthelmintic alone leaves only resistant nematodes with the appearance of clinical disease once the adult nematode population exceeds a certain threshold.

Various strategies have been recommended to delay the progress of anthelmintic resistance; some strategies appear to have been less successful than predicted.

Detection of anthelmintic resistance
The emergence of anthelmintic resistance in a nematode population on a particular sheep enterprise can easily be overlooked because clinical signs may be limited to reduced performance and diarrhoea rather than mortality. The most common technique to detect anthelmintic resistance on a sheep farm is the faecal egg count reduction test. Individual faecal egg counts are undertaken on 10–15 lambs, which are then weighed and drenched with the appropriate volume of anthelmintic. The individual faecal egg counts are repeated ten days later. Failure to effect a reduction in geometric faecal count greater than 85% strongly suggests the presence of resistance to that anthelmintic group.

In-vitro egg hatch assays can be used to identify benzimidazole resistance.

Control strategies

Quarantine treatments
Strict quarantine treatments and appropriate biosecurity on sheep farms are essential in the control of anthelmintic-resistant nematodes. There are a large number of infectious diseases and parasites that can be introduced on to the farm with breeding replacements. Future efforts should be directed at limiting the number of sheep movements on to farms. When purchases become necessary, they should be sourced directly from reputable vendors. All purchased stock should be treated on arrival to avoid importing resistant nematodes on to the farm. The most effective

anthelmintics belong to the 3-AV group. Treated sheep should be held off pasture for 24 hours to avoid contamination with eggs.

Effective treatment

All drenching/injection equipment must be regularly calibrated. Sheep must be weighed and the dose rate calculated for the heaviest group members, not the average. All anthelmintics have a considerable safety margin; slight overdosage will only marginally increase cost. Withholding feed has been recommended when using group 1-BZ and 3-AV drenches because reduced rumen fill delays passage of the drug. This fasted state often exists in sheep transported to market, purchased then transported to their destination; therefore, drenching on arrival is strongly recommended rather than after a few days' delay when pasture contamination could have resulted. Administration of low volume formulations may also increase the likelihood of anthelmintic drench deposition in the rumen.

Annual rotation

Annual rotation amongst the three chemical groups has been recommended but there are few data to support this practice.

Reduction in treatment frequency

A reduction in treatment frequency has been recommended. This approach is based on sound knowledge of the nematode species that has developed resistance. Fewer treatments necessitate a more structured approach than presently operated by many farmers and adoption of more fully integrated grazing programmes. For example, in many UK sheep flocks, ewe treatments could be targeted at eliminating the periparturient rise.

In growing lambs, treatment and movement on to clean grazing can avoid the mid-summer challenge from large numbers of infective larvae on pasture. This practice is causing some concern because of the risk posed by resistant worms remaining after anthelmintic treatment and contaminating the 'safe' or 'clean' grazing. By removing all susceptible strains, resistant helminths would be unopposed in their occupation of the gastrointestinal tract. It has been generally accepted, although never conclusively proven, that anthelmintic-resistant strains are at a disadvantage compared with susceptible strains, such that they do not dominate in number or fecundity. It has further been suggested that 5–10% of lambs could be left untreated to dilute the effects of emerging resistant strains, but this is conjecture. On the majority of sheep farms a review of current practice and grazing management would effect the more significant improvement in parasite control.

Controlled release capsule

Controlled release boluses containing a benzimidazole anthelmintic are available in many countries. They are useful in the face of benzimidazole-resistant strains of nematodes, presumably because of their continuous delivery and hence persistent action and/or greater susceptibility of ingested larval stages compared with established adult worms. A modification of this delivery system is to administer three full drenches with a benzimidazole anthelmintic at 24-hour intervals but this greatly increases handling and labour costs.

FASCIOLOSIS (*Syn*: liver fluke)

Definition/overview

Fasciolosis is a major parasitic disease of sheep in many countries worldwide. This section relates to disease caused by *Fasciola hepatica* as it presents in the UK. Acute and subacute fasciolosis has become a major problem in areas of the country where such infestations have not been seen for decades. In certain countries of the world, *Fasciola gigantica* and *Dicrocoelium dentriticum* assume importance.

Aetiology

F. hepatica has the liver as its site of infection in both cattle and sheep. The intermediate stages involve snails of the genus *Lymnaea*, mostly *L. truncatula*. The important stages of the life cycle of *F. hepatica* necessitate moisture and an environmental temperature above 10°C. Essentially, late spring early/summer infestation of snails by miracidia results in an autumn metacecariae challenge to sheep, with immediate acute disease, subacute disease over the following weeks, or chronic disease apparent some months later, depending on the level of challenge.

Clinical presentation

Acute fasciolosis

During a wet summer, grazing sheep can ingest very large numbers of metacercariae, with invasion of the liver parenchyma by large numbers of immature flukes causing acute disease. Affected sheep die suddenly from haemorrhage and liver damage, with the first evidence of a problem being sudden deaths in previously healthy sheep from August to December. Inspection of others in the group reveals lethargy and reduced grazing activity. Gathering may prove difficult because the sheep are reluctant to run. Closer examination reveals pale mucous membranes. Liver enlargement and ascites have been described.

Subacute fasciolosis

The major presenting clinical findings are very poor body condition score and poor fleece quality despite adequate flock nutrition; this results from ingestion of metacercariae over several weeks/months. Losses typically occur from December onwards but may be much earlier (October) with severe challenge. Affected sheep show marked anaemia, most noticeably affecting the conjunctivae. Liver enlargement is reported but is not easy to appreciate during clinical examination. Ascites cannot usually be appreciated clinically without recourse to ultrasonographic examination (**626**), except in extreme cases (**627, 628**).

Severe illness and death arising from liver damage and associated peritonitis have recently been reported in many parts of the UK where fasciolosis has not been seen before. Typically, some sheep present with severe depression, inappetence and weakness and they may be unable to stand. Body condition is very poor but contrasts with abdominal distension due to fluid accumulation. The sheep have a painful expression and gentle palpation of the anterior abdomen reveals obvious pain, which is

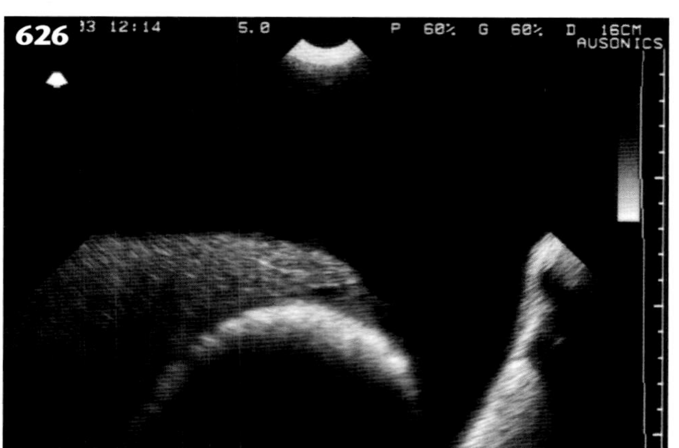

626 Ultrasonographic examination (5 MHz sector scanner) revealing fluid accumulation within the abdomen (anechoic area) extending for up to 20 cm deep. The liver and other abdominal viscera have been displaced dorsally by the fluid away from the probe head situated on the ventral abdominal wall.

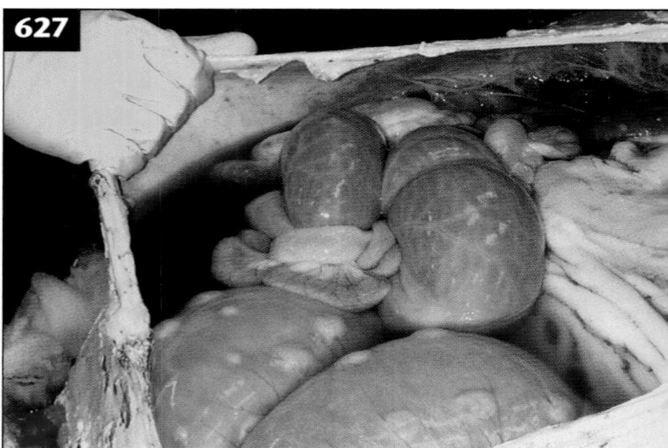

627 Extensive fluid accumulation (about 20 litres already released) within the abdomen of the sheep in **626**.

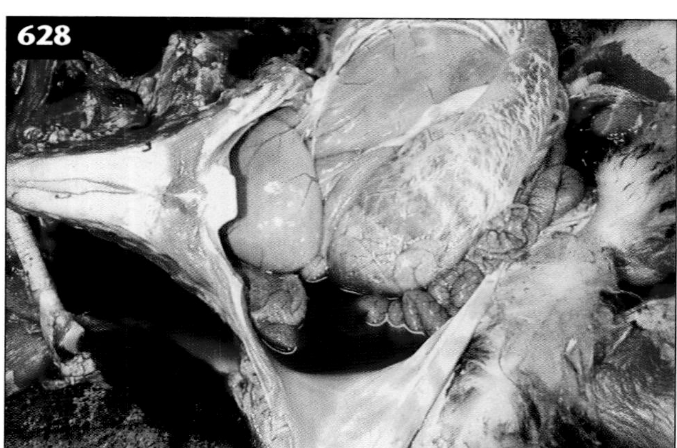

628 Considerable fluid accumulation within the abdomen in a Soay ram with subacute fasciolosis.

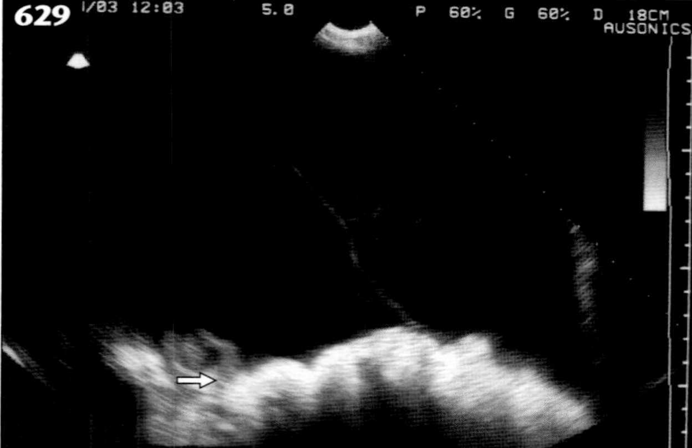

629 Ultrasonographic examination revealing an extensive peritoneal exudate with dorsal displacement of the omentum (arrow) (hyperechoic ribbon-like band).

markedly unusual in sheep where their naturally stoic nature reveals little.

Ultrasonographic examination has revealed dramatic reaction to migrating flukes in some sheep, with considerable peritoneal exudate (629) and extensive fibrinous adhesions between the liver and the body wall (630). The liver capsule has a hyperechoic appearance due to fibrin deposition (631, 632). Necropsy reveals fully the extent of the peritoneal exudate and fibrinous reaction (633, 634). There is severe liver damage in many of the sheep with fibrinous peritonitis (635).

630 Fibrinous adhesions (1) between the liver (2), omentum (3) and body wall. The liver appears more hyperechoic than normal.

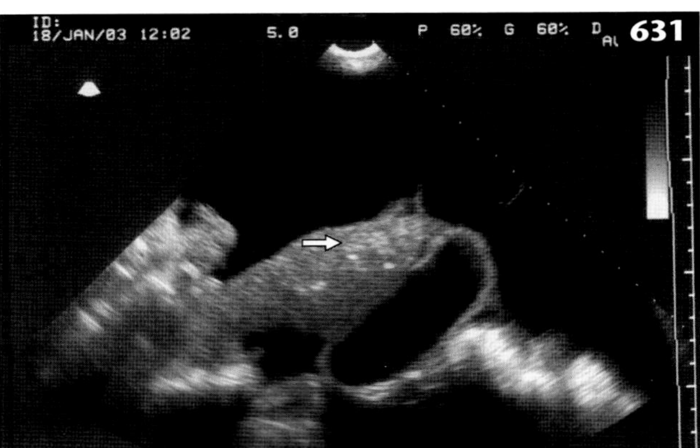

631 The liver (arrow) appears more hyperechoic than normal due to the inflammatory reaction to migrating flukes.

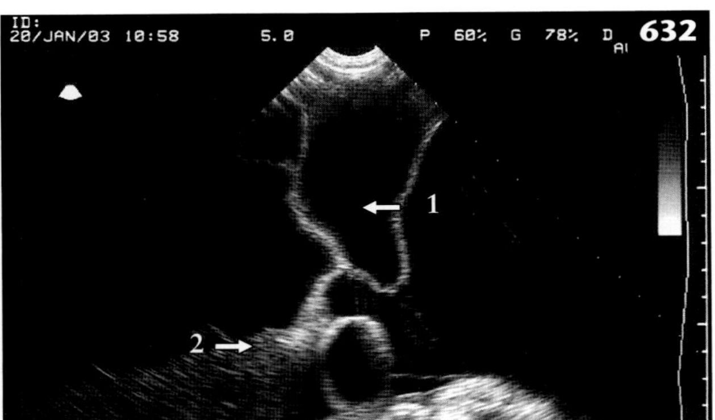

632 Fibrinous adhesions (**1**) between the liver (**2**), omentum and body wall two days after **629–631**.

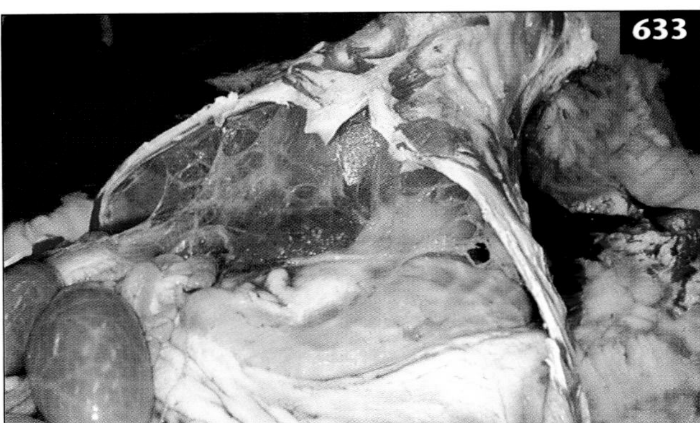

633 Necropsy revealing fibrinous peritonitis and severe liver damage caused by subacute fasciolosis. The peritoneal exudate shown in the sonograms (**629, 630**) has been released.

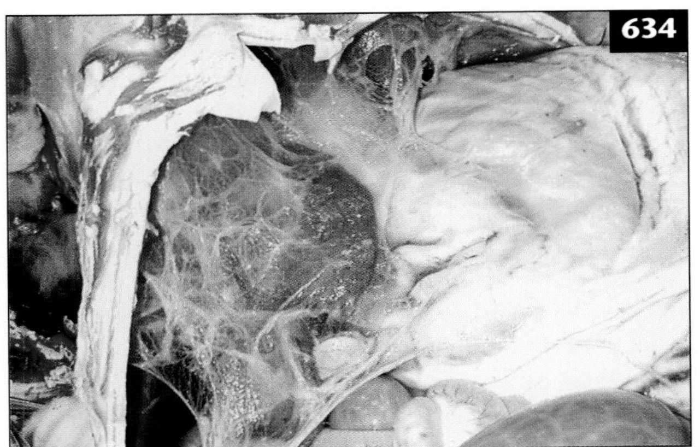

634 Fibrinous peritonitis extending to involve the small intestine.

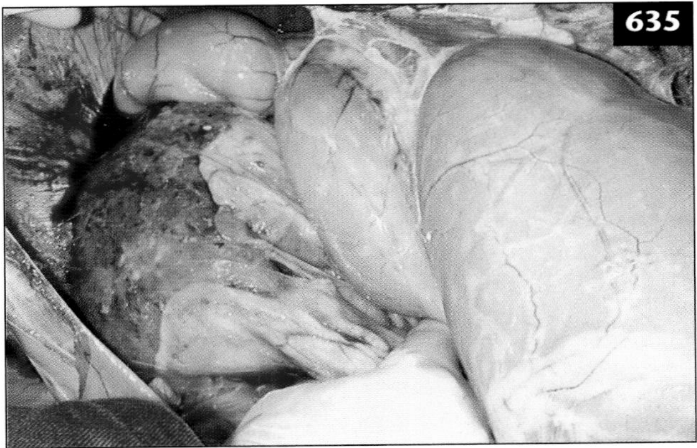

635 Severe liver damage caused by subacute fasciolosis.

Chronic fasciolosis

The major presenting clinical findings are low body condition score and poor fleece quality. There is submandibular oedema in many sheep (**636**). Affected sheep show marked anaemia with PCV values as low as 0.06 l/l. Affected sheep may die in an emaciated state, especially when infestation is compounded by the metabolic demands of advanced gestation/early lactation.

Differential diagnoses

Differential diagnoses of sudden death caused by acute fasciolosis and, less commonly, subacute fasciolosis are:

- Clostridial disease: pulpy kidney disease, blackleg, black disease, braxy.
- Pasteurellosis or other septicaemic disease secondary to tick-borne fever.
- Louping ill.
- Abdominal catastrophe (e.g. volvulus of the abomasum or small intestine).
- Poisoning (e.g. nitrate or ammonia).
- Acidosis if fed grain.

Differential diagnoses of emaciation resulting from subacute and chronic fasciolosis include:

Group problem:

- Poor flock nutrition.
- Virulent footrot.
- Chronic parasitism including anthelmintic-resistant strains.
- Cobalt deficiency (lambs).
- Visceral form of caseous lymphadenitis.

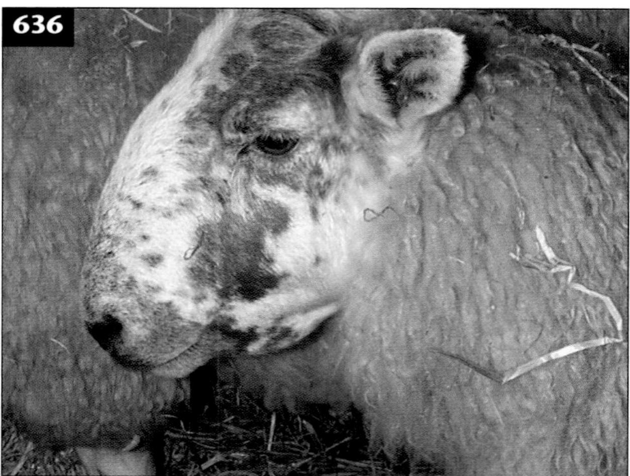

636 Submandibular oedema commonly observed in sheep with chronic fasciolosis.

Individual problem:

- Paratuberculosis.
- Chronic suppurative pneumonia or other septic focus.
- Poor dentition, especially cheek teeth.
- Chronic severe lameness.
- Sheep pulmonary adenomatosis.
- Scrapie.
- Lymphosarcoma.
- Intestinal adenocarcinoma.
- Visna.

Diagnosis

Acute fasciolosis

Diagnosis of acute fasciolosis is based on the epidemiological data (high risk year) and massively raised liver enzymes (e.g. AST), which indicates acute liver insult, and is confirmed at necropsy of sudden deaths.

Subacute fasciolosis

Subacute fasciolosis can be diagnosed by raised serum AST and glutamate dehydrogenase (GLDH) concentrations. Increased serum GGT concentrations, which indicate bile duct damage, are also commonly used to establish the diagnosis. These three liver enzymes are typically increased by 5–30-fold but, in the case of AST, fall to near normal concentrations within 10–14 days of flukacide treatment. Serum GGT and GLDH remain elevated for at least one month after flukacide treatment and are therefore the biochemical determinations of choice for subacute fasciolosis.

The serum albumin concentration is reduced within a range of 12–20 g/l and the serum globulin concentration is massively increased to >65 g/l and often >75 g/l. There are few bacterial infections that give such a dramatic serum protein profile, and certainly none on a group basis; therefore, serum protein analysis should be included with liver enzymes in the biochemistry profile. Immature flukes can be demonstrated within the bile ducts and gall bladder at necropsy.

Chronic fasciolosis

Chronic fasciolosis is diagnosed by demonstration of fluke eggs in faecal samples and by raised serum GGT concentrations but these values may only be increased by 2–3-fold in some cases. Many sheep show profound anaemia, hypoalbuminaemia and hypergammaglobulinaemia. Mature flukes are demonstrated within the bile ducts and gall bladder at necropsy (**637**).

Treatment

Triclabendazole is effective at killing all stages of flukes responsible for acute and subacute fasciolosis. Drenched sheep should be moved to clean pasture or re-treated every three weeks for the next three months at least.

Nitroxynil and oxyclosanide are less effective against immature flukes and should be used for the treatment of chronic fasciolosis. Once again, treated sheep must be moved to clean pastures.

Improved nutrition is essential but significant improvement of body condition score is unlikely because of the increasing demands of pregnancy, especially when chronic fasciolosis is diagnosed from February onwards (i.e. the last trimester).

Prevention/control measures

In areas with endemic fasciolosis, control is founded on strategic flukacide drenches. During low risk years, triclabendazole is given to at-risk sheep in October and January, and either nitroxynil or oxyclosanide is administered in May. In years when epidemiological data indicate a high risk of fasciolosis, an additional triclabendazole treatment should be given in November.

While it may be possible to eradicate fluke from the flock on a farm by strategic drenching, there are risks from wildlife species that harbour flukes. Drenching based on the appearance of clinical disease in a few sheep represents a considerable risk, as serious losses could result in the flock before treatment can be effected. Therefore, it is strongly recommended that strategic drenching is undertaken every year with additional treatments in high-risk years, the latter based upon forecast data.

Fencing off snail habitats (**638**) is rarely practicable and in most situations is cost prohibitive, as these are often extensive sheep enterprises. Drainage is cost prohibitive and many properties are subject to environmental controls.

Economics

Fasciolosis can have a serious financial impact on a sheep farm but infestations can be controlled by strategic drenching with an appropriate flukacide. Losses can result when infested sheep are brought on to a farm, contaminating pasture and infesting snails with subsequent challenge to the home flock. Problems may also arise after a succession of wet summers, which allows snail numbers to increase dramatically, providing an abundance of intermediate hosts for the developing fluke stages.

Welfare implications

There are obvious concerns arising from sheep that die of acute and subacute fasciolosis but the greater concern is the welfare of large numbers of emaciated sheep during late pregnancy. These ewes are more prone to ovine pregnancy toxaemia, have poor colostrum stores and give birth to low birth weight lambs. The latter two factors result in an unacceptably high perinatal lamb mortality rate from starvation and increased susceptibility to environmental pathogens.

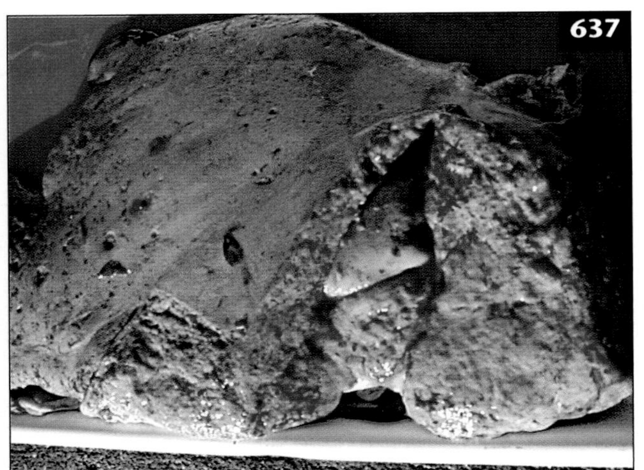

637 Liver damage associated with chronic fasciolosis.

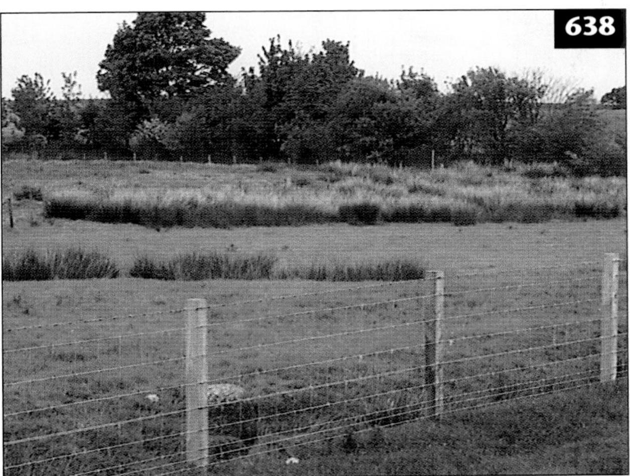

638 Snail habitat fenced off as part of the fluke control programme.

FASCIOLA GIGANTICA

The life cycle of *F. gigantica* is broadly similar to that of *F. hepatica*. The intermediate stages involve the snail *Lymnaea auricula*. Both acute and chronic forms of the disease occur in sheep. Control measures are similar to those for *F. hepatica*.

TICK-BORNE DISEASES

Diseases transmitted by ticks include tick-borne fever, heartwater, louping-ill, tick pyaemia and Lyme disease; however, these diseases are not present in all tick-infested areas.

TICK-BORNE FEVER

Definition/overview

Tick-borne fever can be a sporadic but serious cause of abortion in sheep not previously exposed to the rickettsial infection. It is important in endemically infected flocks because impairment of the immune status predisposes to other infections such as tick pyaemia and louping-ill. Infection is encountered in northern Europe on grazings that provide suitable habitats for ticks.

Aetiology

Tick-borne fever is caused by the rickettsial microorganism *Ehrlichia phagocytophila*. The vector is the nymph and adult stages of the tick *Ixodes ricinus*. A carrier state develops with recurrence of parasitaemia during stressful events. Deer may act as a reservoir for tick-borne fever, with only sporadic exposure of sheep, which may explain the occasional appearance of disease in sheep flocks.

Clinical presentation

Exposure of non-pregnant sheep to infected ticks results in a brief period of malaise with pyrexia, depression and reduced appetite. The resultant leucopenia renders sheep prone to infections such as tick pyaemia in lambs and louping-ill in unvaccinated yearlings. Re-exposure may result in mild transient illness but abortion does not result.

In most situations, lambs and yearlings exposed to tick-borne fever do not encounter infection for the first time when they are pregnant. Exposure of susceptible (purchased) pregnant ewes to tick-borne fever can produce disastrous consequences, with abortion rates >90% reported and high mortality in ewes post abortion. Tick-borne fever may also exacerbate existing respiratory tract infections.

Differential diagnoses

The common causes of abortion:

- *Chlamydophila abortus* infection.
- Toxoplasmosis.
- *Salmonella* serotypes.
- *Campylobacter fetus intestinalis*.
- *Listeria monocytogenes*, *Pasteurella* species.

Diagnosis

Diagnosis is based on the clinical signs and history of recent exposure of susceptible sheep to a tick-infested area. There may be evidence of all three stages of the tick life cycle feeding on the sheep; particular attention should be paid to the groin and axillae when checking sheep for tick infestation. Initially, there is a profound lymphopenia followed by a neutropenia, which slowly return to normal values after 2–3 weeks in uncomplicated cases. Focal bacterial infection will affect these values over time, with a developing mature neutrophilia.

During the first week parasites can be observed microscopically in granulocytes of Giemsa-stained blood films. Seroconversion indicates recent infection and is perhaps of most use in establishing a potential role of tick-borne fever in abortion cases.

Treatment

While uncomplicated cases of tick-borne fever can be successfully treated with oxytetracycline, clinical signs would not be noted unless secondary or associated disease occurred.

Metaphylactic antibiotic injection with long-acting oxytetracycline could be attempted in the face of an abortion problem, in addition to removing sheep from infested pasture and treatment for ticks.

Prevention/control measures

In some countries with extensive management systems it is not possible to avoid tick-infested pastures. Tick activity in spring coincides with the return of ewes and their lambs to hill/mountainous areas such that young lambs are especially susceptible to tick-borne fever and tick pyaemia. Lambs are protected from louping-ill by passively-derived antibody.

Control measures involve the use of synthetic pyrethroid pour-on acaricides such as deltamethrin or flumethrin before turnout to infested areas; these provide control for up to six weeks after topical application. The use of pour-on preparations has numerous advantages over plunge dipping. In some situations the injection of all lambs with long-acting oxytetracycline is used in addition to topical acaricide.

Economics
Application of a synthetic pyrethroid pour-on acaricide costs approximately 0.5% of the value of the ewe. A single injection of long-acting oxytetracycline for a 10 kg lamb costs approximately 1% of the value of the lamb.

Welfare implications
Tick-borne fever has no specific welfare concerns *per se* but the associated condition of tick pyaemia raises serious welfare concerns because of the crippling affects of polyarthritis and vertebral empyema.

TICK PYAEMIA
Definition/overview
Tick pyaemia is typically seen in lambs 10–14 days after exposure to tick-infested pastures where tick-borne fever (*Ehrlichia phagocytophila*) is present; however, not all lambs with tick-borne fever develop tick pyaemia.

Aetiology
Infection of lambs with tick-borne fever causes a leucopenia and this may be followed by bacterial infection of the feeding sites.

Clinical presentation
Lambs are generally turned away to hill (tick-infested) pastures when approximately 1–2 weeks old and infection is observed in lambs 3–4 weeks old. Infection of skin bite wounds with bacteria, commonly *Staphylococcus aureus*, results in large subcutaneous abscesses. Bacteraemia with localization within joints and the vertebral column causes septic joints and eventual paralysis caudal to the affected vertebra, respectively. Severely affected lambs on extensive grazing systems may fall prey to opportunist predators, with the extent of these losses not known until first gathering or weaning. Lambs with polyarthritis are severely lame, non weight-bearing when only one limb is affected, and unable to stand/move if two or more limbs are affected. Unlike most other cases of polyarthritis in young lambs, affected joints become markedly distended with viscous green pus. In many cases the skin overlying aspects of the joint capsule is much thinner than normal, with hair loss typical of an underlying abscess, although the joint contents rarely discharge.

The clinical manifestation of infection of the vertebral column is described in detail in Chapter 7 (Spinal cord lesions, p. 190).

Differential diagnoses
- Other causes of polyarthritis include *Streptococcus dysgalactiae*, typically seen in lambs less than two weeks old, and *Erysipelas rhusiopathiae* in older lambs, which can be differentiated on clinical examination and bacteriology of joint fluid or synovial membrane.
- Vertebral empyema should be differentiated from delayed swayback and, possibly, white muscle disease.

Diagnosis
Diagnosis of tick pyaemia is based on clinical findings and history of tick exposure. It is unlikely that there will be evidence of *E. phagocytophila* in blood films from lambs with chronic bacterial infections.

Treatment
Subcutaneous abscesses can be lanced but lambs with vertebral empyema, and polyarthritis as a consequence of bacteraemia, must be euthanased for welfare reasons.

Prevention/control measures
There are no specific control measures for tick pyaemia. Tick control is described in the section on tick-borne fever.

Economics
Considerable losses can result from mortality associated with tick pyaemia. Preventive measures are relatively inexpensive and topical application of synthetic pyrethroid can be repeated where necessary.

Welfare implications
Crippled lambs with septic joints or vertebral empyema present a serious welfare concern. Many lambs succumb to starvation and/or predation in extensive management systems. When found alive, these lambs must be humanely destroyed for welfare reasons. Treatment is hopeless and merely prolongs suffering.

LOUPING ILL
Definition/overview
Louping-ill is an acute, tick-transmitted viral infection of the central nervous system of sheep and, much less commonly, a range of other species including man. The disease is confined to certain tick-infested areas in certain countries of northern Europe, in particular Scotland, with a seasonal occurrence reflecting tick feeding patterns.

Aetiology

Louping-ill is caused by a flavivirus and is transmitted by the tick *Ixodes ricinus*. The severity of clinical signs is exacerbated following concurrent infection with tick-borne fever. The majority of cases occur during the spring but a distinct autumn feeding population of ticks gives rise to disease much later in the year.

Clinical presentation

All ages of sheep appear susceptible to infection but in endemically-infected areas clinical signs are most common following waning of passive protection; thus disease is seen in weaned lambs associated with an autumn tick quest, and during the following spring as yearlings.

The clinical signs are variable and range from mild ataxia to sudden death. The neurological signs reported include ataxia and seizure activity progressing to opisthotonus. The severity of clinical signs and mortality are increased with concurrent infection with *E. phagocytophila*. It is reported that recovered sheep exhibit posterior paralysis for weeks to months after infection.

Differential diagnoses

- Posterior paresis in weaned lambs could result from delayed swayback and sarcocystis. Numerous sheep may present with sarcocystis over a period of 7–10 days after movement on to pastures contaminated by dog faeces, but no acute deaths result.
- Vertebral empyema of the thoracolumbar column may cause posterior paresis for a few days but this rapidly progresses to paralysis. Such cases occur sporadically and not as an outbreak.
- Oubreaks of acute coenurosis have been reported but would likely differ from louping-ill with respect to epidemiology.
- Acute cases of listerial encephalitis may present with many of the neurological signs of louping-ill, although fewer losses occur and the epidemiology would almost certainly differ.
- Seizure activity and opisthotonus are common presenting signs of polioencephalomalacia.
- Focal symmetrical encephalomalacia should be considered in unvaccinated lambs.
- Sudden death in sheep grazing extensive pasture may result from acute fasciolosis or clostridial disease, in particular black disease. Losses could also result from systemic pasteurellosis and other acute bacterial infections.

Diagnosis

Diagnosis is based on clinical signs affecting a number of susceptible sheep within weeks of moving on to tick-infested pasture. The provisional diagnosis is supported by histopathological examination of brain tissue from carcases and virus isolation. For safety reasons, the sheep's head should be submitted for laboratory examination rather than removing the brain under field conditions. Blood smears may reveal the presence of *E. phagocytophila*. Seroconversion would be evident in recovered sheep.

Treatment

There is no treatment and efforts are directed at prevention by vaccination and tick control.

Prevention/control measures

While tick control programmes using pour-on acaricides may limit all tick-transmitted diseases, these regimens are not completely effective at eliminating tick populations; therefore, control of louping-ill must incorporate a vaccination policy. In endemic areas all replacement breeding stock, including rams, are vaccinated at least 28 days before exposure to tick-infested pastures. Thereafter, vaccination every two years is recommended, which should be given prior to lambing to ensure passive antibody protection of lambs during their first spring.

Economics

Vaccination is relatively expensive (2.5% of the value of the ewe) but is essential on all endemically affected farms.

Welfare implications

Vaccination is indicated on affected farms for both economic and welfare reasons.

HEARTWATER (*Syn*: cowdriosis)

Definition/overview

Heartwater is an important production-limiting disease of sheep in sub-Saharan African countries.

Aetiology

Heartwater is caused by infection with *Cowdria ruminantium* and is transmitted by ticks of the genus *Amblyomma*. The natural tick life cycle may involve non-domesticated ruminants.

Clinical presentation

After an incubation of approximately two weeks, sheep show a marked pyrexia. In mild infections sheep are depressed and inappetent. Respiratory distress, with tachynpoea and an abdominal component to breathing, are present in many cases, resulting from pulmonary oedema and effusion within the chest and pericardium. This rapidly progresses to death. Vague neurological signs may be observed including hyperaesthesia and seizure activity. In peracute situations sheep may simply be found dead. Losses are higher in introduced breeds and may exceed 50%.

Diagnosis
Diagnosis is based on clinical findings and history of exposure to tick-infested pasture, particularly with non-indigenous breeds.

Typical necropsy findings include marked pericardial and pleural effusions and widespread carcase petechiae. Brain smears should be examined carefully for the presence of intracytoplasmic rickettsiae in endothelial cells.

Treatment
Treatment with oxytetracycline is unsuccessful in most cases because of the advanced changes present when sick sheep are identified.

Prevention/control measures
Indigenous breeds have a higher level of resistance to heartwater than introduced breeds. Cross-breeding programmes offer the best compromise to acquiring desired genetic traits whilst still maintaining some degree of resistance to local disease conditions.

A vaccine is reported to be available in South Africa and Zimbabwe but this presents many practical difficulties. Controlled exposure, with oxytetracycline treatment once pyrexia or clinical signs are noted, is one method of acquiring some degree of natural immunization but this is time consuming and not without risk of severe disease from overwhelming challenge.

Control of tick infestation in sheep also involves a programme of intensive acaricide application to cattle, but infestations involving non-domesticated hosts limit the efficacy of this approach.

Economics
Losses accrue not only from deaths involving indigenous breeds but also from limitations to the importation of desirable genetics in other sheep breeds.

Welfare implications
Respiratory distress associated with the more severe presentation of the disease raises obvious welfare concerns; however, these issues are tempered by problems arising from famine and other natural disasters in these areas of the world.

LYME DISEASE

Definition/overview
Lyme disease is a rare tick-transmitted infection of large mammals including sheep, cattle, horses, deer and man. Lyme disease is only of concern because of the remote zoonotic risk.

Aetiology
Lyme disease is caused by the spirochaete *Borrelia burgdorferi* and transmitted by *Ixodes* species ticks.

Clinical presentation
Few, if any, clinical signs have been attributed to Lyme disease; seroconversion has been reported without any ill health. It has been suggested that Lyme disease can give rise to arthritis in lambs. Infection of tick (*I. ricinus*) feeding sites with bacteria, commonly *Staphylococcus aureus*, results in large subcutaneous abscesses and, often, bacteraemia with localization within joints leading to septic joints.

Differential diagnoses
The more common causes of outbreaks of polyarthritis include *Streptococcus dysgalactiae* and *Erysipelas rhusiopathiae*, which can be differentiated on clinical examination and bacteriology of synovial fluid or joint capsule.

Diagnosis
Clinical signs are rarely recognized; seroconversion typically occurs without overt disease.

Treatment
Treatment is not necessary.

Prevention/control measures
Tick control is operated on most farms for the much more important tick-transmitted diseases tick-borne fever and tick pyaemia.

Economics
Lyme disease presents no economic concerns.

Welfare implications
The disease is largely asymptomatic and presents no welfare concerns as recognized to date.

CLINICAL PROBLEM 1

In early autumn a farmer reports the loss of two Blackface gimmers within three weeks of grazing poor hill pasture. The farmer had noted no signs of illness before the death of either gimmer.

What common conditions could cause sudden death in these gimmers?

Differential diagnoses

- Clostridial disease: pulpy kidney disease, blackleg, black disease, braxy.
- Acute fasciolosis.
- Pasteurellosis or other septicaemic disease possibly secondary to tick-borne fever.
- Louping ill.
- Abdominal catastrophe such as volvulus of the abomasum or small intestine.
- Poisoning such as nitrate or ammonia.

Postmortem examination

No ticks were present on the carcases. Postmortem examination revealed multiple haemorrhagic tracts within the liver caused by migrating flukes. No volvulus was detected. The kidneys appeared friable but the gimmers had been dead for approximately 24 hours in 16–18°C daytime temperatures. A urinary dipstick test was negative for glucose. No other abnormalities were found in the carcase. A provisional diagnosis of acute fasciolosis was reached.

Advice

The farmer was advised to remove the sheep from the pasture and treat them with triclabendazole immediately and again with a flukacide in two months' time. More frequent treatment with triclabendazole would be necessary if the new pasture could not be guaranteed free of fluke. The wet areas of the field should either be drained or fenced off.

CLINICAL PROBLEM 2

In mid-winter an 11-month-old Greyface hogg is presented in very poor bodily condition (BCS 1). The farmer reports that many of the group of 98 hoggs are in poor condition (BCS 1.5) despite being lightly stocked on permanent grass supplemented with hay. The farmer reports that the hoggs had been treated with oxfendazole three months previously.

What conditions should be considered?

Clinical examination

The hogg was dull, depressed and emaciated. The rectal temperature was normal. There was obvious pallor of the mucous membranes. Auscultation of the heart and lungs failed to reveal any abnormalities. There was little rumen fill but normal contractions were heard. No other abnormalities were found during clinical examination.

Differential diagnoses

- Chronic internal parasitism, especially trichostrongylosis.
- Chronic fasciolosis.
- Cobalt deficiency.
- Poor grazing/poor hay quality.

Diagnosis

A provisional diagnosis of fasciolosis was based on the clinical examination and epidemiology; the hoggs had been grazing poor pasture during the autumn months.

Laboratory tests

Routine haematological examination revealed a profound anaemia (PCV 0.07 l/l; total RBC count 1.0×10^{12}/l; Hb 20 g/l). The RBCs showed anisocytosis, poikilocytosis and polychromasia. The WBC count was raised at 12.0×10^{9}/l.

The serum GGT concentration was raised at 97 U/l. There was a profound hypoalbuminaemia (9.9 g/l) and increased globulin concentration (60.9 g/l).

A faecal sample from the hogg revealed 1,200 strongyle epg and a fluke egg count of 350 epg; both values are significant. A pooled faecal nematode egg count from ten sheep in the group revealed 800 strongyle epg, and the fluke egg count was 150 epg.

Postmortem examination

The following day a hogg is found dead in the field and is presented for postmortem examination. The carcase is in very poor bodily condition. On skinning, the carcase appears jaundiced. The contents of the chest are unremarkable. The gall bladder has ruptured releasing many mature liver flukes into the abdominal cavity. The liver is enlarged, very friable and bronzed. Cut sections reveal large number of mature flukes.

Outcome

The hoggs were treated with a combined fluke (oxyclozanide) and worm (levamisole) drench. Triclabendazole could have been used as the flukacide but it is considerably more expensive and was thought unnecessary because all the flukes present would be mature. It was recommended that the hoggs should also be treated with a flukacide three and seven months later. The farmer was advised that it was unlikely the hoggs would increase in body condition without supplementary feeding. The farmer fed 250 g of concentrates per head daily as recommended throughout the winter period. At clipping time the hoggs were in very good condition but this had only been achieved by a much higher level of supplementary feeding than usual.

Fencing off wet areas is rarely affordable on many extensive units. Whilst farmers may be tempted to cut costs by not drenching for fluke, the consequences can be considerable.

CLINICAL PROBLEM 3

During late summer a client complains of poor growth in a large group of homebred fattening lambs that had been weaned four weeks ago (**639**). A large number of the lambs show signs of diarrhoea (**640**). The fleeces of some of the lambs are so severely contaminated with faeces that they have had to be dagged.

The pasture has been grazed by ewes and lambs all season (and the previous two years). An anthelmintic was administered when the lambs first showed signs of scouring three weeks ago. The farmer has used a white drench anthelmintic (1-BZ benzimidazoles) for the past five years.

What are the common causes of ill thrift in growing lambs?
How could this problem be investigated?
What control measures should be advised?

Common causes of ill thrift in groups of lambs

- Poor nutrition of ewe, lamb, or both, due to either overstocking or poor pasture management.
- Parasitic gastroenteritis.
- Trace element deficiency (e.g. cobalt or selenium deficiency).
- Virulent footrot.
- Earlier disease episodes leading to poor growth could include coccidiosis and nematodirosis.

Trace element deficiency and virulent footrot may well exacerbate the effects of parasitic gastroenteritis with respect to weight loss and poor performance.

Further investigations

A provisional diagnosis of parasitic gastroenteritis was based on the clinical findings and flock management history. Faeces were collected from six diarrhoeic lambs. The geometric mean faecal egg count was 3,200 epg (range 1,200–4,400 epg): 400 epg = low, 400–1,000 = moderate, >1,000 epg = high.

The high faecal egg count in itself does not indicate benzimidazole resistance; the situation could have simply arisen as a consequence of ill-timed treatment(s). Under the circumstances, testing for the presence of benzimidazole-resistant nematode strains would be prudent. The six lambs were identified for re-sampling in ten days.

Action

The six sampled lambs were weighed and drenched with a benzimidazole anthelmintic. The farmer was instructed to collect faeces from these lambs in ten days and submit them to the surgery.

639 Poor condition in a group of homebred fattening lambs.

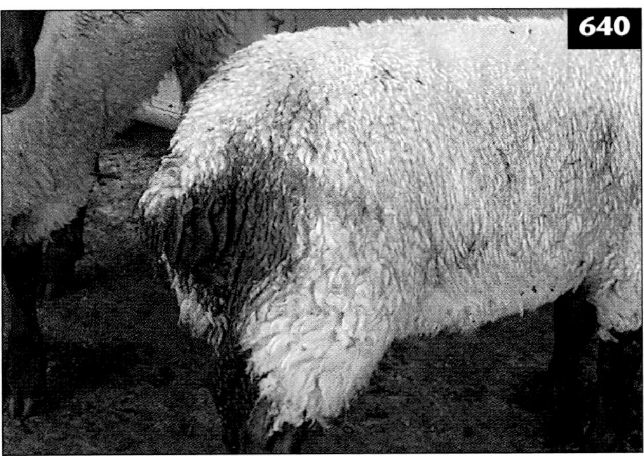

640 A large number of the lambs show signs of diarrhoea.

The remaining lambs in the group were drenched with levamisole that contained a cobalt supplement. The cost of supplementing the whole group with oral cobalt sulphate is much cheaper than assaying serum vitamin B_{12} estimations (30 times less expensive), and can be of doubtful clinical significance anyway.

The lambs were turned on to a field that had been grazed by cattle only since turnout; there was no clean grazing on this farm. The lambs were treated with a topical synthetic pyrethroid preparation to prevent cutaneous myiasis.

Drenching with levamisole containing a cobalt supplement was recommended again in four weeks.

Control

In the absence of a clean grazing system (arable crop/cattle/sheep, rotated annually), parasitic gastroenteritis is controlled by grazing management and strategic anthelmintic treatment to prevent a massive build-up of larvae on the pasture, which can infest susceptible lambs.

Lambs on pasture grazed by lambs during the previous season should be treated with an anthelmintic based on the forecast regarding *N. battus* infestation. Thereafter, the lambs should be re-treated every four weeks until weaning with either levamisole or a benzimadazole anthelmintic (check for resistance in this case) or an avermectin/milbemycin preparation. There is little advantage to be gained from frequent anthelmintic treatments once there has been massive pasture contamination with infective larvae, as has occurred in this case.

Outcome

The diarrhoea stopped almost immediately after drenching. The faecal egg reduction test in the six lambs resulted in a 95% reduction in the counts taken ten days after benzimidazole treatment, implicating mismanagement rather than anthelmintic resistance in this situation. There was a gradual improvement in the lambs' condition over the next ten weeks.

15 Anaesthesia

INTRODUCTION

There are relatively few procedures in sheep that require general anaesthesia. The most common surgical procedures such as caesarean section, vasectomy and digit amputation are generally undertaken using local flank infiltration, spinal analgesia and intravenous regional anaesthesia, respectively. However, in almost all situations the quality of pain management could be improved without adding significantly to the cost of the procedure.

PAIN MANAGEMENT

There are presently few clinical data reporting the positive affects of preoperative NSAID drug administration in sheep but extrapolation from other species warrants their use, even when practice situations result in intravenous administration only 10–20 minutes prior to surgery.

In most situations surgery is undertaken on the farm and veterinarians are rarely able to monitor the sheep afterwards. Many veterinarians would change their views on pain management in sheep if they were to see their caesarean section ewe two hours after surgery. In almost all situations, pain relief should be administered routinely for three days after major surgery. Such medication should not add considerably (approximately 3.0%) to the final professional fee for most surgical procedures.

GENERAL ANAESTHESIA

There are occasions when general anaesthesia is necessary (e.g. abdominal surgery, eye enucleation, radius/ulna fracture necessitating reduction). The problem faced by practitioners worldwide is that few products are licensed for use in sheep. In some countries a standard withdrawal period of 35 days is observed in such situations (e.g. the UK); in some countries the animals must never enter the food chain.

There are inherent risks with general anaesthesia in sheep; for example, regurgitation of rumen content with inhalation giving rise to aspiration pneumonia, and bloat compromising respiratory function and venous return to the heart.

Whenever possible it is advisable to remove concentrate feeding for 24 hours prior to any elective procedure to reduce the likelihood of excess gas production by the rumen microflora, although starvation will not have been possible in emergency situations. Whenever possible the sheep should be positioned in sternal recumbency with the head held lowered to allow drainage of saliva from the buccal cavity.

PENTOBARBITAL

In many emergency field situations there is no ready access to gaseous anaesthesia and the problem has to be dealt with in a cost-effective manner on the farm. The author has had considerable experience of pentobarbital in sheep. Pentobarbital gives acceptable levels of surgical analgesia but recovery is extended for up to two hours, during which time bloat may occur, especially if the sheep becomes cast following attempts to stand. It is acknowledged that pentobarbital is not the best anaesthetic regimen but under field situations it is has the obvious advantages that it is cheap and requires no incremental doses during an average surgery time of 20–40 minutes. Local infiltration can also be used to effect additional analgesia (e.g. a retrobulbar block for enucleation [**641**]).

The dose rate of pentobarbital is 20 mg/kg injected intravenously. Approximately two-thirds of the calculated dose is given intravenously over 20–30 seconds. The depth of anaesthesia is then determined after approximately one minute and the remaining one-third given if necessary. There is little effect of incremental doses given after this induction period. It is important that recovery is supervised until the sheep is able to stand.

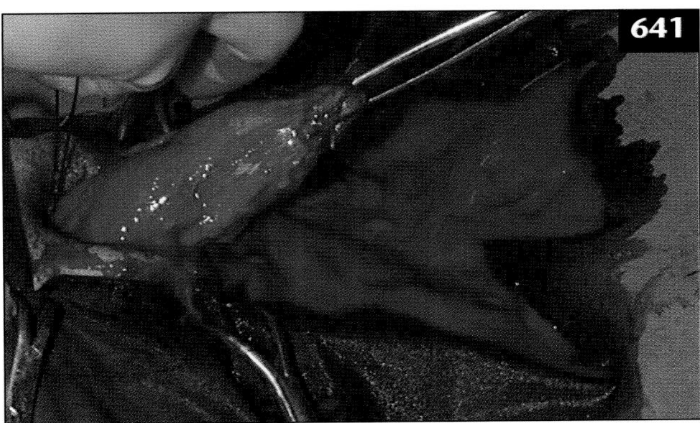

641 Enucleation of the eye performed under pentobarbital anaesthesia supplemented with a retrobulbar block.

XYLAZINE/KETAMINE

Xylazine is very unpredictable as a sedative in sheep, with considerable variation between breeds and individual animals. Poor sedative effects often result if the sheep has been stressed (e.g. gathered) prior to sedation and then isolated in a pen. Whenever possible the sheep to be anaesthetized should be sedated in a pen next to other sheep, with direct vision, if not direct contact, to reduce unnecessary stresses.

Xylazine is best given intramuscularly at a dose rate of 0.05–0.07 mg/kg. Sedation should result within ten minutes but can be very variable. Induction of anaesthesia is then achieved by intravenous injection of 10 mg/kg ketamine, which affords 10–15 minutes surgical anaesthesia. Anaesthesia can be extended following incremental doses of 2–3 mg/kg ketamine intravenously, which give a further ten minutes' surgical anaesthesia.

ALPHAXALONE/ALPHADOLONE COMBINATION

Alphaxalone/alphadolone combination at 2.2–4.4 mg/kg intravenously is very safe in sheep but its short duration of only a few minutes restricts its use to an induction agent when employed in adult sheep. Surgical anaesthesia can then be maintained using halothane or isoflurane and nitrous oxide/oxygen after intubation.

The duration of surgical anaesthesia is longer in neonatal lambs (up to ten minutes after a single injection of 4.4 mg/kg intravenously) where it is the anaesthetic of choice for forelimb fracture reduction and short surgical procedures (e.g. intestine replacement through the umbilicus).

SEDATION WITH XYLAZINE AND LOCAL INFILTRATION WITH LIDOCAINE

Sedation with xylazine and local infiltration with lidocaine is used by some practitioners for some surgical procedures in sheep (e.g. vasectomy), though in this situation lumbosacral extradural lidocaine injection is the better option.

Sedation can be effected in sheep with xylazine (0.05 mg/kg i/m) but care must be undertaken when measuring such small volumes. Alternatively, the 2% xylazine solution can be diluted in distilled water for greater accuracy. During preparation for vasectomy, infiltration of the spermatic cord with 2% lidocaine solution may accidentally result in injection into the pampiniform plexus. Furthermore, it proves difficult to block the noxious stimuli generated when traction is applied to each vas deferens.

CAUDAL ANALGESIA

Effective caudal analgesia is essential before replacement of vaginal, uterine (**642**) and rectal prolapses.

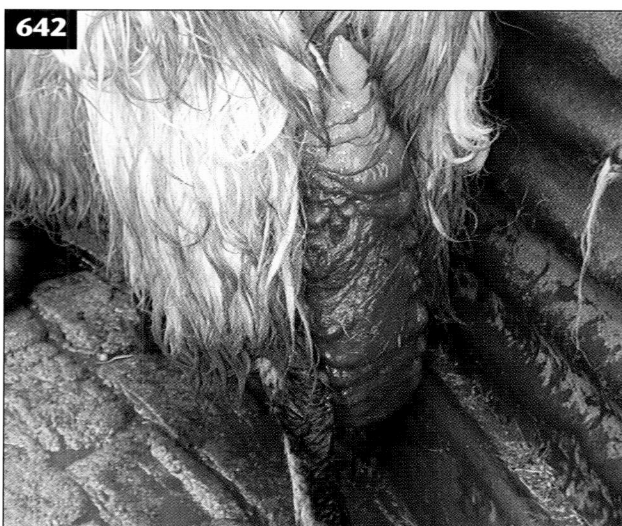

642 Effective caudal analgesia is essential before replacement of a uterine prolapse.

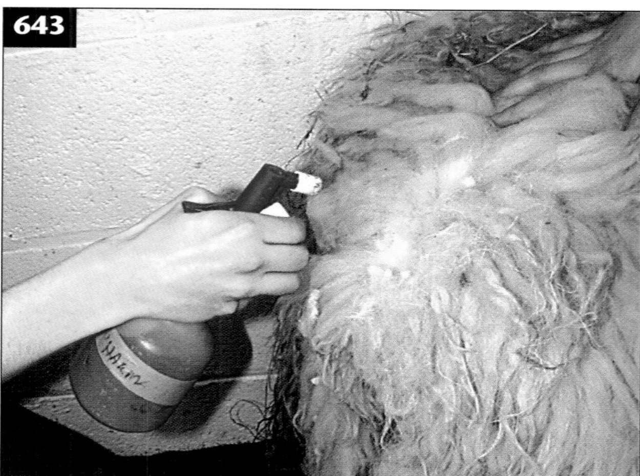

643 The area over the tailhead should be clipped and surgically prepared.

Sacrococcygeal extradural injection

Sacrococcygeal extradural injection is much more easily undertaken in standing sheep than in sheep in sternal recumbency. The area over the tailhead is clipped and surgically prepared (**643**). The first intercoccygeal space can be identified by digital palpation during slight vertical movement of the tail, and a 25 mm 20 gauge needle is directed at 10–20° to the tail, which can either be held horizontally (**644**) or in such a position that the needle point is introduced parallel to the vertebral canal (i.e. in the standing ewe the needle is introduced horizontally). Some veterinarians prefer to use 18 gauge needles for the extradural injection.

Correct position of the point of the needle can be determined by failure to strike bone during travel of the needle point, and lack of resistance to injection of the combined lidocaine and xylazine solution. It is not possible to identify when the point of the needle enters the extradural space by the hanging drop technique because of the shallow angle of the needle. A 40 mm needle may be necessary in sheep >85 kg body weight with high body condition scores (>3.5).

Combined extradural injection of xylazine and lidocaine

Combined extradural injection of xylazine and lidocaine (0.07 mg/kg and 0.5 mg/kg, respectively) at the first intercoccygeal site provides effective analgesia, permitting replacement of rectal, cervical or uterine prolapses after 5–10 minutes, and manipulation of lambs in cases of dystocia. In practical terms, 2 ml of 2% lidocaine and 0.25 ml of 2% xylazine are mixed in the same syringe to administer to adult ewes with live weight ranges from 65–80 kg. A correspondingly reduced volume is used in sheep with live weights from 35–60 kg.

There is loss of tail tone and sensation of the perineum within two minutes of successful sacrococcygeal extradural injection but ten minutes should elapse before vaginal prolapse replacement is attem-pted. It may prove difficult to appreciate loss of tail tone in short-docked breeds and in ewes near full-term where there is considerable slackening of the sacrococcygeal ligaments; therefore, sensation of the tail/anus/vulva should be checked before attempting prolapse replacement.

Inadvertent injection of the combined xylazine and lidocaine solution at the dose rates above into fascia and tissues surrounding the sacrococcygeal or first intercoccygeal site results in mild sedation of the sheep (**645**) for 2–3 hours. If this happens, the sacrococcygeal extradural injection should be attempted again but using only lidocaine. This will avoid further sedation if the second injection also proves unsuccessful. Accidental injection of xylazine at dose rates above 0.07 mg/kg could cause bradycardia and respiratory depression. In some

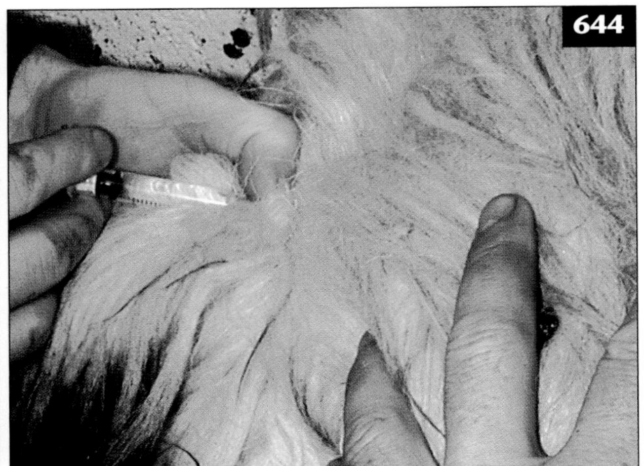

644 The needle is directed at 10–20° to the tail, which can either be held almost horizontally or in such a position that the needle is introduced parallel to the vertebral canal (i.e. in the standing ewe the needle is introduced horizontally).

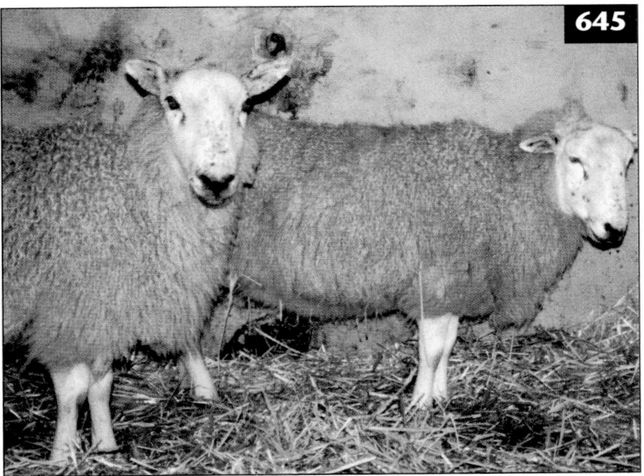

645 Injection of combined xylazine and lidocaine solution into tissue surrounding the sacrococcygeal site causing mild sedation.

sheep mild hindlimb paresis may persist for up to 48 hours after extradural injection (**646**), with periods spent in sternal recumbency (**647**), but these ewes can stand unaided.

Sacrococcygeal extradural xylazine injection

Xylazine, an alpha-2 adrenergic agonist drug, injected into the sacrococcygeal extradural space has been used successfully in cattle, horses, llamas and sheep to provide surgical analgesia of the perineal region, with advantages of extended duration analgesia and less affect on motor innervation compared with lidocaine. In contrast to its effect in cattle, llamas and horses, extradural xylazine does not cause significant sedation in sheep when used at a dose rate of 0.07 mg/kg, and caudal analgesia may extend to 36–48 hours after injection.

While caesarean section can be undertaken in ewes under field infiltration with lidocaine, there are concerns regarding the welfare of the ewe (e.g. when vaginal prolapse has occurred [**648**]) and where there are complicating factors present that necessitate considerable handling during surgery to exteriorize the uterine horn prior to incision (e.g. fetal monster, uterine tear).

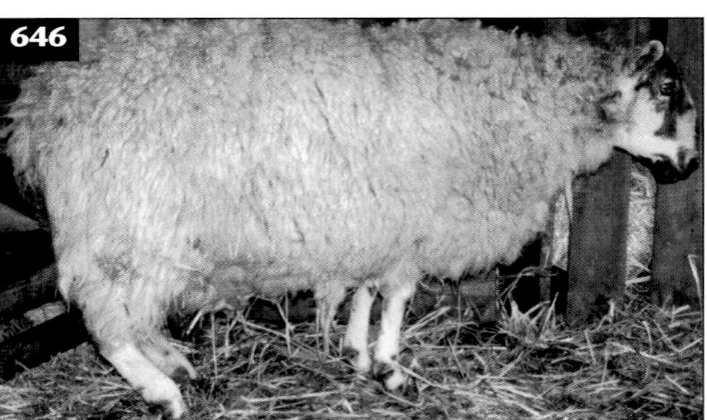

646 Hindlimb weakness after combined xylazine and lidocaine at the sacrococcygeal site.

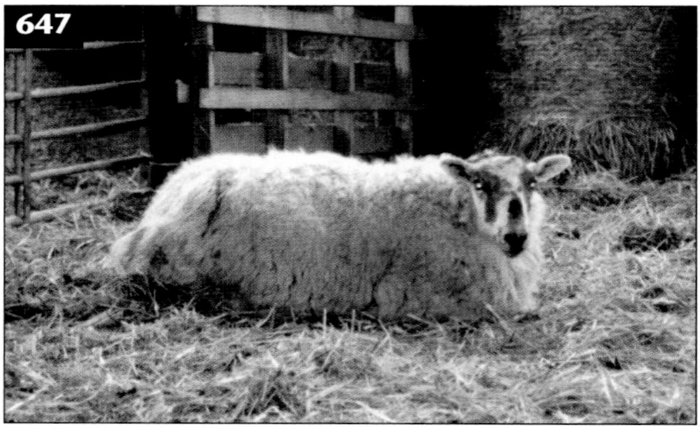

647 Sternal recumbency after combined xylazine and lidocaine at the sacrococcygeal site.

When tested by needle prick 40–50 minutes after injection, analgesia of the flank was present in 12 of 13 ewes and eight of nine ewes following either sacrococcygeal or lumbosacral extradural xylazine injection (0.07 mg/kg to a volume of 2.5 ml), respectively. For welfare reasons the precise interval to onset of surgical analgesia after extradural injection was not determined in this study. Instead, the interval of 40–50 minutes between extradural injection and surgery exceeded the interval to onset of flank analgesia in cattle, perineal skin analgesia in llamas or presence of hindlimb ataxia in sheep after sacrococcygeal injection at a similar xylazine dose rate. As there is no advantage of lumbosacral over sacrococcygeal administration of xylazine, the sacrococcygeal route is recommended because it is the easier technique (see Sacrococcygeal extradural injection).

The minimum 40-minute interval between extradural injection and surgery renders this analgesic impractical for use on farms for caesarean sections. However, it may have potential use in situations where ewes with dystocia are brought to the surgery and other tasks can be undertaken during this interval. For example, when presented with a ewe with dystocia the veterinarian gives a combined extradural injection of xylazine and lidocaine (0.07 mg/kg and 0.5 mg/kg, respectively; see above) at the first intercoccygeal site to provide effective analgesia and permit manipulation of the lamb(s). If, after a brief examination, a caesarean section is deemed necessary, the sheep has already been injected with extradural xylazine. An assistant can then prepare the sheep for surgery while the veterinarian does other work before returning to perform the operation. In all cases the xylazine component of the extradural injection will afford 36–48 hours caudal analgesia after administration.

It is reported that sacrococcygeal injection of 0.4 mg/kg xylazine produces sedation and sufficient

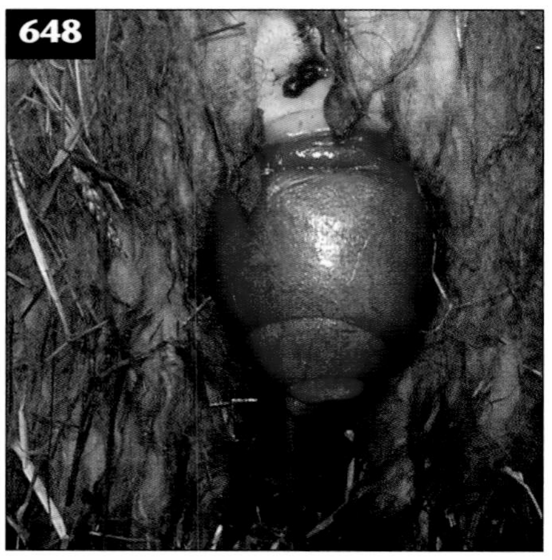

648 Vaginal prolapse during first stage labour.

analgesia for vasectomy without the disadvantage of the hindlimb paralysis associated with extradural lidocaine injection, although individual sheep may exhibit mild paresis for up to 48 hours after injection. Sedation may be marked for up to one hour after extradural xylazine injection at 0.4 mg/kg, with the sheep assuming sternal recumbency with the head rested on the ground.

Experience with this technique to date has sometimes demonstrated marked short duration sedation as outlined above but good to excellent surgical analgesia, although the traction required to remove 4–6 cm of vas deferens and placement of the proximal ligature may cause minor reaction with brief movement of the hindlimbs for up to five seconds while traction is applied. Post surgery the sheep often prefer to remain in sternal recumbency for up to two hours or so but many are able to stand. In some sheep, mild hindlimb paresis may persist for up to 48 hours after injection.

In the author's experience, sheep undergoing this procedure eat enthusiastically within one hour of return to the recovery pen, having had food withheld for 12 hours prior to surgery. The sedation observed at around 15–30 minutes after extradural xylazine injection may at first appear profound but no adverse effects have been observed. This analgesic protocol has the disadvantage of a 30–40 minutes delay between sacrococcygeal extradural injection and surgery; however, two or three sheep can be injected at the same time as surgical analgesia persists for at least two hours, and probably longer.

The duration of spinal analgesia after extradural xylazine injection has yet to be defined but extrapolation from the clinical situation of vaginal and rectal prolapses in sheep suggests that pain relief may be present for 24 hours or longer. Extradural injection at the sacrococcygeal site is easier to perform than at the lumbosacral site in most sheep, especially large fat rams.

The use of extradural xylazine injection does not preclude the use of preoperative injection with an NSAID such as flunixin meglumine (1.1–2.2 mg/kg); indeed, such a combined approach is likely to be additive in terms of analgesia. Neither xylazine nor flunixin are licensed for use in sheep in many countries and a standard withdrawal period before slaughter for human consumption must be strictly observed (35 days in UK but may be longer in other countries).

Lumbosacral extradural lidocaine injection

Excellent analgesia of the flank for caesarean section, and for vasectomy and hindlimb surgery, can be achieved after lumbosacral extradural injection of 4 mg/kg of 2% lidocaine solution. The sheep can be sedated with xylazine (0.05 mg/kg i/m) to facilitate

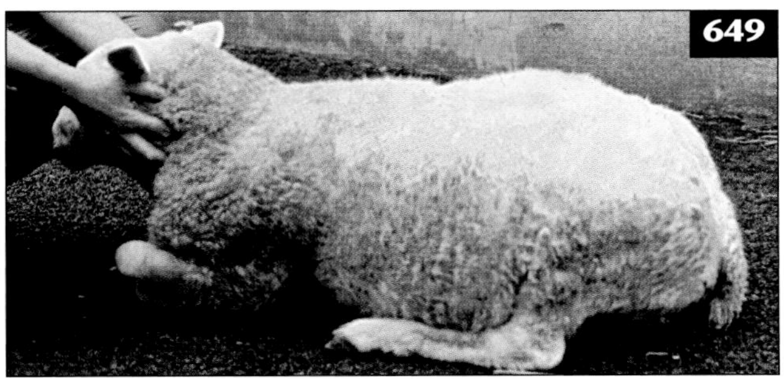

649 Sheep positioned in sternal recumbency for lumbosacral extradural injection. The head is then averted against the chest by an assistant and the hindlimbs drawn forward.

positioning for extradural injection but this is not recommended because the sheep can be adequately restrained in sternal recumbency by an assistant (**649**). The head is averted against the sheep's chest by an assistant and the hindlimbs drawn forward.

This analgesic regimen is also recommended when there is either considerable trauma to the posterior reproductive tract, a fetal monster *in utero* or a concurrent traumatized vaginal prolapse resulting in tenesmus. The ewe must be adequately restrained in sternal recumbency by an assistant to facilitate extradural injection. The lidocaine solution is warmed to body temperature prior to injection. The large volume of 2% lidocaine solution (16 ml for a 80 kg ewe) should be injected slowly over 30–60 seconds with the needle hub firmly anchored between thumb and index finger. The ewe is held in left lateral recumbency with the head elevated for approximately ten minutes after injection, during which time there is onset of hindlimb paralysis. During surgery via the left flank approach the ewe's head should remain elevated relative to the vertebral column. To prevent hypothermia and overlying, lambs delivered by caesarean section must be given colostrum by orogastric tube immediately and placed under a heat lamp or in a warming box until the ewe is ambulatory.

If the point of the needle accidentally punctures the arachnoid mater, CSF will appear within the needle hub. In this event the needle should be withdrawn into the extradural space and the calculated dose rate reduced to two-thirds as a precautionary measure. Further reduction of the dose rate may fail to achieve complete analgesia of the flank. Sheep should be confined to small well-bedded pens until ambulatory, which is usually 2–4 hours after extradural injection. Unfortunately, the duration of hindlimb paralysis after injection and the requirement for precise injection technique has resulted in few veterinarians adopting the lumbosacral extradural lidocaine regimen for potentially difficult caesarean sections.

16 Miscellaneous Diseases

BLUETONGUE

Definition/overview

The geographic distribution of bluetongue is dependent on the *Culicoides* species host and, in the past, was restricted to the African continent. However, bluetongue is now also widespread within the USA, and outbreaks are occasionally reported in southern Europe following introduction from Africa. An outbreak in Holland in summer 2006 highlights an increased risk of its further introduction into northern continental Europe and into the UK, where summer temperatures in southern England are sufficient to support the *Culicoides* species vector. Bluetongue virus has also been identified in Australia but is not associated with overt disease in sheep.

Aetiology

Bluetongue is caused by an arthropod-borne reovirus. Virus may also be transmitted inadvertently by contaminated needles during a vaccination programme.

Clinical presentation

The clinical signs, which vary depending on viral strain and sheep breed, follow an incubation period of 4–12 days. Only a small percentage of viraemic sheep may develop clinical signs. Affected sheep are pyrexic (up to 42.0°C) and appear stiff and very reluctant to move. They often adopt a roached back stance with the neck extended and the head held lowered. There is oedema of the face and ears, and also pulmonary oedema, which may cause dys- pnoea. Erosions may appear on the lips and progress to ulcers. There is often profuse salivation and a serous to mucopurulent nasal discharge. There may be hyperaemia of the coronary band and around the muzzle and mouth. The tongue may become swollen and oedematous and appear cyanotic.

Bluetongue infection during the breeding season may result in a large percentage of early embryonic losses, with sheep returning to oestrus at irregular intervals. Viral infection during early gestation may result in central nervous system defects such as hydranencephaly.

Differential diagnoses

Differential diagnoses include:

- Foot and mouth disease.
- Contagious pustular dermatitis.
- Photosensitizaton including outbreaks of facial eczema.
- Peste des petits ruminants.

Diagnosis

Diagnosis is based on clinical signs, virus isolation and/or seroconversion to bluetongue virus.

Treatment

There is no specific treatment. Antibiotics could be used to treat secondary infections.

Prevention/control measures

Control of bluetongue is very difficult because of the large number of potential hosts and virus serotypes. While control is aimed at keeping susceptible animals away from the vector, this is not always practical. Control of the *Culicoides* species vector can be attempted with pour-on insecticides but this is expensive and does not achieve total freedom from the midge. Co-grazing sheep with cattle affords some protection, as midges feed preferentially on cattle.

Vaccines are used extensively worldwide. Most modified live vaccines produce a viraemia in the vaccinated animal, which affords the opportunity for further spread. Problems may arise with viral reassortment if viraemic animals are vaccinated with a modified live vaccine. The timing of vaccination will depend on local factors, in particular the occurrence of high-risk periods. In certain areas, lambing time may be changed so that waning of passively derived antibody does not coincide with *Culicoides* species activity.

Economics

Bluetongue virus infection has an enormous impact on sheep production in many countries on the African continent and elsewhere. Losses result primarily from mortality, reduced production during protracted convalescence, including poor wool growth, and reduced reproductive performance, including temporary ram infertility.

Welfare implications

Mortality and protracted convalescence with susceptibility to secondary bacterial infections do raise welfare concerns but these may need to be tempered with respect to the impact of bluetongue disease on the agriculture-based community in developing countries.

FOOT AND MOUTH DISEASE

Definition/overview

Foot and mouth disease (FMD) does not occur in Australia, New Zealand or North America because of the very strict quarantine regulations for livestock and strict meat import restrictions. FMD is endemic in many parts of Africa and occurs sporadically in Asia. FMD was reported throughout the UK in 2001.

Aetiology

FMD is caused by a picornavirus that is highly contagious to cattle, sheep and pigs. Disease can be spread readily by aerosol and mechanical vectors. In the UK the widespread dispersal of sheep through markets resulted in rapid distribution of the virus in 2001 FMD epidemic.

Clinical presentation

The author witnessed FMD in sheep during the 2001 epidemic in the UK. The clinical findings observed are described below.

A shepherd suspected FMD when four out of 120 ewes became acutely lame and unable to stand. These ewes could not walk to the feed troughs. The remaining ewes ate less than one half of their concentrate ration that morning. The flock had just started lambing and ten ewes had lambed in the previous four days. Examination of the four ewes revealed severe lameness on all four feet. The ewes were reluctant to stand such that two of the ewes were easily caught where they lay in sternal recumbency. The other two ewes were easily shepherded into a corner of the field. All four ewes showed pyrexia >41.5°C and had not been stressed before being caught. All the ewes had an increased respiratory rate but no abnormal sounds on auscultation of the chest. Examination revealed hyperaemia of the interdigital skin and slight swelling around the coronary band. Two ewes had large vesicles measuring up to 15 mm diameter at the coronary band. There were some small punctate erosions (2–3 mm in diameter) on the dental pad in all four ewes but no lesions on the tongue. Samples were collected from the coronary band vesicles for virus isolation; these subsequently proved positive for FMD.

Four out of 12 lambs were found dead in the lambing field. The lambs were aged from 1–4 days old and were well fleshed. Postmortem examination failed to reveal an obvious cause of death; death was not the result of starvation/exposure or of any of the infectious bacterial diseases common in neonatal lambs.

Differential diagnoses

- The combination of pyrexia and sudden onset of severe lameness with vesicle formation should eliminate other common causes of lameness such as virulent footrot.
- Post-dipping lameness can be ruled out by the clinical examination and the history of the sheep not being recently plunge dipped.
- Pyrexia is not uncommon in sheep when gathering takes more than 30 minutes. During the 2001 epidemic in the UK many flocks were falsely diagnosed as having FMD on the basis of pyrexia alone. Chronic lesions present in the mouths of some sheep can readily be differentiated from FMD by their deep-fissured appearance, paucity and distribution on the dental pad only.
- Sudden death in lambs could be caused by lamb dysentery or septicaemic pasteurellosis and during adverse weather condition. White muscle disease affecting the myocardium causes only sporadic losses.

Diagnosis

Diagnosis is based on clinical signs and confirmed by virus isolation. Retrospective confirmation can be obtained following seroconversion in acute and convalescent samples.

Treatment

Compulsory slaughter of suspected outbreaks of FMD operates in many countries including the UK.

Prevention/control measures

Prevention on a national basis involves strict quarantine of imported livestock. On a farm basis, greatly improved biosecurity is necessary on all farms.

National control schemes

Strict regulations regarding importation of animals, meat and meat products operate in many countries. In the UK, for example, a compulsory slaughter and compensation policy operated during the 2001 epidemic. Other countries have operated a ring vaccination policy to control spread of infection, with subsequent slaughter of all vaccinated cattle.

Economics

Outbreaks of FMD can have serious economic consequences. For example, the 2001 epidemic in the UK cost the Treasury in excess of £2 billion.

Welfare implications

There are no special welfare implications from the disease itself and cattle and sheep do recover from infection, albeit with a protracted convalescence. However, movement restrictions, such as those enforced in the UK in 2001, can cause welfare problems because, for example, cattle and sheep can not be moved across roads or transported home.

PESTE DES PETITS RUMINANTS AND RINDERPEST

Definition/overview

Peste des petits ruminants (PPR) occurs in equatorial Africa, extending into Egypt and, more recently, India and Pakistan. It is not possible to differentiate clinical signs of acute PPR from acute rinderpest. Rinderpest/PPR is not present in the main sheep-producing countries, including Europe, North America, Australia and New Zealand, where strict import controls prevent their introduction.

Aetiology

PPR and rinderpest are caused by a paramyxovirus (genus Morbillivirus). PPR is much more important than rinderpest in sheep and goats. Infection is spread via aerosol.

Clinical presentation

The clinical signs are highly variable, with Indian isolates of PPR causing severe disease in sheep. Susceptible sheep show severe clinical disease with pyrexia (41°C), depression, profuse salivation and serous ocular and nasal discharges that rapidly become purulent. The mucous membranes are congested. There are erosions in the nasal passages and buccal cavity, which coalesce and may ulcerate. There is profuse fetid diarrhoea with occasional colic signs. Affected sheep develop pneumonia with associated dyspnoea. Inability to eat or drink gives a gaunt, pitiful appearance and rapid dehydration. Severely affected sheep die within 7–10 days; those that survive have an extended convalescence but remain immune for life. Pregnant sheep frequently abort.

Clinical signs of PPR are uncommon in areas where the virus is considered to be endemic and are often restricted to mild oral lesions, diarrhoea and mild respiratory signs.

Differential diagnoses

Differential diagnoses include:

- Foot and mouth disease.
- Sheep pox.

Diagnosis

Diagnosis is based on the clinical signs. Severe disease in susceptible sheep populations causes significant losses, with typical histopathological changes in the lungs. Erosions and ulcers are identified in the buccal cavity and there is a viral-type bronchopneumonia with anteroventral consolidation. Virus can be isolated from lymphoid tissue at necropsy, including lymph nodes, Peyer's patches and spleen.

Disease occurring in endemic areas can be confirmed by seroconversion.

Treatment

In many countries affected sheep are slaughtered as part of a control/eradication programme. There is no specific treatment for PPR or rinderpest; efforts are directed to supportive therapy, including antibiotics and oral fluids.

Prevention/control measures

Disease is prevented in many countries by strict quarantine controls. Introduced disease has been eradicated from countries by compulsory slaughter of affected flocks/herds. While live attenuated rinderpest virus has been used successfully in the past, rinderpest control programmes prevent the use of this vaccine in sheep in many endemic countries.

Economics

PPR and rinderpest would have devastating effects on the livestock industry if introduced into disease-free countries; therefore; strict import controls operate.

Welfare implications

Compulsory slaughter would limit any welfare concerns should disease be introduced into many countries.

POISONINGS

Plant poisoning

Plant poisoning is uncommon when sheep are grazing enclosed pastures but it can occur when there is accidental access (rhododendron), poor grazing (bracken) or the sheep are fed exclusively on brassicas.

Prevention is based on maintaining sound perimeter fences and practising good husbandry (e.g. giving sheep ready access to good quality forages when folded on brassica crops).

Rhododendron

Rhododendron poisoning occurs sporadically following accidental access to ornamental gardens during periods of temporary starvation, typically during winter storms with deep snow. Affected sheep are weak, often unable to stand, and present with abdominal pain (bruxism and vocalization) and passive regurgitation of rumen contents. Recumbency, ruminal atony with bloat and rumen fluid around the muzzle lead to confusion with hypocalcaemia. Death can occur within hours (more typically in affected goats). Less severely affected animals recover; symptomatic treatment includes pethidine (3 mg/kg q12h) and NSAIDs.

Bracken

Bracken poisoning causing progressive retinal atrophy (bright blindness) has been described in sheep grazed on moorland for many years.

Brassicas

Toxicity problems may arise when rape, kale, stubble turnips and roots are introduced too quickly, are fed in too high proportion or are fed for too long. The common presenting feature is poor weight gain but acute deaths can occur with sudden and exclusive exposure.

The potentially toxic substances in brassicas include S-methyl-cysteine sulphoxide (precursor of the haemolytic factor), glucosinolates (goitre), nitrate (when reduced to nitrite causes methaemoglobinaemia) and oxalates.

The anaemia, which varies from mild to severe, relates directly to the amount of S-methyl-cysteine sulphoxide, which itself is dependent on variety and stage of growth. Confirmation of the diagnosis is based on demonstration of anaemia with Heinz-Ehrlich bodies. In acute toxicity there is anaemia and jaundice.

Nitrate ingestion in plants (particularly in roots) is converted into nitrite by the rumen microflora. Following absorption, nitrites combine with haemoglobin to form methaemoglobin. Clinical signs include brown mucous membranes, tachypnoea with an abdominal component, weakness progressing to recumbency, and death, which may be precipitated by forced exercise when gathered. Treatment with 10 mg/kg methylene blue injected intravenously has been described but it would present numerous logistic problems if many sheep were involved. Poisoning from ingestion of nitrogenous fertilizers is theoretically possible.

Excessive ingestion of oxalates (particularly in the leaves of beets) can induce acute oxalate poisoning with clinical signs of hypocalcaemia. Long-term ingestion of oxalates can result in deposition of insoluble calcium oxalate in the kidneys, causing chronic renal failure. Sheep should be removed from the crop and acute cases treated as for hypocalcaemia with 20–40 ml of 40% calcium borogluconate.

Inorganic poisons

Inorganic poisons tend to result from industrial pollution and often have a distinct geographical distribution (e.g. chronic lead poisoning from mine workings).

Lead poisoning

Typical features of chronic lead poisoning include chronic lameness affecting growing lambs, with brittle bones leading to multiple fractures and bone abnormalities. Diagnosis is based on lead concentrations in faeces, blood and kidney. Acute lead poisoning following ingestion of lead-based paint is possible but is rare.

Control of chronic disease is based on avoidance of mine workings and other sources of pollution. Treatment of acute cases, where recognized, involves intravenous administration of sodium calcium edetate, repeated two days later.

Appendix: Practice Newsletters

The six fact sheets below have been distributed bi-monthly to sheep clients in a veterinary practice in Scotland in the UK. They are reproduced here as an example of how sheep farmers can be informed about topical subjects and encouraged to keep regular contact with their veterinary practice. Obviously they will need to be adapted to take in to account local conditions and disease prevalence in other sheep-producing countries.

JANUARY (MID-WINTER)

The mild weather in this area until early December may result in problems with parasitic gastroenteritis, especially in store lambs grazing permanent pasture that have not been recently treated with an anthelmintic. *Trichostrongylus vitrinus* is often involved in late season outbreaks of scouring in store lambs and yearling sheep.

Fasciolosis is now common in sheep in this area and farmers must be aware of the risks of fluke infestation. Fluke infestations should now be patent, and the diagnosis can be confirmed by faecal egg counts. Treatment for fasciolosis may have been overlooked, especially if an avermectin/milbemycin product has been used for sheep scab control and displaced one of the combination drenches containing a flukacide from the parasite control programme.

After the service period many rams have lost considerable body weight and these animals should receive up to 750 g/head/day of concentrate feed to restore condition. Foot care in rams is also important at this time.

Ultrasound scanning results provide an opportunity to investigate problems of high (>5%) barren rate in the flock and to review nutrition of multigravid ewes, especially ewes carrying three or more lambs.

There has been a rapid increase in the number of ewes fed using snackers (feed dispensers pulled by a quad bike). These devices greatly facilitate feeding large numbers of ewes but the accuracy of feed delivery should be carefully monitored, especially when the same load of feed is used for two or more fields. It would be prudent to weigh the feed for one group of sheep only into the snacker, returning to the feed hopper for the next load. Alternatively, weighed feedbags can be carried on top of the snacker for the following groups of sheep. Sheep with poor molar dentition will be at a disadvantage when fed cobs compared with more conventional diets containing whole barley and sugar beet shreds etc. Speed of feed delivery must not overlook the need for diligent stock supervision, which is of paramount importance when a shepherd's responsibilities extend to flocks of more than 1,000 ewes.

MARCH (EARLY SPRING)

Ensuring appropriate lamb birth weights and plentiful colostrum accumulation at lambing cannot be overemphasized as these factors remain the major contributors to lamb vitality and ultimate survival. A veterinary visit to your farm to assess ewe nutrition during the critical last six weeks of pregnancy is the most cost-effective advice on flock health. Blood samples are analysed for dietary energy and protein supply.

Vaccination of underfed ewes may not stimulate sufficient antibody production, leaving lambs susceptible to clostridial diseases. The correct amount of vaccine has to be injected subcutaneously 2–6 weeks before the lambing date, the ewe has to mount an appropriate immune response with transfer of immunoglobulin to the udder, and the lamb has to ingest sufficient good quality colostrum within the first 18 hours of life.

Errors can occur at one or all of these important stages of the vaccination programme:

- The vaccination equipment must be sterile and accurately dispense the correct volume of vaccine. Sheep must not be vaccinated when the fleece is wet.
- Timing of the vaccination must be based on keel marks. If the mating period was extended for whatever reason (an infertile ram, for example), it may become necessary to vaccinate later served ewes 10–14 days after the main group.
- The ewe must be in good bodily condition (BCS >2.5) and be receiving an adequate plane of nutrition to mount an effective immune response. Lean, underfed ewes will not produce sufficient colostrum for multiple litters.
- If ewes are to be vaccinated with more than one vaccine (e.g. clostridial vaccine plus either erysipelas or *E. coli* vaccine) it is better to give the vaccines at least one week apart.

- The use of either bovine colostrum or proprietary colostrum supplements indicates that the level of flock nutrition is too low for the level of performance on many sheep farms. Your money would be better spent feeding the ewes correctly rather than buying such supplements.

During the lambing period we offer a free on-farm postmortem service to determine the common causes of neonatal lamb losses (remember, perinatal lamb mortality rates range from 7–25% with an average above 15%). It is usually more valuable to undertake ten gross postmortem examinations on your farm than submit various tissue samples from a single lamb for detailed laboratory examination.

It is essential that ewes are treated with an effective anthelmintic, either during late gestation or within the periparturient period, to prevent pasture contamination. Rams must also be treated with an anthelmintic during lambing time and throughout the grazing season.

MAY (EARLY SUMMER)

Outbreaks of nematodirosis present a perennial problem to young lambs grazing infested pastures during May, when strategically timed anthelmintic drenching, determined by the local climatic conditions, should be practised. This is the first anthelmintic treatment of lambs and provides a useful opportunity for farmers to weigh lambs before drenching, calculate the dose rate based on the heaviest lambs in the group, and check the calibration of the drenching gun.

Coccidiosis has been increasingly reported in young lambs at pasture over the past summers, with poor growth rates reported despite treatment. Preventive measures include regular movement of lamb creep feeders and either inclusion of a coccidiostat in the creep feed or administration of diclazuril.

Teat lesions affecting ewes are often reported by farmers during May, with orf and staphylococcal dermatitis the more common infectious causes. The latter condition responds very well to treatment with intramuscular penicillin for three consecutive days. Teat lesions invariably involve the medial aspect of the teat and are caused by the lamb's incisors during over-vigorous sucking behaviour. It is probable that poor milk yield is an important factor in the development of these lesions, which often predispose to gangrenous mastitis. Unfortunately, while intensive treatment and supportive care may save the lives of ewes suffering from gangrenous mastitis, they cannot be marketed for at least 4–6 months, if ever, and should be euthanased for welfare reasons during the peracute phase of the disease.

Interdigital dermatitis (scald) is commonly seen in lambs during May and June. While formalin footbaths are commonly used by shepherds to treat large numbers of lambs, a much better response is achieved by topical application using oxytetracycline aerosols.

Vaccination against pasteurellosis should be considered in lambs from four weeks old where problems with pneumonia have been encountered in previous years.

JULY (MID-SUMMER)

Weaning time provides an excellent opportunity for farmers to assess flock productivity. Lambing percentage means little unless all lambs turned out to pasture with their dams at two days old survive and grow well. The number of ewes that successfully rear lambs in relation to ewes put to the tup should exceed 96%. This percentage takes into account barren ewes, deaths and ewes that did not rear lambs either due to periparturient illness or poor milk supply. Ultrasound scanning figures in lowland flocks regularly exceed 205% in February, while weaning rates rarely exceed 155% in July. If these figures are correct, they highlight the need for a veterinary flock health programme on your farm.

Farmers often underestimate lamb growth rate potential. Singleton lambs in lowland flocks should reach 40 kg by 12 weeks of age; twin lambs have the potential to reach such live weights by 14 weeks. With these potential growth rates in mind, weaning weights prove a useful indicator of ewe nutrition and flock management during lactation. Ewe nutrition is the major determinant of lactation yield and, therefore, lamb growth rate. If weaning weights are disappointing, the likely cause is ewe nutrition during the first two months of gestation.

Wherever possible weaned lambs should be moved on to clean grazing (areas not grazed by sheep for the previous two seasons). Movement on to silage or hay aftermaths, following appropriate anthelmintic treatment, also removes the challenge from the mid-summer rise in infective larvae on pasture. Continuous grazing of permanent pasture is a recipe for disaster but cannot be avoided on some stock farms.

Farmers should carefully consider the use of pour-on preparations of insect growth regulators to control blowfly strike. Attention should also be given to the control of headfly lesions, which proves very difficult once the skin has been broken and poses a significant welfare problem.

Trace element deficiencies are frequently diagnosed in poorly thriven lambs at this time of year on the basis of low blood concentrations of various trace elements/related enzymes/vitamins. A dose-response trial, with say 20 or so lambs left unsupplemented, can be readily undertaken to establish the role of trace elements as a contributing factor to poor growth in lambs.

Rams must be checked for body condition score and fed accordingly to ensure body condition scores of 3.5 by October. Regular foot care is essential during the summer months. It is important that rams are not returned to the same (infected) small paddock after routine foot care. Footrot vaccination should be carefully considered for rams.

SEPTEMBER (LATE SUMMER)

Breeding replacement ewe lambs and gimmers, draft ewes and rams are purchased during September. Remember to take a cloth tape measure to the ram sales and select rams with maximum scrotal circumference values greater than 36 cm; forget about the ram's bone structure, correct ears and bold head. Scrotal circumference and, therefore, serving capacity has a high heritability, which is of critical importance, especially to the pedigree breeder.

A large number of diseases can be introduced into a flock with purchased sheep, especially draft ewes, and strict quarantine must be observed for at least one month. Treatment on arrival for sheep scab and internal parasites must be undertaken; examination for lice is important because treatment, in addition to an avermectin or milbemycin product, would be necessary. It is important to check on the vaccination status of purchased stock. Female breeding stock should be vaccinated against chlamydial abortion and toxoplasmosis.

Store lambs are also purchased during the late summer/early autumn. The vaccination status of these lambs can rarely be guaranteed and it would be prudent to commence a clostridial vaccination programme on their arrival on the farm in addition to those measures detailed above. The importance of poor nutrition prior to weaning as a cause of poor lamb growth (otherwise they would have been fat lambs months ago) must not be underestimated. It may take up to six weeks' good nutrition before weight gain can be appreciated in such lambs. Trace element deficiency as a potential contributory factor to ill thrift in these lambs can prove difficult to determine by interpretation of blood metabolites alone. As a general rule, poor quality store lambs should receive either vitamin B_{12} injection or oral cobalt supplementation on arrival, with the latter supplementation given every 2–3 weeks on at least two further occasions. Selenium status can be determined in blood samples.

All ewes should be checked for molar teeth problems and udders must be checked prior to breeding. The former group can be identified amongst those ewes with body condition scores 1–2 units less than the group average, which should be 3 or slightly higher during September. Broken mouth problems can largely be overcome by preferential feeding of high levels of concentrates during pregnancy but the trend is towards reducing concentrates and making greater use of silage and other forages, such that these sheep are at risk from twin lamb disease.

The provision of a good grass sward for up to one month before mating (flushing) is a farming tradition that may be difficult to justify with the trend towards lower concentrate inputs during late gestation. Improved nutrition to increase ovulation rate and embryo implantation rate makes physiological sense, but take a careful look at your orphan lambs and you will see that the majority rarely reach slaughter weights before Christmas. On many farms rearing orphans lambs is a chore and rarely are these lambs well managed. It should also be remembered that triplet-bearing ewes are more prone to pregnancy toxaemia, vaginal prolapse and rupture of the prepubic tendon. Compare your scanning rates in February (often 205% for lowland flocks) to weaning rates (often 155%) and then ask do you really need these lambs that simply die? Reducing perinatal mortality is much more important than producing even more 3 kg triplet lambs on a cold wet March night to a ewe with insufficient milk. Flushing ensures good ewe body condition scores at mating but this can be achieved by other means.

Prophylactic treatment for acute fluke using triclabendazole may be necessary on some farms in October and again 4–6 weeks later.

NOVEMBER (EARLY WINTER)

The reproductive capacity of sheep is often greatly underestimated. The first service conception rate target should exceed 95%. There are many advantages to a system of using three rams per 100–120 ewes in lowland and upland situations compared with one ram to 30–40 ewes. These include more multiple services, which increases ovulation and fertilization rates and litter size, and compensation for a ram of reduced fertility. Groups of rams should be rotated after 17 days and all rams removed after five weeks (two oestrous cycles). Ewes lambing during May invariably have large singletons. At the same time, supervision is often limited to 6–8 hourly intervals with consequent dystocia problems. These late lambs never thrive and it may prove more beneficial to sell such ewes at scanning during February when cull prices are at a seasonal high. Sheep that do not breed should be culled and not given a second opportunity next season. A compact lambing period allows more efficient use of seasonal labour and reduces disease build-up over the shorter lambing period.

Brisket sores caused by ill fitting harnesses are all too common in rams; keel paint prevents such problems and more clearly identifies correct ram service behaviour. Daily feeding of all rams is essential to prevent excessive loss of condition, and it also gives an opportunity for the keel paint to be replenished. Veterinary examination of ram(s) is indicated when more than 20% of ewes return to service. Rams must be rested for a minimum of five days before attempting semen collection.

It is common practice to administer an anthelmintic to ewes immediately prior to the mating period. Late season anthelmintic treatment may be necessary in areas where mild autumn weather has resulting in large numbers of infective *Trichostrongylus vitrinus* larvae on pasture. Re-treatment of sheep with triclabendazole to kill immature fluke may be indicated on certain farms. Black disease may result in unvaccinated stock, especially store lambs.

Store lambs must be treated with an anthelmintic before turning on to crops such as kale and stubble turnips. Mountain breeds are especially susceptible to acidosis and concentrates must be slowly introduced in to the ration. Careful hoof inspection of all store lambs and appropriate treatment prior to housing significantly reduces problems caused by footrot during the 6–8 week intensive fattening period.

Index

Note: Page numbers in **bold** refer to major discussions of a topic

abdomen
  disorders **109–18**
  examination **100–2**, 103
abdominal contractions, reflex 40–1
abdominal distension
  ascites 158, 159, 163, 164, 304
  differential diagnoses 112
  in lambs 89, 90, 117
abdominocentesis 95, **101**, 159, 164
abomasum
  bloat **113**
  emptying defect **113–14**
  lamb postmortem examination 96
  palpation in neonate 86
  ulceration 136
  ultrasonography 102, 103
abortion 33, **60–9**
  border disease **67–8**
  Brucella **68–9**
  Campylobacter **66–7**
  causes 60, 61
  chlamydial 31, **60–2**
  in OPT 280, 286
  salmonella **64–6**
  sample collection 60
  toxoplasmosis **62–4**
abscess
  actinobacillosis 107
  brain **173–4**
  liver 94, 102
  lung/pleura 106, 107, 140, **151–3**, 156–9
  pharynx **108–9**
  scrotum 76–7
  subcutaneous **248–9**
  udder 156, 157, 274–5
  white line **207–8**
accreditation
  C. abortus 62
  MVV 151
acidosis **109–12**, 129
actinobacillosis **107**, 247
Actinobacillus lignieresi 107
Actinobacillus seminis/H. ovis 76, 79
Actinomyces bovis 108
actinomycosis **108**
adenocarcinoma, intestinal **114–15**
adhesions
  abdominal 102, 103, 115, 136
  thoracic 159
agalactia, contagious **277**
allantochorion 37–8
alpha-tocopherol concentrations, plasma 292
alphaxalone/alphadolone 118, 214, 220, 222, 230, **316**
alveld, *see* photosensitization
Amblyomma spp. 310
ammonium chloride 236, 237, 239
ammonium tetrathiomolybdenate 295, 296
amnion, rupture 38
amputation, digital 211, 212
anaemia
  brassica poisoning 323
  cobalt deficiency 288
  copper toxicity 294, 296
  cow colostrum-induced 88
  fasciolosis 306, 312
  nematode infestation 299
anaesthesia, general 118, **315–16**
anaesthetic agents 220, 222
analgesia **315**
  atresia ani correction 116
  caesarean section 55, 318
  castration 29
  caudal 40, 53, 116, 214, 220, 221, 222, **316–19**
  dystocia 36, 40, 45
  foot 211
  hindlimbs 222, 230
  joints 214, 228
  long bone fractures 230
  NSAIDs 65, 211, 214, 218, 228, 273, 274, 315
  rectal prolapse 54
  uterine prolapse 53, **316–19**
  vaginal prolapse 48–9, **316–19**
anisocoria 168
ankylosis
  distal interphalangeal joints 211–12
  phalangeal joints 208–9
anterior uveitis **267–8**
anthelmintics 31, 288, **300–303**
Arcanobacterium pyogenes 152, 153, 177, 190, 220, 248, 274
arthritis
  MVV infection 151, **228–9**
  septic pedal **208–12**
  see also osteoarthritis; polyarthritis
arthrocentesis **200–1**, 210, 214, 227
artificial rearing of lambs **26–7**
arytenoid cartilages 154–5
ascites
  fasciolosis 304
  pleural abscess 158, 159
  ultrasound assessment 101–2, 103
  vegetative endocarditis 163, 164
ataxia 166, 192
  enzootic, *see* swayback, delayed
  hindlimb 131, 183, 185, 188, 190
atlanto-occipital joint, infection 213
atresia ani/coli **117**
avermectins 255, 256, **300**
axial collateral ligament, rupture 210

'baboon bum' (perivulval oedema) **69**
bacteraemia
  endocarditis 161–2
  growing lambs 209
  mastitis 157, 275
  neonatal lambs 212
  respiratory disease 138, 152–3, 157
balance, loss of 177–8
balanoposthitis 239
barley feeding 109, 110
barren ewe 33, 291
basilar empyema 174
bedding 20, 89, 205, 215
benzimadazole anthelmintics 288, **300**, 302, 313
birth injuries 44, **85–6**
birth weights 84, **88–9**, 96, 98, 324
black disease **128–9**
blackleg **129–30**
bladder
  distension 235–6, 237, 238, 239
  emptying 48
  ultrasonography 101, 235–6
blepharospasm 265, 266, 268, 270, 277
blindness
  cerebral abscess 173, 174, 175
  cerebral dysfunction 166
  coenurosis 187
  keratoconjunctivitis 266, 267
  OPT 279, 280
  periorbital eczema 251
blink response, loss 179
bloat 100, **112**
  abomasal **113**
blowfly, *see* cutaneous myiasis
bluetongue **320**
body condition score (BCS) **14**, 324
  and lamb mortality 84
  loss 122, 123, 272, 278
  rams 72, 73
border (hairy shaker) disease **67–8**
Borrelia burgdorferi 311
'bottle brush' lesions 244
botulism **132**
Bovicola ovis 262
bovine virus diarrhoea (BVD) 67, 68
brachial intumescence lesions 192

bracken poisoning 323
brain abscessation **173–4**, 196
brassicas, feeding 292, **323**
braxy **128**
breech presentation **44–5**
brisket sores 73, 199, 327
broken mouth **102–4**
bronchitis, parasitic **150**
bronchoalveolar lavage 138
Brucella melitensis **68–9**
Brucella ovis 76, 79
bruxism 38, 45, 110, 186, 233, 280
buccal cavity **99–100, 106–9**
Buhner suture **50**, 51, 54, 69, 70, 238
3-OH butyrate concentration **16–17**, 18, 88, 98, 280, 281, 286

caesarean section **55–8**, 115, 281, 318
calcium 281, 282, 283, 284, 287, 323
calculi, urinary 232, **233–8**, 242
Calliphora erythrocephala 256
campylobacteriosis **66–7**
cardiovascular system 161–4
carpal joint, *see* knee joint
carpal valgus 229
caseous lymphadenitis (CLA) 32, 102, **246–8**
cast, Plaster of Paris 221–2
casting tape 222
castration 9, **27–30**
  bloodless (Burdizzio) method 30
  elastrator ring **28–9**, 217, 257
  reasons for 28
  surgical 29
caudal analgesia 40, 53, 116, 214, 220, 221, 222, **316–19**
cellulitis
  cervical spine 108, 192
  skin 108, 131, 200, 213, **248–9**
central nervous system, examination 165
cerebellar abiotrophy **190**
cerebellar syndrome **166**
cerebral hypoplasia 67
cerebral syndrome **166**
cerebrocortical necrosis, *see* polioencephalomalacia
cerebrospinal fluid (CSF)
  analysis **170**, 174, 181, 196
  collection **169–70**
cervical spine lesions 108, **191–2**
cervicovaginal prolpase 238
cervix, dilation 37, **40–1**, 52
chlamydial abortion **60–2**
Chlamydophila psittaci 149, 265, 270
chloride, rumen fluid 114
choke 100, 112
chondroprotective agents 228
circling behaviour 166, 174, 178, 187
cirrhosis 250
clinical problems
  cardiorespiratory disease 155–60
  digestive system 134–6
  eye disease 270
  female reproductive system 70–1
  male reproductive system 81–2
  mastitis 278
  metabolic disorders 285–7
  musculoskeletal disorders 229–31
  neonatal lamb disease 97–8
  neurological disorders 195–8
  parasitic diseases 312–14
  peritonitis 135–6
  skin disorders 263–4
  urinary tract disease 242
closantel 300
clostridial diseases **125–32**, 310
  vaccination 18, 125–6, 131
Clostridium botulinum 132
Clostridium chauvoei 129
Clostridium novyi type B 128
Clostridium perfringens 126–7
Clostridium tetani 131
cobalt
  defiency **287–9**
  supplementation 289, 314
coccidiosis 26, **119–21**, 159–60, 234, 240, 288, 325
Codes of Recommendation for the Welfare of Livestock 10
coenurosis 178, **186–8**, 196, 310
Coenurus cerebalis 186
colostrum 85, 86, 126, 214
  assessing ingestion 86, 102, 103
  bovine 87, 88
  ensuring ingestion 87, 88
coma, lambs **87–8**
concentrates, feeding 106, 109, 111
conception rate **15**, 326
conjunctivitis 266
constipation 282, 283
contagious pustular dermatitis (CPD/orf) 27, **243–5**, 272
copper
  antagonist 295, 296
  deficiency 171, **289–90**
  liver reserves 171, 289, 290
  plasma levels 289–90, 296
  supplementation 171–2, 290
  toxicity **293–6**
corium, damage 200, 204, 206, 208
cornea, ulceration 266, 269
coronary band
  cellulitis 218–19
  CPD **243–4**
  sinus 209, 210
  'strawberry' footrot 244
  vesicles 321
Corynebacterium pseudotuberculosis 102, 247
Corynebacterium renale 232, 239
cough
  atypical pneumonia 149
cough (*continued*)
  SPA 147
Cowdria ruminantium 310
cowdriosis (heartwater) **310–11**
crackles 138
cranial nerves **167–9**
crutching 258–9
cryptosporidiosis **118–19**, 127
Cryptosporidium parvum 118, 119
Culicoides spp 320
culling 14, 30
cutaneous myiasis 27, 204, 238, 239, 246, **256–60**
cis cypermethrin 255–6, 259, 261
cyromazine 259–60
cystitis 236, 239

'dagging' 258–9
Dandy-Walker malformation **189**
decoquinate 64, 121, 160
dehydration
  acidosis 110
  cryptosporidiosis 119
  E. coli enteritis 91–2
  haematology 158, 164
  nematode infestation 297
  treatment 111, 119, 133, 181
dentigerous cysts **104, 105**
dentition, correct 99
depression, causes 272
dermatitis
  contagious pustular (orf) 27, **243–5**
  facial 244, 245, **249–51**
  interdigital **201–2**, 217, 218, 325
  mycotic, *see* dermatophilosis
  periorbital 131, 244, **251**
dermatophilosis **245–6**
Dermatophilus congolensis 244, **245–6**
dextrose solution 88, 281
diarrhoea
  acidosis 110
  bovine virus (BVD) 67, 68
  causes in lambs 89, 91–2, 118, 119–20, 132–3
  control 258
  copper toxicity 294
  green/black 135, 136
  nematode infestations 120, 297, 298, 299
  salmonellosis 92, 132, 133
Dichelobacter nodosus 202, 203
diclazuril 26, 121, 188
Dicrocoelium dentriticum 303
Dictyocaulus filaria **150**
dicyclanil 260
diet
  brassicas 292, **323**
  cattle feeds 295
  concentrates 106, 109, 111
  ewe energy requirements **16–17**, 279, 286
  fibrous 99, 100, 106, 111

diet (*continued*)
history 99
legumes 112, 292
mineral content 233, 296
digestive system **99–102**
digital amputation 211, 212
digital dermatitis 204
dimpylate (diazinon) 255, 259
dipping
cutaneous myiasis 259–60
dermatophilosis 246
flock replacements 31
lameness following **218–19**, 321
plunge 31, 255–6, 259
sheep scab 255–6
shower 248, 259
dip wash, contamination 218, 219
disorientation 282
docking, hygiene 217
dog-sitting posture 190, 192–3, 196, 233
doramectin 255, **300**
dosing gun injuries 106, 108, 109, 191
dysentery, lamb 92, **126–7**
dyspnoea, severe 154–5
dystocia 34, **40–5**
analgesia 40, 45
birth injuries 44, **85–6**
caesarean section **55–8**
clinical problem 70–1
Dandy-Walker malformation 189
fetal presentation/postural abnormalities **41–5**, 70–1
hygiene 35, 58, 60
repelling lamb 43, 44–5, 71
unskilled assistance 38, 39, 58
veterinary assistance 8, 11, 35, 36, **38–40**

Eales clips 269
ear drop 166, 167, 168, 179, 180
ears
haematoma 255
swelling 250
tip necrosis 250
economics, and welfare 10
see also under named diseases and conditions
ectoparasites
blowfly (myiasis) 27, 204, 238, 239, 246, **256–60**
control 248
keds 262–3
lice **262**
Psoroptes ovis 186, **253–6**, 263–4
ticks 310, 311
eczema
facial (photosensitization) 244, **249–51**
periorbital 131, 244, **251**
Eimeria spp. 120, 121
elastrator rings **28–9**, 217, 257
elbow joint 223
elbow joint (*continued*)
enthesophyte formation 200, 201, 226, 227, 228
infective arthritis 212, 213
osteoarthritis 199, **224–8**
trauma 223, 228
electroejaculation 74–5, 76
electrolyte therapy 88, 90, 92, 133
embryo
flushing 33
implantation 15
loss, *see* abortion
empyema
basilar 174
vertebral body **190–1**, 194, 196–7, 291, 310
encephalitis, listeric **178–81**, 310
endectocides, systemic 255
endocarditis, vegetative **161–4**, 199, 213, 227
endotoxaemia 90
enemas, soapy water 90
energy requirements, ewe **16–17**, 279, 286
enteritis, *E. coli* **91–2**
enteropathy, protein-losing 124
enthesitis 223
entropion **268–9**
epididymitis **76–80**, 81–2
epiphora 265, 268, 270, 277
erysipelas 18–19, 202, **217–18**, 230–1, 291
Erysipelothrix rhusiopathiae 200, 212, 214, 215, **217–18**, 231
Escherichia coli 89, 119, 212, 274
evisceration, vaginal tear 54
ewe mortality 7, 34
exercise intolerance 146, 150–1
extradural injection 220, 221, 222, 230, **317–19**
eye
discharge 268
enucleation 315
pink, *see* keratoconjunctivitis, infectious
silage (anterior uveitis) **267–8**
eye drop 174, 178
eyelid, dropped 166, 168, 178, 179, 180

facial abscesses 107
facial nerve 166, **168**, 178, 179–80
facial swelling 130–1, 244, 250, 320
faecal egg counts
fluke 312
nematodes 297, 300, 302, 312, 313
faecal egg reduction test 302, 314
faecal staining, prevention 258–9
Fasciola gigantica 303, 308
Fasciola hepatica 303
fasciolosis (liver fluke) 116, 124, 128, 142, 279, **303–8**, 312–13
chronic 306
fasciolosis (liver fluke) (*continued*)
subacute 102, 103, 304–5, 306
treatment and prevention 307, 324, 326
fat reserves, lambs 96–7
feed storage 63, 66
feet **200–208**
female reproductive system
clinical problems 70–1
examination 33–4
fertility
ewes 33, 291
ram **74–6**
fetal number, determination 33–4
fetlock joint
infection 214, 215
knuckling 179, 184
fetus
growth and development **16–17**
loss, *see* abortion
mummified 63
oversize 37, 55
posture 37
presentation/postural abnormalities 36, **41–5**, 70–1, 85–6
repelling 43, 44–5, 71
retained 34, **46**, 116, 130
fibroma, toe 200, 205, **206–7**
fighting behaviour 131
fighting injuries 177
Five Freedoms 8–10
fleece
faecal staining 258–9, 298
loss 185, 254–5, 257, 282, 286
meconium staining 86, 96
pigmentation 246
poor condition 122, 185, 289
flies
causing cutaneous myiasis 256–7
headfly **260–2**
flock
culling 14, 30
health plans 11, 31, 98, 325
replacements **30–2**, 248, 326
selection 14
fluid therapy
acidosis 110–11
intravenous 90, 110–11
oral 65, 111, 119
flukacides 307, 312–13
flumethrin 255, 256
flunixin 58, 90, 91, 211, 214, 218, 228, 274, 319
'flushing' (ewe) 15, 326
fly strike, *see* cutaneous myiasis
focal symmetrical encephalomalacia (FSE) **131–2**, 310
food impaction, cheeks 99, 105
footbaths 13, 205, 206
formalin 32, 202, 204
zinc sulphate 32, 202, 204
foot and mouth disease 244, **321–2**

footrot **202–6**
benign (scald) 202
prevention/control 205–6
'strawberry' 244
virulent 200, 202–3, 206, 209, 299
fostering **23–6**
fractures
long bone **220–3**, 229–31, 289
reduction and realignment 222, 230
ribs 44
frontal bone, softening 187
Fusobacterium necrophorum 82, 93, 201, 202, 203
buccal cavity infection **106–7**, 152
inhalation 151–3

gait abnormalities
cerebellar syndrome 166
kangaroo gait 194–5
scrapie 185–6
gall bladder 102, 103, 163
gangrene, postparturient (blackleg) **129–30**
gastroenteritis
copper toxicity 294
E. coli **91–2**
parasitic 258, 288, **298–302**, 313–14, 324
genetic disorders, *see* inherited disorders
gid (coenurosis) 178, **186–8**, 196, 310
gingivitis, acute 102
glass bolus, soluble 289
glossopharyngeal nerve 169
gloves, disposable 35, 40
glucose, plasma levels 90, 286
glucose (dextrose) solution 88, 281
glucosinolates 323
glutamate dehydrogenase 306
goats 122, 277
goitre 293
goitrogens 292, 293
grain
feeding 109, 111
overload (acidosis) **109–12**, 129
propionic acid-treated 291
granulation tissue, exuberant 207, 244
granuloma, toe (toe fibroma) **206–7**
griseofulvin 252
growth plate, infection **219–20**
growth problems
causes in individuals 120
cobalt deficiency 288

haematoma, aural 255
haemoglobinuria, bacillary **129**
haemolysis 293–4, 296
haemonchosis **299–301**
Haemonchus contortus 298
hairy shaker (border) disease **67–8**
handling facilities **12–13**, 199
'hardbag' (lymphocytic mastitis) 277
head
oedema/swelling 154
trauma 130, 131, 177, 257
head carriage, lowered 191
headfly **260–2**
head pressing behaviour 174, 175, 176, 280
head tilt 177, 180, 183, 187
heart disease
congenital 161
vegetative endocarditis **161–4**, 199, 213, 227
heart failure, right-sided 158, 159, 161, 162, 163–4
heartwater **310–11**
hemicastration 80
hemiparesis 179, 180
hepatic encephalopathy 132
hepatic necrobacillosis 93, **94–5**
hepatitis, infectious necrotic (black disease) **128–9**
hepatomegaly 102, 159, 162–3, 304–5
hernia
inguinal/scrotal 29, **133**
umbilical **118**
hindlimbs
ataxia 131, 183, 185, 188, 190
detection of lameness 199
erysipelas 217
infective arthritis 230–1
paralysis, MVV infection 183–4
paralysis/paresis following analgesia 50, 222, 230, **319**
paresis 50, 71, 171, 188
stiffness 131
hip joint, arthritis 224, 225
Histophilus ovis 76, 78, 79
hock joint
infective arthritis 230–1, 277
septic physitis 220
Horner's syndrome 166, **168**
housing **20–2**
at night 20
bedding and drainage 20, 89, 205, 215
pen dimensions 20, 21–2, 83–4
hunger, neonatal lambs 84, 85
'hung' lamb **43**
hydrocephalus 189
hydronephrosis 235–6, 238
Hydrotea irritans 260
hygiene
bedding materials 20, 215
castration/docking procedures 217
coccidiosis prevention 119–20
cryptosporidiosis prevention 119
epididymitis 79
feed storage 63, 66
lambing difficulties 35, 36, 40, 58, 60, 83
navel dressing 71, 87, 95, 98, 215
hyperaemia, interdigital skin 202, 203
hyperaesthesia 185, 282
hyperimmune serum 126
hypoalbuminaemia 18, 123, 124, 134, 240
hypocalcaemia 18, 116, 130, 281, **282–4**, 286–7, 323
diagnosis/misdiagnosis 142, 287
treatment and prevention 8, **283–4**, 323
hypoglycaemia 88
hypomagnesaemia 8, **284–5**
hypometria 183
hypopyon 269
hypothalamic syndrome 169
hypothermia 88

ileum, thickening 124–5
ill-thrift
causes in growing lambs 291, 313, 326
causes in young lambs 120, 297
immunosuppression 288
implantation 15
infertility, ewe 33, 291
inguinal hernia **133**
inherited disorders
cerebellar abiotrophy **190**
Dandy-Walker malformation **189**
entropion **268–9**
interdigital dermatitis **201–2**, 217, 218, 325
interdigital growths **208**
interdigital infection 210
interdigital space, widening 209, 210
intestinal adenocarcinoma **114–15**
intestinal atresia **117**
intussusception 234
iodine
deficiency 292–3
navel dressing 71, 87, **95**, 98, 215
iritis (anterior uveitis) **267–8**
ivermectin 255, **300**
Ixodes spp. 310, 311

jaagsiekte retrovirus (JSRV) 146
jaundice 129, 294, 295–6
jetting wands 259
Johne's disease (paratuberculosis) 32, **121–5**, 134
joint aspiration **200–1**, 214
joint capsule, fibrous thickening 213, 214, 216, 227
joint effusions 223, 227, 277
endocarditis 162–3
polyarthritis 212–13, 214
joint ill, *see* polyarthritis, infectious
joints
analgesia 218, 220
arthrocentesis **200–1**, 210, 214, 227
bacterial infection 162

joints (*continued*)
clinical examination **200**, 217, 227
crepitus 213, 227, 228
imaging **201**
injuries 213, 223, 228
lavage 214, 215
septic physitis **219–20**
synovial fluid 200–1

kangaroo gait **194–5**
keds **262–3**
keel harness 73
keel paint 74
keratitis 266, 269
exposure 179
keratoconjunctivitis 277
infectious (pink eye) **265–7**, 270
ketamine **316**
ketoprofen 118, 214, 218, 228, 274
kidney disease
nephrosis **240–1**
pulpy **127–8**
kidneys
biopsy 233
copper toxicity 294, 296
fat deposits around 96
ultrasonography 235–6
knee joint
grazing on 199
infective arthritis 213, **217**, 230–1, 277

labour (staffing) requirments 19, 119, 206
Lactobacillus spp. 91, 109
lambing
definitions 36–7
difficult, *see* dystocia
easy-care system 35
ewe mortality rates 7, 34
facilities **19–22**
indoors 119–20
outdoor 19, 88, 97
veterinary attention 8, 19
lambing sheds
hygiene standards 35, 36, 40, 58, 60, 83
individual pens 20, 21–2, 83–4
lamb mortality, perinatal 7, 15, 16, **83–9**, 97–8
aetiology **84–7**, 97
postmorten examinations 96–7
prevention **88–91**
rates 83
lameness
causes 213, 221, 226–7
causes of sudden onset 129, 321
clinical examination 200–1
in contagious agalactia 277
detection 199, 218
in endocarditis 162, 199, 227
erysipelas 217
in footrot 203, 204
lameness (*continued*)
in infectious polyarthritis 212, 213
in interdigital dermatitis 201
in mastitis 272
in osteoarthritis 224–6
post-dipping **218–19**, 321
rams 72, 202, 208
scoring 200
in septic pedal arthritis 209
lameness, limb fractures 220
laminitis 109, 110
laparoscopy 33
laryngeal chondritis **153–5**
larynx, compression 107
lead poisoning 168, **323**
legumes, feeding 112, 292
levamisole 31, 244, 312, 314
lice **262**
lidocaine
extradural injection 55, 70, 117, 220–2, 230, **319**
digit amputation 211
sedation 316
limbs, swelling 129
Linognathus ovillus 262
Linognathus pedalis 262
lip, flaccid 179
Listeria monocytogenes 178, 181, 267
listeriosis 165, 174, **178–83**, 195–6, 310
liver
abscess 94, 102
copper reserves 171, 289, 290
copper toxicity 293, 294, 296
enlargement 159, 304–5
in fasciolosis 103, 304–5, 307
imaging 101, 102, 103, 163–4
in vegetative endocarditis 163–4
vitamin B_{12} concentrations 288
liver enzymes, raised 164, 247, 250, 293, 306
liver fluke, *see* fasciolosis
long bones
fracture **220–3**, 229–31, 289
septic physitis **219–20**
louping ill 129, 131, 132, **309–10**
lower motor neuron disease 191
Lucilia cuprina 256–7
Lucilia sericata 256
lumpy wool (dermatophilosis) **245–6**
lung abscesses 106, 107, **151–3**, 156–9
'lungers' 247
lungs
clinical examination 138
neonatal lamb necropsy 97
ultrasonography **139–41**, 156
lymphadenitis, caseous 32, 102, **246–8**
lymph nodes
enlargement 200, 219–20, 230
infection 247–8
maedi-visna virus (MVV) infection 32, 149
arthritis 151, **228–9**
mammary gland 151, **277–8**
prevention/control 184
respiratory **150–1**
visna **183–4**
magnesium
dietary intake 233
hypomagnesaemia 8, **284–5**
male reproductive system **72–82**
malignant oedema **130–1**
malnutrition 160
mammary gland
antibiotics 276
examination 271
trauma 276–7
mandible
examination 100
swellings 100, 105, 108
Mannheimia haemolytica 132, 142, 147
respiratory disease **142–4**
Mannheimia spp. 271, 278
mastitis 87, 243, **271–6**, 278
acute **273–4**
bacteraemia 157, 275
chronic 156–7, **274–6**
gangrenous **271–3**, 325
maedi-visna virus 151, **277**
mating
identification of ewes 72–3
timing of **13–15**, 80
meconium
retention 89–90
staining of fleece 71, 86, 96
Melophagus ovinus 262–3
menace response
interpretation 167–8
reduced/absence 172, 176, 187, 280, 285, 287
meningitis 165, 168, **169**
meningoencephalitis 67, 131, **172–3**
mental state, alteration 185
methylmalonic acid (MMA) 288
metritis 34, 42, **58–60**, 116, 130
midbrain syndrome 169
milbemycins 255, 256
milk-producing sheep 274
milk replacers, artificial 88
mineral deficiencies **287–93**, 299
miosis 168
mismothering 22, 87
molasses, liquid 281
molybdenum 295, 296
monensin sodium 64
Monezia 302
mouth, *see* buccal cavity; teeth
mouth breathing (panting) 146, 151, 154, 282
mucous membranes
jaundice 294, 295–6
toxic 272, 278
Muellerius capillaris **150**

Mules mutilation 253
muscle fasciculations 190, 280
muscle tremors 284
muscle wastage 199, 200, 209
muscular dystrophy 213
musculoskeletal system
  clinical examination **200–1**
  clinical problems 229–31
muzzle, deviation 168, 179
Mycobacterium avium ssp. *paratuberculosis* 122, 125
Mycoplasma agalactiae 277
Mycoplasma conjunctivae 265, 270
Mycoplasma ovipneumoniae 149
mycotic dermatits (dermatophilosis) **245–6**

narcolepsy 185
nasal bot (*Oestrus ovis*) **141–2**
nasal discharge 141, 142, 147, 152, 157
nasal tumour, enzootic **141**
natamycin, topical 252
navel, *see* umbilicus
neck, dorsiflexion 280
Nematodirus spp. 120, 258, 297, 298, 314
nematodirosis 92, 120, 240, **297–301**, 313–14
  faecal egg counts 300, 302, 312, 313
  treatment and control 258, **297–8**
Nematodirus battus 120, 258, 297, 298, 314
Nematodirus fillicolis 297
nephrosis 132, **240–1**
nerve blocks 201
neurological disease
  border disease **67–8**
  clinical problems 195–8
  genetic **189–90**
  history and examination 165
  visna **183–4**
neurological syndromes **166–9**
nibble response 185, 186
nitrate ingestion 323
nitroxynil 300, 307
notifiable diseases 122, 184
NSAIDs 50, 65, 211, 214, 218, 228, 273, 274
  preoperative injection 315, 319
nutrition
  minerals 284, **287–93**, 295
  pasture assessment **17–18**
  pregnant ewe 7, **17–18**, 88–9, 98, 126, 281, 286, 325
nystagmus 169, 175, 177–8

oculomotor nerve **168**
oedema
  face/ears 130–1, 244, 250, 320
  head 154
  malignant **130–1**
  perivulval **69**
oedema (*continued*)
  pulmonary 311, 320
  scrotum 234
oesophagus, examination **100**
oestrous 15
  synchronization 80
Oestrus ovis infestation **141–2**
omphalophlebitis **93–6**
opisthotonus 131, 284, 310
optic nerve *167*, **167–8**
orf (CPD) 27, **243–5**
organic food schemes 125–6
organophosphate insecticides 258, 259, 262, 263
orphan lambs **22–7**
  respiratory disease 27, 159–60
osteoarthritis **223–8**
osteophyte formation 213, 216
osteoporosis 289
otitis media/externa 178
ovine pregnancy toxaemia (OPT) 88, 165, **279–82**
  aetiology 266, 279
  clinical presentation 195, 279–80
  clinical problem 285–6
  diagnosis 175, 280
  prevalence 279
  treatment and prevention 8, 281
oxyclozanide 307, 312–13

pain management **315**
  see also anaesthesia; analgesia
pampiniform plexus 78
panniculus reflex 193
panting (mouth breathing) 146, 151, 154, 282
parainfluenza 3 virus 149
paralysis
  facial 166–7, 168, 178, 179–80
  hindlimbs following analgesia 50, 222, 230, **319**
  hindlimbs in MVV infection 183–4
  radial nerve 180
  spastic 191
parasitic disease
  bronchitis **150**
  coccidiosis 26, **119–21**, 159–60, 234, 240, 288, 325
  cryptosporidiosis **118–19**, 127
  fasciolosis (liver fluke) 102, 103, 116, 124, 128, 142, 279, **303–7**
  gastrointestinal nematodes 92, 120, 258, 288, **297–302**, 313–14
  tick-borne 190, 215, **308–11**
paratuberculosis 32, **121–5**, 134
paresis
  hemiparesis 179, 180
  hindlimbs 50, 71, 171, 188
  tetraparesis 108, 191, 192, 213
parturition
  assessment of ewe 38–40
  ewe mortality rates 7, 34
  normal process **37–8**
Pasteurella spp. 177, 271, 278
Pasteurella multocida 142
Pasteurella trehalosi 142
pasteurellosis 19, 127, 128, 137, **142–6**
pasture
  cattle grazing 206
  contamination with coccidia 120, 121
  ewe and lamb turnout 89
  lush 284, 285
  nematode control 297, **300–1**, 303
  nutritional value 15, **17–18**, 326
pedal arthritis, septic **208–12**
pediculosis (lice) **262**
penis
  exteriorization 232, 242
  rupture 233–4
pens, lambing 20, 21–2, 83–4
pentobarbital **315**
pericardial effusion 163, 311
peripheral vestibular disease **177–8**, 196
perirenal fat 96
peritoneal fluid 101
peritonitis **115–16**, 135–6
  clinical presentation 162
  fibrinous 115, 305
  localized fibrinous 94, 95
  septic 60, 93–4, 116
perivulval oedema **69**
pestes des petits ruminants **322**
pH
  rumen 109–11
  silage 182
  urine 232
pharynx
  abscesses **108–9**
  examination **100**
phenylbutazone 228
phimosis 239
Phormia terrae-novae 256
phosphate, dietary intake 233
phospholipase D (PLD) 248
photophobia 266, 270
photosensitization **249–51**
physitis, septic **219–20**
'pine'(cobalt defiency) **287–9**
pink eye, *see* keratoconjunctivitis, infectious
Pithomyces chartarum 249, 250
pituitary abscessation 174
pizzle-rot 239
placenta, development **16**
plants
  photosensitization 249
  poisonous 22, **322–3**
Plaster of Paris cast 221–2
pleural abscesses 106, 107, 140, **151–3**, 156–9

pleural effusion 311
pleuritis, fibrinous 140
plochteach (photosensitization) **249–51**
pneumonia
  atypical **149–50**
  chronic suppurative **151–3**, 159–60
poisonings
  lead 168, 323
  plants 22, **322–3**
polioencephalomalacia (PEM) 67, 131, 132, 165, **174–6**, 310
  clinical problem 197–8
polyarthritis 162
  erysipelas 18–19, 202, **217–18**, 230–1, 291
  infectious (joint ill) **212–16**
  Lyme **311**
pontomedullary syndrome **166–9**
posthitis, ulcerative (sheath rot) **239–40**
potassium aluminium sulphate 246
potassium iodide 293
potassium selenate 292
povidone iodine 118
pox, *see* sheep pox
pox viruses 243
practice newsletters **324–7**
pregnancy **15–17**
  diagnosis/assessment 16, 33–4
  ewe nutrition 7, **17–18**, 88–9, 98, 126, 281, 286, 325
  toxaemia **279–82**
prepubic tendon, rupture **41**
prepuce
  hygiene 76
  oedema 234
presentation (fetus) **41–5**, 70–1
  anterior **42–3**, 85–6
  defined 36
  posterior **43–5**
  two lambs 45
prolapse
  cervicovaginal 238
  rectal 54
  see also uterine prolapse; vaginal prolapse
propetamphos 255, 256, 259
propionic acid, in grain 291
proprioceptive deficits 183–4, 192, 193
  unilateral 187
propulsive tendency 179
propylene glycol 181, 281
protein
  CSF 170, 172, 174, 181
  serum 18, 86, 123, 124, 134, 164, 240, 306
  synovial fluid 201
protein status, assessment 18, 98
Protostrongylus rufescens **150**
Psoroptes cuniculi 255
Psoroptes ovis (sheep scab) **253–6**, 263–4
ptosis 166, 168, 178, 179, 180
pulmonary oedema 311, 320
pulmonary valve, vegetations 162
pulpy kidney disease **127–8**
pulses, peripheral 161
pupils, diameter 168
pyaemia, tick 152, 190, 215, 309
pyelonephritis 236
pyothorax 106, 107
pyrethroids, synthetic 258, 259, 262, 263
pyrexia 162, 274, 278
  differential diagnosis 321
pyrimethamine 63

quarantine 32
quidding 105

raddles, ram 72–3
radial nerve paralysis 180
radiography
  abdomen **100–1**
  jaw/teeth 99, 104, 105
  joints **201**, 210, 226
  limb fractures 201, 221, 223
  thorax **138–9**, 152–3
  urinary tract 232
rain scald, *see* dermatophilosis
rams 324, 326–7
  body condition score 72, 73
  brisket sores 73, 199, 327
  epididymitis **76–80**, 81–2
  fertility assessment **74–6**
  fighting behaviour/injuries 130, 131, 177, 257
  inguinal/scrotal hernia **133**
  lameness 72, 202, 208
  laryngeal chondritis **153–5**
  malignant oedema **130–1**
  service marking of ewe **72–4**
  vaccinations 126
  vasectomy 33, 80–1, 316
rectal prolapse 54
redgut 110, **112–13**
redwater (bacillary haemoglobinuria) **129**
reflex arc 191
rehydration 111, 119, 133, 181
renal biopsy 233
renal failure, copper toxicity 295, 296
respiratory disease
  clinical problems 155–60
  history and examination 137–40
  laryngeal chondritis **153–5**
  maedi-visna virus **150–1**
  orphan lambs 27
  see also pasteurellosis; pneumonia; sheep pulmonary adenomatosis
respiratory rate, raised 146, 151, 154, 156, 157, 282, 311
rhododendron poisoning 323
rib fracture 44
right ventricle, dilatation 161, 164
rinderpest **322**
ringwomb **40–1**, 52
ringworm **252–3**
root crops 112
rope halters 25–6
Ruakura probe 75
rumen
  acidosis 109–11
  bloat 100, **112**
  examination **100**
rumen fluid
  chloride 114
  collection and analysis 100, 114
rumenotomy 111
rumen sounds 100, 114

sacrococcygeal extradural injection **317–19**
salivation, excessive 179, 180
Salmonella spp. 65–66, 92, 220
Salmonella abortus ovis 64–5
Salmonella brandenburg 65
Salmonella dublin 65, 92
Salmonella infections
  abortion **64–6**
  enteric **132–3**
  neonatal lambs **92–3**
Salmonella montevideo 65, 92
Salmonella typhimurium 65, 92, 93, 132
Sarcocystis spp. 188
sarcocystosis 108, **188**, 310
scabby mouth, *see* contagious pustular dermatitis
sclera, injection 145, 266, 272
scour, *see* diarrhoea
scrapie **184–6**
scrotal hernia **133**
scrotal swelling
  differential diagnosis 78
  epididymitis 76–7, 81–2
  urolithiasis 233–4, 236
scrotum, examination 74, 75
sedation **316**
seizure activity 131, 172, 173, 175, 255, 284, 310
selenium deficiency **291–2**
self-trauma, headfly 260, 261
semen
  collection method 75
  evaluation **74–6**
service returns, causes 291
sewage 92, 132
shearing
  equipment hygiene 248
  and summer dipping 259
  wounds 247
sheath rot (ulcerative posthitis) **239–40**
sheep pox 244
sheep pulmonary adenomatosis (SPA) 32, 138, **146–9**
  thoracic ultrasound 140–1

sheep scab 186, **253–6**, 263–4
shelter 267
silage
  feeding 181–2, 267
  listeriosis risk 181–2
silage eye (anterior uveitis) **267–8**
skeletal abnormalities **229**
skin
  discolouration in mastitis 272
  keratinization 254
  photosensitization **249–51**
  in urinary tract obstruction 234
skinning of lambs 24
skin scrapings 255
skull, doming 189
S-methyl-cysteine sulphoxide 323
snackers 324
snails 303, 307
snare rope 43
'snow blindness' 265
sodium lauryl sulphate 202, 204
SPA, *see* sheep pulmonary adenomatosis
spastic paralysis 191
sperm
  abnormalities 76
  motility and morphology 75–6
spermatic cord, incision 80–1
sperm granuloma 80, 81
spider syndrome **229**
spinal cord lesions **190–4**, 196–7
  brachial intumescence 192
  cervical spine 108, 191–2
  diagnosis 194
  thoracolumbar 192–3
  treatment 194
spirochaetes, role in footrot 203
splints, fracture stabilization 222, 230
sporidesmin 249
squamous cell carcinoma **253**
'staggers' 8, 284
stance, abnormal
  crab-like 212
  in elbow arthritis 199, 225
  kneeling 135, 136
  roached-back 116, 162, 233, 320
  wide-based 233
standing, inability 282, 321
Staphylococcus spp. 190–1
Staphylococcus aureus 244, 251, 271, 272, 276, 278, 309, 311
'star-gazing' behaviour 175, 280
starvation, neonatal lambs 84–5, 97, 127
'stealing' behaviour 22, 23
'steely wool' 289
stertor 107, 154
stiffness, sudden-onset, causes 291
stifle joint
  infective arthritis 216, 224, 230–1
  osteoarthritis 224, 227
stomatitis, *F. necrophorum* **106–7**
strabismus 168, 172, 175
'strawberry footrot' 244
Streptococcus spp. 177, 274
Streptococcus dysgalactiae 157, 200, 212, 213, 214, 215, 311
Streptococcus faecium 91
stricture, urinary tract **238–9**
stridor 141, 142, 282
Strongyloides westeri 120
struvite calculi 233
stupor 123, 176, 180, 282, 283
sublumbar fossa, sunken 123
sudden death 112, 306, 310, 321
  causes in lambs 92, 127, 128, 133, 142, 297, 321
  causes in older sheep 142, 284
sulphonamides 63, 119, 121
sulphur toxicity **176–7**
superoxide dismutase 290
swayback 67, **170–2**, 289
  congenital form 171
  delayed 108, 131, 170, 171, 213
  prevention 171–2, 290
synovial fluid, normal 200–1

tachypnoea 146, 151, 154, 156, 157, 311
Taenia multiceps 186
tail docking **27–30**, 47, 260
  and cutaneous myiasis 27–8, 257
  and rectal prolapse 54
  welfare concerns 8, 9, 29
tapeworm infestations 186, **302**
tear-staining 265, 270
teat lesions 243, **276–7**, 325
teat-searching 87
teeth 326
  cheek teeth problems 99, **104–6**
  correct dentition 99
  dentigerous cysts **104, 105**
  examination **99–100**
  grinding (bruxism) 38, 45, 110, 186, 233, 280
  incisor loss (broken mouth) **102–4**, 326
Teladosagia (*Ostertagia*) 298
teladosagiosis **299–301**
tenesmus
  dystocia 38, 39
  rectal 92, 120, 127
  rectal prolapse 54
  urinary 232, 233
  uterine prolapse 52, 53
testicles, examination 74, 75, 76, 77, 82
tetanus 126, **131**
tetraparesis 108, 191, 192, 213
thiamine 111, 174, 176, 177
'thin ewe syndrome' 247
thoracocentesis 138
thorax
  clinical examination **138**
  imaging **138–40**, 156, 158, 163
tibia, fracture 229–30
tick-borne disease
  heartwater **310–11**
  louping ill 129, 131, 132, **309–10**
  Lyme disease **311**
  pyaemia 152, 190–1, 215, 309
tilmicosin 276, 277
toe fibroma 200, 205, **206–7**
tongue
  Fusobacterium necrophorum lesions 106, 152
  innervation 169
  oedema 320
toxaemia
  gangrenous mastitis 272
  post-parturition 130
  weaned lambs 110
toxicities
  copper **293–6**
  neurological signs 168
  sulphur **176–7**
Toxoplasma gondii 62–3
toxoplasmosis **62–4**, 67
trace element deficiencies **287–93**, 299, 326
transmissable spongiform encephalopathies (TSEs) **184–6**
trauma
  dosing gun 106, 108, 109, 191
  during delivery **44, 85–6**
  head in rams 130, 131, 177, 257
  joints 213, 223, 228
  long bone fractures **220–3**, 229–31, 289
  mammary gland 276–7
  self in headfly 260, 261
Trichophyton verrucosum 252
trichostrongylosis **299–301**, 324
Trichostrongylus spp. 298
triclabendazole 307, 312
tricuspid valve, vegetative lesions 161, 162
trigeminal motor nucleus 166–7
trigeminal nerve 166–7, 168, 179, 180
trocharization 112
tuberculosis 247
tumours
  intenstinal adenocarcinoma **114–15**
  mandible 100
  nasal enzootic **141**
  SPA 32, 138, **146–9**
  squamous cell carcinoma **253**
turning crates 200, 204
twin lamb disease, *see* ovine pregnancy toxaemia (OPT)
tylosin 277

udder
  examination 271
  infections 87
  teat lesions **276–7**
  see also mastitis

ultrasonography
  abdomen **101–2**, 103, 163–4, 304–5
  cellulitis lesions 249
  copper toxicity 296
  dystocia 58
  endocarditis 163
  ewe infertility 33
  fasciolosis **304–5**
  joints **201**, 224, 227
  neonatal lamb abomasum 86
  osteoarthritis 228
  pleural abscesses 153
  pregnancy assessment/diagnosis 7, 16, **33–4**
  SPA 147–8
  testicles 74, 75, 76, 77, 82
  thorax **139–41**, 156, 158, 163–4
  transrectal 101
  udder 271
  urinary tract 232, **235–6**, 238
  vaginal prolapse 48
umbilicus (navel)
  dressing 71, **87**, **95**, 98, 215
  herniated intestines **118**
  infection **93–6**, 97–8
  thickened 212
urea, blood (BUN) 90, 98
  copper toxicity 295, 296
  nephrosis 240
  protein status 18, 98
  urolithiasis 234–5
urease 239
urethra
  obstruction in urolithiasis 233–8
  rupture 233–4, 236–7
urethrostomy, subischial 236, 238
urinary system
  examination **232–3**
  infection 236, 239
  stricture **238–9**
urination, observation 232
urine
  acidification 236, 237, 239
  bacteriology 232
  biochemistry 232, 234–5, 240
  dark red 129, 294, 296
  scald 257
  specific gravity 232
urolithiasis 232, **233–8**, 242
uroperitoneum 233–4
uterine inertia 41
uterine prolapse 34, **52–4**, 70
  analgesia 53, **316–19**
  prevention and welfare issues 54
  treatment 8, 52, 53, 54
uterine rupture **45–6**, 130
uterine torsion 41

vaccination **18–19**, 32, 324
  bluetongue 320
  border disease 68
  caseous lymphadenitis 248
  chlamydial abortion 62
  clostridial diseases 18, 125–6, 131
  CPD 245
  erysipelas 218, 231
  FMD 321
  footrot 205–6
  heartwater 311
  listeriosis 182
  paratuberculosis 125
  pasteurellosis 144–5, 146, 160, 325
  rams 126
  S. abortus ovis 64
  salmonellosis 133
  statistics of use 7
  toxoplasmosis 64
  watery mouth disease 92
vagal nerve 169
vagina, dorsal wall tear 54
vaginal prolapse 34, **46–52**
  analgesia 48–9, **316–19**
  treatment 8, 48–51, 52
vas deferens, incision 80–1
vasectomy 33, **80–1**, 316
vermiform appendix
  calculus 234, 242
  excision 234, 242
vermin 63
vertebral empyema **190–1**, 194, 196–7, 291
vestibular disease **177–8**, 196
vestibular syndrome **166**
vestibulocochlear nerve 169
visna **183–4**
visual pathway, testing 167–8
vitamin B_1 (thiamine) 111, 174, 176, 177
vitamin B_{12} 288–9, 314
vitamin E deficiency **291–2**
vulval discharge 59, 61

warming box 88
water intake, encouraging 237
watery mouth disease 7, 86, **89–91**
weight loss
  causes in adult sheep 115, 123, 134, 152, 247
  causes in flocks 123, 299, 306
  in young lambs 120, 297
welfare concerns **8–10**
  castration and tail docking 8, 9, 29
  Codes of Recommendation 10
  Five Freedoms 8–10
  see also under individual diseases and conditions
'wheelbarrow' test **147**, 156, 158
wheezes 138
white cells
  CSF 170, 172, 174, 181
  joint aspirate 201
  peritoneal fluid 101
  semen 75, 76, 79
white line abscess 204, **207–8**, 210
white liver syndrome 288
white muscle disease 291
wool loss/wool slip 185, 254–5, 257, 282, 286
wounds
  cellulitis/abscess formation **248–9**
  fly strike 257
  shearing 247
  see also trauma

xanthochromia 170, 171
xylazine
  extradural injection 55, 70, **317–19**
  sedation **316**

yellowses (photosensitization) **249–51**

zoonoses 60, 62–3, 65, 118, **243–5**, 252, 311